PHARMACOTHERAPY OF OBESITY

Options and Alternatives

PHARMACOTHERAPY

OF

OBESITY

Options and Alternatives

Karl G. Hofbauer
Ulrich Keller
Olivier Boss

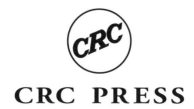

CRC PRESS

Boca Raton   London   New York   Washington, D.C.

Library of Congress Cataloging-in-Publication Data

Pharmacotherapy of obesity: options and alternatives / edited by Karl G. Hofbauer, Ulrich Keller, Olivier Boss.
p. ; cm.
Includes bibliographical references and index.
ISBN 0-415-30321-4 (alk. paper)
1. Obesity—Chemotherapy. 2. Weight loss preparations. I. Hofbauer, Karl G. II. Keller,
U. (Ulrich) II. Boss, Olivier.
[DNLM: 1. Obesity—drug therapy. 2. Anti-Obesity Agents—therapeutic use. 3. Diet,
Reducing. 4. Health Behavior. WD 210 P5366 2004]
RC628.P47 2004
616.3'98061—dc22   2003070272

Visit the CRC Press Web site at www.crcpress.com

© 2004 by CRC Press LLC

No claim to original U.S. Government works
International Standard Book Number 0-415-30321-4
Library of Congress Card Number 2003070272
Printed in the United States of America 1 2 3 4 5 6 7 8 9 0
Printed on acid-free paper

Preface

Drug treatment of obesity is a controversial topic. Opinions in the public and medical communities range from advocating life-long treatment of obesity with a single drug or a drug combination to opposing treatment of obesity with "life-style" drugs. This book was designed to present the current and future options for drug treatment of obesity in the context of pathophysiology and clinical requirements and to put them into perspective against available alternative treatments. The value of antiobesity drugs can only be assessed when their risks are compared with the benefits of weight loss — a comparison that also includes their effects on the diseases associated with obesity.

The book is primarily intended for physicians and health care professionals who are treating obese patients. However, readers from other disciplines such as pharmacists, scientists in academia or industry, and students of life sciences should also find information relevant to their daily work. The book is organized in six sections that cover a wide range of topics from pathophysiology of obesity to the benefits of weight loss. The core sections on pharmacotherapy deal with currently available drugs and drugs in preclinical or clinical development. These sections are complemented with sections on nondrug treatment and general therapeutic aspects. Taken together, these sections and the chapters contained therein should provide an integrated view of therapeutic approaches to the treatment of obesity and its associated diseases as illustrated in the figure below. Obviously, a certain

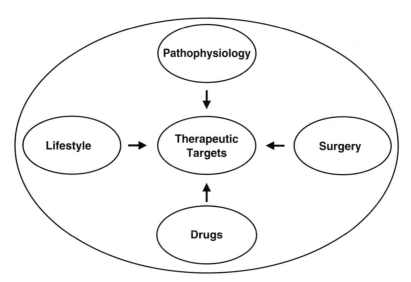

An integrated view of therapeutic approaches to the treatment of obesity and associated diseases. The process of drug discovery starts with identification of a molecular target amenable to pharmacological manipulation. Such targets are usually derived from an understanding of the pathophysiology of the disease. During recent years, numerous central and peripheral targets for the treatment of obesity have emerged and intense efforts are ongoing in preclinical drug discovery in many pharmaceutical companies. However, the value of the currently available and possible future drugs must be seen in the context of other treatment options. Permanent changes in life-style are the basis for any attempt to treat obesity, while surgery is, at least for the time being, the most efficacious intervention to lose excessive weight. In any case, it must be considered that the ultimate therapeutic goal of antiobesity treatment is not only to achieve significant weight loss but also to eliminate the associated metabolic, cardiovascular, and other risk factors.

overlap exists between the individual chapters within and between sections. The index may guide the readers to the parts of the book most relevant for their specific interests.

Many distinguished scientists and clinical investigators agreed to write chapters for this book and thus have provided state-of-the-art reviews of the individual topics. The editors would like to thank all the authors and co-authors for their valuable contributions, as well as the publishers for expert editorial guidance and advice. The editors acknowledge with particular gratitude the excellent secretarial assistance provided by Jny Wittker, who was responsible for all administrative and organizational work during all stages of the preparation of this volume.

Books in a fast-moving field such as obesity carry the risk of becoming quickly outdated. For this reason, the editors have installed a Website (www.endo-diabase.ch/bookanti-obesitydrugs.htm) where important new developments related to the pharmacotherapy of obesity are made accessible until a new edition of this book may provide the opportunity for a general update.

Karl G. Hofbauer
Ulrich Keller
Olivier Boss

Editors

Karl G. Hofbauer holds the Chair for Applied Pharmacology at the Medical Faculty of the University of Basel. He received his M.D. degree from the University of Vienna, Austria, and specialized in experimental pharmacology at the University of Heidelberg, Germany. He spent more than 20 years in preclinical research at Ciba, later Novartis, in Basel, Switzerland, where he became interested in the search for antiobesity drugs. He has continued to work on this subject after moving back to academia.

Most relevant publications include:

Chiesi, M., Huppertz, C., Hofbauer, K.G., Pharmacotherapy of obesity — targets and perspectives. *Trends Pharmacol. Sci.*, 22: 247–254, 2001.

Hofbauer, K.G. and Huppertz, C., Pharmacotherapy and evolution. *Trends Ecol. Evol.*, 17: 328–334, 2002.

Hofbauer, K.G., Molecular pathways to obesity. *Int. J. Obesity*, 26, Suppl. 2: S18–27, 2002.

Ulrich Keller received his training in endocrinology and internal medicine in Zurich; Basel; Nashville, Tennessee; and Rochester, Minnesota. He is currently head of the division of endocrinology, diabetes, and clinical nutrition; since 1988, he has held the position of professor of medicine at the University of Basel. His main clinical activities are diabetology (type 1 and type 2 diabetes) and obesity and lipid disorders. This can only be achieved in close collaboration with other services of the hospital (diabetes and nutrition counseling; nephrology; gynecology; ophthalmology; cardiology; and others). Interdisciplinary consultations are specifically devoted to the assessment of morbidly obese subjects.

Keller is head of a research group in the Department of Research that is interested in the field of metabolism and adipocyte biology. His research has been devoted to the hormonal regulation of ketogenesis, as well as to studies on substrate effects on protein and lipid metabolism in man.

Olivier Boss received his training in medical biochemistry, exercise physiology, and endocrinology of energy metabolism from the University of Geneva (Switzerland) and Harvard Medical School and Beth Israel Deaconess Medical Center (Boston, Massachusetts).

He is currently head of a pharmacology laboratory involved in target discovery and validation, diabetes and metabolism at the Novartis Institutes for Biomedical Research, Cambridge, Massachusetts. He is also head of a project team at Novartis working on the mechanisms of insulin resistance associated with obesity and type 2 diabetes. His research has been devoted to control of energy metabolism, and his current activities are focused on development of treatments for obesity and insulin resistance/diabetes.

Contributors

Rexford S. Ahima
University of Pennsylvania, Division of
  Endocrinology, Diabetes, and
  Metabolism
Philadelphia, Pennsylvania

Trino Baptista
Los Andes University Medical School
Merida, Venezuela

Esther Biedert
Institut für Psychologie
Basel, Switzerland

John E. Blundell
University of Leeds
Leeds, United Kingdom

Olivier Boss
Novartis Institutes for Biomedical
  Research, Inc.
Cambridge, Massachusetts

Philippe Boutin
Institut Biologie de Lille, Institut Pasteur de
  Lille
Lille, France

George A. Bray
Pennington Biomedical Research Center
Baton Rouge, Louisiana

L. Arthur Campfield
Colorado State University
Fort Collins, Colorado

Vivion E. F. Crowley
Addenbrooke's Hospital, University of
  Cambridge
Cambridge, United Kingdom

Robert Dent
Ottawa Hospital
Ottawa, Ontario, Canada

James D. Douketis
McMaster University
Hamilton, Ontario, Canada

Abdul G. Dulloo
Institute of Physiology
Fribourg, Switzerland

Philippe Froguel
Pasteur Institute
Lille, France

Frank Greenway
Pennington Biomedical Research Center
Baton Rouge, Louisiana

Jason C. G. Halford
University of Liverpool
Liverpool, United Kingdom

Michael Hamilton
Pennington Biomedical Research Center
Baton Rouge, Louisiana

Mary-Ellen Harper
University of Ottawa
Ottawa, Ontario, Canada

Hans Hauner
Else-Kröner-Fresenius-Center for
  Nutritional Medicine
Technical University Munich
Munich, Germany

Karl G. Hofbauer
Biozentrum/Pharmazentrum
Basel, Switzerland

Alexandra Kazaks
University of California
Davis, California

Ulrich Keller
Kantonsspital Basel
Basel, Switzerland

Jaroslaw Kolanowski
Catholic University of Louvain
Brussels, Belgium

Leslie P. Kozak
Pennington Biomedical Research Center
Baton Rouge, Louisiana

Stephan Krähenbühl
Abt. Klinische Pharmakologie
Basel, Switzerland

Michael E. J. Lean
University of Glasgow
Glasgow, United Kingdom

Jürgen Margraf
Institut für Psychologie
Basel, Switzerland

Ruth McPherson
University of Ottawa
Ottawa, Ontario, Canada

Suzette Y. Osei
University of Pennsylvania
Philadelphia, Pennsylvania

F. Xavier Pi–Sunyer
St. Luke's-Roosevelt Hospital Center
New York, New York

Tobias Pischon
Franz Volhard Clinic — Charité and Max
    Delbrück Center for Molecular
    Medicine
Berlin, Germany

Eric Ravussin
Pennington Biomedical Research Center
Baton Rouge, Louisiana

Donna H. Ryan
Pennington Biomedical Research Center
Baton Rouge, Louisiana

André J. Scheen
Division of Diabetes, Nutrition and
    Metabolic Disorders, CHU Liège
Liège, Belgium

Arya M. Sharma
McMaster University, Hamilton General
    Hospital
Hamilton, Ontario, Canada

Françoise J. Smith
Colorado State University
Fort Collins, Colorado

Judith S. Stern
University of California
Davis, California

Rolf Stöckli
Kantonsspital Basel
Basel, Switzerland

Paolo M. Suter
Universitätsspital Zürich
Zürich, Switzerland

Frederique Tesson
University of Ottawa
Ottawa, Ontario, Canada

Antonio J. Vidal–Puig
University of Cambridge
Cambridge, United Kingdom

Contents

Part VII Appendix

Part I

Pathophysiology of Obesity

1

Energy Homeostasis

Eric Ravussin and Leslie P. Kozak

CONTENTS

ABSTRACT   The increasing prevalence of obesity worldwide has prompted the World Health Organization (WHO) to classify it as a global epidemic. Around the globe, almost 1 billion people are overweight or obese, and the chronic disease of obesity represents a major threat to health care systems in developed and developing countries. The major health hazards associated with obesity are the risks of developing diabetes; cardiovascular disease; stroke; osteoarthritis; and some forms of cancer. This chapter first reviews the relative contribution of environmental conditions and genetic make-up to the development of obesity and then the metabolic factors favoring weight gain in an "obesigenic" environment. Although weight gain results from a sustained imbalance between energy intake and energy expenditure, only recently have studies identified important new mechanisms involved in regulation of body weight. The etiology of the disease is presented as a feedback model in which afferent signals inform the central controllers in the brain as to the state of the external and internal environment and elicit responses related to regulation of food intake and energy metabolism. Some of the newly discovered molecular mechanisms underlying the variability in energy expenditure and fat oxidation are presented. Because pharmacological agents may intervene at different levels of the feedback model, new potential targets for generation of drugs that may assist people in increasing total energy expenditure and fat oxidation are discussed.

1.1   Is Obesity a Disease?

The question as to whether obesity is a disease has been vigorously debated over the past two decades. Acute diseases such as pneumonia and injury are usually curable and may not recur once healed. On the other hand, chronic diseases such as hypertension and obesity may go into remission and have undulating courses, but of long duration. Obesity is a chronic disease, whether it is judged from the standpoint of personal suffering endured by affected individuals or by the cost to public health systems and societies. Obesity results from chronic disruption of the energy balance. The long-term balance between energy intake and energy expenditure primarily determines the amount of energy stored in the body. When energy intake chronically exceeds energy expenditure, the resulting imbalance causes expansion of fat cells and, in some cases, increased numbers of fat cells. Hypertrophy and hyperplasia of fat cells represent the one and unique pathology of obesity. The enlarged fat cells are then likely to induce other metabolic disturbances leading eventually to other chronic diseases.

Whether the culprit is increased food intake or decreased energy expenditure is generally unknown and probably varies from case to case. It is likely that obesity results from impaired energy expenditure and an inability to control food intake in an environment not conducive to physical activity and in which highly palatable food is widely and easily available. Regardless, the consequence of this long-lasting imbalance is the obvious accumulation of fat. One of the most important questions is why the increasing fat stores provide a signal to the brain to reduce food intake in some people, but not in others. Another question is why some people are not able to increase their metabolic rates or discretionary physical activity to match their inappropriately high levels of caloric intake.

Since the discovery of leptin and its receptors 8 years ago, it is now better recognized that obesity is not only a lack of willpower leading to "sloth and gluttony," but can also be the consequence of metabolic defects. However, prejudice and discrimination still plague the lives of the obese. The stigma often derives from the society's "thinness" cult and, especially among women, a general dissatisfaction with one's body weight. Regardless of whether the impact of obesity is judged by the personal dissatisfaction of obese individuals and their families with their weight and shape, or by the cost to public health care systems, the problem needs to be taken seriously. Obesity must therefore be considered as a chronic disease with considerable personal and societal ill consequences that should be treated with efficacious and safe pharmacological agents.

1.2   "Essential" Obesity in an "Obesigenic" Environment

Although lifestyle and environmental influences on obesity are readily accepted, it is now recognized that human obesity has an important genetic component as well. Obesity is characterized by a strong familial aggregation pattern. However, except for some rare Mendelian disorders, the vast majority of obese patients do not exhibit a clear pattern of

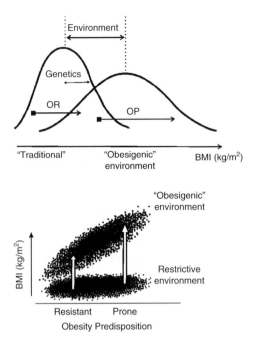

FIGURE 1.1
The potential effects of gene and environment on adiposity assessed here by body mass index (BMI). Genetic susceptibility to obesity can be defined as a variable resulting from allelic variations at a set of obesity genes in low-risk (traditional, left distribution) and high-risk (obesigenic, right distribution) environments. Top panel: In a restrictive environment in which caloric availability is limited and physical activity is high, individuals with a low genetic susceptibility (*obesity resistant*, OR) will have a very low body mass index. In contrast, those with a high genetic susceptibility (*obesity prone*, OP) will have a higher BMI (higher degree of adiposity), but still relatively low compared to the BMI distribution in an obesigenic environment. When these individuals move into an environment replete with high-fat foods and low demand for physical activity, the overall distribution of adiposity will shift to the right. Obesity-resistant subjects will gain some weight but much less than obesity-prone subjects, who will become frankly obese. Bottom panel: The same scenario is represented, showing the presence of a gene x environment interaction. The obesigenic environment amplifies the effects of genetic susceptibility in obesity-prone individuals compared to obesity-resistant individuals.

Mendelian inheritance. The susceptibility to obesity is determined to a significant extent by genetic factors, but a favorable "obesigenic" environment is necessary for its phenotypic expression. In other words, in the presence of a genetic predisposition to obesity, lifestyle and environmental conditions largely determine the severity of the disease.

Figure 1.1 illustrates these synergistic relationships between genes and environment. The variability of the distribution of body mass index (or adiposity) in a given environment ("restrictive" in the left distribution or obesigenic in the right distribution) is mostly attributable to genes, whereas the average of the distributions is primarily determined by environmental conditions. An example can be derived from a population extremely susceptible to obesity and diabetes, such as the Pima Indians. Those living in a restrictive environment in the remote Mexican Sierra Madre Mountains have a much lower prevalence of obesity and type-2 diabetes mellitus than Pima Indians living in Arizona in the Southwestern U.S. (Ravussin et al., 1994). The Mexican Pimas would fit the left distribution in the top panel of Figure 1.1.

In contrast, U.S. Pima Indians have the highest prevalence of type 2 diabetes in the world (Knowler et al., 1990) and one of the highest for obesity (Knowler et al., 1991). They are a reasonable fit to the distribution on the right. Figure.1.1 also depicts the potential interaction between genes and environment in the development of obesity. For example, it is

likely that when individuals from a population living in a restrictive environment characterized by a traditional lifestyle evolves toward an obesigenic environment, such as that
found in industrialized countries, most individuals from this population are likely to gain
weight. However, those with a high genetic predisposition for obesity will gain the most
weight whereas those resistant to obesity will gain little weight (Figure 1.1, bottom panel).

Considerable speculation surrounds the reasons why the human genome could harbor
genes predisposing to positive energy balance and obesity and at such a high frequency
if one takes the genetic epidemiology estimates of heritability at face value. The most
frequently stated theory is that of the "thrifty genotype hypothesis" (Neel, 1962), which
is essentially as follows: during mankind's history, individuals and populations have
evolved in restrictive environments in which food was not abundant and required much
physical work to obtain. Thus, survival mechanisms have evolved to confer a protection
against periods of food scarcity. Often cited examples of such populations include the
aboriginal populations of Australia; navigators of the Pacific Islands; and the Pima Indians
of the U.S., who were typically exposed to alternating periods of feast and famine. The
thrifty genotype hypothesis states that evolution in such restrictive environments has
progressively (or through genetic bottlenecks) selected for a thrifty genotype, conferring
survival advantages in periods of famine but resulting in liabilities in an affluent environment (Neel, 1962, 1998). The hypothesis is not unreasonable because abundance of food
and lack of the necessity for physical exercise to acquire food are fairly recent phenomena.

One implication of the thrifty genotype hypothesis is that it should not be surprising
to observe that highly industrialized populations are now struggling with the problem of
obesity due to rapid changes in environmental conditions. This has led to a second
hypothesis, which states that obesity in the present environment is an essential condition,
and only those with fewer obesity susceptibility genes (the former nonsurvivors) are now
apt to resist the obesigenic environment and remain at normal weight without conscious
effort (Ravussin and Bogardus, 1992). However, many individuals overcome the development of obesity but at the cost of constant dietary restrictions and regular physical activity
regimens. The common thread between these two hypotheses is that what was an asset
in early mankind has now rapidly become a liability.

1.3 Etiology of Obesity and Risk Factors for Weight Gain

Weight gain results from a sustained imbalance between energy intake and energy expenditure favoring positive energy balance. However, this simple statement belies the complex, multifactorial nature of obesity and the numerous biological and behavioral factors
that can affect both sides of the energy balance equation. These pathways and factors have
been reviewed elsewhere (Ravussin and Swinburn, 1993; Rosenbaum et al., 1997; Salbe
and Ravussin, 2000).

In the context of a discussion on the implications of recent progress for potential drug
targets for obesity, it is useful to consider the etiology of the disease as a feedback model
as illustrated in Figure 1.2 (Bray, 1991, 1998; Bray and Greenway, 1999). In this model,
afferent signals indicate to the central controllers in the brain the state of the external and
internal environments as they relate to food, metabolic rates, and activity behavior, to name
but a few. In turn, these central controllers transduce these messages into efferent signals
governing the behavioral search for acquisition of food, as well as modulating its subsequent deposition into such energy storage compartments as adipose tissue, liver, and
muscle and by modulating metabolic rates. Finally, a component of the system regulates

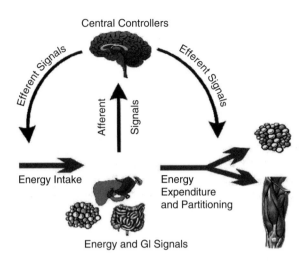

Central Controllers

Efferent Signals

Efferent Signals

Afferent Signals

Energy Intake

Energy Expenditure and Partitioning

Energy and GI Signals

FIGURE 1.2
A negative feedback model for regulation of body weight. In this model, peripheral signals from energy stores (adipose tissue, liver, and probably muscle) as well as hormonal and gastrointestinal signals provide afferences to the central controllers in the brain, indicating the state of the external and internal environment as they relate to food, metabolic rates, and activity behavior. In turn, the central controllers integrate all the signals and transduce these messages into efferent signals governing the behavioral search for acquisition of food (energy intake) as well as modulating its subsequent deposition (partitioning) into energy storage compartments, such as adipose tissue, liver, and muscle, by modulating energy expenditure. Afferent signals, efferent signals, and central controllers can be targeted for new potential antiobesity drugs (see text Section 1.5).

ingestion, digestion, absorption, transport, and storage of the ingested foods, as well as other related metabolic and behavioral functions. Each of these components of the system can be targeted for the development of drugs. New potential targets in pathways involved in the regulation of energy expenditure and fat oxidation are discussed later in Section 1.5.

Cross-sectional studies that compare lean and obese individuals have not provided true insights on the metabolic predictors of human obesity. Such studies have commonly reported that obesity is associated with high absolute energy expenditure; low respiratory quotient; high fat oxidation; insulin resistance; high sympathetic nervous system activity; and elevated plasma leptin concentrations (Ravussin and Gautier, 1999). In contrast, longitudinal studies that follow the same individuals over time have indicated that, relative to body size, low metabolic rate; high respiratory quotient; insulin sensitivity; low sympathetic nervous system activity; and low plasma leptin concentrations predict weight gain over time (Table 1.1).

Upon gaining weight, the original "abnormal" metabolic state becomes "normalized" (Weyer et al., 2000). Such "normalization" with weight gain explains why cross-sectional studies have not led to identification of metabolic risk factors for obesity. Weight gain thus

TABLE 1.1

Metabolic Characteristics of Obese and Preobese Individuals

	Obese (Factors Associated with Obesity)	Pre- or Postobese (Factors Predicting Weight Gain)
Relative resting metabolic rate	High or normal	Low
Energy cost of activity	Normal	Low
Fat oxidation	High	Low
Sympathetic nervous system activity	High	Low
Insulin sensitivity	Low	High
Relative leptin concentration	High	Low

causes an increase in metabolic rate; a decrease in respiratory quotient; a decrease in insulin sensitivity; an increase in sympathetic nervous activity; and an increase in plasma leptin concentrations — all of which serve to counteract further weight gain. Therefore, it is not surprising that weight loss plateaus after a few months of therapy. Based on these observations, one could hypothesize that not only drugs inhibiting food intake but also drugs increasing energy expenditure and/or increasing fat oxidation will be efficacious in prevention and treatment of obesity.

An understanding of the etiology of human obesity demands longitudinal studies. Cross-sectional studies have added little to understanding of the physiological mechanisms predisposing to weight gain (Ravussin and Swinburn, 1993). Cross-sectional studies can only provide associations, whereas longitudinal studies reveal predictors or risk factors. Several studies have examined these predictors in Pima Indians, a population prone to obesity (Knowler et al., 1991).

1.3.1   Low Metabolic Rate

A low absolute metabolic rate is unlikely to cause obesity because obese individuals have high metabolic rates, in resting (lying on a bed) and sedentary (during a day in a respiratory chamber) conditions (Ravussin et al., 1986; Weyer et al., 1999). Many investigators who have studied energy expenditure in humans have therefore suggested that, in the absence of a clear defect in energy expenditure in obese subjects, obesity can only be the result of excessive energy intake. However, the scatter around the regression line between metabolic rate and body size suggests that, at any given body size, individuals can have a "high," "normal," or "low" relative metabolic rate (RMR). Our studies in adult nondiabetic Pima Indians found that a low relative metabolic rate adjusted for differences in fat-free mass, fat mass, age, and sex was a risk factor for body weight gain (Ravussin et al., 1988). After 4 years of follow-up, the risk of gaining 10 kg was approximately eight times greater in subjects with the lowest RMR (lower tertile) compared with those with the highest RMR (higher tertile). According to a meta-analysis of published studies, formerly obese subjects have a 3 to 5% lower mean RMR than control subjects, which likely contributes to the high rate of weight regain in formerly obese persons (Astrup et al., 1999).

Nevertheless, these data need to be interpreted with caution because

- Variability of baseline energy expenditure accounted for only 16% of the variability of weight gain.
- Theoretical estimates suggest that only 30 to 40% of the increase in body energy stores in people who gained weight can be attributed to the baseline deficit in energy expenditure.
- Relatively low energy expenditure does not seem to be a predictor of weight gain in other adult populations (Weinsier et al., 1995; Amatruda et al., 1993).

Together, the results may suggest that a low metabolic rate may be a direct risk factor for body weight gain and also a marker for hyperphagia or inactivity.

1.3.2   Low Physical Activity

Another component of 24-h energy expenditure is the energy cost of spontaneous physical activity, which accounts for 8 to 15% of total daily expenditure (Ravussin et al., 1986).

Consistent with the cross-sectional observation of a decrease in spontaneous physical activity in obese subjects, longitudinal studies showed that even in the confined environment of a respiratory chamber, spontaneous physical activity is a familial trait and that a low level of spontaneous physical activity is associated with subsequent weight gain in males, but not in females (Zurlo et al., 1992). A recent study found that resistance to the development of obesity might be due to the ability of increasing spontaneous physical activity (also defined as nonexercise activity thermogenesis or NEAT) in response to overfeeding (Levine et al., 1999).

Prospective studies in which ambulant physical activity is measured (doubly labeled water technique) are absolutely needed to assess objectively what most scientists believe, i.e., that a low level of physical activity is a major predisposing factor for weight gain in individuals and in populations (Sundquist and Johansson, 1998). Studies from Schoeller's group indicate that patients successful at maintaining weight loss are those engaging in a considerable amount of physical activity up to 80 min per day (Schoeller et al., 1997). However, in longitudinal studies in Pima Indian children, it was observed that decrease in physical activity level (measured by doubly labeled water) seems to follow, not precede, development of obesity (Salbe et al., 2002).

1.3.3 Low Rates of Fat Oxidation

The composition of nutrient intake has been shown to be an important factor in the genesis of obesity; consequently, one might expect that the composition of nutrient oxidation would also play a role. The nonprotein respiratory quotient is an index of the ratio of carbohydrate to fat oxidation ranging from a value of about 0.80 after an overnight fast when fat is the main oxidative substrate (McNeill et al., 1988) to values close to 1.00 after a large carbohydrate meal when glucose is the major substrate (Astrup et al., 1995). Apart from the effect of diet composition, the respiratory quotient is also influenced by recent energy balance (negative balance causing more fat oxidation); sex (females tend to have reduced fat oxidation); adiposity (higher fat mass leads to higher fat oxidation); and family membership, suggesting genetic determinants (Zurlo et al., 1990; Toubro et al., 1998).

In a longitudinal study in Pima Indians, a high 24-h respiratory quotient predicted weight gain (Zurlo et al., 1992). Those in the 90th percentile for respiratory quotient (low fat oxidizers) had a 2.5 times larger risk of gaining 5 kg or more body weight than those in the 10th percentile (high fat oxidizers). This effect was independent of a relatively low or high 24-h metabolic rate. Similar results were found in Caucasian volunteers participating in the Baltimore Longitudinal Study on Aging (Seidell et al., 1992). In support of these observations, others have demonstrated that weight-reduced obese volunteers have high respiratory quotients, i.e., low rates of fat oxidation (Astrup et al., 1995; Larson et al., 1995), and those who are able to maintain weight loss have lower respiratory quotients compared to those experiencing weight relapse (Froidevaux et al., 1993).

1.3.4 Low Sympathetic Nervous Activity

The activity of the sympathetic nervous system (SNS) is positively related to the three major components of energy expenditure (resting metabolic rate; (Spraul et al., 1993); thermic effect of food (Schwartz et al., 1988); and spontaneous physical activity (Christin et al., 1993). SNS activity is negatively related to 24-h respiratory quotient (Snitker et al., 1998). Further indications of the possible role of SNS activity in the regulation of energy balance in humans comes from a study showing that a low SNS activity is associated with a poor weight loss outcome in obese subjects treated with diet (Astrup et al., 1995).

Furthermore, Pima Indians, who are prone to obesity, have low rates of muscle sympathetic nerve activity compared to weight-matched Caucasians (Spraul et al., 1993). In a prospective study, it was found that baseline urinary excretion rate of norepinephrine, a global index of SNS activity, was negatively correlated with body weight gain in male Pima Indians (Tataranni et al., 1997). Thus, low activity of the SNS is associated with the development of obesity.

1.3.5   Low Plasma Concentration of Leptin

Leptin, the product of the *OB* gene, is a hormone produced by the adipose tissue that inhibits food intake and increases energy expenditure (Caro et al., 1995). To investigate whether individuals prone to weight gain are hypoleptinemic, fasting plasma leptin concentrations were measured in two groups of weight-matched, nondiabetic Pima Indians followed for approximately 3 years, 19 of whom subsequently gained weight (average weight gain 23 kg) and 17 of whom maintained their weight within 0.5 kg. After adjustment for initial percent body fat, mean plasma leptin concentration was lower in those who gained weight than in those whose weight was stable (Ravussin et al., 1997). Despite the leptin resistance apparent in obesity (Caro et al., 1996), these data indicate that relatively low plasma leptin concentrations may play a role in development of obesity. However, relative hypoleptinemia was not a risk factor for obesity in other studies (Lissner et al., 1999; McNeely et al., 1999).

1.4   Molecular Mechanisms of Energy Metabolism

As described previously, the positive energy balance that leads to excessive deposition of fat results from excessive food consumption together with reduced total energy expenditure. Understanding the molecular mechanisms by which variation in energy expenditure contributes to the development of obesity has been an elusive goal. Energy expenditure includes many components, such as physical activity; fidgeting; the thermic effect of food; ambient temperature; fever; shivering; and the efficiency of basal metabolism. The effects of some of these factors, such as physical exercise and ambient temperature, are obvious; however, what determines "metabolic efficiency" is extremely complex. All components of energy expenditure, whether simple or complex, are most likely influenced by variations in the genetic constitution of an individual.

Based upon the "thrifty gene" hypothesis, one would predict that mutations changing the efficiency of energy metabolism should exist. Yet spontaneous or induced mutations that can cause obesity without increased food consumption in mice or humans are not known. In mouse and man, single gene mutations in the genes for leptin, leptin receptor, or melanocortin receptors, act directly on the CNS to affect food intake and indirectly on peripheral tissues to affect energy expenditure (Friedman and Halaas, 1998). Recent evidence suggests that leptin administered to mice can acutely stimulate directly lipid oxidation in skeletal muscle (Minokoshi et al., 2002) and the expression of genes of lipid oxidation in the liver (Zhou et al., 1997). Peripheral metabolism including adipocyte, muscle, and liver metabolism accounts for a major portion of the obesity phenotype of ob/ob mice. In other words, food restricted ob/ob mice remain fat even though total body weight is diminished to the level of wild-type controls (Alonso and Maren, 1955; Levin et al., 1996).

Whether genetic variations exist that modulate, but do not totally inactivate, the leptin signaling system among obese individuals is not known. Suggestive data of the importance of leptin on peripheral metabolism are now emerging in humans (Petersen et al., 2002; Rosenbaum et al., 2002; Ravussin et al., 2002). Evidence is that, in addition to inhibition of food intake, leptin can stimulate energy expenditure by its action on muscle (Minokoshi et al., 2002) and by stimulation of sympathetic activity (Haynes et al., 1997). Accordingly, it remains a mystery why this regulatory circuit fails in maintaining energy balance in a large number of obese individuals.

An obesity genetic model in which the primary effect is on the efficiency of energy expenditure alone would therefore improve understanding on how variations in energy expenditure contribute to the development of obesity. This part of the review will examine the genetic evidence related to obesity phenotypes that appear to be acting at the level of energy expenditure.

Here, the consideration is of mutations related to energy metabolism at two levels: those that affect the generation of fuels for thermogenesis and those that directly affect the thermogenic mechanisms. The goal in this categorization is to determine at which level lie the rate limiting steps for a given energy homeostasis. Put another way, it is conceivable that the capacity for thermogenesis, that is, mechanisms that consume ATP by substrate cycling or generate heat by uncoupling respiration from ATP synthesis, is not limiting and is always in excess. In this case, simply increasing the availability of oxidizable fuel, preferentially lipids, would reduce obesity. Alternatively, if thermogenic mechanisms are rate limiting, then no matter how active fatty acid oxidation may be, the low mitochondrial uncoupling or ATPase will prevent combustion of calories and obesity cannot be reduced.

Examples of substrate cycling that could function as futile ATPases to "waste" energy include the phoshpofructokinase/fructose diphosphatase cycle; the glycerol phosphate cycle; and the Cori cycle. Variants for the fructose phosphate cycle have not been reported, but spontaneous and induced mutations for the cytoplasmic and mitochondrial glycerol 3-phosphate dehydrogenases have been characterized (Prochazka et al., 1989; Brown et al., 2002). Mice deficient in the cytoplasmic enzyme have no obesity phenotype even though muscle ATP levels are reduced during exercise. Mice deficient in the mitochondrial enzyme are slightly smaller, but not obese. Similarly, mutations to a putative substrate cycle, which is also inducible in liver by thyroid hormone (Lee and Lardy, 1965), have no significant effects on obesity. Evidence supports the existence of a substrate cycling system, formed by lipolysis of triacylglycerol and reesterification of fatty acids, that can be stimulated by leptin (Reidy and Weber, 2002).

Genetic variation can alter energy expenditure not only at the level of substrate cycles, ATPases, or uncoupling proteins, but also at any of the steps at which the organism manages its nutrients. Can genetic studies (gene knockout or gene overexpression) help in elucidating the thermogenic mechanisms underlying interindividual variability in energy expenditure? For example, mice with inactive long- or short-chain acyl CoA dehydrogenase genes are cold sensitive like mice with an inactive UCP1 gene. The acyl CoA dehydrogenases are not thermogenic per se, but their absence affects the ability of the mouse to provide fuel for thermogenesis through fatty acid oxidation. Thus, modulations of the thermogenic mechanism (i.e., UCP1 inactivation) or supportive mechanisms can have significant effects on energy expenditure. This distinction between true thermogenic mechanisms and those that are supportive is important for understanding the mechanisms controlling energy expenditure. Therefore, reviews have been attempted of variations in genes believed to be associated directly with thermogenic mechanisms as well as some closely associated with fuel partitioning.

1.4.1   Insulin Receptor

Through its effects on mobilization of cellular fuels at the metabolite, enzymatic, and gene expression levels, the insulin pathway plays a pivotal role in the control of fuels available for thermogenesis. Although unexpectedly normal at birth (only slight growth retardation), mice homozygous for a deletion of the insulin receptor quickly develop severe hyperglycemia and hyperinsulinemia and die shortly after of β-cell failure, severe diabetes, and ketosis (Joshi et al., 1996; Accili et al., 1996). Therefore, to define the function of the insulin receptor in different insulin-responsive tissues and its contribution to type 1 and type 2 diabetes, a strategy was developed based upon Cre/lox technology for conditional inactivation of the insulin receptor gene in specific tissues (Kitamura et al., 2002). This experimental approach was expected to provide a clear, unambiguous picture of the role of selective insulin responsive-tissues in glucose and fat homeostasis.

To the contrary, a very confusing picture has emerged that is difficult to interpret. The muscle-specific knockout causes dyslipidemia with no effects on glucose metabolism (Bruning et al., 1998). On the other hand, muscle/adipose knockout mice have impaired glucose tolerance whereas the adipose-specific knockout mice are lean and have improved glucose tolerance with no insulin resistance (Kitamura et al., 2002). Even more surprising, brown fat insulin receptor knockout mice have defective β-cell insulin secretion (Guerra et al., 2001). In summary, this experimental approach designed to identify the contribution of the insulin receptor in insulin responsive tissues has not been conclusive.

1.4.2   Adrenergic Receptor Activation of Nonshivering Thermogenesis

Adrenergic activation of the nonshivering thermogenesis in adult animals is mediated by the fat-specific β3-adrenergic receptor via induction of UCP1 expression (Arch et al., 1984). The inactivation of the UCP1 gene causes cold sensitivity in mice and a targeted inactivation of dopamine β-hydroxylase (Dbh); preventing the animal from synthesizing catecholamines makes the mice even more sensitive to cold (Enerback et al., 1997). Furthermore, neither the UCP1 –/– mice nor the Dbh –/– mice show any evidence of increased obesity compared to wild-type mice despite reduced capacity for thermogenesis (Thomas and Palmiter, 1997). Accordingly, neither the inability to synthesize catecholamines nor the absence of UCP1 causes obesity in mice.

Lowell and colleagues have approached this problem of thermogenesis and susceptibility to obesity by selective inactivation of the beta adrenergic receptors by gene targeting (Susulic et al., 1995). They first inactivated the β3-adrenergic receptor and found that the mice had normal levels of UCP1 mRNA, normal cold sensitivity, but showed only a mild obesity with increasing age (Susulic et al., 1995). The normal levels of UCP1 expression in β3-deficient mice indicated that other β-adrenergic receptors might be compensatory. The mild obesity, even though UCP1 expression was unaffected, suggested that a reduction in adrenergically stimulated lipolysis occurred, probably in the white fat. Mice with an inactivated β1-adrenergic receptor died perinatally, although some survived, depending on the background genotype (Rohrer et al., 1996). On the contrary, β2-AR-deficient mice appeared normal, but weighed about 10% less than wild-type mice (Chruscinski et al., 1999). Thus, none of the three β-adrenergic receptor mutants produced significant obesity.

However, Lowell and his colleagues carried this analysis further by inactivating all three β-adrenergic receptor genes in the same mouse (Bachman et al., 2002). Remarkably, these animals survived and had the very intriguing phenotype of being sensitive to cold exposure and very prone to diet-induced obesity. Thus, one is faced with the conundrum that UCP1- and dopamine β-hydroxylase-deficient mice have a phenotype of cold sensitivity but resistance to obesity, whereas the β-adrenergic receptor mice are also cold sensitive, but susceptible to diet-induced obesity. Taken together, these results suggest that other adrenergic receptors, i.e., the α-receptors, are important in the etiology of obesity. Indeed, β3-adrenergic receptor deficient mice expressing the human α2-adrenergic receptor as a transgene are obese because of adipocyte hyperplasia (Valet et al., 2000). In addition, the presence of the β-adrenergic receptors in the UCP1-deficient mice may enable the mice to utilize alternative mechanisms of thermogenesis (Liu et al., 2003).

1.4.3 Mutations in Fatty Acid Oxidation Pathways

- *Acetyl CoA Carboxylase.* Acetyl CoA Carboxylase 2 (ACC2) catalyzes the rate-limiting step in fatty acid biosynthesis from acetyl-CoA. Mice deficient in ACC2 are fertile and have a normal life span, but weigh less and have smaller fat depots than wild type mice (Abu–Elheiga et al., 2001). These mice consume up to 30% more food, suggesting increased energy expenditure. In the absence of ACC2, malonyl CoA is decreased and fatty acid oxidation is stimulated in muscle to serve as a sink for fatty acids that would normally be deposited in the liver and adipose tissue. Although the effects of ACC2 deficiency on adiposity are striking, some important questions remain unanswered.

  In the face of a major increase in β-oxidation in muscle, what is the heat producing mechanism, because there is a reduction in fat depots in the mice despite increased food intake? The enhanced generation of NADH and FADH2 by fatty acid oxidation is dissipated by mitochondrial respiration as long as the supply of ADP is continual or the muscle mitochondria are uncoupled by one of the uncoupling proteins. If the mitochondria are coupled to ATP synthesis, then energy must be expended by a futile ATPase or by muscle activity. This would become evident experimentally by increased oxygen consumption at rest or through increased physical activity. Similarly, if the mitochondria were dissipating the membrane potential by an uncoupling mechanism, then increases in oxygen consumption and heat production would be observed. It is hoped that these determinations will be reported in the near future.

  An encouraging aspect of this model is that the capacity for increased energy expenditure exists in response to increased fuel oxidation due to a shift in metabolism caused by blocking fatty acid synthesis and reducing malonyl CoA levels, an inhibitor of fatty acid uptake by the mitochondria. Whether the mice are generating heat or have increased physical activity remains to be shown.

- *Acyl CoA Dehydrogenase Deficiency.* A spontaneous mutation in the short chain of the acyl CoA dehydrogenase gene (Acads) of BALB/cByJ mice and a targeted mutation in the long chain acyl CoA dehydrogenase gene (Acadl) cause a phenotype characterized by extreme sensitivity to cold (Guerra et al., 1998). Although UCP1 mRNA levels are similar in mutant and wild-type controls maintained at an ambient temperature of 23°C, the rate of induction of UCP1 and type 2 deiodinase levels lags in the mutant mice when housed at near thermoneutrality. The basis for this difference in mRNA inductions for these two genes is unknown. Although not proven, it has been hypothesized that the inability of the mice to mount a thermogenic response that would maintain body temperature is due to deficiency in β-oxidation of fatty acids in the brown fat. Histological examination of interscapular brown fat shows an accumulation of fat in the Acads-deficient mice similar to that previously found in UCP1 deficient mice. The effects of Acyl

CoA dehydrogenase deficiency on adiposity and other parameters of energy metabolism have not been fully studied.

- *Diacylglycerol acyltransferase* (DGAT). Mice with the targeted inactivation of the DGAT gene are leaner than wild-type mice when fed a high-fat diet (Smith et al., 2000). In addition, DGAT deficiency causes reduced obesity in Ay mice but not in ob/ob mice. Chen et al. (2002) found that reduced obesity in fat-fed mice and Ay mice leads to improved glucose tolerance and insulin sensitivity in DGAT −/− mice. The authors propose that DGAT −/− mice have increased energy expenditure; however, the evidence for this is not strong yet. It is possible that the difference in oxygen consumption would not be as apparent if the data had been calculated on the basis of lean body mass, rather than body weight. Chen and colleagues failed to express their results using the appropriate method of normalizing energy expenditure data using regression analysis instead of ratios (Ravussin and Bogardus, 1989; Poehlman, 2003).

   Because the DGAT −/− mice are more active physically, it is necessary to consider the increased energy expenditure from activity before making conclusions about energy efficiency. Furthermore, it has been proposed that increased leptin sensitivity in DGAT −/− mice is associated with a mechanism for increased energy expenditure (Chen et al., 2002). At this time, one can conclude that DGAT −/− mice are leaner than wild-type controls, probably because of reduced capacity of triglyceride synthesis; however, the energy expenditure phenotype needs to be better studied. Because DGAT could be part of a thermogenic substrate cycle of triacylglycerol and fatty acids (see earlier discussion), it is puzzling that the absence of DGAT would stimulate energy expenditure. Interestingly, a genetic polymorphism in the promoter of the DGAT1 gene was found to be associated with body mass index in a Turkish population (Ludwig et al., 2002).

1.4.4   Mitochondria-Uncoupling Protein UCP1 and Brown Fat Thermogenesis

It is well established from analysis of transgenic mice that an increase in UCP1 expression in brown adipose tissue or an increase in the number of brown adipocytes (induced by the conversion of white adipocytes to brown adipocytes) can reduce obesity, insulin resistance, and diabetes. Transgenic mice have been created in which the UCP1 gene has been placed under the control of a promoter that causes ectopic expression in tissues such as white adipose and skeletal muscle (Kopecky et al., 1995, 1996; Li et al., 2000; Cederberg et al., 2001). In addition, genetic variation among inbred strains of mice causes a variation in the induction of brown fat in traditional white fat depots (Koza et al., 2000; Guerra et al., 1998). These mice provide some of the strongest experimental proof of principle for the idea that increased uncoupling of mitochondria by genetic manipulation can reduce obesity and the development of type 2 diabetes (Li et al., 2000; Clapham et al., 2000).

   However, practical application of this experimental approach to humans by pharmacological activation of the UCP1 gene seems remote. It is less far-fetched to think that induction of brown adipocytes in white fat depots of humans can be achieved pharmacologically (Champigny et al., 1991; Himms–Hagen et al., 1994). Given the effectiveness of increased brown adipocyte number in white fat depots on reducing obesity in rats and mice, such an approach clearly represents a promising strategy in humans. Much evidence has accumulated showing that UCP1 is present in white adipose depots of adult humans

(Lean, 1992); however, whether the expression of UCP1 can achieve a level sufficient to reduce obesity remains to be answered.

Excluding the obvious difference that mice have major depots of brown fat around several vital organs and in the interscapular region, important features of brown adipocyte expression in white fat depots are relevant to the characteristics of the brown adipocyte phenotype in humans:

- In the absence of sympathetic stimulation (cold or adrenergic agonists), mice 2 months of age or older have very low levels of UCP1 expression in white fat (Guerra et al., 1998). Chronic exposure to cold is a rare occurrence among humans because they use behavioral strategies rather than physiological adaptative thermogenesis to protect themselves from the cold.

- The amount of UCP1 that can be induced by adrenergic stimulation varies by approximately two orders of magnitude in different white fat depots of the same animal (Guerra et al., 1998). Although several morphological and a few molecular studies have identified small numbers of brown adipocytes in humans under standard conditions (Esterbauer et al., 1998), none of these studies has attempted to map out relative expression among different fat depots.

- Large genetic variation in the induction of brown adipocytes is found among inbred strains of mice, with some strains highly resistant to induction and others showing that the majority of adipocytes in a white fat depot have acquired brown adipocyte morphology (Guerra et al., 1998).

To assess the potential for brown adipocyte induction in humans confidently, it will be necessary to establish appropriate environmental conditions, sample the right fat depots, and determine genetic haplotypes that carry variant genes for induction. Genetic studies should be undertaken to identify the range of haplotypes for regulatory genes implicated in brown adipocyte induction from genetic studies in mice.

1.4.5 Mechanisms Controlling Induction of Brown Adipocytes

Mechanisms controlling the induction of brown adipocytes can be identified in two ways. The first is based upon transgenic and gene knockout models that cause an increase in the number of brown adipocytes in white fat depots (Cederberg et al., 2001 ; Soloveva et al., 1997; Tsukiyama–Kohara et al., 2001). The discoveries of these genes (including the FoxC2 transcription factor; Cederberg et al., 2001), 4BP translation inhibitor (Tsukiyama–Kohara et al., 2001), and the protein kinase A RIIβ regulatory subunit (Cummings et al., 1996) have been largely serendipitous, because the initial phenotype of the genetically altered mouse was reduced body weight. Only subsequent analysis revealed increased numbers of brown adipocytes in white fat and increased UCP1 expression. Overexpression of the β1-adrenergic receptor also increases brown adipocytes in white fat depots (Soloveva et al., 1997). The mechanism of the induction of new brown adipocytes is unknown but, in most cases, the genetic manipulations cause an increase in cAMP levels in the white adipocytes, which seems to be essential for subsequent induction of brown adipocytes.

1.4.6 Other Potential Thermogenic Mechanisms: UCP2 and UCP3

Following the discovery of two genes with homology to brown fat-specific UCP1, there was great excitement that these genes could become targets for the induction of thermogenesis in the human. Their structural similarity to UCP1 also suggested that they could serve an uncoupling function in the mitochondria. Indeed, expression of UCP2 and UCP3 in yeast and in reconstituted proteoliposomes supports an uncoupling function. Moreover, these genes are broadly expressed in humans and, in particular, UCP3, is abundantly expressed in skeletal muscle, an important tissue for thermogenesis (Zurlo et al., 1990). As evidenced by recent literature (Ricquier and Bouillaud, 2000; Kozak and Harper, 2000), a huge effort has been made to establish a function for UCP2 and UCP3 in the regulation of body weight.

However, the phenotypes of mice in which the UCP2 and UCP3 genes have been inactivated do not indicate that these homologues have a function in regulating body temperature or body weight (Gong et al., 2000; Vidal–Puig et al., 2000; Arsenijevic et al., 2000; Zhang et al., 2001). In one study in which UCP3 was overexpressed in skeletal muscle of transgenic mice, the mice showed a resistance to diet-induced obesity and an improvement in insulin sensitivity (Clapham et al., 2000). Because the amount of UCP3 in the muscle of the transgenic mice was at a level shown previously (by the same group of investigators) to be toxic to the mitochondria of mammalian cells, it is possible that the mitochondria of the transgenic mice were leaky due to toxicity from the high levels of UCP3 (Stuart et al., 2001). Consequently, the effects of the UCP3 transgene expression were not indicative of a normal physiological function. A recent study in which UCP3 was induced in human muscle by a high-fat diet and then the rate of recovery of energy stores, i.e., creatine phosphate, was determined failed to find an effect, suggesting that UCP3 in humans does not uncouple muscle mitochondria (Hesselink et al., 2003).

Although no genetic evidence exists for variation in genes encoding ion transporters other than the UCPs, the human genome project has revealed a huge number of genes that could function in thermogenic mechanisms. The known possibilities for energy dissipation by ion transport-related processes are huge and becoming even larger as mining of human and mouse genomic databases continues (see databases being compiled by the Alliance for Cellular Signaling, http://www.signaling-gateway.org). However, evidence that these mechanisms actually limit the development of obesity by stimulating energy expenditure must be demonstrated. Ultimately, proof that a putative mechanism of energy expenditure actually has a role in maintaining caloric homeostasis must come through genetic studies in animal models and then through discovery of genetic variability for these mechanisms in humans.

1.5 Potential Targets for Obesity Drugs

According to the negative feedback model presented in Figure 1.2, pharmaceutical agents may intervene at three different levels. First, small molecules can reinforce the afferent signals from the periphery. Second, such molecules can target the central pathways involved in the regulation of food intake and energy expenditure. Third, agents can directly increase peripheral energy expenditure and increase energy partitioning toward muscle. Some of these targets have been reviewed elsewhere (Halford and Blundell, 2000). This review will concentrate on the potential targets relevant to energy expenditure and fat oxidation.

A number of features are desirable in a next-generation obesity medication. The first is obviously safety because the history of the pharmacological treatment of obesity has been marked by several disasters (Bray, 1998). This is particularly important because many

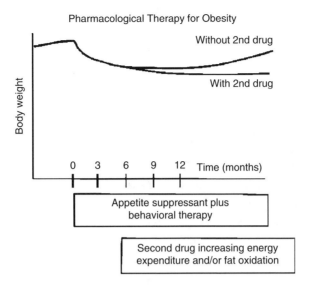

Pharmacological Therapy for Obesity

FIGURE 1.3
A scenario for using two drugs with different modes of action to treat obese patients. In a first phase, patients combine an appetite suppressant with behavioral modifications to lose weight rapidly. However, after a few months, due to counteracting mechanisms (decrease in energy expenditure and decrease in fat oxidation), a thermogenic agent is added to avoid the resistance to weight loss that is often manifested by a relapse in weight gain.

people will seek pharmacological treatment for obesity, even if they have no clinical indication for drug therapy. Of course, an equally important feature for a new generation of drugs is efficacy. Future pharmacotherapy should be potent enough to induce a weight loss of at least 15% of initial body weight on average and maintain the weight loss. The mechanism of action will also be very important. Almost all previous drugs were acting centrally and associated with side effects, so it would be preferable if some drugs of the next generation acted peripherally. Finally, because pharmacological treatment of obesity requires lifelong therapy, the cost of such an agent should be affordable. If the cost of treating obesity exceeds the cost of treating its co-morbidities, then these new drugs are bound to fail on the market.

An important issue is that the pharmacological treatment of the future will not cure obesity. Weight loss reaches a plateau after a few months of treatment as a result of many compensatory mechanisms coming into play and re-equilibrating the energy balance (see etiology section and Table 1.1). This reality must be understood by patients and health care providers to avoid the vicious cycles of frustration that often occur between parties when realistic expectations are not clearly established at the onset of treatment (Garrow, 1992). Because of this, combination therapy targeting different mechanisms is likely to be more efficacious.

For instance, during the first phase of a weight loss program, an appetite suppressant, in association with behavioral therapy, may be the most relevant approach (Figure 1.3). However, after 2 or 3 months of weight loss, an agent that increases energy expenditure and/or fat oxidation could be added to counteract the decrease in metabolic rate and sustain negative energy balance conditions. Together, an appetite suppressant and a stimulator of metabolic rate should be helpful in preventing some of the regained weight so commonly observed. Finally, further away in the future, anticipated advances in human genomics and proteomics should make it possible to prescribe drugs designed to alleviate specific genetic deficiencies identified by genotyping for mutations at relevant genes. These advances will allow development of an "à la carte" approach to treatment.

TABLE 1.2

Potential Targets (Pathways) for Increasing Energy Expenditure or Fat Oxidation
or for Inhibiting Adipose Tissue Proliferation

Pathway	Activation (+) or Inhibition (–) to Decrease Obesity
Acetyl CoA carboxylase β (ACC2)	(–)
Adrenergic (β3) receptor	(+)
Carnitine palmitoyltransferase 1 (MCPT1)	(+)
Diacylglycerol acyltransferase (DGAT)	(–)
Hmgic	(–)
Leptin (LEPR)	(+)
Peroxisome proliferator-activator receptor α (PPAR-α)	(+)
PPAR γ	(–)
PPAR γ coactivator1 (PGC1)	(+)
Sterol regulatory element binding protein (SREBP)	(–)
Thyroid hormones; (thyroid β receptor)	(+)
Uncoupling proteins (UCP)	(+)

The ideal molecule to target energy metabolism at the periphery would be one that could increase resting energy expenditure and fat oxidation. Table 1.2 presents some potential targets or pathways involved in an increase in energy expenditure and/or fat oxidation via central mechanisms or directly on peripheral tissues. At the present time, development of selective β_3-adrenoreceptor agonists targeting the human receptor is receiving the most attention (Weyer et al., 1999). Previous compounds were generated against the rat receptor and have typically shown problems of bioavailability or lack of selectivity in humans. Leptin remains an attractive target because of the dual effect on food intake and energy metabolism. Whether a small agonist molecule of the leptin receptor can be generated remains to be shown. Alternatively, molecules causing an allosteric enhancement of endogenous leptin action may be a viable strategy because obese patients already have high plasma and cerebrospinal fluid leptin concentrations.

Thyroid hormones have always represented an attractive target for stimulating energy expenditure. However, because of the well-known side effects on the cardiovascular system, molecules acting predominantly on the thyroid β-receptor in the muscle may be a potential means to increase energy expenditure (Weiss et al., 1998) without unwanted effects. If uncoupling proteins can be activated only in desirable tissues, then they are likely to represent good targets for obesity (Ricquier and Bouillaud, 2000). Recent data from knockout of the protein tyrosine phosphatase 1B indicate that inhibitors of this phosphatase may represent a viable way of increasing energy expenditure with a concomitant improvement of insulin sensitivity (Elchebly et al., 1999; Klaman et al., 2000). Among other proposed potential obesity targets are

- Diacylglycerol acyltransferase (DGAT) (Smith et al., 2000)
- Peroxisome proliferator-activated receptor-α (PPAR-α) (Kubota et al., 1999)
- PPAR-γ (Guerre–Millo et al., 2000; Willson et al., 2000)
- Peroxisome proliferator-activated receptor γ-coactivator 1 (PGC1) (Wu et al., 1999)
- Carnitine palmitoyltransferase (Cohen et al., 1998)
- High-mobility group protein (HMGIC) (Anand and Chada, 2000)
- Sterol regulatory element-binding protein (SREBP) (Boizard et al., 1998; Kakuma et al., 2000)

However, most of these pathways may need more validation before they are considered true obesity targets.

With growing understanding of the biology of the human genome, it is very likely that new targets will be identified and prioritized on the basis of their validation. New generations of drugs with different mechanisms of action will be developed and used in combination therapy to treat the complex disease of obesity. Moreover, in the future, it is likely that the treatment of obesity will be characterized by growing individuality and sophistication. Regardless, it is certain that the next 5 years will see an explosion of research on target identification and target validation for the pharmacological treatment of obesity. However, given the epidemic nature of obesity at this time, only public health measures and drastic public policy changes can modify the "obesigenic" environment (Egger and Swinburn, 1997). Without major societal changes, it is almost certain that the obesity epidemic will continue to spread around the world in the present century.

References

Abu–Elheiga, L. et al. Continuous fatty acid oxidation and reduced fat storage in mice lacking acetyl-coa carboxylase 2. *Science* 291.5513 (2001): 2613–2616.

Accili, D. et al. Early neonatal death in mice homozygous for a null allele of the insulin receptor gene. *Nat. Genet.* 12.1 (1996): 106–109.

Alonso, L.G. and T.H. Maren. Effect of food restriction on body composition of hereditary obese mice. *Am. J. Physiol.* 183 (1955): 284–290.

Amatruda, J.M., M.C. Statt, and S.L. Welle. Total and resting energy expenditure in obese women reduced to ideal body weight. *J. Clin. Invest.* 92.3 (1993): 1236–1242.

Anand, A. and K. Chada. *In vivo* modulation of hmgic reduces obesity. *Nat. Genet.* 24.4 (2000): 377–380.

Arch, J.R.S. et al. Atypical β-adrenoreceptor on brown adipocytes as targets for antiobesity drugs. *Nature* 309 (1984): 163–165.

Arsenijevic, D. et al. Disruption of the uncoupling protein-2 gene in mice reveals a role in immunity and reactive oxygen species production [in process citation]. *Nat. Genet.* 26.4 (2000): 435–439.

Astrup, A. et al. Failure to increase lipid oxidation in response to increasing dietary fat content in formerly obese women. *Am. J. Physiol.* 266.4 Pt. 1 (1994): E592–599.

Astrup, A. et al. Prognostic markers for diet-induced weight loss in obese women. *Int. J. Obes. Relat. Metab. Disord.* 19.4 (1995): 275–278.

Astrup, A. et al. Meta-analysis of resting metabolic rate in formerly obese subjects. *Am. J. Clin. Nutr.* 69.6 (1999): 1117–1122.

Bachman, E.S. et al. Beta Ar-signaling required for diet-induced thermogenesis and obesity resistance. *Science* 297.5582 (2002): 843–845.

Boizard, M. et al. Obesity-related overexpression of fatty-acid synthase gene in adipose tissue involves sterol regulatory element-binding protein transcription factors. *J. Biol. Chem.* 273.44 (1998): 29164–29171.

Bray, G.A. (1998) *Contemporary Diagnosis and Management of Obesity.* Newton, PA: Handbooks in Health Care Co.

Bray, G.A. Obesity, a disorder of nutrient partitioning: the Mona Lisa hypothesis. *J. Nutr.* 121.8 (1991): 1146–1162.

Bray, G.A. and F.L. Greenway. Current and potential drugs for treatment of obesity. *Endocr. Rev.* 20.6 (1999): 805–875.

Brown, L.J. et al. Normal thyroid thermogenesis, but reduced viability and adiposity in mice lacking the mitochondrial glycerol phosphate dehydrogenase. *J. Biol. Chem.* 277 (2002): 32892–32898.

Bruning, J.C. et al. a muscle-specific insulin receptor knockout exhibits features of the metabolic syndrome of NIDDM without altering glucose tolerance. *Mol. Cell* 2.5 (1998): 559–569.

Caro, J.F. et al. Decreased cerebrospinal-fluid/serum leptin ratio in obesity: a possible mechanism for leptin resistance. *Lancet* 348.9021 (1996): 159–161.

Caro, J.F. et al. Leptin: The tale of an obesity gene. *Diabetes* 45.11 (1996): 1455–1462.

Cederberg, A. et al. Foxc2 is a winged helix gene that counteracts obesity, hypertriglceridemia, and diet-induced insulin resistance. *Cell* 106 (2001): 563–573.

Champigny, O. et al. Beta 3-adrenergic receptor stimulation restores message and expression of brown-fat mitochondrial uncoupling protein in adult dogs. *Proc. Natl. Acad. Sci. USA* 88.23 (1991): 10774–10777.

Chen, H.C. et al. Increased insulin and leptin sensitivity in mice lacking acyl coa:diacylglycerol acyltransferase 1. *J. Clin. Invest.* 109.8 (2002): 1049–1055.

Christin, L. et al. Norepinephrine turnover and energy expenditure in Pima Indian and white men. *Metabolism.* 42.6 (1993): 723–729.

Chruscinski, A.J. et al. Targeted disruption of the β2 adrenergic receptor gene. *J. Biol. Chem.* 274.24 (1999): 16694–16700.

Clapham, J.C. et al. Mice overexpressing human uncoupling protein-3 in skeletal muscle are hyperphagic and lean. *Nature* 406.6794 (2000): 415–418.

Cohen, I. et al. The *N*-terminal domain of rat liver carnitine palmitoyltransferase 1 mediates import into the outer mitochondrial membrane and is essential for activity and malonyl-coa sensitivity. *J. Biol. Chem.* 273.45 (1998): 29896–29904.

Cummings, D.E. et al. Genetically lean mice result from targeted disruption of the RII β subunit of protein kinase A [see comments]. *Nature* 382.6592 (1996): 622–626.

Egger, G. and B. Swinburn. An ecological approach to the obesity pandemic. *Br. Med. J.* 315.7106 (1997): 477–480.

Elchebly, M. et al. Increased insulin sensitivity and obesity resistance in mice lacking the protein tyrosine phosphatase-1β gene. *Science* 283.5407 (1999): 1544–1548.

Enerback, S. et al. Mice lacking mitochondrial uncoupling protein are cold-sensitive but not obese [see comments]. *Nature* 387.6628 (1997): 90–94.

Esterbauer, H. et al. Uncoupling protein-1 MRNA expression in obese human subjects: the role of sequence variations at the uncoupling protein-1 gene locus. *J. Lipid Res.* 39.4 (1998): 834–844.

Friedman, J.M. and J.L. Halaas. Leptin and the regulation of body weight in mammals. *Nature* 395.6704 (1998): 763–770.

Froidevaux, F. et al. Energy expenditure in obese women before and during weight loss, after refeeding, and in the weight-relapse period. *Am. J. Clin. Nutr.* 57.1 (1993): 35–42.

Garrow, J.S. Treatment of obesity. *Lancet* 340.8816 (1992): 409–413.

Gong, D.W. et al. Lack of obesity and normal response to fasting and thyroid hormone in mice lacking uncoupling protein-3. *J. Biol. Chem.* 275 (2000): 16251–16257.

Guerra, C. et al. Abnormal nonshivering thermogenesis in mice with inherited defects of fatty acid oxidation. *J. Clin. Invest.* 102.9 (1998): 1724–1731.

Guerra, C. et al. Emergence of brown adipocytes in white fat in mice is under genetic control. Effects on body weight and adiposity. *J. Clin. Invest.* 102.2 (1998): 412–420.

Guerra, C. et al. Brown adipose tissue-specific insulin receptor knockout shows diabetic phenotype without insulin resistance. *J. Clin. Invest.* 108.8 (2001): 1205–1213.

Guerre–Millo, M. et al. Peroxisome proliferator-activated receptor alpha activators improve insulin sensitivity and reduce adiposity. *J. Biol. Chem.* 275.22 (2000): 16638–16642.

Halford, J.C. and J.E. Blundell. Pharmacology of appetite suppression. *Prog. Drug Res.* 54 (2000): 25–58.

Haynes, W.G. et al. Receptor-mediated regional sympathetic nerve activation by leptin. *J. Clin. Invest.* 100.2 (1997): 270–278.

Hesselink, M.K. et al. Increased uncoupling protein 3 content does not affect mitochondrial function in human skeletal muscle *in vivo*. *J. Clin. Invest.* 111.4 (2003): 479–486.

Himms–Hagen, J. et al. Effect of Cl-316,243, a thermogenic beta 3-agonist, on energy balance and brown and white adipose tissues in rats. *Am. J. Physiol.* 266.4 Pt. 2 (1994): R1371–1382.

Joshi, R.L. et al. Targeted disruption of the insulin receptor gene in the mouse results in neonatal lethality. *Embo. J.* 15.7 (1996): 1542–1547.

Kakuma, T. et al. Leptin, troglitazone, and the expression of sterol regulatory element binding proteins in liver and pancreatic islets. *Proc. Natl. Acad. Sci. USA* 97.15 (2000): 8536–8541.

Kitamura, T., C.R. Kahn, and D. Accili. Insulin receptor knockout mice. *Annu. Rev. Physiol.* 65 (2003): 8.1–8.20.

Klaman, L.D. et al. Increased energy expenditure, decreased adiposity, and tissue-specific insulin sensitivity in protein-tyrosine phosphatase 1β-deficient mice. *Mol. Cell Biol.* 20.15 (2000): 5479–5489.

Knowler, W.C. et al. Diabetes mellitus in the Pima Indians: incidence, risk factors and pathogenesis. *Diabetes Metab. Rev.* 6.1 (1990): 1–27.

Knowler, W.C. et al. Obesity in the Pima Indians: its magnitude and relationship with diabetes. *Am. J. Clin. Nutr.* 53.6 Suppl. (1991): 1543S–1551S.

Kopecky, J. et al. Expression of the mitochondrial uncoupling protein gene from the Ap2 gene promoter prevents genetic obesity. *J. Clin. Invest.* 96.6 (1995): 2914–2923.

Kopecky, J. et al. Reduction of dietary obesity in Ap2-UCP transgenic mice: physiology and adipose tissue distribution. *Am. J. Physiol.* 270.5 Pt. 1 (1996): E768–E775.

Koza, R.A. et al. Synergistic gene interactions control the induction of the mitochondrial uncoupling protein (UCP1) gene in white fat tissue. *J. Biol. Chem.* 275.44 (2000): 34486–34492.

Kozak, L.P. and M.-E. Harper. Mitochondrial uncoupling proteins in energy expenditure. *Annu. Rev. Nutr.* 20 (2000): 339–363.

Kubota, N. et al. Ppar gamma mediates high-fat diet-induced adipocyte hypertrophy and insulin resistance. *Mol. Cell* 4.4 (1999): 597–609.

Larson, D.E. et al. Energy metabolism in weight-stable postobese individuals. *Am. J. Clin. Nutr.* 62.4 (1995): 735–739.

Lean, M.E.J. Evidence for brown adipose tissue in humans. In *Obesity.* Ed. B.N. Brodoff. Philadelphia: J.B. Lippincott. (1992) 117–129.

Lee, Y.-P., and H.A. Lardy. Influence of thyroid hormones on L-α-glycerophosphate dehydrogenases and other dehydrogenases in various organs of the rat. *J. Biol. Chem.* 240 (1965): 1427–1436.

Levin, N. et al. Decreased food intake does not completely account for adiposity reduction after Ob protein infusion. *Proc. Natl. Acad. Sci. USA* 93 (1996): 1726–1730.

Levine, J.A., N.L. Eberhardt, and M.D. Jensen. Role of nonexercise activity thermogenesis in resistance to fat gain in humans. *Science* 283.5399 (1999): 212–214.

Li, B. et al. Skeletal muscle respiratory uncoupling prevents diet-induced obesity and insulin resistance in mice. *Nat. Med.* 6.10 (2000): 1115–1120.

Lissner, L. et al. Birth weight, adulthood BMI, and subsequent weight gain in relation to leptin levels in Swedish women. *Obes. Res.* 7.2 (1999): 150–154.

Liu, X. et al. Paradoxical resistance to diet-induced obesity in UCP1-deficient mice. *J. Clin. Invest.* 111.3 (2003): 399–407.

Ludwig, E.H. et al. Dgat1 promoter polymorphism associated with alterations in body mass index, high density lipoprotein levels and blood pressure in Turkish women. *Clin. Genet.* 62.1 (2002): 68–73.

McNeely, M.J. et al. Association between baseline plasma leptin levels and subsequent development of diabetes in Japanese Americans. *Diabetes Care* 22.1 (1999): 65–70.

McNeill, G. et al. Inter-individual differences in fasting nutrient oxidation and the influence of diet composition. *Int. J. Obes.* 12.5 (1988): 455–463.

Minokoshi, Y. et al. Leptin stimulates fatty-acid oxidation by activating Amp-activated protein kinase. *Nature* 415 (2002): 339–343.

Neel, J.V. Diabetes mellitus: a thrifty genotype rendered detrimental by progress? *Bull. World Health Organ.* 77.8 (1999): 694–703; discussion 692–693.

Neel, J.V. Diabetes mellitus: a thrifty genotype rendered detrimental by progress? *Am. J. Hum. Genet.* 14 (1962): 353–363.

Neel, J.V. The thrifty genotype in 1998. *Nutr. Rev.* 57.5 Pt. 2 (1999): S2–9.

Petersen, K.F. et al. Leptin reverses insulin resistance and hepatic steatosis in patients with severe lipodystrophy. *J. Clin. Invest.* 109.10 (2002): 1345–1350.

Poehlman, E.T. Reduced metabolic rate after caloric restriction — can we agree on how to normalize the data? *J. Clin. Endocrinol. Metab.* 88.1 (2003): 14–15.

Prochazka, M., U.C. Kozak, and L.P. Kozak. A glycerol-3-phosphate dehydrogenase null mutant in Balb/Chea mice. *J. Biol. Chem.* 264.8 (1989): 4679–4683.

Ravussin, E. and C. Bogardus. A brief overview of human energy metabolism and its relationship to essential obesity. *Am. J. Clin. Nutr.* 55.1 Suppl. (1992): 242S–245S.

Ravussin, E. and C. Bogardus. Relationship of genetics, age, and physical-fitness to daily energy-expenditure and fuel utilization. *Am. J. Clin. Nutr.* 49.5 (1989): 968–975.

Ravussin, E. et al. Effects of human leptin replacement of food intake and energy metabolism in 3 leptin–deficient adults (Abstract). *Int. J. Obesity* 26.S1 (2002): S136.

Ravussin, E. and J.F. Gautier. Metabolic predictors of weight gain. *Int. J. Obes. Relat. Metab. Disord.* 23 Suppl. 1 (1999): 37–41.

Ravussin, E. et al. Determinants of 24-hour energy expenditure in man. Methods and results using a respiratory chamber. *J. Clin. Invest.* 78.6 (1986): 1568–1578.

Ravussin, E. et al. Reduced rate of energy expenditure as a risk factor for body-weight gain. *N. Engl. J. Med.* 318.8 (1988): 467–472.

Ravussin, E. et al. Relatively low plasma leptin concentrations precede weight gain in Pima Indians. *Nat. Med.* 3.2 (1997): 238–240.

Ravussin, E. and B.A. Swinburn. Metabolic predictors of obesity: cross-sectional versus longitudinal data. *Int J. Obes. Relat. Metab. Disord.* 17 Suppl. 3 (1993): S28–31; discussion S41–42.

Ravussin, E. et al. Effects of a traditional lifestyle on obesity in Pima Indians. *Diabetes Care* 17.9 (1994): 1067–1074.

Reidy, S.P. and J.M. Weber. Accelerated substrate cycling: a new energy-wasting role for leptin *in vivo*. *Am. J. Physiol. Endocrinol. Metab.* 282.2 (2002): E312–317.

Ricquier, D. and F. Bouillaud. The uncoupling protein homologues: UCP1, UCP2, UCP3, Stucp and Atucp. *Biochem. J.* 345 Pt. 2 (2000): 161–179.

Rohrer, D.K. et al. Targeted disruption of the mouse β-adrenergic receptor gene: developmental and cardiovascular effects. *Proc. Natl. Acad. Sci. USA* 93.14 (1996): 7375–7380.

Rosenbaum, M., R.L. Leibel, and J. Hirsch. Obesity. *N. Engl. J. Med.* 337.6 (1997): 396–407.

Rosenbaum, M. et al. Low dose leptin administration reverses effects of sustained weight-reduction on energy expenditure and circulating concentrations of thyroid hormones. *J. Clin. Endocrinol. Metab.* 87.5 (2002): 2391–2394.

Salbe, A.D. and E. Ravussin. The determinants of obesity. In Bouchard, C. (Ed.) *Physical Activity and Obesity.* Champaign, IL: Human Kinetics Publishers, Inc., 2000.

Salbe, A.D. et al. Assessing risk factors for obesity between childhood and adolescence: II. energy metabolism and physical activity. *Pediatrics* 110.2 Pt. 1 (2002): 307–314.

Schoeller, D.A., K. Shay, and R.F. Kushner. How much physical activity is needed to minimize weight gain in previously obese women? *Am. J. Clin. Nutr.* 66.3 (1997): 551–556.

Schwartz, R.S., L.F. Jaeger, and R.C. Veith. Effect of clonidine on the thermic effect of feeding in humans. *Am. J. Physiol.* 254.1 Pt. 2 (1988): R90–94.

Seidell, J.C. et al. Fasting respiratory exchange ratio and resting metabolic rate as predictors of weight gain: the Baltimore longitudinal study on aging. *Int. J. Obes. Relat. Metab. Disord.* 16.9 (1992): 667–674.

Smith, S.J. et al. Obesity resistance and multiple mechanisms of triglyceride synthesis in mice lacking Dgat. *Nat. Genet.* 25.1 (2000): 87–90.

Snitker, S., P.A. Tataranni, and E. Ravussin. Respiratory quotient is inversely associated with muscle sympathetic nerve activity. *J. Clin. Endocrinol. Metab.* 83.11 (1998): 3977–3979.

Soloveva, V. et al. Transgenic mice overexpressing the β1-adrenergic receptor in adipose tissue are resistant to obesity. *Mol. Endocrin.* 11 (1997): 27–38.

Spraul, M. et al. Reduced sympathetic nervous activity. A potential mechanism predisposing to body weight gain. *J. Clin. Invest.* 92.4 (1993): 1730–1735.

Stuart, J.A. et al. Physiological levels of mammalian uncoupling protein 2 do not uncouple yeast mitochondria. *J. Biol. Chem.* 276.21 (2001): 18633–18639.

Sundquist, J. and S.E. Johansson. The influence of socioeconomic status, ethnicity and lifestyle on body mass index in a longitudinal study. *Int. J. Epidemiol.* 27.1 (1998): 57–63.

Susulic, V.S. et al. Targeted disruption of the β3-adrenergic receptor gene. *J. Biol. Chem.* 270 (1995): 29483–29492.

Tataranni, P.A. et al. A low sympathoadrenal activity is associated with body weight gain and development of central adiposity in Pima Indian men. *Obes. Res.* 5.4 (1997): 341–347.

Thomas, S.A., and R.D. Palmiter. Thermoregulatory and metabolic phenotypes of mice lacking noradrenaline and adrenaline. *Nature* 387.6628 (1997): 94–97.

Toubro, S. et al. Twenty-four-hour respiratory quotient: the role of diet and familial resemblance. *J. Clin. Endocrinol. Metab.* 83.8 (1998): 2758–2764.

Tsukiyama–Kohara, K. et al. Adipose tissue reduction in mice lacking the translational inhibitor 4e-Bp1. *Nat. Med.* 7.10 (2001): 1128–1132.

Valet, P. et al. Expression of human α2-adrenergic receptors in adipose tissue of β3-adrenergic receptor-deficient mice promotes diet-induced obesity. *J. Biol. Chem.* 275.44 (2000): 34797–34802.

Vidal–Puig, A.J. et al. Energy metabolism in uncoupling protein 3 gene knockout mice. *J. Biol. Chem.* 275 (2000): 16258–16266.

Weinsier, R.L. et al. Metabolic predictors of obesity. Contribution of resting energy expenditure, thermic effect of food, and fuel utilization to four-year weight gain of post-obese and never-obese women. *J. Clin. Invest.* 95.3 (1995): 980–985.

Weiss, R.E. et al. Thyroid hormone action on liver, heart, and energy expenditure in thyroid hormone receptor β-deficient mice. *Endocrinology* 139.12 (1998): 4945–4952.

Weyer, C., J.F. Gautier, and E. Danforth, Jr. Development of β3-adrenoceptor agonists for the treatment of obesity and diabetes — an update. *Diabetes Metab.* 25.1 (1999): 11–21.

Weyer, C. et al. Energy expenditure, fat oxidation, and body weight regulation: a study of metabolic adaptation to long-term weight change. *J. Clin. Endocrinol. Metab.* 85.3 (2000): 1087–1094.

Weyer, C. et al. Determinants of energy expenditure and fuel utilization in man: effects of body composition, age, sex, ethnicity and glucose tolerance in 916 subjects. *Int. J. Obes. Relat. Metab. Disord.* 23.7 (1999): 715–722.

Willson, T.M. et al. The PPARs: from orphan receptors to drug discovery. *J. Med. Chem.* 43.4 (2000): 527–550.

Wu, Z. et al. Mechanisms controlling mitochondrial biogenesis and respiration through the thermogenic coactivator Pgc-1. *Cell* 98.1 (1999): 115–124.

Zhang, C.Y. et al. Uncoupling Protein-2 negatively regulates insulin secretion and is a major link between obesity, beta cell dysfunction, and type 2 diabetes. *Cell* 105.6 (2001): 745–755.

Zhou, Y.-T. et al. Induction by leptin of uncoupling protein-2 and enzymes of fatty acid oxidation. *Proc. Natl. Acad. Sci. USA* 94 (1997): 6386–6390.

Zurlo, F. et al. Spontaneous physical activity and obesity: cross-sectional and longitudinal studies in Pima Indians. *Am. J. Physiol.* 263.2 Pt. 1 (1992): E296–300.

Zurlo, F. et al. Skeletal muscle metabolism is a major determinant of resting energy expenditure. *J. Clin. Invest.* 86.5 (1990): 1423–1427.

Zurlo, F. et al. Low ratio of fat to carbohydrate oxidation as predictor of weight gain: study of 24-H Rq. *Am. J. Physiol.* 259.5 Pt. 1 (1990): E650–E657.

2

The Pathophysiology of Appetite Control

Jason C. G. Halford and John E. Blundell

CONTENTS

2.1 Appetite Regulation and Expression

Appetite is expressed by the tendency to seek food and consume it. Traditionally, it has been thought that appetite is influenced solely by bodily components or by metabolism. These influences are commonly referred to as the glucostatic, aminostatic, thermostatic, or lipostatic hypotheses. Each suggests that a single variable, such as glucose, amino acids, heat generation, or adipose tissue stores, plays the major role in modulating the expression of appetite. It can be accepted that these four variables can be monitored and each can exert some influences over food consumption.

However, in the last few years, research has given renewed support to lipostatic ideas. Specifically, identification of the adipose signal leptin and discovery of the inhibitory effect of leptin on hypothalmic neuropeptide Y (NPY) (which potently stimulates feeding) have contributed greatly to understanding how tonic energy balance can modulate appetite. Thus, a mechanism by which long-term, tonic energy status-altered episodes of feeding behaviors has been identified. However, the short-term consequences of food ingestion generated by a meal also powerfully inhibit further intake (satiety). The monoamine serotonin (5-HT) has been closely implicated with the inhibitory process of within-meal satiation and postmeal satiety. More recently, it has become apparent that various hypothalamic peptides, including the melanocortins, may be responsive to short-term satiety signals (episodic) and/or long-term energy status signals (tonic). It is noteworthy that the agonism of the leptin and certain melanocortin and 5-HT receptors appear to block NPY-induced hyperphagia.

Over the next 10 years, the exact nature of the integration of these key appetite control systems may be understood. A distinction can be drawn between short-term satiety signals generated by physiological consequences of meal intake (episodic), and long-term signals generated by the body's constant metabolic need for energy (tonic). This distinction may be a useful starting point in an examination of the integration of the CNS systems ultimately responsible for expression of appetite.

The expression of appetite is determined by various component homeostatic subsystems that maintain the body's levels of energy, and the environment from which that energy is acquired. Energy need initiates the drive to acquire energy (hunger). The environment determines the source and availability of food and, ultimately, the satisfaction of the drive (satiation). In the developed world, vast amounts of pleasurable food items are "freely" available. The appetite system defends well against energy deficit (brought about by underconsumption), but not against energy excess (overconsumption). Signals of energy surplus appear less potent than those of energy deficit. The biopsychological system underlying the expression of appetite can be conceptualized as containing three domains (Figure 2.1):

- Psychological events (e.g., subjective sensations of hunger, satiety, hedonics, and cravings) accompanying observable behavioral operations (meal intake, snacking behavior, food choice) and their measurable consequences (energy intake and macronutrient composition of food consumed)
- Peripheral physiology and metabolic events related to the effect of absorbed nutrients and their utilization or subsequent conversion for storage (i.e., the changes in the body due to energy intake and/or energy deficit)
- Neurochemical (classic neurotransmitters, neuropeptides, and hormones) and metabolic interactions within the CNS (i.e., how various signals of the body's energy status are detected in the brain)

The expression of appetite reflects the synchronous operation of events and processes in all three domains.

2.2 Hunger and Satiety, and Longer-Term Factors in Appetite Regulation

Hunger can be defined as the motivation to seek and consume food that initiates a period of feeding behavior. The process that brings this period of eating (or meal) to an end is termed satiation. Satiation processes ultimately lead to the state of satiety in which the hunger drive, and thus eating behavior, is inhibited. The processes of satiation determine meal size and the state of satiety determines length of the postmeal interval. The net effect of these systems can be considered before (preprandial or cephalic phase), during (prandial), and after (postprandial) a meal (see Figure 2.2).

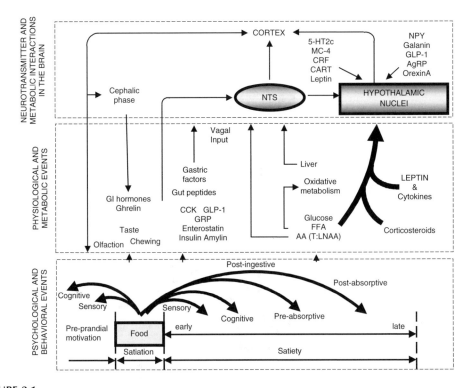

FIGURE 2.1
The psychobiological expression of appetite and the three levels of operation; *i.* psychological and behavioral events; *ii.* physiological and metabolic operations; and *iii.* neurochemical and metabolic interactions within the CNS. (Abbreviations: 5-HT, serotonin; AA, amino acids; AgRP, agouti related peptide; CART, cocaine and amphetamine regulated transcript; CCK, cholecystokinin; CRF, corticotropin releasing factor; FFA, free fatty acids; GI, gastrointestinal; GLP-1, glucagon like peptide-1; GRP, gastric releasing peptide; MC, melanocortin; NPY, neuropeptide Y; NTS, nucleus tractus solitarius; T/LNAA, tryptophan large neutral amino acids ratio.)

Preconsumption physiological signals are generated by the sight and smell of food that prepare the body to ingest it. Such afferent sensory information, carried to the brainstem via cranial nerves, stimulates hunger before eating and into the initial stages of consumption (the prandial phase). During the prandial phase, the CNS receives postingestive sensory afferent input from the gut reflecting the amount of food eaten and earliest representations of its nutrient content. Mechanoreceptors in the gut detect the distension of gut lining caused by the presence of food, thus aiding the estimation of the volume of food consumed. Gut chemoreceptors detect the chemical presence of various nutrients in the gastrointestinal tract and thus provide information on the composition (and possible energy content) of the food consumed. Prandial and postprandial signals are generated by detection of nutrients absorbed from the gastrointestinal tract that have entered the circulation in the periphery (postabsorptive satiety signals). Circulating nutrients metabolized in the periphery (e.g., liver) activate CNS receptors (e.g., in brain stem), or they enter and affect the brain directly and act as postabsorptive metabolic satiety signals (Blundell, 1991).

Appetite is not only derived from the daily flux of physiology associated with meals and eating behavior, but also must respond to the long-term (tonic) energy status of the organism. Factors derived from the processes of energy storage and the status of the body's energy stores must also contribute to appetite and its expression (e.g., indicators of glucose metabolism and fat storage). Blood carries various substances (other than nutrients) generated in organs implicated in nutrient metabolism and energy storage, such as the liver

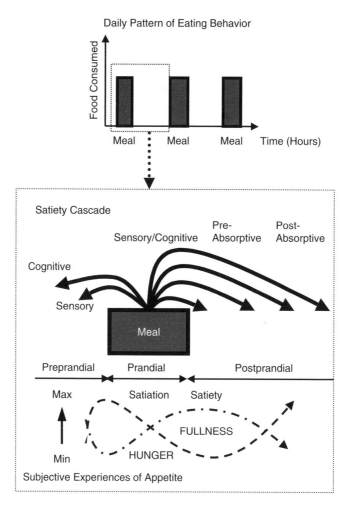

FIGURE 2.2
The satiety cascade. The signals generated prior to (preprandial), during (prandial), and after (postprandial) consumption of a meal critical to short-term (episodic) meal-by-meal appetite regulation throughout the day.

and pancreas and in adipose tissue layers, that reflect the body's energy status and have been shown to have potent effects on food intake (insulin, glucagon, and leptin). The number of potential active metabolites and byproducts produced by energy metabolism of differing nutrients is vast, providing a wide range of potential indicator substances (e.g., satietin, adipsin, or cytokine signals such as interleukins and tumor-necrosis factors). These may provide the most potent determinants of food intake and expression of appetite in the long term (promoting satiety and potently inhibiting food intake, or stimulating hunger and initiating food intake).

2.3   Neural Structures in Assessment of Appetite

The CNS receives information generated by the sensory experience of eating as well as from the periphery indicating the ingestion, absorption, metabolism, and storage of energy.

To regulate appetite, a variety of structures within the CNS integrate multiple signals in order to assess the biological need for energy; to generate or inhibit conscious experiences of hunger; and subsequently to initiate the appropriate behavioral action. Information reaches the CNS via three main routes.

- Signals from the periphery: peripheral receptors in the gut (distension and chemoreceptors) and metabolic changes in the liver (energy conversion and energy status) send afferent signals via vagus nerve to area postrema/nucleus of the solitary tract (AP/NTS) complex in the brain stem.
- Signals from specific receptors within the brain, particularly in the brain stem, that detect circulating levels of nutrients, their metabolites, and other factors within the periphery.
- Substances, such as neurotransmitter precursors, cross the blood–brain barrier to enter the brain and directly alter CNS neurochemical activity, particularly in key hypothalamic nuclei and associated limbic areas.

Original theories of the neural control of appetite conceptualized food intake to be controlled by the opposing action of two hypothalamic centers: lateral hypothalamus (LH) and ventral medial hypothalamus (VMH). However, with later precision technologies, numerous hypothalamic and nonhypothalamic nuclei have been implicated in the control of hunger and satiety. For instance, infusions of various agents in or near the paraventricular nucleus (PVN), a key hypothalamic site, produce marked increases or decreases in the intake of specific macronutrients. Other key limbic sites identified as playing critical roles in appetite regulation include the arcuate nucleus (ARC); nucleus accumbens (NAc); amygdala; posterior hypothalamus; and dorsal medial hypothalamus.

In considering the role of nonhypothalamic/limbic sites as the key to the expression of appetite, much attention has been paid to tracts that run from the brain stem into the limbic system. The NTS/AP (nucleus of the solitary tract/area postrema) adjacent areas in the hindbrain relay vagal afferent satiety signals from the periphery (particularly receptors in the gastrointestinal tract and liver) to the hypothalamus. This area of the brain stem appears to possess receptors sensitive to levels of circulating nutrients. Additionally, afferent sensory information from the mouth, including taste (carried by cranial nerves), is relayed to the cortex via the NTS. The NTS sends neural projections into key hypothalamic and other limbic sites associated with appetite control. These interlinked sites contain the key neurotransmitters and numerous neuropeptides now associated with expression of appetite.

2.4   Initiation and Stimulation of Eating

The intimate contact of mainly chemical, but also physical, stimuli with receptors in the mucosa of the nose and mouth sets up orosensory effects of food stimuli. This is transmitted to the brain by afferent fibers of primary olfactory, gustatory, and somatosensory neurons of cranial nerves I, V, VII, IX, and X. These peripheral inputs appear to make contact with dopamine and opioid neurotransmitters in the brain. The cephalic phase of appetite control refers to physiological responses engendered by the sight or smell of food, which are anticipatory and serve to prepare the system for the imminent ingestion of food. Cephalic phase responses occur in the mouth (anticipatory secretion of saliva), stomach, and small intestine and represent preprandial changes that are precursors for the onset of a meal.

In addition, it has been proposed that changes in blood glucose may serve as a signal for meal initiation. Although many chemicals can induce feeding when injected into the brain, it has been difficult to demonstrate the specific pattern of physiological events that proceeds eating in animals or man. Some years ago it was proposed that a small fall in blood glucose was correlated with meal initiation in rats. Recent evidence provides some support for a role for "transient declines" in blood glucose in humans leading to increased expression of hunger and initiation of eating. Potent feeding responses can also be obtained by microinjection of peptides into the brains of animals. A number of peptides, including β-endorphin; dynorphin; neuropeptide Y (NPY); orexins (OX-A and OX-B); galanin; ago-uti-related peptide (AGRP); and melanin-concentrating hormone (MCH), increase food intake. For example, when injected into the PVN, NPY can induce rats to eat 50% of their normal daily food intake within hours.

Classic research of a decade ago indicated how projections between the brainstem and hypothalamic nuclei were involved in neuroendocrine regulation. This pattern of projections is also important for feeding; peptides such as NPY and galanin appear to originate (in part) in adrenergic (C1, C2) or noradrenergic (A1, A2, A6) nuclei in the brain stem. Thus, various peptides and monoamines appear to act in concert to influence the organization of expression of appetite and energy balance more generally. These actions are generated in response to visceral and metabolic information that reflects the immediate past history of feeding and the body's nutritional status. At the present time, experimental evidence favors a role for NPY in overall energy balance expressed by changes in appetite and insulin-mediated metabolic activity.

2.4.1   CNS "Hunger" Peptides

NPY is found throughout the CNS and in abundance in the PVN of the hypothalamus. Hypothalamic NPY neurons implicated in appetite regulation project from the ARC to the PVN (Dryden and Williams, 1996). Infusing NPY directly into the CNS or increasing release of NPY within the PVN promotes meal initiation and produces an immediate and marked increase in food intake, delaying the onset of satiety (Bouali et al., 1993; Lynch et al., 1994; Bivens et al., 1998). Central administration of NPY agonists has also been shown to increase food intake (Corp et al., 2001), while NPY antagonists block the NPY- or deprivation-induced feeding response (Myers et al., 1995; Ishihara et al., 1998). A number of studies employing specific NPY receptor ligands or antagonists have demonstrated that the NPY Y1 receptor (Leibowitz and Alexander, 1991; Stanley et al., 1992; Lopez–Valpuesta et al., 1996; Kask et al., 1998a; Wieland et al., 1998; Kanatani et al., 1998; Larsen et al.,1999; Polidori et al., 2000) and NPY Y5 receptor (Hu et al., 1996; Haynes et al., 1998; Criscione et al., 1998; Marsh et al., 1998; Hwa et al., 1999; McCrea et al., 2000; Balasubramaniam et al., 2002) mediate the hyperphagic effects of NPY.

NPY is sensitive to a variety of peripherally generated signals; the pancreatic hormone amylin blocks its hyperphagic effects (Balasubramaniam et al., 1991; Morris and Nguyen, 2001). The hyperphagic gut factor ghrelin increases neuronal c-Fos expression in the ARC, an effect associated with an increase in NPY mRNA, thus suggesting that ghrelin effects are mediated by endogenous NPY (Wang et al., 2002). Moreover, the hyperphagic effects of centrally infused ghrelin on food intake in rats can be blocked by NPY1 antagonists (Lawrence et al., 2002a). Evidence is also strong that the adiposity signal leptin reduces food intake, at least in part, through interaction with the endogenous NPY system. For instance, leptin-deficient ob/ob mice, also bred to be deficient in endogenous NPY, are significantly less obese compared to ob/ob mice deficient in endogenous leptin alone

(Erickson et al., 1996). Peripheral leptin administration to ob/ob mice not only reduces food intake and body weight but also decreases NPY mRNA expression in the ARC (Schwartz et al., 1996). Central leptin administration to normal weight rats also reduces food intake, body weight, and hypothalamic NPY expression (Thorsell et al., 2002). Moreover, exogenous NPY-induced hyperphagia is blocked by prior leptin infusions (Smith et al., 1998b).

Thus, hypothalamic NPY appears sensitive to episodic and tonic signals generated in the periphery. NPY also interacts with other CNS appetite regulatory systems. Serotonin (5-HT) activation suppresses the levels of NPY within the PVN while blocking 5-HT synthesis, or antagonizing 5-HT receptors increases NPY functioning in the PVN (Dryden et al., 1995, 1996a, b; Gutierrez et al., 2002). A series of studies have suggested that activation of the 5-HT_{1B} and/or 5-HT_{2A} receptor (rather than 5-HT_{2C}) is critical to the serotonergic inhibition of NPY-induced hyperphagia (Grignaschi et al., 1996; Currie et al., 1997, 1998, 1999, 2002).

In 1998, two groups (de Lecea et al., 1998; Sakurai et al., 1998) independently identified a closely related pair of novel neuropeptide molecules located in brain areas such as the perifornical, dorsal hypothalamus, LH, VMH, and PVN associated with appetite regulation (Rodgers et al., 2002). Two peptides, termed orexin-A and orexin-B, were described along with two orexin receptors, orexin-1(OX1) and orexin-2 (OX2); orexin-A had the higher affinity for the OX1 receptor and orexin-B had the higher affinity for the OX2 receptor.

The endogenous orexin system is integrated with other critical hypothalamic energy regulatory systems and responds to insulin-induced hypoglycaemia and food restriction (Moriguchi et al., 1999; Lopez et al., 2000; Yamamoto et al., 2000; Kurose et al., 2002). Leptin reduces orexin-A concentration in the LH and also blocks fasting-induced changes in hypothalamic prepro-orexin mRNA and orexin OX1 receptor mRNA (Beck and Richy, 1999; Lopez et al., 2000). Moreover, leptin preadministration partially blocks orexin-A-induced changes in feeding behavior (Zhu et al., 2002). Although both orexins have been shown to stimulate feeding behavior, the stronger and more reliable effects on food intake are produced by orexin-A.

Intracerebroventricular administration of orexin-A in rats or mice produces a dose-dependent increase in food intake during the light phase of the light/dark cycle (Lubkin and Stricker–Krongrad, 1998; Yamanaka et al., 1999; Haynes et al., 1999; Rodgers et al., 2000; Szekely et al., 2002). Infusion of orexin-A directly into the LH and the perifornical hypothalamus of rats also produces a marked increase in food intake during the light phase (Sweet et al., 1999; Mullett et al., 2000; Kotz et al., 2002). Orexin-A induced-hyperphagia can be blocked by NPY Y1 (Ida et al., 2000; Jain et al., 2000; Yamanaka et al., 2000) and NPY Y5 receptor antagonists (Dube et al., 2000), suggesting that orexin may stimulate feeding via the NPY system. Intracerebroventricular orexin-A increases NPY expression in the ARC of the rat hypothalamus (Lopez et al., 2002).

Like NPY, galanin-induced hyperphagia has been well documented over the past 15 years. Early studies demonstrated that direct infusion of galanin into the hypothalamus stimulated feeding behavior (Kyrkouli et al., 1986; Crawley et al., 1990; Schick et al., 1993). High concentrations of galanin and its receptors are found in the hypothalamus and are associated with appetite regulation (Leibowitz, 1995; Crawley, 1999). Central infusions of GALP, a novel galanin-like peptide, produce short-term hyperphagia similar to that produced by galanin (Matsumoto et al., 2002; Lawrence et al., 2002a). Galanin-induced increases in food intake can be stimulated by direct infusion of the peptide into the AP/NTS, the amygdala, and the PVN (Kyrkouli et al., 1990; Koegler and Ritter, 1998). These infusions produce an increase in intake without disrupting other behaviors, suggesting a selective effect on appetite (Kyrlouli et al., 1990). Some authors have further suggested that natural galanin functioning in the PVN may selectively stimulate the intake of dietary fat (Leibowitz, 1995; Leibowitz et al., 1998; Lin et al., 1996). Rats overexpressing galanin mRNA in the PVN and other hypothalamic areas show a marked preference for a lipid diet (Odorizzi et al., 1999).

Ghrelin is an endogenous growth hormone secretagogue receptor ligand that appears responsive to nutritional status. For instance, human plasma ghrelin immunoreactivity increases during fasting and decreases after food intake (Inui et al., 2001; Ariyasu et al., 2001). Unlike the other gut-derived factors detailed in the review, ghrelin *stimulates* rather than inhibits feeding behavior. Peripheral and central infusions of ghrelin have been shown to stimulate food intake in rats and mice (Asakawa et al., 2000; Wren et al., 2000). Chronic peripheral and central infusions of ghrelin increase cumulative food intake and body weight gain in rats (Wren et al., 2001a; Kamegai et al., 2001; Nakazato et al., 2001).

The acute effect of central ghrelin on food intake in the rat can be blocked with NPY1 receptor antagonists (Lawrence et al., 2002b). Moreover, a single peripheral infusion of ghrelin increases c-Fos expression in NPY-synthesizing neurons in mouse ARC (Wang et al., 2002), strongly suggesting that CNS NPY mediates ghrelin-induced hyperphagia. In lean humans, endogenous plasma ghrelin levels rise markedly before a meal (Cummings et al., 2001) and are suppressed by food intake (Caixas et al., 2001). In lean healthy volunteers, ghrelin infusions increase food intake, premeal hunger, and prospective consumption (Wren et al., 2001b). The obese, however, have lower levels of endogenous ghrelin, and these are not suppressed by food intake (Tschop et al., 2001; Geliebter et al., 2002; English et al., 2002).

2.5   Satiety: Peripheral Physiological Influences

The structure of feeding behavior consists of discrete units of feeding behavior (meals and snacks). The physiological events and psychological experiences occurring before, during, and after feeding can be conceptualized in the satiety cascade (Figure 2.2.). The satiety cascade is a temporal account of factors that lead to the initiation and termination of a meal, and the postmeal factors that determine subsequent intake. Sensory and cognitive factors serve first to stimulate and then to inhibit meal intake. Preabsorptive and postabsorptive factors are generated postingestively to terminate the meal and inhibit postmeal intake.

Intake of energy can only be achieved (in mammals) through the gastrointestinal tract, and energy intake is limited by the capacity of the tract. In humans, the gastrointestinal tract can be regarded as a food processor with the capacity to hold three or four meals per day. Humans are periodic feeders and usually meals are separated by periods (intermeal intervals) of 3 to 5 hours in which little food it eaten. (However, it should be noted that, with the advent of snacking and freely available food outlets, this meal-taking pattern is being transformed by modern society into a semicontinuous or grazing pattern of eating.) It can be noted that the periodicity of meal eating is compatible with the time taken by the gastrointestinal tract to process a meal. After the ingestion of a meal, the stomach homogenizes the meal and delivers the mixture at a steady rate into the small intestine for further chemical digestion and absorption. At the end of 4 hours, most of the meal has left the stomach and the majority has been absorbed.

It seems obvious that the stomach must be involved in the termination of eating (satiation). Indeed, stomach distension is regarded as an important satiety signal. A good deal of experimental evidence indicates that gastric distension can arrest eating behavior, but the effect may be short lived. By itself, gastric distension does not appear to produce the sensation of satiety; therefore, gastric distension cannot be the only factor controlling meal size. It seems likely that chemicals released by gastric stimuli or by food processing in the gastrointestinal tract are involved in the control of appetite.

Many of these chemicals are peptide neurotransmitters and many peripherally administered peptides cause changes in food consumption. There is evidence for an endogenous role for cholecystokinin (CCK); pancreatic glucagon; bombesin; and somatostatin. Much recent research has confirmed the status of CCK as a hormone-mediating meal termination (satiation) and possibly early-phase satiety. Food consumption (mainly protein and fat) stimulates the release of CCK (from duodenal mucosal cells), which in turn activates CCK-A type receptors in the pyloric region of the stomach. This signal is transmitted via afferent fibers of the vagus nerve to the nucleus tractus solitarii (NTS) in the brain stem. From here the signal is relayed to the hypothalamic region where integration with other signals occurs. Other potential peripheral satiety signals include peptides such as enterostatin, neurotensin, and glucagon-like-peptide (GLP-1).

Researchers are continually searching for components of peripheral metabolism that could provide information to the brain concerning the pattern of eating behavior. Considerable interest is currently focused on a peptide called enterostatin formed by the cleavage of procolipase that produces colipase and this 5 amino acid activation peptide. The administration of enterostatin reduces food intake and, because it is increased after high-fat feeding, it has been suggested that enterostatin could be a specific fat-induced satiety signal.

One further source of biological information relevant for the control of appetite concerns fuel metabolism. The products of food digestion may be metabolized in peripheral tissues or organs or may enter the brain directly. Most research has involved glucose metabolism and fatty acid oxidation in the hepatoportal area. The main hypothesis suggests that satiety is associated with an increase in fuel oxidation. Indirect evidence is provided by the use of antimetabolites that block oxidation pathways or impair fuel availability and lead to increases in food intake. It is argued that membranes or tissues sensitive to this metabolic activity modulate afferent discharges relayed to the brain via the vagus nerve. Researchers have begun to map out pathways in the CNS that are sensitive to this metabolic signaling.

It is difficult to identify specific CNS mechanisms that integrate short-term satiety signals alone into appetite regulation. As stated previously, a vast number of CNS neurotransmitters, gut peptides, and neuropeptides, when administered in the CNS, decrease food intake (5-HT, CART [cocaine and amphetamine regulated transcript]; CRF [corticotropin releasing factor]; CCK; GLP-1 [glucagon like peptide-1]; GRP [gastric releasing peptide]; enterostatin; α-melanocyte-stimulating hormone; leptin). The contribution of neuropeptides to within-meal satiation and postmeal satiety has, for the best part, not been assessed. The role of the various gut peptides in generating satiety has been well established in animal and recent human research. Generally, the peripheral release and detection of these peptides could account for their satiety function. However, direct entry into, and action on, receptors in the CNS may also contribute to their satiety action. The one central factor clearly associated with episodic satiety, rather than tonic energy status, is serotonin (5-HT). The role of 5-HT in satiety will be reviewed later.

2.6 Satiety Peptides

The endogenous gastrointestinal peptide cholecystokinin (CCK) is released from cells in the intestinal tract (Polak et al., 1975) into the blood stream in response to the detection of ingested nutrients (specifically protein and fat) (Hopman et al., 1985). Animal data suggest that endogenous CCK release mediates the preabsorptive satiating effect of intestinal fat infusions and may, in turn, be critical in regulating fat intake (Greenberg et al., 1992; Greenberg, 1993). Early studies demonstrated that direct infusions of CCK dose dependently reduce food intake in mice, rats, and monkeys; this gave rise to the notion that CCK was a critical peripheral satiety factor (Gibbs et al., 1973, 1976). In human volunteers it has been reliably shown that the infusion of the CCK octapeptide CCK-8 reduces food intake and enhances satiety (Kissileff et al., 1981; Geary et al., 1992; Greenough et al., 1998, Gutzwiller et al., 2000). Animal studies indicate that the effects of CCK-8 administration are mediated by CCK-A receptors in the periphery, rather than by CCK receptors found in the CNS (Corp et al., 1997; Brenner and Ritter, 1998). Peripheral CCK-8 administration has also been shown to increase the release of serotonin in the hypothalamus, a neurotransmitter implicated in the integration of episodic satiety signals (Esfanhani et al., 1995; Voigt et al., 1998).

Glucagon-like peptide (GLP)-1 is an incretin hormone released from the gut into the blood stream in response to intestinal nutrients. Endogenous GLP-1 levels increase after meals; the largest increase is in response to carbohydrate ingestion. In lean men, infusions of glucose directly into the gut produce corresponding decreases in appetite and increases in blood GLP-1 (Lavin et al., 1998). Oral carbohydrate induces an endogenous plasma GLP-1 response in lean women (Ranganath et al., 1996).

These studies suggest a role for GLP-1 in mediating the effects of carbohydrate (specifically glucose) on appetite. Infusion of GLP-1$_{(7-36)}$ amide into the CNS of fasted rats dose dependently reduces food intake (Turton et al., 1996). In healthy, normal weight men, infusions of synthetic human GLP-1$_{(7-36)}$ enhance ratings of fullness and satiety and reduce food intake at a later *ad libitum* meal (Flint et al., 1998). Intravenous GLP-1 also dose dependently reduces spontaneous food intake and adjusts appetite in lean male volunteers (Gutzwiller et al., 1999a) and overweight/obese male patients (Gutzwiller et al., 1999b; Naslund et al., 1998, 1999; Flint et al., 2001). These data demonstrate that exogenous GLP-1 reduces food intake and enhances satiety in humans, both lean and obese. Recently, research has begun to focus on glucagon-like peptide (GLP)-2, because it has been demonstrated that central infusion of GLP-2 also potently inhibits fasting and NPY-induced feeding in rats (Tang–Christensen et al., 2001).

Endogenous enterostatin levels in the periphery rise in response to a high-fat meal. The administration of exogenous enterostatin reduces food intake per se when the diet contains a significant level of fat and selectively reduces the intake of high-fat diets when rats are offered a choice (Erlanson–Albertsson and Larson, 1988; Erlanson–Albertsson et al., 1991; Okada et al., 1991; Lin et al., 1993, 1998; Mei and Erlanson–Albertsson, 1996; Ookuma et al., 1997; Lin and York, 1998). Peripheral enterostatin activates neurons in the NTS, PVN, and VMH via afferent vagal mechanisms; centrally administered enterostatin directly acts on the PVN and the amygdala to reduce intake (Okada et al., 1991; Lin and York, 1994, 1997a, b; Mei and Erlanson–Albertsson, 1996).

The hypophagic effect of enterostatin appears to be moderated centrally by 5-HT and opioidergic systems (Lin and York, 1994; Koizumi and Kimura, 2002). When administered chronically, enterostatin inhibits weight gain in rats maintained on high-fat diets (Okada et al., 1991). In choice diet paradigms, chronic enterostatin selectively reduced intake of the high-fat diet, sparing consumption of the low-fat diet (Lin et al., 1997). Early studies examining the effects of intravenous enterostatin on food intake and appetite did not yield any significant results (Rossner et al., 1995, Smeets et al., 1999). It is probable that the effects of peripherally administered enterostatin are weak and fairly short lived in humans.

The effect of exogenous infusion of the intestinal hormone bombesin provided initial evidence for the role of bombesin-like peptides in satiety (Gibbs et al., 1979). Peripheral administration and central infusions of bombesin, gastric releasing peptide (GRP), and neuromedin B reduce food intake (McCoy et al., 1989; Bado et al., 1989; Dietze and Kulkosky, 1991; Kirkham et al., 1995). High concentrations of endogenous bombesin are found in a number of key CNS sites associated with feeding control including the hypothalamus and the amygdala (Vigh et al., 1999a, b). Moreover, definitive meal-related flux in endogenous levels of bombesin-like peptides has been observed in a number of hypothalamic sites, confirming the role of bombesin as one indicator of episodic satiety (Stuckley and Gibbs, 1982; De Caro et al., 1998; Merali et al., 1998).

Human studies confirm the hypophagic effects of bombesin-like peptide administration. In healthy male volunteers bombesin infusions have been shown to reduce the meal intake and subjective experiences of appetite (Muurahainen et al., 1993; Gutzwiller et al., 1994). Although infusion of bombesin has also been shown to inhibit food intake and increases satiety in lean women (Lieverse et al., 1994, 1998), it failed to influence these parameters in obese women. Thus, the obese may be insensitive to peripheral bombesin induced satiety.

Another gut factor stimulated by ingestion of dietary fat is intestinal glycoprotein apolipoprotein A-IV produced in the human small intestine and released into intestinal lymph in response to dietary lipids (Fujimoto et al., 1993). In rats, the administration of exogenous apo A-IV reduces intake and meal size in a manner consistent with satiety. Chronic exposure to high-fat diets blunts endogenous A-IV secretion (Tso et al., 2001; Kalogeris and Painter, 2001). Recent research has also focused on amylin, a pancreatic hormone, which also has a potent effect on food intake and body weight (Reda et al., 2002). Peripheral administration of amylin reduces food intake in mice and rats, and meal size in rats (Morley and Flood, 1991; Lutz et al., 1994; Arnelo et al., 1997). Central infusions of amylin, directly into the lateral hypothalamus, into the third ventricle, or NAc, also reduce food intake (Lutz et al., 1998; Balbo and Kelly, 2001; Rushing et al., 2002). Amylin administration blocks the hyperphagic effects of NPY (Balasubramaniam et al., 1991; Morris and Nguyen, 2001) and amylin antagonism blocks the hypophagic effects of bombesin and CCK (Lutz et al., 2000). Peripherally administered amylin induces c-Fos expression in the AP, and lesioning the AP blocks amylin-induced hypophagia (Riediger et al., 2001, 2002; Lutz et al., 2001).

2.7 Appetite Signals from Adipose Tissue

As noted earlier, one of the classical theories of appetite control concerns the notion of a so-called long-term regulation involving a signal that informs the brain about the state of adipose tissue stores (Kennedy, 1953). This idea has given rise to the notion of a lipostatic or ponderostatic mechanism. Indeed, this is a specific example of a more general class of peripheral appetite (satiety) signals believed to circulate in the blood reflecting the state of depletion or repletion of energy reserves that directly modulate brain mechanisms. Such substances may include satietin, adipsin, or cytokine signals such as interleukin-6 (IL-6) tumor-necrosis factors (such as TNFα) (Mohamed-Ali et al., 1998).

Moreover, other circulating hormones, for example gonadal steroids, have potent effects (increasing and reducing) on food intake; meal size and frequency; body weight; and, specifically, percent body fat (Schwartz and Wade, 1981; Palmer and Gray, 1985; Dubac, 1985; Geary, 2000). Because circulating levels of gonadal steroids (androgens, estrogens, and progesterone) reflect the body fat mass, and thus its energy status, it is not surprising that appetite may respond to their fluctuations. Gonadal steroids may alter food intake, body mass, and body composition by directly modulating brain energy regulation systems such as NPY and the melanocortin systems, as well as by regulating leptin production (Mystkowski and Schwartz, 2000).

2.7.1 Leptin (ob-Protein)

For 40 years, scientists searched for a mechanism by which the brain could monitor bodily fat deposition in order to keep an animal's body weight constant. In 1994, a gene that controlled the expression of a protein produced by adipose tissue was identified. Circulating levels of this protein (the ob-protein) could be measured in normal weight mice. However, in obese ob/ob mice, which display marked overeating, this protein was absent due to a mutation of the ob-gene (Zhang et al., 1994). A series of studies demonstrated that the absence of this protein was responsible for overconsumption and obesity in the obese ob/ob mice (Pelleymounter et al., 1995). Administration of the ob-protein dramatically reversed the hyperphagia and obesity of the ob/ob mouse, but also the obesity and intake of mice rendered obese though exposure to highly palatable high fat diets (Halaas et al., 1995; Campfield et al., 1995). Moreover, the observation that peripheral and central administration of the ob-protein reduced intake in lean mice (Rentsch et al., 1995; Campfield et al., 1996) also demonstrated that the ob-protein did act in the brain.

Very soon a number of researchers had identified, characterized, and located ob-protein receptors in the chorioid plexus and hypothalamus (Tartaglia et al., 1995; Devos et al., 1996; Lynn et al., 1996). Because the ob-protein reduces food intake and increases metabolic energy expenditure, both of which would result in weight loss, it was named *leptin* from the Greek *leptos*, meaning thin. In general, circulating levels of leptin appear to reflect the current status of body fat deposition and increase with the level of adiposity, demonstrating the responsiveness of endogenous leptin to weight gain and energy status (Maffei et al., 1995; Considine et al., 1996; Blum et al., 1997). In animals whose obesity is induced by diet or genetic mutation other than that of the ob/ob gene (such as the db/db mouse), and in the vast majority of obese humans, plasma leptin levels are higher than in their lean counterparts. It soon became clear that these animals and humans were insensitive to the leptin adiposity signal.

Since the identification of leptin and its receptor, researchers have isolated numerous CNS hypothalamic neuropeptide systems, which mediate the hypophagic action of leptin (Inui, 1999). NPY, the melanocortins, CRF, CART, and the orexins may all be part of the circuit linking adipose tissue with central appetite regulatory mechanisms with metabolic activity. Certainly, the fact that leptin has multiple effects on complex hypothalamic appetite systems consisting of wide ranging but integrated regulatory neuropeptides would appear to support the view that leptin is a major factor in body weight regulation. Tonic leptin could act on short-term appetite regulation by restraining hunger (through inhibition of CNS levels of NPY, galanin, orexins, agouti-related peptide, or any other stimulatory "hunger" peptides) and by augmenting signals of satiety (boosting effects of peripherally generated satiety systems through the activation of CNS intake inhibitory systems such as melanocortin, CRF, and CART). By such action, tonic signals generated by energy storage, such as leptin, can moderate episodic meal-by-meal appetite regulation.

As already noted, leptin has been shown to reduce food intake in lean, ob/ob, and, in some studies, dietary obese, mice and rats. This evidence suggests that some form of leptin treatment could be used to treat human obesity. In rats, the central administration of mouse leptin dose dependently decreases food intake (Hulsey et al., 1998; Flynn et al., 1998). This is accompanied by increases in intermeal interval and decreases in meal size and eating rate, suggesting a strengthening of postmeal satiety and within-meal satiation (Hulsey et al., 1998; Flynn et al., 1998). Central leptin administration significantly increases the c-Fos response to a gastric nutrient preload within the NTS (leptin alone having no effect). Leptin alone, like the preload, induces c-Fos expression in the PVN; the combination of both produces the greatest c-Fos response. These data suggest that central leptin acts on the NTS and the PVN to enhance within-meal signals of satiety selectively (Emond et al., 2001).

As stated previously, there is evidence of synergy between leptin and the short-term, meal-generated satiety factor CCK. Systemic administration of CCK enhances leptin-induced decreases in food intake at 24 and 48 hours, and augments weight loss in rodents (Matson et al., 1997, 2002; Matson and Ritter, 1999). However, the same dose of CCK alone produces a comparatively transitory reduction in food intake and has little or no effect on body weight. Prior administration of low doses of leptin into the CNS enhances CCK-induced c-Fos expression in the PVN (Wang et al., 1998). At these doses, leptin alone produces little or no hypophagia or c-Fos PVN expression. These data again suggest that central leptin acts in the PVN to enhance within-meal signals of satiety, such as CCK, selectively.

2.8   Integration of Hunger and Satiety, and Signals of Adipose Status

As stated previously, certain brain stem sites, hypothalamic, and other limbic sites appear critical in the regulation of food intake and feeding behavior. Within these sites numerous neurochemicals, first neurotransmitters and then neuropeptides, have been identified as potent inhibitors and stimulators of feeding behavior. These include all the monoamine neurotransmitters and a growing number of neuropeptides of which the currently most prominent include NPY, melanocortins, orexins, CART, and CRF (see Figure 2.3). Although it is not possible to describe all these systems in detail, it is justifiable to describe two key systems here. Serotonin (5-HT) has been implicated as a critical CNS satiety factor in the short-term regulation of food intake. Specifically, the 5-HT system appears to be sensitive to meal-generated satiety factors such as CCK, enterostatin, and ingested macronutrients. Moreover, 5-HT drugs appear to enhance satiety, suppress CNS NPY release, and inhibit hunger. 5-HT appears to mediate the effects of episodic meal-generated satiety on appetite. The second CNS system is the melanocortins, which appear integral in the action of circulating leptin on intake and (like serotonin) also inhibit NPY functioning. Thus, the melanocortins may mediate the effects of tonic energy status on appetite.

2.9   CNS Systems of Integration

2.9.1   Serotonin (5-HT)

Of all the monoamines, serotonin (5-HT) has been most closely linked with the process of satiation and the state of satiety (Blundell, 1977). Moreover, it has been known for a long time that serotoninergic drugs reliably reduce food intake and body weight in animals and humans (Blundell and Halford, 1998). The earliest studies to demonstrate a link between 5-HT and food intake were performed over 25 years ago and first reviewed by Blundell (1977). Increasing 5-HT levels by administering 5-HT or its precursors (such as tryptophan or 5-hydroxytryptophan [5-HTP]) not only reduced food intake but also

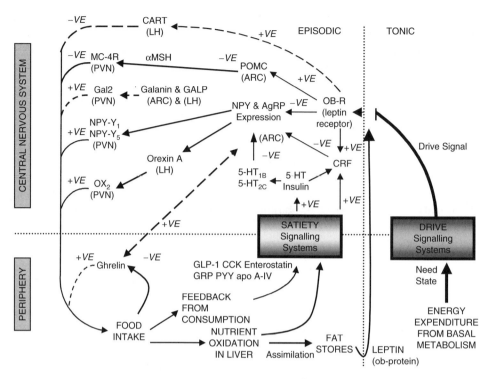

FIGURE 2.3
The integration of peripherally generated episodic and tonic signals critical to the expression of appetite. Signals generated by meal consumption and fat deposition are integrated into a complex hypothalamic system of neuropeptides, which in turn stimulate or inhibit subsequent food intake. (Abbreviations: 5-HT, serotonin; αMSH, alpha melanocortin stimulating hormone; AgRP, agouti related peptide; A-IV, apoliproprotein-IV; ARC, arcuate nucleus; CART, cocaine and amphetamine regulated transcript; CCK, cholecystokinin; CRF, corticotropin releasing factor; GAL, galanin; GLP-1, glucagon like peptide-1; GRP, gastric releasing peptide; LH, lateral hypothalamus; MC, melanocortin; NPY, neuropeptide Y; OX, orexin; PVN, paraventricular hypothalamus; POMC, pre-pro-opiomelanocortin; PYY, peptide YY.)

slowed eating rate and reduced meal size, indicating a selective action on processes of satiation. Drugs that increase synaptic 5-HT (by release and reuptake inhibition) produce the same effects. Because the number of meals did not increase or intermeal intervals shorten to compensate for the change in meal size, this demonstrated that the postmeal state of satiety was also strengthened (Blundell and Halford, 1998). Confirming the critical role of 5-HT in appetite control, inhibition of 5-HT synthesis or neurochemical lesioning of 5-HT neurons resulted in a significant increase in food intake in rodents.

Given the distribution of 5-HT neurons within the CNS and numerous 5-HT receptor subtypes, much subsequent research was devoted to the identification of precise receptors and exact location of the 5-HT satiety mechanism. The earliest studies employed "selective" 5-HT receptor antagonists to block the hypophagia induced by the 5-HT releasing drug fenfluramine, and by 5-HT reuptake inhibitors such as fluoxetine and sertraline. These early antagonists lacked specificity for any one 5-HT receptor subtype; however, a number of researchers identified the critical role of 5-HT_1 and 5-HT_2 receptors, specifically, 5-HT_{1B} and 5-HT_{2C} in satiety effect of 5-HT.

Direct agonists of the 5-HT_{1B} and 5-HT_{2C} were later shown to reduce intake and to produce changes in feeding behavior consistent with the operation of satiety (Blundell and Halford, 1998; Blundell, 1992; Halford et al., 2000). Early studies with selective 5-HT_{1B} and 5-HT_{2C} agonists in humans confirmed their satiety-enhancing properties. Transgenic animal studies also confirmed the role of 5-HT$_{1B}$ and 5-HT$_{2C}$ receptors in feeding behavior. Knockout mice lacking either one of these receptors overconsume and become obese (Tecott et al., 1995; Bouwknecht et al., 2001). Moreover, the hypophagic effects of 5-HT drugs such as *d*-fenfluramine are blunted in mice lacking 5-HT$_{2C}$ receptors (Vickers et al., 1999).

Hypothalamic areas, including the PVN, have been implicated in 5-HT hypophagia (Hutson et al., 1988; Coscina et al., 1994; Fletcher and Coscina, 1993). Activation of 5-HT suppressed levels of the appetite stimulatory peptide NPY within the PVN. Conversely, blocking 5-HT synthesis or antagonizing 5-HT receptors increased NPY functioning in the PVN (Dryden et al., 1995, 1996a, b). This interaction between 5-HT and NPY may be one of the critical mechanisms in short-term (episodic) appetite determining the generation of hunger or satiety.

As mentioned previously, 5-HT function has been linked to peripheral signals triggered by fat ingestion, such as CCK and enterostatin. Moreover, CNS levels of the 5-HT precursor tryptophan are directly affected by dietary carbohydrate through its action on the tryptophan/large neutral amino acid competition to cross the blood brain–barrier (Fernstorm, 1987). Thus, CNS 5-HT is sensitive to fat and carbohydrate ingestion; additionally, the 5-HT drug *d*-fenfluramine does seem to suppress the intake of high-fat foods in fat-preferring rats (Blundell et al., 1995; Smith et al., 1998a, 1999). This drug has also been shown to exert its greatest hypophagic effect in humans on the intake of high-fat snack foods, an effect also produced by other 5-HT drugs in humans (see Halford et al., 2000, for review).

The effects of serotonergic enhancing drugs have been well documented in humans, with most of the initial studies conducted with fenfluramine or *d*-fenfluramine. Both drugs reduced food intake and produced pronounced sustainable weight loss in the obese (Halford and Blundell, 2000a). Along with the reduction in energy intake, fenfluramine and *d*-fenfluramine reduced the urge to eat; suppressed between-meal intake; reduced the frequency of snacking; reduced the consumption of dietary fat; and increased the satiating potency of food (Halford and Blundell, 2000a). Similarly, the selective serotonin reuptake inhibitor fluoxetine reduces food intake in humans, an effect accompanied by reductions in hunger and the number of eating occasions (Lawton et al., 1995; Foltin et al., 1996, Ward et al., 1999); for reviews see Halford and Blundell (2000b) and Haddock et al. (2002). The selective 5-HT$_{2C}$ agonist mCPP has been shown to reduce intake and/or hunger in the lean (Walsh et al., 1994; Cowen et al., 1995) and the obese, with the effect in the obese accompanied by weight loss (Sargent et al., 1997). Similarly, the 5-HT$_{1B/1D}$ agonist sumatriptan has been shown to reduce food intake — specifically, the intake of dietary fat in healthy women (Boeles et al., 1997). These studies indicate the critical role of 5-HT$_{1B}$ and 5-HT$_{2C}$ receptors in human appetite regulation.

2.9.2 Melanocortins

The melanocortins comprise one of the inhibitory systems through which the tonic adiposity signal leptin inhibits food intake. Like leptin, the role of CNS melanocortins was revealed through investigation of a genetic mouse model of obesity. The agouti (A $^y/_a$) syndrome in mice, linked to fur depigmentation, revealed a critical role of CNS melanocortin receptors in energy regulation. These animals were obese, displayed marked hyperphagia, and produced excessive amounts of agouti, an endogenous antagonist of melanocortin receptors (Fan et al., 1997). Agouti caused the lack of pigmentation leading to the yellow fur color and the marked hyperphagia, obesity, and resulting metabolic abnormalities (Fan et al., 1997; Ollmann et al., 1997; Schwartz, 1999; Moussa and Claycomber, 1999). The hyperphagia was linked specifically to the blockade of the melanocortin

MC4 receptor. Notably, it was also discovered that an inability to synthesize endogenous melanocortin receptor ligands such as the alpha melanocyte stimulating hormone (αMSH) from the melanocortin precursor pre-pro-opiomelanocortin (POMC) was linked to a severe, early-onset obesity syndrome in children (Krude et al., 1998). These children displayed phenotypic abnormal eating patterns and red-hair pigmentation. It became apparent that the melanocortin receptor MC4R, as well as a number of its endogenous agonists (such as αMSH) and antagonists (such as agouti-related peptide-AgRP), was part of the endogenous body weight regulation system.

MC4 receptors are expressed widely throughout the CNS; in the hypothalamus, they are found in the PVN, dorsal hypothalamus, and LH. Central infusions of MC4R agonists (such as αMSI I or MTII) into the third ventricle and into the brain stem have been shown to reduce food intake dose dependently and to block NPY or fasting-induced hyperphagia (Murphy et al., 1998; Grill et al., 1998). Infusion of the agonist MTII directly into the PVN also produces a marked decrease in food intake (Giraudo et al., 1998; Wirth et al., 2001). MC4R agonist-induced decreases in food intake and body weight are accompanied by increases in c-Fos expression in appetite regulatory centers such as the PVN and the NTS/AP complex (Benoit et al., 2000). Chronic infusions of αMSH decrease food intake and body weight while increasing c-Fos expression in the PVN (McMinn et al., 2000). Alpha-MSH neurons in the ARC show increased c-Fos expression at the end of a meal.

Hypothalamic αMSH neurons and AgRP neurons, implicated in appetite regulation, project from the location of POMC cell bodies to the arcuate nucleus. These systems appear to mediate the effects of a number of factors such as leptin and insulin (see McNeil et al., 2002, for a review). The hyperphagic effects of selective MC4R antagonists can be fully or partially blocked by NPY Y_1 receptor antagonists (Kask et al., 1998b, 1999). MC4R antagonist studies have also confirmed the contribution of the brain stem MC system in the control of feeding (Grill et al., 1998) and long-term weight regulation (Kask et al., 1998c). Selective MC4R antagonists inhibit the action of CNS leptin on food intake and body weight. This suggests that endogenous leptin inhibits food intake and lowers body weight via the melanocortin system. Moreover, hypothalamic POMC mRNA is stimulated by leptin (Schwartz et al., 1997; Mizuno et al., 1998). The interaction with leptin suggests that the melanocortin system is sensitive to tonic signals of energy status. Whether the melanocortins are equally reactive to the fluxes of episodic meal-derived satiety signals remains to be determined (Halford and Blundell, 2000a; Blundell et al., 2001).

2.10 Tonic Signals and Hunger and Satiety

Even if tonic signals are generated independently from episodic signals, they must feed back to reduce intake by altering subjective experiences of hunger and satiety. Therefore, it should not be surprising if increases or decreases in endogenous circulating leptin have an effect on modulating subjective experiences of hunger. Moreover, endogenous leptin levels may fluctuate across the day, in part as a consequence of meal consumption and its effects on metabolism. Strong evidence for the role of tonic signals in appetite regulation comes from examining the effects of their absence in individuals with gene mutations.

Individuals with an inability to produce leptin experience constant hunger because, without the tonic leptin signal, the constant drive for energy is unleashed and leads to continuous and voracious food-seeking behavior (Montague et al., 1997). Treatment with recombinant leptin appears to bring about a significant decrease in hunger and food intake and, eventually, marked weight loss (Farooqui et al., 1997). Similarly, specific deficits in a system that responds to circulating leptin — in this case, the absence of functional melanocortin MC4 receptors — produce similar effects on appetite and intake (Krude et al., 1998). These extreme examples demonstrate the inability of short-term, meal-generated episodic signals alone to block the overriding demand for energy (expressed as continuous hunger) generated by basal metabolism. Evidence exists that leptin does have an effect on hunger in individuals without such gene mutations.

During an 84-day weight loss trial in obese women, levels of food intake were reduced and levels of exercise were increased (Keim et al., 1998). This decrease in intake and increase in exercise was accompanied by corresponding decreases in body weight, body fat, and circulating leptin. As leptin decreased during the trial, hunger increased — a significant negative correlation. Those whose leptin levels dropped the most experienced the greatest increase in perceived hunger (Keim et al., 1998). Moreover, these correlated changes demonstrated that the depletion of energy stores does increase hunger. In a 35-day weight loss trial in overweight women, levels of CCK, insulin, and leptin were monitored, as were subjective perceptions of appetite (hunger and satiety) (Heine et al., 1998). CCK, leptin, and insulin levels declined with body weight during the trial; however, only changes in leptin levels correlated with changes in the intensity in perceived hunger.

The contribution to satiety of changes in circulating leptin or diet-induced falls in leptin production remains to be determined. However, the studies do suggest that leptin concentrations are nutrient sensitive and not merely a reflection of adiposity. This is consistent with the observation that leptin concentrations are elevated in high-fat phenotypes (Cooling et al., 1998). These are individuals whose energy intake is driven up by a habitual diet of an energy-dense, high-fat intake. Leptin appears to be operating to regulate body weight in the face of a potential weight-increasing energy intake and is thus closely involved with storage and nutrient metabolism in translating "need" into "drive."

2.11 Summary: Episodic and Tonic Factors in Regulation of Appetite

This chapter has proposed that endogenous 5-HT and leptin represent two aspects of negative feedback integral to the appetite control system. Both systems appear to inhibit NPY functioning, with the effect of leptin partly mediated by melanocortins and other excitatory and inhibitory neuropeptides. Endogenous 5-HT mediates the effect of meal-derived satiety factors derived from pre- and postingestive processes, promotes meal termination, and prolongs the intermeal interval. By such a mechanism, the body deals with the daily physiological fluxes that result from meal intake, ensuring an approximately appropriate daily energy intake. Circulating leptin accurately reflects the current status of the body's energy store. Leptin levels continually modify total daily food intake to maintain a sufficient, but not excessive, level of energy deposition.

Thus, 5-HT and leptin represent two classes of feedback signals: short-term episodic and long-term tonic, respectively. The net result of the actions of episodic and tonic signals will be an adjustment in the expression of appetite, adjusting subsequent feeding behavior to compensate for previous intake and energy stored (Halford and Blundell, 2000a; Blundell et al., 2001). Eventually, other mechanisms, some already identified as important in regulation of appetite, may be classified as signals of short-term episodic or long-term tonic feedback. This distinction may be a useful starting point in future examination and understanding of the appetite system.

Acknowledgments

The authors thank Lisa D. M. Richards for her help in preparing this manuscript and Terence M. Dovey for his assistance in preparing the figures.

References

Ariyasu, H., Takaya, K., Tagamis, T., Ogawa, Y., Hosoda, K., Akamizu, T., Suda, M., Koh, T., Natsui, K., Toyooka, S., Shirakami, G., Usui, T., Shimatsu, A., Doi, K., Hosoda, H., Kojima, M., Kangawa, K., and Nakao, K. (2001) Stomach is a major source of circulating ghrelin, and feeding state determines plasma ghrelin-like immunoreactivity levels in humans, *J. Clin. Endcrin. Metab.*, 86: 4753–4758.

Arnelo, U., Permert, J., Larsson, J., Reidelberger, R.D., Amelo C., and Adrian, T.E. (1997) Chronic low dose islet amyloid polypeptide infusion reduces food intake, but does not influence glucose metabolism, in unrestrained conscious rats: studies using a novel aortic catheterization, *Endocrinology*, 138: 4081–4085.

Asakawa, A., Inui, A., Kaga, T., Yuzuriha, H., Nagata, T., Ueno, N., Makino, S., Fujimiya, M., Niijima, A., Fujino, M.A., and Kasuga, M. (2000) Ghrelin is an appetite stimulatory signal from the stomach with structural resemblance to moltin, *Gastroenterology*, 120: 337–345.

Bado, A., Lewin, M.J.M., and Dubrasquet, M. (1989) Effects of bombesin on food intake and gastric acid secretion in cats, *Am. J. Physiol.*, 256: R181–186.

Balasubramaniam, A., Renugopalakrishnan, V., Stein, M., Fischer, J.E., and Chance, W.T. (1991) Synthesis, structures and anorectic effects of human and rat amylin, *Peptides*, 6: 919–924.

Balasubramaniam, A., Sheriff, S., Zhai, W.X., and Chance W.T. (2002) Bis(31/31'){[Cys(31),Nva(34)] NPY(27-36)-NH2}: a neuropeptide Y (NPY) Y-5 receptor selective agonist with a latent stimulatory effect on food intake in rats, *Peptides*, 23:1485–1490.

Balbo, B.A. and Kelley, A.E. (2001) Amylin infusion into rat nucleus accumbens potently depresses motor activity and ingestive behavior, *Am. J. Physiol.*, 281: R1232–1242.

Beck, B. and Richy, S. (1999) Hypothalamic hypocretin/orexin and neuropeptide Y: divergent interaction with energy depletion and leptin, *Biochem. Biophys. Res. Comm.*, 258: 119–122.

Benoit, S.C., Schwartz, M.W., Lachey, J.L., Hagan M.M., Rushing, P.A., Blake, K.A., Yagakoff, K.A., Kurylko, G., Franco, L., Danhoo, W., and Seeley, R.J. (2000) A novel selective malanocrotin-4 receptor agonist reduces food intake in rats and mice without producing aversive consequences, *J. Neurosci.* 20, 3442–3448.

Bivens, C.L.M., Thomas, W.J., and Stanley, B.G. (1998) Similar feeding patterns are induced by perifornical neuropeptide Y injection and by food deprivation, *Brain Res.*, 782: 271–280.

Blum, W., Englaro, P., Heiman, M., Juul, A., Attanasio, A.M., and Kiess, W. (1997) Clinical studies of serum leptin, in Blum, W.F., Kiess, W., and Rascher, A. (Eds.) *Leptin — The Voice of Adipose Tissue*, Bath Verlag, Switzerland.

Blundell, J.E. (1977) Is there a role for serotonin (5-hydroxytryptamine) in feeding? *Int. J. Obesity*, 1: 15–42.

Blundell, J.E. (1991) Pharmacological approaches to appetite suppression, *Trends Pharm. Sci.*, 12: 147–157.

Blundell, J.E. (1992) Serotonin and the biology of feeding, *Am. J. Clin. Nutr.*, 55: 1555–1595.

Blundell, J.E., Goodson, S., and Halford, J.C.G. (2001) Regulation of appetite; role of leptin in signaling systems for drive and satiety, *Int. J. Obesity*, 25(s1): s29–34.

Blundell, J.E. and Halford, J.C.G. (1998) Serotonin and appetite regulation: implications for the pharmacological treatment of obesity, *CNS Drugs*, 9: 473–495.

Blundell, J.E., Lawton, C.L., and Halford, J.C.G. (1995) Serotonin, eating behavior and fat intake, *Obesity Res.*, 3: 471–476.

Boeles, S., Williams, C., and Campling, G.M. (1997) Sumatriptan decreases food intake and increases plasma growth hormone secretion in women, *Psychopharmacology*, 129, 179–182.

Bouali, S.M., Fourbier, A., St-Pierre, S., and Jolivcoeur, F.B. (1993) Effects of NPY and NPY2-36 on body temperature and food intake following administration onto hypothalamic nuclei, *Brain Res. Bull.*, 36: 131–135.

Bouwknecht, J.A., van der Gutgten, J., Hijzen, T.H., Maes, R.A.A., Hen, R., and Olivier, B. (2001) Male and female 5-HT1B receptor knock out mice have higher body weights than wild type, *Physiol. Behav.*, 74: 507–516.

Brenner, L.A. and Ritter, R.C. (1998) Type A CCK receptors mediate satiety effects of intestinal nutrients, *Physiol. Behav.*, 63, 711–716.

Caixas, A., Bashore, C., Trause, A., Pi-Sunyer, F.X., and Laferrere, B. (2001) Feeding acutely suppresses ghrelin levels in normal weight human subjects, *Obesity Res.*, 9 (sup. 3), 73s.

Campfield, L.A., Smith, F.S., Guisez, Y., Devos, R., and Burn, P. (1995) Recombinant mouse OB protein: evidence for peripheral signal linking adiposity and central neural networks, *Science*, 269: 546–549.

Campfield, L.A., Smith, F.S., Guisez, Y., Devos, R., and Burn, P. (1996) Ob protein: a peripheral signals linking adiposity and central neural networks, *Appetite*, 26: 302.

Considine, R.V., Sinda, M.K., Heiman, M.L., Kriauciunas, A., Stephens, T.W., Nyce, M.R., Ohanne-sian, J.P., Marco, C.C., McKee, L.J., Baur T.L., and Caro, J.F. (1996) Serum immunoreactive-leptin concentrations in normal weight and obese humans, *New Engl. J. Med.*, 334: 292–295.

Cooling, J., Barth, J., and Blundell, J.E. (1998) The high-fat phenotype: is leptin involved in the adaptive response to a high fat (high energy) diet? *Int. J. Obesity*, 22: 1132–1139.

Coscina, D.V., Feifel, D., and Norbrega, J.N. (1994) Intraventricular but not intraparaventricular nucleus metergoline elicits feeding in satiated rats, *Am. J. Physiol.*, 266: R1562–1567.

Corp, E.S., Curcio, M., Gibbs, J., and Smith, G.P. (1997) The effect of centrally administered CCK-receptor antagonists on food intake, *Physiol. Behav.*, 61: 823–827.

Corp, E.S., McQuade, J., Krasnicki, S., and Conze, D.B. (2001) Feeding after fourth ventricular administration of neuropeptide Y receptor agonists in rats, *Peptides*, 2:, 493–499.

Cowen, P.J., Sargent, P.A., Williams, C., Goodall, E.M., and Orlikov, A.B. (1995) Hypophagic, endocrine and subjective responses to *m*-chlorophenylpiperazine in healthy men and women, *Hum. Psychopharmacol.*, 10, 385–391.

Crawley, J.N. (1999) The role of galanin in feeding behavior, *Neuropeptides*, 33: 369–375.

Crawley, J.N., Austin, S.M., Fiske, B., Martin, S., Consolo, S., Berthold, U., Langel, U., Fisone, G., and Bartfai, T. (1990) Activity of centrally administered galanin fragments on stimulation of feeding-behavior and on galanin receptor binding in the rat hypothalamus, *J. Neurosci.*, 10: 3695–3700.

Criscione, L., Rigollier, P., Batzl–Hartmann, C., Rueger, H., Sticker–Krongrad, A., Wyss, P., Brunner, L., Whitebread, S., Yamaguchi, Y., Gerald, C., Heurich, R.O., Walker, M.W., Chiesi, M., Schilling, W., Hofbauer, K.G., and Levens, N. (1998) Food intake in free-feeding and energy-deprived lean rats is mediated by the neuropeptide Y-5 receptor, *J. Clin. Invest.*, 102: 2136–2145.

Cummings, D.E., Purnell, J.Q., Frayo, R.S., Schmidova, K., Wisse, B.E., and Weigle, D.S. (2001) A pre-prandial rise in plasma ghrelin levels suggests a role in meal initiation in humans, *Diabetes*, 50: 1714–1719.

Currie, P.J. and Coscina, D.V. (1997) Stimulation of 5-HT2A/2C receptors within specific hypothalamic nuclei differentially antagonizes NPY-induced feeding, *Neuroreport*, 8: 3759–3762.

Currie, P.J. and Coscina, D.V. (1998) 5-hydroxytryptaminergic receptor agonists: effects on neuropeptide Y potentiation of feeding and respiratory quotient, *Brain Res.*, 803: 212–217.

Currie, P.J., Coiro, C.D., Niyomchai, T., Lira, A., and Farahmand, F. (2002) Hypothalamic paraventricular 5-hydroxytryptamine: Receptor-specific inhibition of NPY-stimulated eating and energy metabolism, *Pharmacol. Biochem. Behav.*, 71, 709–716.

Currie, P.J., Saxena, N., and Tu, A.Y. (1999) 5-HT2A/(2C) receptor antagonists in the paraventricular nucleus attenuate the action of DOI on NPY-stimulated eating, *Neuroreport*, 10: 3033–3039.

De Caro, G., Polidori, C., Beltz, T.G., and Johnson. A.K. (1998) Area postrema, lateral parabrachial nucleus, and the antinatriorexic effect of bombesin, *Peptides*, 19: 1399–1406.

De Lecea, L., Kilduff, T.S., Peyron, C., Gao, X-B., Foye, P.E., Danielson, P.E., Fukuhara, C., Battenberg, E.L.F., Gautvik, V.T., Bartlett, F.S., Frankel, W.N., van den Pol, A.N., Bloom, F.E., Gautvik, K.M., and Sutcliffe, J.G. (1998) The hypocretins: hypothalamus-specific peptides with neuroexcitatory activity, *Proc. Natl. Acad. Sci.*, 95: 322–327.

Devos, R., Richards, J.G., Campfield, L.A., Tartaglai, L.A., Guisez, Y., Van det Heyden, J., Travernier, J., Plaetinck, G., and Burn, P. (1996) OB protein binds specifically to the choroids plexus of mice and rats, *Proc. Nat. Acad. Sci.*, 93: 567–573.

Dietze, M.A. and Kulkosky P.J. (1991) Effects of caffeine and bombesin on ethanol and food intake, *Life Sci.*, 48: 1837–1844.

Dryden, S., Frankish, H.M., Wang, Q., Pickavance, L., and Williams, G. (1995) The serotonergic agent fluoxetine reduces neuropeptide Y levels and neuropeptide Y secretion in the hypothalamus of lean and obese rats, *Neuroscience*, 72: 557–566.

Dryden, S., Frankish, H.M., Wang, Q., and Williams, G. (1996a) Increased feeding and neuropeptide Y (NPY) but not NPY mRNA levels in the hypothalamus of the rat following central administration of the serotonin synthesis inhibitor *p*-chlorophenylalanine, *Brain Res.*, 724: 232–237.

Dryden, S., Wang, Q.O., Frankish, H.M., and Williams, G. (1996b) Differential effects of the 5-HT1B/2C receptor agonist mCPP and the 5-HT1A agonist flesinoxan on hypothalamic neuropeptide Y in the rat: evidence that NPY may mediate serotonin's effects on food intake, *Peptides*, 17: 943–949.

Dryden, S. and Williams, G. (1996) The role hypothalamic peptides in the control of energy balance and body weight, *Curr. Opin. Endocrin. Daib.*, 3: 51–58.

Dubac, P.U. (1985) Effects of estrogen on food intake, body weight and temperature of male and female obese mice, *Proc. Soc. Exper. Biol. Med.*, 180: 468–473.

Dube, M.G., Horvath, T.L., Kalra, P.S., and Kalra, S.P. (2000) Evidence of NPYY5 receptor involvement in food intake elicited by orexin A in sated rats, *Peptides*, 21: 1557–1560.

Emond, M., Ladenheim, E.E., Schwartz, G.J., and Maron, T.H. (2001) Leptin amplifies the feeding inhibition and neural activation arising from a nutrient preload, *Physiol. Behav.*, 72: 123–128.

English, P.J., Ghatei, M.A., Malik, I.A., Bloom, S.R., and Wilding, J.P.H. (2002) Food fails to suppress ghrelin levels in obese humans, *J. Clin. Endocrinol. Metab.*, 87: 2984–2987.

Erickson J.C., Hollpeter, G., and Palmiter, R. (1996) Attenuation of the obesity syndrome of ob/ob mice by the loss of neuropeptide Y, *Science*, 274: 1704–1707.

Erlanson–Ablertsson, C. and Larsson, A. (1988) The activation peptide of pancreatic procolipase decreases food intake in rats, *Reg. Peptides*, 22: 325–331.

Erlanson–Ablertsson, C., Mei, J., Okada, S., York, D.A., and Bray, G.A. (1991) Pancreatic procolipase propeptide, enterostatin, specifically inhibits fat intake, *Physiol. Behav.*, 49, 1191–1194.

Esfanhani, N., Bedner, I., Quershi, G.A., and Sodersten, P. (1995) inhibition of serotonin synthesis attenuates inhibition of ingestive behavior by CCK-8, *Pharmacol. Biochem. Behav.*, 51: 9–12.

Fan, W., Boston, B.A., Kesterson, R.A., Hruby, V.J., and Cone, R.D. (1997) Role of melanocortinergic neurons in agouti obesity syndrome, *Nature*, 385: 1645–1648.

Farooqui, I.S., Jebb, S.A., and Landmack, G. (1997) Recombinant leptin induced weight loss in human congenital leptin, *Nature*, 341: 879.

Fernstorm, J.D. (1987) Food induced changes in brain serotonin, *Appetite*, 8: 163.

Fletcher, P.J. and Coscina, D.V. (1993) Injecting 5-HT into the PVN does not prevent feeding induced by 8-OH-DPAT in then raphe, *Pharmacol. Biochem. Behav.*, 46: 487–491.

Flint, A., Raben, A., Astrup, A., and Holst, J. (1998) Glucagon like peptide 1 promotes satiety and suppresses energy intake in humans, J. *Clin. Invest.*, 101: 515–520.

Flint, A., Raben, A.,. Ersbøll, A.K., Holst, J.J., and Astrup, A.A. (2001) The effect of physiological levels of glucagon like peptide 1 on appetite, gastric emptying, energy and substrate metabolism in obesity, *Int. J. Obesity*, 25: 781–792.

Flynn, M.C., Scott, T.R., Pritchard, T.C., and Plata–Salaman, C.R. (1998) Mode of action of OB protein (leptin) on feeding, *Am. J. Physiol.*, 275: R174–179.

Foltin, R.W., Haney, M., Comer, S.D., and Fischman, M.W. (1996) Effect of fluoxetine on food intake of humans living in a residential laboratory, *Appetite*, 27: 165–181.

Fujimoto, K., Machidori, H., Iwakiri, R., Yamamoto, K., Fukagawa, K., Sakata, T., and Tso, P. (1993) Effect of intravenous administration of apolipoprotein A-IV on patterns of feeding, drinking and ambulatory activity of rats, *Brain Res.*, 608: 233–237.

Geary, N. (2000) Estradiol and appetite, *Appetite*, 35: 273–274.

Geary, N., Kissileff, H.R., Pi–Sunyer, F.X., and Hinton, V. (1992) Individual, but not simultaneous, glucagon and cholecystokinin infusions inhibit feeding in men, *Am. J. Physiol.*, 262: R975–80.

Geliebter, A., Gluck, M.E., Yahav, A., Hashim, Y.E., Ednie, M., and Strauss, C., (2002) Fasting and postprandial ghrelin in binge eating disorder, *Int. J. Obesity*, 26(s1): s76.

Gibbs, J., Falasco, J.D., and McHugh, P.R. (1976) Cholecystokinin decreased food intake in Rhesus monkeys, *Am. J. Physiol.*, 230, 12–18.

Gibbs, J., Fauser, E.A., Rolls, B.J., Rolls, E.T., and Maddison, S.P. (1979) Bombesin suppresses food intake in rats, *Nature*, 282: 208–210.

Gibbs, J., Young, R., and Smith, G.P. (1973) Cholecystokinin decreases food intake in rats, *J. Comp. Physiol. Psychol.*, 84: 488–493.

Giraudo, S.Q., Billington, C.J., and Levine, A.S. (1998) Feeding effects of hypothalamic injection of melanocortin 4 receptor ligands, *Brain Res.*, 809: 302–306.

Greenberg, D. (1993) Is cholecystokinin the peptide that controls fat intake? *Nutr. Rev.*, 51, 181–183.

Greenberg, D., Smith, G.P., and Gibbs, J. (1992) Cholecystokinin and the satiating effect of fat. *Gastroenterology*, 102: 1801–1803.

Greenough, A., Cole, G., Lewis, J., Lockton, A., Blundell, J.E. (1998) Untangling the effects of hunger, anxiety and nausea on food intake during intravenous cholecystokinin octapeptide (CCK-8) infusions, *Physiol. Behav.*, 65: 303–310.

Grignaschi, G., Sironi, F., and Samanin, R. (1996) Stimulation of 5-HT2A receptors in the paraventricular hypothalamus attenuates neuropeptide Y-induced hyperphagia through activation of corticotropin releasing factor, *Brain Res.*, 708: 173–176.

Grill, H.J., Gindberg, A.B., Seeley, R.J., and Kaplan, J.M. (1998) Brainstem application of melanocortin receptor ligands produces long-lasting effects on feeding and body weight, *J. Neurosci.*, 18: 10128–10135.

Gutierrez, A., Saracibar, G., Casis.L., Echevierria, E., Rodriguez, V.M., Macarulla, M.T., Abecia, L.C., and Portillo, M.P. (2002) Effects of fluoxetine administration on neuropeptide Y and orexins in obese Zucker rat hypothalamus, *Obesity. Res.*, 10: 532–540.

Gutzwiller, J.P., Drewe, J., Goke, B., Schmidt, H., Rohrer, B., Lareide, J., and Beglinger, C. (1999b) Glucagon like peptide promotes satiety and reduced food intake in patients with diabetes mellitus, *Am. J. Physiol.*, 276: R1541–1544.

Gutzwiller, J.P., Drewe, J., Hildebrand, P., Rossi, R., Lauper, J.Z., and Beglinger, C. (1994) Effect of intravenous human gastrin releasing on food intake in humans, *Gastroenterology*, 106, 1163–1173.

Gutzwiller, J.P., Drewe, J., Ketter, S., Hildebrand, P., Krautheim, A., and Beglinger, C. (2000) Interaction between CCK and a preload on food intake is mediated by CCK-A receptors in humans, *Am. J. Physiol.*, 279, R189–195.

Gutzwiller, J.P., Goke, B., Drewe, J., Hildebrand, P., Ketterer, S., Handschin, D., Winterhalder, R., Conen, D., and Beldlinger, C. (1999a) Glucagon-like peptide-1: a potent regulator of food intake in humans, *Gut*, 44: 81–86.

Haddock, C.K., Poston, W.S.C., Dill, P.L., Foreyt, J.P., and Ericsson, M. (2002) Pharmacotherapy for obesity: a quantitative analysis of four decades of published randomised clinical trials, *Int. J. Obesity*, 26, 262–273.

Halaas, J.L., Gajwala, K.S., Maffie, M., Cohen, S.L., Chait, B.T., Raninowtiz, D., Lallone, R.L., Burley, S.K., and Friedmans, J.M. (1995) Weight reducing effected of the plasma protein encoded by the obese gene, *Science*, 269: 543–546.

Halford, J.C.G. and Blundell, J.E. (2000a) Separate systems for serotonin and leptin in appetite control, *Ann. Med.*, 32: 222–232.

Halford, J.C.G. and Blundell, J.E. (2000b) Serotonin drugs and the treatment of obesity, in *Obesity: Pathology and Therapy.* Lockwood, D.H. and Heffner, T.C. (Eds.), Springer–Verlag, Berlin.

Halford, J.C.G., Smith, B.K., and Blundell, J.E. (2000) Serotonin (5-HT) and serotoninergic receptors in the regulation of macronutrient intake, in *Neural Control of Macronutrient Selection*, 425–444, Berthoud, H.R. and Seely, J.R. (Eds). CRC Press, Boca Raton, FL.

Haynes, A.C., Arch, J.R.S., Wilson, S., McClue, S., and Buckingham, R.E. (1998) Characterization of the neuropeptide Y receptor that mediates feeding in the rat: a role for the Y5 receptor? *Reg. Peptides*, 75–76: 355–361.

Haynes, A.C., Jackson, B., Overend, P., Buckingham, R.E., Wilson, S., Tadayyon, M., and Arch, J.R.S. (1999) Effects of single and chronic Intracerebroventricular administration of the orexins on feeding in the rat, *Peptides*, 20: 1099–1115.

Heine, A.F., Lara–Castro, C., Kirkam, K.A., Considine, R.V., Caro, J.F., and Weinsier, R.L. (1998) Association of leptin and hunger-satiety ratings in obese women, *Int. J. Obesity*, 22: 1084–1087.

Hopman, W.P.M., Jansen, J.B., and Lamers, C.B. (1985) Comparative study on the effects of equal amounts of fat, protein and carbohydrate on plasma cholecystokinin in man, *Scand. J. Gastroenterol.*, 20, 843–847.

Hu, Y., Bloomquist, B.T., Cornfield, L.J., DeCarr, L.B., Flores–Riveros, J.R., Friedman, L., Jiang, P.L., Lewis–Higgins, L., Sadlowski, Y., Schaefer, J., Velazquez, N., and McCaleb, M.L. (1996) Identification of a novel hypothalamic neuropeptide Y receptor associated with feeding behavior, *J. Biol. Chem.*, 42: 26315–26318.

Hulsey, M., Lu, H., Wang, T., Martin, R.J., and Baile, C.A. (1998) Intracerebroventricular (i.c.v.) administration of mouse leptin in rats: behavioral specificity and effects on meal patterns, *Physiol. Behav.*, 65: 445–455.

Hutson, P.H., Donohoe, T.P., and Curzon, G. (1988) Infusions of the 5-hydroxytryptamine agonists RU-24969 and TFMPP into then paraventricular nucleus of the hypothalamus induces hypophagia, *Psychopharmacology*, 97: 550–552.

Hwa, J.J., Witten, M.B., Williams, P.M., Ghibaudi, L., Gao, J., Salisbury, B.G., Mullins, D., Hamud, F., Strader, C.D., and Parker, E.M. (1999) Activation of the NPYY5 receptor regulates both feeding and energy expenditure, *Am. J. Physiol.*, 277: R1428–1434.

Ida, T., Nakahara, K., Kuroiwa, T., Fukui, K., Nakazato, M., Murakami, T., and Murakami, N. (2000) Both corticotropin releasing factor and neuropeptide Y are involved in the effect of orexin (hypocretin) on the food intake in rats, *Neursci. Lett.*, 293, 119–122.

Inui, A. (1999) Feeding and body-weight regulation by hypothalamic neuropeptides — mediation of the actions of leptin, *Trends Neurosci.*, 22: 62–67.

Inui, A. (2001) Ghrelin: an orexigenic and somatotrophic signal from the stomach, *Nat. Neurosci. Rev.*, 2: 551–560.

Ishihara, A., Tanaka, T., Kanatani, T., Fukami, M., Ihara, M., and Fuckuroda, T. (1998) A potent neuropeptide Y antagonist, 1229U91, suppressed spontaneous food intake in Zucker fatty rats, *Am. J. Physiol.*, 274: R1500–1504.

Jain, M.R., Horvath, T.L., Kalra, P.S., and Kalra, S.P. (2000) Evidence that NPYY1 receptors are involved in stimulation of feeding by orexins (hypocretins) in sated rats, *Reg. Peptides*, 87: 19–24.

Kamegai, J., Tamura, H., Shimizu, T., Ishii, S., Sugihare, H., and Wakabayashi, I. (2001) Chronic central infusion of ghrelin increases hypothalamic neuropeptide Y and agouti-related protein mRNA levels and body weight in rats, *Diabetes*, 50: 2438–24343.

Kask, A., Rago, L., and Harro, J. (1998a) Evidence for involvement of neuropeptide Y receptors in the regulation of food intake: studies with Y-1-selective antagonist BIBP3226, *Brit. J. Pharmacol.*, 124: 1507–1515.

Kask, A., Rägo, L., Korrovits, P., Wikberg, J.E.S., and Schiöth, H.B. (1998b) Evidence that orexigenic effects of melanocortin 4 receptor antagonist HS014 are mediated by neuropeptide Y, *Biochem. Biophys. Res. Comm.*, 248: 245–249.

Kask, A., Rago, L., Wikberg, J.E.S., and Schioth, H.B. (1998c) Evidence for involvement of the melanocortin MC4 receptor in the effects of leptin on food intake and body weight, *Eur. J. Pharmacol.*, 360: 15–19.

Kask, A., Schiöth, H.B., Harro, J., Wikberg, J.E.S., and Rägo L. (1999) Orexigenic effect of the melanocortin MC4 receptor HS 014 is inhibited only partially by neuropeptide Y Y1 receptor selective antagonist, *Can. J. Physiol. Pharmacol.*, 78: 143–149.

Kalogeris, T.J. and Painter, R.G. (2001) Adaptation of intestinal production of apolipoprotein A-IV during chronic feeding of lipid, *Am. J. Physiol.*, 280: R1151–1161.

Kanatani, A., Ito, J., Ishihara, A., Iwaasa, H., Fukuroda, T., Fukami, T., and MacNeil, D.J. (1998) A potent neuropeptide Y antagonist, 1229U91, suppressed spontaneous food intake in Zucker fatty rats, *Reg. Peptides*, 75–76: 409–415.

Keim, N.L., Stern, J.S., and Haval, P.J. (1998) Relation between circulating leptin concentrations and appetite during a prolonged, moderate energy deficit in women, *Am. J. Clin. Nutr.*, 68: 794–801.

Kennedy, J.C. (1953) The role of a fat depot in the hypothalamic control of food intake in the rat, *Proc. R. Soc. London (Biol.)*, 140: 578.

Kirkham, T.C., Perez, S., and Gibbs, J. (1995) Prefeeding potentiated anorectic actions of neuromedin B and gastrin releasing peptide, *Pharmacol. Biochem. Behav.*, 48: 809–811.

Kissileff, H.R., Pi–Sunyer, X., Thornton, J., and Smith, G.P. (1981) C-terminal octapepide of cholecystokinin decreases food intake in man, *Am. J. Clin. Nutr.*, 34:154–160.

Koegler, F.H. and Ritter, S. (1998) Galanin injection into the nucleus of the solitary tract stimulates feeding in rats with lesions of the paraventricular nucleus of the hypothalamus, *Physiol. Behav.*, 63: 521–527.

Koizumi, M. and Kimura, S. (2002) Enterostatin increases extracellular serotonin and dopamine in the lateral hypothalamic area in tats measured by *in vivo* microdialysis, *Neurosci. Lett.*, 329, 96–98.

Kotz, C.M., Teske, J.A, Levine, J.A., and Wang, C-F. (2002) Feeding and activity induced by orexin A in the lateral hypothalamic in rats, *Reg. Peptides*, 10: 27–32.

Krude, H., Biebermann, H., Luck, W., Horn, R., Brabant, G., and Grüters, A. (1998) Severe early onset obesity, adrenal insufficiency and red hair pigmentation caused by POMC mutations in humans, *Nat. Genet.*, 19: 155–157.

Kurose, T., Ueta, Y., Yamamoto, Y., Serino, R., Ozaki, Y., Saito, J., Nagata, S., and Yamashita, H. (2002) Effects of restricted feeding on the activity of hypothalamic orexin (OX)-A containing neurons and OX2 receptor mRNA level in the paraventricular nucleus of rats, *Reg. Peptides*, 104: 145–151.

Kyrkouli, S.E., Stanley, B.G., and Leibowitz, S.F. (1986) Galanin — stimulation of feeding induced by medial hypothalamic injection of this novel peptide. *Eur. J. Pharmacol.*, 122: 159–160.

Kyrkouli, S.E., Stanley, B.G., Seirafi, R.D., and Leibowitz, S.F. (1990) Stimulation of feeding by galanin — anatomical localization and behavioral specificity of this peptides effect in the brain, *Peptides*, 11: 995–1001.

Larsen, P.J., Tang–Christensen, M., Stidsen, C.E., Madsen, K., Smith, M.S., and Cameron, J.L. (1999) Activation of central neuropeptide Y Y1 receptors potently stimulates food intake in male rhesus monkeys, *J. Clin. Endocrinol. Metab.*, 84: 3781–3791.

Lavin, J.H., Wittert, G.A., Andrews, J., Yeap, B., Wishart, J.M., Morris, H.A., Morley, J.E., Horowitz, M., and Read, N.W. (1998) Interaction of insulin, glucagon-like peptide 1, gastric inhibitory polypeptide, and appetite in response to intraduodenal carbohydrate, *Am. J. Clin. Nutr.*, 68: 591–598.

Lawrence, C.B., Baudoin, F.M.H., and Luckman, S.M. (2002a) Centrally administered galanin-like peptide modifies food intake in the rat: a comparison with galanin, *J. Neuroendocrinol.*, 14: 853–860.

Lawrence, C.B., Snape, A.C., Baudoin, F.M.H., and Luckman, S.M. (2002b) Acute central ghrelin and GH secretagogues induce feeding and activate brain appetite centres, *Endocrinology*, 143: 55–62.

Lawton, C.L., Wales, J.K., Hill, A.J., and Blundell, J.E. (1995) Serotoninergic manipulation, meal-induced satiety and eating pattern: effect of fluoxetine in obese female subjects, *Obesity Res.*, 3: 345–356.

Leibowitz, S.F. (1994) Specificity of hypothalamic peptides in the control of behavioral and physiological processes, *Ann. NY Acad. Sci.*, 739: 12–35.

Leibowitz, S.F., Akabayashi, A., Alexander, J.T., and Wang, J. (1998) Gonadal steroids and hypothalamic galanin and neuropeptide Y: Role in eating behavior and body weight control in female rats, *Endocrinology*, 139, 1771–1780.

Leibowitz, S.F. and Alexander, J.T. (1991) Analysis of neuropeptides Y induced feeding — dissociation of Y1-receptor and Y2 receptor effects on natural meal patterns, *Peptides,* 12:1251–1260.

Lieverse, R.J., Jansen, J.M.B.J., Van de Zwan, A., Samson, L., Masclee, A.A.M., Rovati, L.C., and Lamers, C.B.H.W. (1994) Significant satiety effect of bombesin in lean but not in obese subjects, *Int. J. Obesity,* 18: 579–583.

Lieverse, R.J., Mascle, A.A.M., Jansen, J.B.M.J., Lam, W.F., and Lamers, C.B.H.W. (1998) Obese women are less sensitive for the satiety effects of bombesin that lean women, *Eur. J. Clin. Nutr.,* 52: 207–212.

Lin, L., Chen, J., and York, D.A. (1997) Chronic ICV enterostatin preferentially reduced fat intake and lowered body weight, *Peptides,* 18: 657–661.

Lin, L., McClanahan, S., York, D.A., and Bray, G.A. (1993) The peptide enterostatin may produce early satiety, *Physiol. Behav.,* 53, 789–794.

Lin, L., Umahara, M., York, D.A., and Bray, G.A. (1998) Beta casomorphins stimulate and enterostatin inhibits the intake of dietary fat in rats, *Peptides,* 19: 325–331.

Lin, L. and York, D.A. (1994) Metergoline blocks the feeding response to enterostatin, *Appetite,* 23: 313.

Lin, L. and York, D.A. (1997a) Enterostatin actions in the amygdala and the PVN to suppress feeding in the rat, *Peptides,* 18, 1341–1347.

Lin, L. and York, D.A. (1997b) Comparison of the effects of enterostatin on food intake and gastric emptying in rats, *Brain Res.,* 745, 205–209.

Lin, L. and York, D.A. (1998) Chronic ingestion of dietary fat is a prerequisite for inhibition of feeding by enterostatin, *Am. J. Physiol.,* 44: R619–R623.

Lin, L., York, D.A., and Bray, G.A. (1996) Comparison of Osborne–Mendel and S5B/PL strains of rat: central effects of galanin, NPY, beta-casomorphin and CRH on intake of high-fat and low-fat diets, *Obesity Res.,* 4: 117–123.

Lopez, M., Seoane, L.M., Garcia, M.D., Dieguez, C., and Senaris, R. (2002) Neuropeptide Y, but not agouti-related peptide or melanin-concentrating hormone, is a target peptide for orexin-A feeding actions in the rat hypothalamus, *Neuroendocrinology,* 75: 34–44.

López, M., Seoane, L., García, M.C., Lago, F., Casanueva, F.F., Señarís, R., and Dieguez, C. (2000) Leptin regulation of prepro-orexin and orexin receptor mRNA levels in the hypothalamus, *Boichem. Biophys. Res. Comm.,* 269: 41–45.

Lopez–Valpuesta, F.J., Nyce, J.W., and Myers, R.D. (1996) NPY-Y1 receptor antisense injected centrally in rats causes hyperthermia and feeding, *Neuroreport,* 7: 2781–2784.

Lubkin, M. and Stricker–Krongrad, A. (1998) Independent feeding and metabolic actions of orexins in mice, *Biochem. Biophys. Res. Comm.,* 253: 241–245.

Lutz, T.A., Delprete, E., and Scharrer, E. (1994) Reduction of food intake in rats by intrapritoneal injections of low doses of amylin, *Physiol. Behav.,* 55: 891–895.

Lutz, T.A., Rossi, R., Akthaus, J., Del Prete, E., and Scharrer, E. (1998) Amylin reduces food intake more potently than calcitonin gene related peptide (CGRP) when injected into the lateral brain ventricle in rats, *Peptides,* 19: 1533–1540.

Lutz, T.A., Tschudy, S., Mollet, A., Geary, N., and Scharrer, E. (2001) Dopamine D2 receptors mediated amylin's acute satiety effect, *Am. J. Physiol.,* 280, R1697–1703.

Lutz, T.A., Tschudy, S., Rushing, P.A., and Scharrer, E. (2000) Attenuation of the anorectic effects of cholecystokinin and bombesin by the specific amylin antagonist AC 253, *Physiol. Behav.,* 70, 533–536.

Lynch, W.C., Hart, P., and Babcock, A.M. (1994) Neuropeptide-Y attenuates satiety — evidence from a detailed analysis of patterns of ingestion, *Brain Res.,* 636: 28–34.

Lynn, R.B., Cao, G.Y., Considine, R.V., Hyde, T.M., and Caro, J.F. (1996) Autoradiographic localization of leptin binding in the choroids plexus of ob/ob and db/db mice, *Biochem. Biophysic. Res. Comm.,* 219: 884–889.

MacNeil, D.J., Howard, A.D., Guann, X., Fong, T.M., Nargund, R.P., Bednarek, M.A., Goulet, M.T., Weinebrg, D.H., Strack, A.M., Marsh, D.J., Vhen, H.Y., Shen, C-P., Chen, A.S., Rosenblum, C.I., MacNeil, T., Tota, M., MacIntyre, E.D., and Van der Ploeg, L.H.T. (2002) The role of melanocortins in body weight regulation: opportunities for the treatment of obesity, *Eur. J. Pharmacol.,* 450: 91–108.

Maffei, M., Halaas, J., Ravussin, E., Partley, R.E., Lee, G.H., Zhang, Y., Fei, H., Kim, S., Lallone, R., Ranganathan, S., Kern, P.A., and Friedman, J.M. (1995) Leptin levels in humans and rodents: measurement of plasma leptin and ob mRNA in obese and weight-reduced subjects, *Nat. Med.*, 1: 1155–1161.

Marsh, D.J., Hollopeter, G., Kafer, K.E., and Palmiter, R.D. (1998) Role of the Y5 neuropeptide Y receptor in feeding and obesity, *Nat. Med.*, 4: 718–721.

Matson, C.A., Reid, D.F., and Ritter, R. (2002) Daily CCK injection enhances reduction of body weight by chronic intracerebroventricular leptin infusion, *Am. J. Physiol.*, 282: R1369–1373.

Matson, C.A. and Ritter, R.A. (1999) Long-term CCK-leptin synergy suggests a role for CCK in the regulation of body weight, *Am. J. Physiol.*, 276: R1038–1045.

Matson, C.A., Wiater, M.F., Kuijper, J.L., and Weigle, D.S. (1997) Synergy between leptin and Cholecystokinin (CCK) to control daily caloric intake, *Peptides*, 18: 1275–1278.

Matsumoto, Y., Watanabe, T., Adachi, Y., Itoh, T., Ohtaki, T., Onda, H. Kurokawa, T., Nishimura, O., and Fujino, M. (2002) Galanin-like peptide stimulates food intake in the rat, *Neurosci. Lett.*, 322: 67–69.

Mays, G.G., Woolf, E.A., Monroe, C.A., and Tepper, R.I. (1995) Identification and expression cloning of a leptin receptor, OB-R, *Cell*, 83: 1263–1271.

McCoy, J.G., Stunp, B., and Avery, D.D. (1989) Intake of individual macronutrients following IP injections of BBS and CCK in rats, *Peptides*, 11: 221–225.

McMinn, J.E., Wilkinson, C.W., Havel, P.J., Woods., S.C., and Schwartz, M.C. (2000) Effect of intracerebroventricular α-MSH on food intake, adiposity, c-Fos induction, and neuropeptide expression, *Am. J. Physiol.*, 279: R695–703.

Mei, J. and Erlanson–Albertsson, C. (1996) Plasma insulin in response to enterostatin and effect of adrenalectomy in rats, *Obesity. Res.*, 4: 61–165.

Merali, Z., McIntosh, J., Kent, P., Michard, D., and Anisman, H. (1998) Aversive and appetitive events evoke the release of corticotropin-releasing hormone and bombesin-like peptide at the central nucleus of the amygdala, *J. Neurosci.*, 18: 4758–4766.

Mizuno, T.M., Kleopoulos, S.P., Bergen, H.T., Roberts, J.L., Priest, C.A., and Mobbs, C.V. (1998) Hypothalamic pro-opiomelanocortin mRNA is reduced by fasting in ob/ob and db/db mice, but is stimulated by leptin, *Diabetes*, 47: 294–297.

Mohamed–Ali, V., Pinkney, J.H., and Coppack, S.W. (1998) Adipose tissue as an endocrine and paracrine organ, *Int. J. Obesity*, 22: 1145–1158.

Montague, C.T., Farooqi, I.S., Whitehead, J.P., Soos, M.A., Rau, H., Wareham, N.J., Sweter, C.P., Digby, J.E., Hurst, J.A., Cheetham, C.H., Early, A.R.E., Barnett, A.H., Prins, J.B., and O'Rahilly, S. (1997) Congenital leptin deficiency is associated with severe early onset obesity in humans, *Nature*, 387: 903–908.

Morley, J.E. and Flood, J.F. (1991) Amylin decreases food intake in mice, *Peptides*, 12: 865–869.

Moriguchi, T., Sakurai, T., Nambu, T., Yanagisawa, M., and Goto, K. (1999) Neurons containing orexin in the lateral hypothalamic area of the adult rat brain are activated by insulin-induced acute hypoglycaemia, *Neurosci. Lett.*, 264: 101–104.

Morris, M.J. and Nguyen, T. (2001) Does neuropeptide Y contribute to the anorectic action of amylin? *Peptides*, 22: 541–546.

Moussa, N.M. and Claycomber, K.J. (1999) The yellow mouse obesity syndrome and mechanisms of agouti induced obesity, *Obesity Res.*, 7: 506–514.

Mullett, M.A., Billington, C.J., Levine, A.S., and Kotz, C.M. (2000) Hypocretin I in the lateral hypothalamus activates key feeding-regulatory brain sites, *Neuroreport*, 11: 103–108.

Murphy, B., Nuners, C.N., Ronan, J.J., Harper, C.M., Beall, M.J., Hanaway, M. et al. (1998) Melanocortins mediated inhibition of feeding behavior in rats, *Neuropeptides*, 32: 491–497.

Muurahainen, N.E., Kissileff, H.R., Xavier, P., and Sunyer, F. (1993) Intravenous infusion of bombesin reduced food intake in humans, *Am. J. Physiol.*, 264: R350–354.

Myers, R.D., Wooten, M.H., Ames, C.D., and Nyce J.W. (1995) Anorexic action of a new potential neuropeptide Y antagonists D-TYR(27,36), D-THR(32)]-NPY(27-36) infused into the hypothalamus of the rat, *Brain Res. Bull.*, 37: 237–245.

Mystkowski, P.M. and Schwartz, M.D. (2000) Gonadal steroids and energy homeostasis in the leptin era, *Nutrition*, 16: 937–949.

Nakazato, M., Murakami, N., Date, Y., Kojima, M., Matsuo, H., Kangawa, K., and Matsukura, S. (2001) A role for ghrelin in the central regulation of feeding, *Nature*, 409: 194–198.

Näslund, E., Gutniak, M., Skogar, S., Rössner, S., and Hellström, P.M. (1998) Glucagon-like peptide 1 increase the period of postprandial satiety and slows gastric emptying in obese men, *Am. J. Clin. Nutr.*, 68: 525–530.

Näslund, E., Barkelin, B., King, N., Gutniak, M., Blundell J.E., Holst, J.J., Rössner, S., and Hellström, P.M. (1999) Energy intake and appetite are suppressed by glucagon like peptide 1 (GLP-1) in obese men, *Int. J. Obesity*, 23: 304–311.

Odorizzi, M., Max, J.P., Tankosic, P., Burlet, C., and Burlet, A. (1999) Dietary preferences of Brattleboro rats correlated with an over expression of galanin in the hypothalamus, *Eur. J. Neurosci.*, 11: 3005–3014.

Okada, S., York, D.A., Bray, G.A., and Erlanson Albertsson, C. (1991) Enterostation (Val-Pro-Asp-Prop Arg), the activation peptide of procolipase, selectively reduces fat intake, *Physiol. Behav.*, 49: 1185–1189.

Ollmann M.M., Wilson, B.D., Yang, Y-K., Kerns, J.A., Chen, Y., Gantz, I., and Barsh, G.S. (1997) Antagonism of central melanocortin receptors *in vitro* and *in vivo* by agouti related protein, *Science*, 278: 135–138.

Ookuma, K., Barton, C., York, D.A., and Bray, G.A. (1997) Effect of enterostatin and kappa-opioids on macronutrients selection and consumption, *Peptides*, 18: 785–791.

Palmer, K. and Gray, J.M. (1985) Central vs. peripheral effects of estrogen on food intake and lipoprotein lipase activity in ovariectomized rats, *Physiol. Behav.*, 37: 187–189.

Pelleymounter, M.A., Cullen, M.J., Baker, M.B., Hecht, R., Winters, D.W., Boone, T., and Collins, F. (1995) Effects of the obese gene product on the body weight regulation in ob/ob mice, *Science*, 269: 540–543.

Polak, J.M., Bloom, S.R., Rayford, P.L., Pearse, A.G.E., Buchan, A.M.J., and Thompson, J.C. (1975) Identification of cholecystokinin secreting cells, *Lancet*, Nov. 22, 1016–1020.

Polidori, C., Ciccocioppo, R., Regoli, D., and Massi, M. (2000) Neuropeptide Y receptor(s) mediating feeding in the rat: characterization with antagonists, *Peptides*, 21: 29–33.

Ranganath, L.R., Beety, J.M., Morgan, L.M., Wright, W., Howland, R., and Marks, V. (1996) Attenuated GLP-1 secretion in obesity: cause or consequence?, *Gut*, 38: 916–919.

Reda, T.K., Geliebter, A., and Pi–Sunyer, F.X. (2002) Amylin, food intake, and obesity, *Obesity Res.*, 10: 1087–1091.

Rentsch, J., Levens, N., and Chiesi, M. (1995) Recombinant OB-Gene product reduces food intake in fasted mice, *Biochem. Biophys. Res. Commun.*, 214: 131–136.

Riediger, T., Schmid, H.A, Lutz, A., and Simon, E. (2001) Amylin potently activates AP neurons possibly via formation of the excitory second messenger cGMP, *Am. J. Physiol.*, 281: R1833–1843.

Riediger, T., Schmid, H.A, Lutz, A., and Simon, E. (2002) Amylin and glucose co activate area postrema neurons of the rat, *Neurosci. Lett.*, 328: 121–124.

Rodgers, J., Halford, J.C.G., Nunes de Souza, R.L., Canto de Souza, A.L., Piper, D.C., Arch, J.R.S., and Blundell, J.E. (2000) Dose–response effects of orexin-A on food intake and the bahavioural satiety sequence in rats, *Reg. Peptides*, 96: 71–84.

Rodgers, R.J., Ishii, Y., Halford, J.C.G., and Blundell, J.E. (2002) Orexins and appetite regulation, *Neuropeptides*, 36: 303–326.

Rössner, S., Barkeling, B., Erlanson–Albertsson, C., Larsson, P., and Wåhlin–Boll, E. (1995) Intravenous enterostatin does not affect single meal food intake in man, *Appetite*, 24, 37–42.

Rushing, P.A., Seely, R.J., Air, E.L., Lutz, T.A, and Woods, S.C. (2002) Acute 3rd ventricular amylin infusion potently reduces food intake but does not produce aversive consequences, *Peptides*, 23: 985–988.

Sakurai, T., Amemiya, A., Ishii, M., Matsuzaki, I., Chemelli, R.M., Tanaka, H., Williams, S.C., Richardson, J.A., Kozlowski, G.P., Wilson, S., Arch, J.R.S., Buckingham, R.E., Haynes, A.C., Carr, S.A., Annan, R.S., McNulty, D.E., Liu, W.S., Terrett, J.A., Elshourbagy, N.A., Bergsma, D.J., and Yanagisawa, M. (1998) Orexins and orexin receptors: A family of hypothalamic neuropeptides and G protein-coupled receptors that regulate feeding behavior, *Cell*, 92: 573–585.

Sargent, P.A., Sharpley, A.L., and Williams, C. (1997) 5-HT2C activation decreases appetite and body weight in obese subjects, *Psychopharmacology*, 133: 309–312.

Schick, R.R., Samsami, S., Zimmermann, T., Eberl, C., Enders, C., and Schusdziarra, V. (1993) Effect of galanin on food-intake in rats-involvement of lateral and ventromedial hypothalamic sites, *Am. J. Physiol.*, 264: R355–361.

Schwartz, M.W. (1999) Mahogany adds color to the evolving story of body weight regulation, *Nat. Med.*, 5: 374–376.

Schwartz, M.W., Baskin, D.G., Bukowski, T.R., Kuijper, J.L., Foster, D., Lasser, G., Prunkard, D.E., Porte, D., Woods, S.C., Seeley, R.J., and Weigle, D.S. (1996) Specificity of leptin action on elevated blood glucose levels and hypothalamic neuropeptide Y gene expression in ob/ob mice, *Diabetes*, 45: 531–535.

Schwartz, M.W., Seeley, R.J., Woods, S.C., Weigle, D.S., Campfield, L.A., Burn, P., and Baskin, D.G (1997) Leptin increases hypothalamic pro-opiomelanocortin mRNA expression in the rostal arcuate nucleus, *Diabetes*, 46: 2119–2125.

Schwartz, S.M. and Wade, G.N. (1981) Effects of estradiol and progesterone on food intake, *Am. J. Physiol.*, 240: E499–503.

Smeets, M., Geiselman, P., Bray, G.A., and York, D.A. (1999) The effect of oral enterostatin on hunger and food intake in human volunteers, *FASEB J.*, 13(5): A871.

Smith, B.K., York, D.A., and Bray, G.A. (1998a) Chronic d-fenfluramine treatment reduces fat intake independent of macronutrient preference, *Pharmacol. Biochem. Behav.*, 60: 105–112.

Smith, B.K., York, D.A., and Bray, G.A. (1999) Effects of intrahypothalamic infusions of serotonin and serotonin receptor agonists on macronutrient selection, *Am. J. Physiol.*, 43, R802–811.

Smith, F.J., Campfield, L.A., Moschera, J.A., Bailon, P.S., and Burn, P. (1998b) Brain administration of OB protein (leptin) inhibits neuropeptide-Y-induced feeding in ob/ob mice, *Reg. Peptides.*, 75: 433–439.

Stanley, B.G., Magdaline, W., Seirafi, A., Nguyen, M.M., and Leibowitz, S.F. (1992) Evidence for neuropeptide Y mediation of eating produced by food deprivation for a variant of the Y1 receptor mediated this peptides effect, *Peptides*, 13: 581–587.

Stuckley, J.A. and Gibbs, J. (1982) Lateral hypothalamic injection of bombesin decreases food intake in rats, *Brain Res. Bull.*, 8, 617–621

Sweet, D.C., Levine, A.S., Billington, C.J., and Kotz, C.M. (1999) Feeding response to central orexins, *Brain Res.*, 821: 535–538.

Székely, M., Pétervári, E., Balaskó, M., Hernádi, I., and Uzsoki, B. (2002) Effects of orexins on energy balance and thermoregulation, *Reg. Peptides*, 104: 47–53.

Tang–Christensen, M., Vrang, N., and Larsen, P.J. (2001) Glucagon like peptide containing pathways in the regulation of feeding behavior, *Int. J. Obesity*, 25 (suppl 5): s24–47.

Tartaglia, L.A., Dembski, M., Weng, X., Deng, N., Culpepper, J., Richards, G.J., Campfeild, L.A., Clark, F.T., Deeds, J., Muir, C., Sanker, S., Moriarty, A., Moore, K.J., Sumtko, J.S., Mays, C.G., Woolf, E.A., Monroe, C.A., and Tepper, R.I. (1995) Identification and expression cloning of a leptin receptor, OB-R, *Cell*, 83: 1263–1271.

Tecott, L.H., Sum, L.M., and Akana, S.F. (1995) Eating disorder and epilepsy in mice lacking 5-HT2C receptors, *Nature*, 374: 542–546.

Thorsell, A., Caberlotto, L., Rimondini, R., and Heilig, M. (2002) Leptin suppression of hypothalamic NPY expression and feeding, but not amygdala NPY expression and experimental anxiety, *Pharmacol. Biochem. Behav.*, 71: 425–430.

Tschöp, M., Weyer, C., Tataranni, A., Devenarayan, V., Ravussin, E., and Heiman, M.L. (2001) Circulating ghrelin levels are decreased in human obesity, *Diabetes*, 50: 707–709.

Tso, P., Liu, M., Kalogeris, T.J., and Thomson, A.B.R. (2001) The role of apolipoprotein A-IV in the regulation of food intake, *Ann. Rev. Nutr.*, 21: 231–254.

Turton, M.D., Oshea, D., Gunn, I., Beak, S.A., Edwards, C.M.B., Meeran, K., Choi, S.J., Taylor, G.M., Heath, M.M., Lambert, P.D., Wilding, J.P.H., Smith, D.M., Ghatei, M.A., Herbert, J., and Bloom, S.R. (1996) A role for glucagon like peptide 1 in the central regulation of feeding, *Nature*, 379: 69–72.

Vickers, S.P., Clifton, P.G., Dourish, C.T., and Tecott, L.H., (1999) Reduced satiating effect of d-fenfluramine in serotonin 5-HT2C receptor mutant mice, *Psychopharmacology*, 143: 309–314.

Vígh, J., Lénárd, L., Fekete, É., and Hernádi, I. (1999a) Bombesin injection into the central amygdala influences feeding behavior in the rat, *Peptides*, 20: 437–444.

Vígh, J., Lénárd, L., and Fekete, É. (1999b) Bombesin microinjection into the basolateral amygdala influences feeding behavior in the rat, *Brain Res.*, 847, 253–261.

Voigt, J.P., Sohr, R., and Fink, H. (1998) CCK-8S facilitates 5-HT release in the rat hypothalamus, *Pharmacol. Biochem. Behav.*, 59: 179–182.

Walsh, A.E., Smith, K.A., and Oldman, A.D. (1994) *m*-Chhlorophenylpiperazine decreases food intake in a test meal, *Psychopharmacology*, 116: 120–122.

Wang, L., Martinez, V., Barrachina, M.D., and Tache, Y. (1998) Fos expression in the brain induced by peripheral injection of CCK or leptin plus CCK in fasted lean mice, *Brain Res.*, 791: 157–166.

Wang, L.X., Saint–Pierre, D.H., and Tache, Y. (2002) Peripheral ghrelin selectively increases Fos expression in neuropeptide Y-synthesizing neurons in mouse hypothalamic arcuate nucleus, *Neurosci. Lett.*, 325: 47–51

Ward, A.S., Comer, S.D., Haney, M., Fischman, M.W., and Foltin, R.W. (1999) Fluoxetine maintained obese humans: effect on food intake and body weight, *Physiol. Behav.*, 66: 815–821.

Wieland, H.A., Engel, W., Eberlein, W., Rudolf, K., and Dodds, H.N. (1998) Subtype selectivity of the novel non-peptide neuropeptide Y Y1 receptor antagonist BIBO 3304 and its effect on feeding in rodents, *Br. J. Pharmacol.*, 125: 549–560.

Wirth, M.M., Olszewski, P.K., Yu, C., Levine, A.S., and Giraudo, Q.Q. (2001) Paraventricular hypothalamic α-melanocyte-stimulation hormone and MTII reduced feeding without causing aversive effects, *Peptides*, 22: 129–134.

Wren, A.M., Small, C.J., Abbott, C.R., Dhillo, W.S., Seal, L.J., Cohen, M.A., Batterham, R.L., Taheri, S., Stanley, S.A., Ghatei, M.A., and Bloom, S.R. (2001a) Ghrelin causes hyperphagia and obesity in rats, *Diabetes*, 50: 2540–2547.

Wren, A.M., Seal, L.J., Cohen, M.A., Brynes, A.E., Frost, G.S., Murphy, K.G., Dhillo, W.S., and Ghatei, M.A. (2001b) Ghrelin enhances appetite and increases food intake in humans, *J. Clin. Encocrinol. Metab.*, 86: 5992–5995.

Wren, A.M., Small, C.J., Ward, H.L., Murphy, K.G., Dakin, C.L. Taheri, S., Kennedy, A.R., Roberts, G.H., Morgan, D.G.A., Ghatei, M.A., and Bloom, S.R. (2000) The novel hypothalamic peptide ghrelin stimulates food intake and growth hormone secretion, *Endocrinology*, 141: 4325–4328.

Yamamoto, Y., Ueta, Y., Serino, R., Nomura, M., Shibuya, I., and Yamashitia, H. (2000) Effects of food restriction on the hypothalamic prepro-orexin gene expression in genetically obese mice, *Brain Res. Bull.*, 51: 515–521.

Yamanaka, A., Sakuria, T., Katsumoto, T., Yanagisawa, M., and Goto, K. (1999) Chronic intracerebroventricular administration of orexin-A to rats increases food intake in daytime, but has no effect on body weight, *Brain Res.*, 849: 248–252.

Yamanaka, A., Kunii, K., Nambu, T., Tusjino, T., Sakai, A., Matsuzaki, I., Miwa, Y., Goto, K., and Sakurai, T. (2000) Orexin-induced food intake involves neuropeptide Y pathway, *Brain Res.*, 859: 404–409.

Zhang, Y., Proenca, R., Maffei, M., Barone, M., Leopold, L., and Friedman, J.M. (1994) Positional cloning of the mouse obese gene and its human homologue, *Nature*, 372: 425–432.

Zhu, Y., Yamanaka, A., Kunii, K., Tsujino, N., Goto, K., and Sakuri, T. (2002) Orexin-mediated feeding behavior involves both leptin-sensitive and -insensitive pathways, *Physiol. Behav.*, 77: 251–257.

3

Genetics of Obesity

Philippe Boutin and Philippe Froguel

CONTENTS

ABSTRACT Environmental risk factors related to a sedentary lifestyle and unlimited access to food apply constant pressure in subjects with a genetic predisposition to gain weight. The fact that genetic defects can result in human obesity has been unequivocally established over the past years with the identification of the genetic defects responsible for different monogenic forms of human obesity: the leptin gene and its receptor; pro-opiomelanocortin (POMC); prohormone convertase 1 (PC1); and, more frequently, mutations in the melanocortin receptor 4 (1 to 4% of very obese cases). All these obesity genes encode proteins that are strongly connected as part of the same loop of the regulation of food intake. They all involve the leptin axis and one of its hypothalamic targets: the melanocortin pathway. The common forms of obesity are, however, polygenic. The examination of specific genes for involvement in the susceptibility to common obesity has not yet yielded convincing results. Approaches involving the candidate genes and the positional cloning of major obesity-linked regions will be discussed.

3.1 Introduction

Obesity is a common disease that has become more prevalent in all countries over the past few years (WHO, 1997). About 8 to 10% of the French population, 17 to 20% of the English and Welsh, and over 25% of North Americans are obese (Maillard et al., 2000; Prescott–Clarke et al., 1998; Mokdad et al., 2003). In Europe, although obesity is less prevalent in adults than in the U.S., the prevalence of overweight is increasing among children and teenagers. In France, the latest data showed that 16% of children and teenagers are overweight and the number of obese children has increased fivefold in the last 10 years (Maillard et al., 2000). Obesity is a risk factor for early mortality and a wide range of metabolic and cardiovascular complications (Lean et al., 1998).

Although rapid globalization of the westernized way of life is responsible for the rise in the number of cases of obesity (about 1 billion individuals are now overweight, or frankly obese), obesity is a typical common multifactorial disease because environmental and genetic factor interaction lead to a disease state (Bouchard, 1991). Strong evidence for a genetic component to human obesity exists — for example, familial clustering (relative risk of 3 to 7 among siblings) (Allison et al., 1996), and the high concordance of body composition in monozygotic twins (Maes et al., 1997). However, the role of genetic factors in common obesity is complex because it is determined by the interaction of several genes (polygenic), each of which may have relatively small effects (i.e., they are susceptibility genes) and work in combination with the others, as well as with environmental factors (such as nutrient intake, physical activity, and smoking). As complex traits arise through the concerted action of multiple genetic factors (through a network implying genetic heterogeneity and epistatic interactions) with different and strong environmental factors, the task of identifying any single susceptibility factor remains problematic.

The aim of this review is to describe methodologies to identify obesity genes and to summarize some of the results obtained in genetic studies. It will also emphasize the power of the genetic approach to provide clues for therapeutic intervention in obesity.

3.2   Syndromic Forms of Obesity

Most of the syndromic forms of obesity, like Prader-Willi, Cohen, Alstrom, and Bardet–Biedl have been genetically mapped. Bardet–Biedl syndrome (BBS) is known to map to at least seven loci: 11q13 (BBS1); 16q21 (BBS2); 3p13-p12 (BBS3); 15q22.3-q23 (BBS4); 2q31 (BBS5); 20p12 (BBS6); and 4q27 (BBS7). Causative genes have only been identified in five distinct BBS loci. BBS6 is caused by mutations in the MKKS (McKusick–Kaufman syndrome) gene (Katsanis et al., 2000; Slavotinek et al., 2000), which presents homologies with a bacterial chaperonin. Genes responsible for BBS2 (Nishimura et al., 2001); BBS4 (Mykytyn et al., 2001); and BBS1 (Mykytyn et al., 2002) code for proteins with unknown function. BBS1 and BBS4 sequences exhibit weak similarity to the BBS2 protein sequence and to TPR (tetratricopeptide repeat)-containing proteins (O-linked N-acetylglucosamine), respectively. Two new genes, BBS2L1 and BBS2L2, that show homologies with regions of BBS2 have defined the BBS7 locus (Badano et al., 2003). In some cases, a combination of three mutant alleles at two loci (triallelic inheritance) was shown to be necessary for development of BBS, in favor of an oligogenic rather than a recessive model of disease transmission (Beales et al., 2003).

The Prader–Willi syndrome results from deletions of the paternal copies of the imprinted *SNRPN* (small nuclear ribonucleoprotein polypeptide N) gene on chromosome 15q11–q13 (Meguro et al., 2001). A Prader–Willi-like syndrome was shown to be caused by deletions on chromosome 6q16 at the transcription factor *SIM1* gene (Faivre et al., 2002). Holder et al. reported that a girl with early-onset obesity and excessive food intake presented a balanced translocation between 1p22.1 and 6q16.2, with disruption of the *SIM1* gene (Holder at al., 2000). Authors hypothesize that haploinsufficiency of *SIM1* (single-minded

1) could cause severe obesity of this girl by acting upstream or downstream of the melanocortin 4 receptor in the paraventricular nuclei of the hypothalamus.

Alstrom syndrome (ALMS), an autosomal recessive disorder characterized by childhood obesity and type 2 diabetes, was shown to be caused by mutations in the ALMS1 gene (Collin et al., 2002; Hearn et al., 2002). Understanding the function of the genes involved in BBS, Prader–Willi syndrome, and Alstrom disease could allow identification of new pathways involved in the control of food intake, which may possibly contribute to the physiopathology of common forms of obesity as well.

3.3 Monogenic Forms of Human Obesity

A successful strategy was to screen extremely obese individuals for mutations in candidate genes selected on the basis of the mouse genetic studies. One limitation of this approach is that it only investigates previously suspected genes. Nevertheless, the findings of mutations in these homologous genes underscored the role of the underlying pathways in energy homeostasis. Although the prevalence is infrequent, the opportunity to cure certain patients of their genetic obesity phenotype has important implications for the development of similar therapies for the more common forms of obesity.

Several different obesity genes have been found. The first gene found in the mouse was the *agouti* gene, dominant mutations of which confer an obese phenotype with increased linear growth and a yellow coat color. Other mouse mutations are recessive and lead to composite phenotypes, associating obesity with endocrine and metabolic dysfunction (leptin, leptin receptor, Cpe fat mutation) or multiple sensory deficits (*tubby* mutation). Mutations in genes with homology to the mouse obesity genes or in genes acting in the same metabolic pathways have been identified in humans. These include genes encoding leptin and its receptor; pro-opiomelanocortin (*POMC*); melanocortin-4 receptor (*MC4R*); and the prohormone convertase 1 enzyme (*PC1*) (Montague et al., 1997; Clement et al., 1998; Krude et al., 1998; Vaisse et al., 1998; Yeo et al., 1998; Jackson et al., 1997). All the proteins encoded by these five genes are part of the same pathway regulating food intake.

Interestingly, no mutation in genes involved in the other numerous pathways regulating energy intake was found in human obesity cases. This suggests that the leptin pathway may be the pre-eminent regulator of energy balance in humans or may reveal our ignorance of most of the complex network of proteins regulating body weight. Supporting the latter, one may argue that, despite initial success, human genetics still only explain a minority of mendelian forms of obesity. Animal studies, as well as new genomic approaches, will probably reveal new candidate genes that also cause monogenic human obesity.

The human genes causing monofactorial obesity fall into two categories. The first includes the gene coding for leptin, leptin receptor, and POMC. Mutations in those genes induce very rare, recessive forms of obesity associated with multiple endocrine dysfunctions. Two kindreds with defects in the leptin gene were reported with loss-of-function mutations (Montague et al., 1997; Strobel et al., 1998). Homozygous carriers consistently exhibit a similar phenotype of morbid obesity with onset in the first weeks of life, with associated severe hyperphagia, hypogonadotropic hypogonadism, and central hypothyroidism.

One family has been identified with a leptin receptor mutation (Clement et al., 1998). In the three individuals with the homozygous mutation, a truncation of the receptor before the transmembrane domain completely abolishes leptin signaling, leading to a phenotype that, although more severe, is similar to that of individuals with leptin deficiency. The three sisters bearing the leptin receptor mutation also display significant growth retardation because of impaired growth hormone secretion. These obese individuals, as well as their heterozygous healthy parents, presented very high levels of leptin. Chromatography of the circulating leptin revealed that the hormone was bound to the truncated leptin receptor, leading to an increased plasma leptin half-life, although leptin expression in fat remains correlated to the fat mass. The full knockout of the leptin pathway in humans is not responsible for compensatory hypersecretion of leptin. Interestingly, the two surviving affected siblings were not diabetic or hyperlipidemic.

The key role of the melanocortin system in the control of body weight in humans is evidenced by the discovery of mutations in *POMC* and *MC4R* genes that also result in severe obesity. The *POMC* gene, expressed in human brain, gut, placenta, and pancreas, is involved in the leptin/melanocortin pathway (O'Donohue et al., 1982). Furthermore, POMC is the precursor of other peptides, including adrenocorticotropin (ACTH) and melanocyte-stimulating hormones (MSH) involved in energy homeostasis (Woods et al., 1998). *POMC* knockout mice have obesity, a defective adrenal development, and an altered pigmentation (Yaswen et al., 1999). These are similar to the phenotypes of patients with mutations in the coding region of the *POMC* gene (Krude et al., 1998). Indeed, two children with homozygous or compound heterozygous loss-of-function mutations in *POMC* exhibited a phenotype reflecting the lack of pituitary neuropeptides derived from the *POMC* gene. The absence of αMSH was responsible for the ensuing obesity (as a result of the absence of the melanocortin ligand for MC4R), and altered pigmentation and red hair (resulting from the absence of the ligand for the melanocortin-1 receptor [MC1R]). The absence of ACTH led to adrenal deficiency through melanocortin-2 receptor (MC2R) signal deficiency.

The second group of monogenic forms of obesity is related to nonsyndromic obesity related to numerous mutations in the *MC4R* gene (Vaisse et al., 1998, 2000; Yeo et al., 1998). The most prevalent obesity gene, the *MC4R* gene, is involved in 1 to 4% of cases of severe obesity (Vaisse et al., 2000). *MC4R* mutations generally segregate in families under an autosomal dominant mode of inheritance with variable penetrance. In some consanguineous pedigrees, *MC4R* mutations with relatively modest loss of function appear to be co-dominantly or even recessively associated with obesity; 81.3% of childhood obesity-associated heterozygous *MC4R* mutations lead to intracellular retention of the receptor (Lubrano–Berthelier et al., 2003). Loss of function mutations are associated with a more severe phenotype (Farooqi et al., 2003) and binge-eating disorder is a major phenotypic component for the *MC4R*'s mutation bearers in a severely obese cohort, suggesting that *MC4R* modulates eating behavior (Branson et al., 2003).

The *MC4R*-associated human obesity phenotypes are similar to those found in mice lacking *MC4R*. These rodents show moderate to severe co-dominant obesity that is more severe in homozygous than in heterozygous knockout mice. The neuroendocrine function with regard to adrenals, growth, reproduction, and thyroid is not altered. Human obesity caused by *MC4R* mutations is similar to the more common forms of obesity, but with an earlier onset age and a trend for hyperphagia in infancy, a trait that seems to disappear with age. Recent data obtained in mice as well as in humans suggest that impaired *MC4R* signaling could be involved in hyperinsulinemia through impaired negative neuronal control of insulin secretion (Cone, 2000). In this respect, *MC4R* might be considered a "thrifty" gene (i.e., a gene whose product promotes energy efficiency) serving as a primary target for small, antiobesity molecules (regardless of the proximate cause of the obesity) and possibly as a target for drugs treating the metabolic syndrome.

3.4 Genomic Approach to Common Human Obesity

3.4.1 The Candidate Gene Approach

Two general approaches are used in the search for genes underlying common polygenic obesity in humans. The first one is focused on "candidate" genes, that is, genes with some plausible role in obesity based on their known or presumed biologic role in energy homeostasis. Beta-adrenoceptor (β-*AR*) and uncoupling protein (*UCP*) genes are discussed here as examples of candidate gene studies, but many other genes tested in linkage or association studies are described by Chagnon et al. (2003).

Some of the first efforts to identify candidate genes for obesity were concentrated on adipose tissue. In brown adipose tissue, regulation of thermogenesis by the sympathetic nervous system is mediated by β-AR (Nonogaki, 2000). In humans, the β3-AR is modestly expressed in adipocytes lining the gastrointestinal tract (Krief et al., 1993). A Trp64 → Arg mutation located in the first transmembrane domain of the receptor was first correlated with obesity, body weight gain, and insulin resistance in Pima Indians, the French, and Finns (Walston et al., 1995; Clement et al., 1995; Widen et al., 1995). Discordant associations as well as functional studies were then published (Buettner et al., 1998; Ghosh et al., 1999) indicating that the role, if any, of this candidate gene in human obesity is modest, or should be considered in combination with other actors of the same pathway.

In mature brown adipocytes, stimulation of β3-AR by norepinephrine activates uncoupling protein 1 (UCP-1) via the cyclic adenosine monophosphate (cAMP) signaling pathway. UCPs are inner mitochondrial membrane transporters that dissipate the proton gradient, thus releasing stored energy in the form of heat (Klingenberg, 1990). An A to G variation in UCP-1 at position −3826 (−3826A/G) was associated with a gain in fat mass in a Quebec family study (Oppert et al., 1994). Additional effects of the UCP-1 −3826G allele with the Trp64 → Arg mutation of β3-AR gene occurred in the French morbid obese population (Clement et al., 1996). Synergistic effects of UCP-1 with β3-AR polymorphisms in decreasing sympathetic nervous system activity were also observed in a Japanese population (Shihara et al., 2001).

Polymorphisms in other members of the uncoupling protein, UCP-2 and UCP-3, were associated with variation in energy metabolism in Pima Indians contributing to overall body fat (Walder et al., 1998). A common polymorphism in the promoter of UCP-2 is associated with increased mRNA expression and decreased risk of obesity (Esterbauer et al., 2001), while no effect was described with other genetic variations in Caucasians (Otabe et al., 1998). Recent data from UCP-2 knockout mice (Arsenijevic et al., 2000) showed no effect on body weight, but these mice exhibit hyperinsulinemia. Further studies showed that UCP-2 is a potent inhibitor of insulin secretion (Zhang et al., 2001).

All these uncertainties have illustrated the complexity of the candidate gene approach. Because of their potential involvement in obesity and energy balance regulation, many other susceptibility genes have been analyzed for presence of an association with BMI, body fat, and other obesity-related genes. The results of theses studies are carefully reported annually in a review paper in *Obesity Research* (Chagnon et al., 2003). Readers are directed to look at this report of the "obesity gene map" for details. The candidate genes are primarily involved in three pathways relating to obesity. These include:

- Food intake regulation by the central nervous system and gastrointestinal factors including leptin; peptide YY; GABA; serotonin; dopamine; cannabinoid and ghrelin; glucagon-like peptide-1; and cholecystokinin pathways

- Modulation of insulin action and glucose metabolism in target tissues that may contribute to the excess of fat deposition and development of obesity-induced insulin resistance (sulfonylurea receptors; fatty acid-binding proteins; tumor necrosis factor α, etc.)

- Regulation of energy expenditure; lipid metabolism including lipid oxidation; lipolysis; lipogenesis; and, more generally, adipose tissue metabolism

The latter group includes genes encoding the lipoprotein lipase (*LPL*) that provides fatty acids for fat storage in adipose tissue and interacts with a co-activator apoprotein C2 (*apo*C2), the hormone-sensitive lipase (*HSL*), which is one of the enzymes determining whole-body fuel availability by catalyzing the rate-limiting step of adipose tissue lipolysis, and the peroxisome proliferator-activated receptor γ (*PPAR* γ), an important transcription factor activated by fatty acids that transactivates several genes involved in adipocyte metabolism and is critical for adipocyte differentiation. These studies usually showed small or uncertain effects, depending on the population studied.

Studies of interactions between polymorphisms in candidate genes and environmental factors have also been undertaken. In this regard, a polymorphism in the UCP-3 gene was shown to alter the benefit of physical activity on body weight (Otabe et al., 2000). The role of physical activity in the relationships between the phenotypic expression of obesity and a genetic variation in the β2-AR was also described in males of a French cohort (Meirhaeghe et al., 1999). Extensive gene targeting experiments in mice and functional genomic studies (expression profiles in different tissues of interest for energy balance in intervention studies) — together with completion of the Human Genome Project — provide a new generation of candidate genes for obesity. The choice of an ideal candidate gene may be based on several criteria, including (but not limited to):

- Chromosomal localization near an obesity–linked locus in human or in animal models

- Expression profile in response to modification of the environment (e.g., in adipocyte, hypothalamus, or muscle)

- Regulation of its expression by food intake, nutrients, or physical activity

- Targeted gene disruption or overexpression modifying body weight in animal models (see for review Fruhbeck and Gomez–Ambrosi, 2003, who describe the numerous knockout and transgenic models leading to obesity or to "lean" phenotypes conferring resistance to obesity)

Selected candidates for gene screening in large populations should fulfill at least two of these criteria.

3.4.2   Genome-Wide Scans in Obesity

The second approach used for identifying genes underlying common polygenic obesity utilizes genome-wide scans in order to detect chromosomal regions showing linkage with obesity in large collections of nuclear families. Linkage analysis, by using polymorphic markers (microsatellites) evenly spaced across the entire genome, identifies chromosomal regions with statistically significant co-segregation with the disease. This strategy requires no assumptions regarding the function of genes at the susceptibility loci because it attempts to map genes purely by position. Such susceptibility genes for obesity may then be positionally cloned in the intervals of linkage.

Study samples and phenotypes used for linkage analyses have been diversely chosen. Depending on the population, researchers have decided to focus on severe obese phenotypes in sibling pairs (French and American Caucasians; Hager et al., 1998; Lee et al., 1999; Stone et al., 2002; Feitosa et al., 2002) or on prospectively phenotyped general populations (Rice et al., 2002) to study the genetic influence on several obesity-related phenotypes. Family collections with the same ethnicity as study groups with extreme obesity phenotypes may be enriched in the same genetic background, thus lowering the genetic complexity and heterogeneity and increasing the statistical power to detect the gene effect on the development of disease. Importantly, the same susceptibility genes could also be involved in more modest forms of obesity and overweight, depending of the susceptibility haplotype prevalence, of the genetic background and interacting environmental factors. In this regard, the extreme forms of obesity (very severe and/or occurring very early) may be considered a paradigm for genetic studies. Until now, genome-wide scans for obesity genes have been carried out in (Figure 3.1):

- Mexican American families (Comuzzie et al., 1997; Mitchell et al., 1999)
- French pedigrees (Hager et al., 1998)
- Pima Indians (Norman et al., 1997; Hanson et al., 1998; Lindsay et al., 2001)
- White Americans (Lee et al., 1999; Kissebah et al., 2000; Rice et al., 2002; Stone et al., 2002; Feitosa et al., 2002)
- Amish (Hsueh et al., 2001)
- African–Americans (Zhu et al., 2002)
- Nigerians (Adeyemo et al., 2003)

Comuzzie et al. (1997) and Hager et al. (1998) reported a candidate region on chromosome 2p21 that could explain a significant part of the variance of leptin levels in humans. This linkage was replicated in a cohort of African–American families (Rotimi et al., 1999). Other major loci for obesity and leptin levels were identified on chromosome 10p11 and on 5cen-q in French families. This 10p locus may account for 20 to 30% of the genetic risk for obesity in this population (Hager et al., 1998).

The involvement of this chromosomal region in obesity was recently confirmed in a cohort of young Germans with obesity (Hinney et al., 2000; Saar et al., 2003), as well as in white Caucasians and African–Americans (Price et al., 2001) and old order Amish (Hsueh et al., 2001). A significant linkage on chromosome 10p12 was recently identified in bulimia nervosa, a psychiatric disorder characterized by overeating and self-induced vomiting (Bulik et al., 2003). In addition to this 10p locus, a genome scan performed in white Americans showed evidence for linkage on chromosome 20q13 and 10q (Lee et al., 1999). In Pima Indians, the most interesting region was shown on chromosome 11q21-22 (Norman et al., 1997), a region also linked with BMI in Nigerians (Adeyemo et al., 2003). In addition, a predisposition locus for severe obesity (female only) in a Utah pedigree was identified at 4p15-p14 (Stone et al., 2002).

Subsequently, the U.S. biotechnology company Myriad Genetics made a public announcement claiming that they had identified the obesity susceptibility gene mapping in this region. They named it human obesity gene 1 (HOB 1) but no article showing this discovery has been published so far. Strong evidence of linkage with BMI was shown on 7q32.3 in families from the National Heart, Lung, and Blood Institute Family Heart Study (Feitosa et al., 2002). Kissebah et al., (2000) described a locus at 3q27 that was linked to various quantitative traits characterizing the metabolic/insulin resistance syndrome. This 3q27 locus was previously identified as a type 2 diabetes mellitus locus in the French

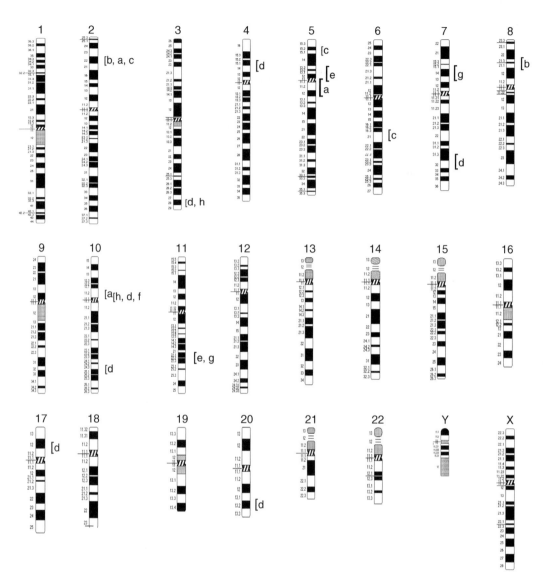

[a] **French Caucasian** (Hager et al., 1998)
[b] **Mexican American** (Comuzzie et al., 1997; Mitchell et al., 1999
[c] **African American** (Rotimi et al., 1999; Zhu et al., 2002)
[d] **American Caucasian** (Lee et al., 1999; Kissebah et al., 2000;
　　　Stone et al., 2002; Feitosa et al., 2002)
[e] **Pima Indian** (Norman et al., 1997; Hanson et al., 1998; Lindsay et al., 2001)
[f] **Amish** (Hsueh et al., 2001)
[g] **Nigerian** (Adeyemo et al., 2003)
[h] **German young obese** (Hinney et al., 2000)

FIGURE 3.1
Positive linkages in adult obesity. Chromosomal location of obesity loci identified in genome-wide screens.
(Updated from *Baillière's Best Practice and Research: Clinical Endocrinology and Metabolism.* 2001 Sep; 15(3): 391–404.)

population (Vionnet et al., 2000) and was replicated in African–Americans for BMI and percentage of body fat (Zhu et al., 2002). Several candidate genes map to this region, including the *APM1* gene encoding the differentiated adipocyte-secreted protein ACRP30/ adiponectin, which is abundantly present in the plasma.

The purified C-terminal domain of adiponectin has been reported to protect mice on a high-fat diet from obesity. It rescued obese or lipoatrophic mice from severe insulin resistance by decreasing levels of plasma free fatty acids (FFA) and enhancing lipid oxidation in muscle (Fruebis et al., 2001). Plasma levels of adiponectin were shown to be decreased in obese patients with diabetes mellitus (Arita et al., 1999). Decreased adiponectin is implicated in the development of insulin resistance in mouse models of obesity and lipoatrophy (Yamauchi et al., 2001), which makes *ACRP30* an attractive candidate gene for fat-induced metabolic syndrome and type 2 diabetes mellitus. SNPs located in the coding and the 5′ sequences of the gene defined an at-risk haplotype for type 2 diabetes which also reduced adiponectinemia in diabetic and normoglycemic populations (Vasseur et al., 2002; Menzaghi et al., 2002).

Some concerns have been raised about the heterogeneity and reliability of genetic data in multifactorial diseases in general (i.e., mostly the lack of replication). Numerous genome-wide searches for obesity genes have failed to identify major regions of linkage. These data suggest that few major loci may contribute to the genetic risk for obesity and related phenotypes in humans. A working hypothesis based on available data is that obesity is an oligogenic disease whose development can be modulated by various polygenic factors (modifier genes) and by environmental influences. The challenge now is to identify the true etiologic gene variants, explaining those genome wide scan results.

3.4.3 The Positional Cloning Strategy

To identify genes associated with an enhanced risk for overweight, chromosomal regions of linkage should be first refined using a dense map of biallelic single-nucleotide polymorphisms (SNPs). The state of the art in positional cloning of complex-disorder susceptibility genes utilizes SNP markers systematically for linkage disequilibrium (LD) mapping (Terwilliger et al., 1998; Zollner and Von Haeseler, 2000; Abecasis et al., 2001). DNA polymorphisms located at a distance from the true functional variant can be associated with the affection or variation of an obesity-associated trait. Different studies have shown that the LD extends between 10 and 30 kb for common alleles (Ardlie et al., 2002), whereas other studies show that it can extend to 60 kb in a U.S. population of Northern Europe descent (Reich et al., 2001). It has been postulated that working with "isolated" populations will significantly increase LD expectancy, but recent evidence has shown that even working in the Finnish or Icelandic populations is not a solution (Eaves et al., 2000).

The recent identification of the NIDDM1 (non-insulin-dependent diabetes mellitus 1) gene (calpain 10) for type 2 diabetes mellitus on 2q confirmed that LD mapping could be a successful strategy to unravel other polygenic diseases (Horikawa et al., 2000). This work also illustrated the complexity of the search because, in this case, the disease was associated with an intronic *NIDDM1* polymorphism (UCSNP-43) in the study population (Mexican Americans). In fact, three noncoding polymorphisms, including UCSNP-43, have been identified as defining an at-risk haplotype. In other ethnic groups, such as French Caucasians, the rarity of this high-risk haplotype complicates the assignment of a definite role for calpain 10 in type 2 diabetes mellitus. Moreover, because the function of this protease is still unclear, this study emphasized the limitation of genetic studies to prove a functional relation from solely statistic-based methods.

LD mapping should be integrated in a complex positional cloning strategy combining extensive family resources; genotyping technologies; bioinformatics and transcriptional profiling to assess biologic candidacy of regional transcripts; and molecular epidemiology. Clinical and methodological resources are, therefore, key issues for success in the positional cloning of major obesity-linked regions. Technological developments and new information sources (e.g., genome annotation) will allow increased efficiency for LD mapping. For example, tissue expression profiling may provide the most direct way to improve overall understanding of the molecular circuitry maintaining energy homeostasis. Therefore, expression profiling in humans, on the one hand, and genetic analysis of populations on the other, will provide complementary tools to advance understanding of the complex network of gene–gene and gene–environment interactions underlying susceptibility to obesity.

Following identification of genetic variations, exploration of the consequences at the level of tissue (tissue expression profiling), organism, and population (molecular epidemiology) will clarify the role of these variants in disease pathogenesis and their implications for diagnostic and therapeutic developments. Recent studies in patients with prostate cancer (Tavtiglian et al., 2001); inflammatory bowel disease (Hugot et al., 2001); and psoriasis (Asumalahti et al., 2002) show evidence of the resolution of linkage to identify a candidate gene. An improved understanding of the genetic and environmental predictors of risk factors for complex diseases provides a rational basis for stratification of the disease risk and response to treatment, allowing effective targeting of preventive and therapeutic tools.

3.5 Conclusion

Given the strong association of adiposity with cardiovascular, metabolic, and other morbidities, the current epidemic of obesity represents a major public health concern. Preventive and therapeutic approaches are hampered by lack of fundamental understanding of the mechanisms controlling human body fat mass and disturbance of this control in obese states. Human geneticists have pioneered the understanding of the genetic basis of obesity through their discovery of the first monogenic defects leading to extreme childhood obesity. The more challenging problem is identification of genetic variants that underlie susceptibility to the common forms of human obesity. Based on high-quality family material and recent widely confirmed genome-wide scan results, putative etiological variants in candidate genes will emerge. The success of these studies will require a multidisciplinary approach that combines genomics; bioinformatics; expression profiling; biochemistry; human physiology; and molecular epidemiology. Although the task is considerable, the breadth and depth of expertise now available in human genetics of complex traits provide unique scientific opportunities for significant advances.

Acknowledgments

This work was supported by the CNRS, a grant from Eli Lilly, and the NUGENOB European consortium.

References

Abecasis, G.R., Noguchi, E., Heinzmann, A. et al. (2001) Extent and distribution of linkage disequi-librium in three genomic regions. *Am. J. Hum. Genet.* 68(1): 191–197.

Adeyemo, A., Luke, A., Cooper, R., Wu, X., Tayo, B., Zhu, X., Rotimi, C., Bouzekri, N., and Ward, R.A. (2003) Genome-wide scan for body mass index among Nigerian families. *Obes. Res.* 11(2): 266–273.

Allison, D.B., Faith, M.S., and Nathan, J.S. (1996) Risch's lambda values for human obesity. *Int. J. Obes.* 20: 990–999.

Ardlie, K.G., Kruglyak, L., and Seielstad, M. (2002) Patterns of linkage disequilibrium in the human genome. *Nat. Rev. Genet.* 3(4): 299–309.

Arita, Y., Kihara, S., Ouchi, N. et al. (1999) Paradoxical decrease of an adipose-specific protein, adiponectin, in obesity. *Biochem. Biophys. Res. Commun.* 257: 79–83.

Arsenijevic, D., Numa, H., Pecqueur, C. et al. (2000) Disruption of the uncoupling protein-2 gene in mice reveals a role in immunity reactive oxygen species production. *Nat. Genet.* 26: 435–439.

Asumalahti, K., Veal, C., Laitinen, T. et al. (2002) Coding haplotype analysis supports HCR as the putative susceptibility gene for psoriasis at the MHC PSORS1 locus. *Hum. Mol. Genet.* 11(5): 589–597.

Badano, J.L., Ansley, S.J., Leitch, C.C., Lewis, R.A., Lupski, J.R., and Katsanis, N. (2003) Identification of a novel Bardet–Biedl syndrome protein, BBS7, that shares structural features with BBS1 and BBS2. *Am. J. Hum. Genet.* 72: 650–658.

Beales, P.L., Badano, J.L., Ross, A.J., Ansley, S.J., Hoskins, B.E., Kirsten, B., Mein, C.A., Froguel, P., Scambler, P.J., Lewis, R.A., Lupski, J.R., and Katsanis, N. (2003) Genetic interaction of BBS1 mutations with alleles at other BBS loci can result in non-Mendelian Bardet–Biedl syndrome. *Am. J. Hum. Genet.* 72(5): 1187–1199.

Bouchard, C. (1991) Current understanding of aetiology of obesity genetic and non genetic factors. *Am. J. Clin. Nutr.* 53: 1561–1565.

Branson, R., Potoczna, N., Kral, J.G., Lentes, K.U., Hoehe, M.R., and Horber, F.F. (2003) Binge eating as a major phenotype of melanocortin 4 receptor gene mutations. *N. Engl. J. Med.* 348(12): 1096–1103.

Buettner, R., Schaffler, R.D., and Arndt, H. et al. (1998) The Trp64Arg polymorphism of the beta3-adrenergic receptor gene is not associated with obesity or type 2 diabetes mellitus in a large population-based caucasian cohort. *J. Clin. Endocrinol. Metab.* 83(11): 2892–2897.

Bulik, C.M., Devlin, B., Bacanu, S.A., Thornton, L., Klump, K.L., Fichter, M.M., Halmi, K.A., Kaplan, A.S., Strober, M., Woodside, D.B., Bergen, A.W., Ganjei, J.K., Crow, S., Mitchell, J., Rotondo, A., Mauri, M., Cassano, G., Keel, P., Berrettini, W.H., and Kaye, W.H. (2003) Significant linkage on chromosome 10p in families with bulimia nervosa. *Am. J. Hum. Genet.* 72: 200–207.

Chagnon, Y.C., Rankinen, T., Snyder, E.E., Weisnagel, S.J., Perusse, L., and Bouchard, C. (2003) The human obesity gene map: the 2002 update. *Obes. Res.* 11(3): 313–367.

Clement, K., Vaisse, C., Manning, B.S.J. et al. (1995) Genetic variation in the beta 3 adrenergic receptor gene and an increased capacity to gain weight in patients with morbid obesity. *N. Engl. J. Med.* 333: 352–354.

Clement, K., Ruiz, J., Cassard–Doulcier, A.M. et al. (1996) Additive effects of polymorphims in the uncoupling protein gene and the beta-3 adrenergic receptor gene on gain weight in morbid obesity. *Int. J. Obes.* 20: 1062–1066.

Clement, K., Vaisse, C., Lahlou, N. et al. (1998) A mutation in the human leptin receptor gene causes obesity and pituitary dysfunction. *Nature* 392: 398–401.

Collin, G.B., Marshall, J.D., Ikeda, A., So, W.V., Russell–Eggitt, I., Maffei, P., Beck, S., Boerkoel, C.F. Sicolo, N., Martin, M., Nishina, P.M., and Naggert, J.K. (2002) Mutations in ALMS1 cause obesity, type 2 diabetes and neurosensory degeneration in Alstrom syndrome. *Nat. Genet.* 31(1): 74–78.

Comuzzie, A.G., Hixson, J.E., Almasy, L. et al. (1997) A major quantitative trait locus determining serum leptin levels and fat mass is located on human chromosome 2. *Nat. Genet.* 15(3): 273–276.

Cone, R.D. (2000) Haploinsufficiency of the melanocortin-4 receptor: part of the thrifty genotypes? *J. Clin. Invest.* 106: 185–187.

Eaves, I.A., Merriman, T.R., Barber, R.A. et al. (2000). The genetically isolated populations of Finland and Sardinia may not be a panacea for linkage disequilibrium mapping of common disease genes. *Nat. Genet.* 25: 320–323.

Esterbauer, D., Schneitler, C., Oberkofler, H. et al. (2001) A common polymorphism in the promoter of UCP2 is associated with decreased risk of obesity in middle-aged humans. *Nat. Genet.* 28: 178–183.

Faivre, L., Cormier–Daire, V., Lapierre, J.M., Colleaux, L., Jacquemont, S., Genevieve, D., Saunier, P., Munnich, A., Turleau, C., Romana, S., Prieur, M., De Blois, M.C., and Vekemans, M. (2002) Deletion of the SIM1 gene (6q16.2) in a patient with a Prader–Willi-like phenotype. *J. Med. Genet.* 39(8): 594–596.

Farooqi, I.S., Keogh, J.M., Yeo, G.S., Lank, E.J., Cheetham, T., O'Rahilly, S. (2003) Clinical spectrum of obesity and mutations in the melanocortin 4 receptor gene. *N. Engl. J. Med.* 348(12): 1085–1095.

Feitosa, M.F., Borecki, I.B., Rich, S.S. et al. (2002) Quantitative trait loci influencing body mass index reside on chromosomes 7 and 13: the national heart lung and blood institute family heart study. *Am. J. Hum. Genet.* 70: 72–82.

Fruebis, J., Tsao, T., Javorschi, S. et al. (2001) Proteolytic cleavage product of 30-kDa adipocyte complement-related protein increases fatty acid oxidation in muscle and causes weight loss in mice. *Proc. Natl. Acad. Sci. USA* 98: 2005–2010.

Frühbeck, G. and Gomez–Ambrosi, J. (2003) Control of body weight: a physiologic and transgenic perspective. *Diabetologia* 46: 143–172.

Ghosh, S., Langefeld, C.D., Ally, D. et al. (1999) The W64R variant of the beta3-adrenergic receptor gene is not associated with type 2 diabetes or obesity in a large Finnish sample. *Diabetologia.* 42(2): 238–244.

Hager, J., Dina, C., Francke, S. et al. (1998) A genome-wide scan for human obesity genes shows evidence for a major susceptibility locus on chromosome 10. *Nat. Genet.* 20: 304–338.

Hanson, R.L., Ehm, M.G., Pettitt, D.J. et al. (1998) An autosomal genomic scan for loci linked to type II diabetes mellitus and body-mass index in Pima Indians. *Am. J. Hum. Genet.* 63: 1130–1138.

Hearn, T., Renforth, G.L., Spalluto, C., Hanley, N.A., Piper, K., Brickwood, S., White, C., Connolly, V., Taylor, J.F., Russell–Eggitt, I., Bonneau, D., Walker, M., and Wilson, D.I. (2002) Mutation of ALMS1, a large gene with a tandem repeat encoding 47 amino acids, causes Alstrom syndrome. *Nat. Genet.* 31(1): 79–83.

Hinney, A., Ziegler, A., Oeffner, F. et al. (2000) Independent confirmation of a major locus for obesity on chromosome 10. *J. Clin. Endocrinol. Metab.* 85(8): 2962–2965.

Holder, J.L., Jr., Butte, N.F., and Zinn, A.R. (2000) Profound obesity associated with a balanced translocation that disrupts the SIM1 gene. *Hum. Mol. Genet.* 9(1):101–108.

Horikawa, Y., Oda, N., Cox, N.J. et al. (2000) Genetic variation in the gene encoding calpain-10 is associated with type 2 diabetes mellitus. *Nat. Genet.* 26: 163–175.

Hsueh, W.C., Mitchell, B.D., Schneider, J.L. et al. (2001) Genome-wide scan of obesity in the old order Amish. *J. Clin. Endocrinol. Metab.* 86(3): 1199–1205.

Hugot, J.P., Chamaillard, M., Zouali, H. et al. (2001) Association of NOD2 leucine-rich repeat variants with susceptibility to Crohn's disease. *Nature* 31(411): 599 603.

Jackson, R.S., Creemers, J.W., Ohagi, S. et al. (1997) Obesity and impaired prohormone processing associated with mutations in the human prohormone convertase 1 gene. *Nat. Genet.* 16: 303–306.

Katsanis, N. et al. (2000) Mutations in MKKS cause obesity, retnal distrophy and renal malformations associated with Bardet–Biedl syndrome. *Nat. Genet.* 26: 67–70.

Kissebah, A.H., Sonnenberg, G.E., Myklebust, J. et al. (2000) Quantitative trait loci on chromosome 3 and 17 influence phenotypes of the metabolic syndrome. *Proc. Natl. Acad. Sci. USA* 97: 14478–14483.

Klingenberg, M. (1990) Mechanism and evolution of the uncoupling protein of brown adipose tissue. *Trends Biochem. Sci.* 15: 108–112.

Krief, S., Lonnqvist, F., Raimbault, S. et al. (1993) Tissue distribution of beta3-adrenergic receptor nRNA in man. *J. Clin. Invest.* 91: 344–349.

Krude, H., Biebermann, H., Luck, W. et al. (1998) Severe early-onset obesity, adrenal insufficiency and red hair pigmentation caused by POMC mutations in humans. *Nat. Genet.* 19(2): 155–157.

Lean, M.E.J., Hans, T.S., and Seidell, J.C. (1998) Impairment of health and quality life in people with large waist circumference. *Lancet* 351: 853–856.

Lee, J.H., Reed, D.R., Li, W.D. et al. (1999) Genome scan for human obesity and linkage to markers in 20q13. *Am. J. Hum. Genet.* 64(1): 196–209.

Lindsay, R.S., Kobes, S., Knowler, W.C., Bennett, P.H., Hanson, R.L. (2001) Genome-wide linkage analysis assessing parent-of-origin effects in the inheritance of type 2 diabetes and BMI in Pima Indians. *Diabetes* 50(12): 2850–2857.

Lubrano–Berthelier, C., Durand, E., Dubern, B., Shapiro, A., Dazin, P., Weill, J., Ferron, C., Froguel, P., and Vaisse, C. (2003) Intracellular retention is a common characteristic of childhood obesity-associated MC4R mutations. *Hum. Mol. Genet.* 12(2):145–153.

Maes, H.H., Neale, M.C., and Eaves, L.J. (1997) Genetic and environmental factors in relative body weight and human adiposity. *Behav. Genet.* 27: 325–351.

Maillard, G., Charles, M.A., Tibult, N. et al. (2000) Trends in the prevalence of obesity in children and adolescent in France between 1980 and 1991. *Int. J. Obes.* 24(12): 1608–1617.

Meguro, M., Mitsuya, K., Nomura, N., Kohda, M., Kashiwagi, A., Nishigaki, R., Yoshioka, H., Nakao, M., Oishi, M., and Oshimura, M. (2001) Large-scale evaluation of imprinting status in the Prader–Willi syndrome region: an imprinted direct repeat cluster resembling small nucleolar RNA genes. *Hum. Mol. Genet.* 10(4): 383–394.

Menzaghi, C., Ercolino, T., Di Paola, R., Berg, A.H., Warram, J.H., Scherer, P.E., Trischitta, V., and Doria, A. (2002) A haplotype at the adiponectin locus is associated with obesity and other features of the insulin resistance syndrome. *Diabetes* 51(7): 2306–2312.

Meirhaeghe, A., Helbecque, N., Cottel, D. et al. (1999) Beta2-adrenoceptor gene polymorphism, body weight and physical activity [letter]. *Lancet* 13: 896.

Mitchell, B.D., Cole, S.A., Comuzzie, A.G. et al. (1999) A quantitative trait locus influencing BMI maps to the region of the beta-3 adrenergic receptor. *Diabetes* 48(9): 1863–1867.

Mokdad, A.H., Ford, E.S., Bowman, B.A., Dietz, W.H., Vinicor, F., Bales, V.S., and Marks, J.S. (2003) Prevalence of obesity, diabetes, and obesity-related health risk factors, 2001. *JAMA* 289(1): 76–79.

Montague, C.T., Farooqi, I.S., Whitehead, J.P. et al. (1997) Congenital leptin deficiency is associated with severe early-onset obesity in humans. *Nature* 387: 903–908.

Mykytyn, K., Braun, T., Carmi, R. et al. (2001) Identification of the gene that, when mutated, causes the human obesity syndrome BBS4. *Nat. Genet.* 28: 188–191.

Mykytyn, K., Nishimura, D.Y., Searby, C.C., Shastri, M., Yen, H., Beck, J.S., Braun, T., Streb, L.M., Cornier, A.S., Cox, G.F., Fulton, A.B., Carmi, R., Luleci, G., Chandrasekharappa, S.C., Collins, F.S., Jacobson, S.G., Heckenlively, J.R., Weleber, R.G., Stone, E.M., and Sheffield, V.C. (2002) Identification of the gene (BBS1) most commonly involved in Bardet–Biedl syndrome, a complex human obesity syndrome. *Nat. Genet.* 31: 435–438.

Nishimura, D.Y., Searby, C.C., Carmi, R. et al. (2001) Positional cloning of a novel gene on chromosome 16q causing Bardet–Biedl syndrome (BBS2). *Hum. Mol. Genet.* 10: 865–874.

Nonogaki, K. (2000) New insights into sympathetic regulation of glucose and fat metabolism. *Diabetologia* 43: 533–549.

Norman, R.A., Thompson, D.B., Foroud, T. et al. (1997) Genome-wide search for genes influencing percent body fat in Pima Indians: suggestive linkage at chromosome 11q21-q22. *Am. J. Hum. Genet.* 60: 166–173.

O'Donohue, T.L. and Dorsa, D.M. (1982) The opiomelanotropinergic neuronal and endocrine systems. *Peptides* 3: 353–395.

Oppert, J.M., Vohl, M.C., Chagnon, Y.C. et al. (1994) DNA polymorphism in the uncoupling protein (UCP) gene and human body fat. *Int. J. Obes.* 18: 526–531.

Otabe, S., Clement, K., Rich, N. et al. (1998) Mutation screening of the human UCP2 gene in normoglycemic and NIDDM morbidly obese patients. *Diabetes* 47: 840–842.

Otabe, S., Clement, K., Dina, C. et al. (2000) A genetic variation in the 5′ flanking region of the UCP3 gene is associated with body mass index in humans in interaction with physical activity. *Diabetologia* 43(2): 245–249.

Prescott–Clarke, P. and Primatesta, P. (1998) Health survey for England 1996. London: HMSO.

Price, R.A., Li, W.D., Bernstein, A. et al. (2001). A locus affecting obesity in human chromosome region 10p12. *Diabetologia* 44: 363–366.

Reich, D.E., Cargill, M., Bolk, S., Ireland, J., Sabeti, P.C., Richter, D.J., Lavery, T., Kouyoumjian, R., Farhadian, S.F., Ward, R., Lander, E.S. (2001) Linkage disequilibrium in the human genome. *Nature* 10(411): 199–204.

Rice, T., Chagnon, Y.C., Perusse, L. et al. (2002) A genomewide linkage scan for abdominal subcutaneous and visceral fat in black and white families: the HERITAGE family study. *Diabetes* 51(3): 848–855.

Rotimi, C.N., Comuzzie, A.G., Lowe, W.L. et al. (1999) The quantitative trait locus on chromosome 2 for serum leptin levels is confirmed in African–Americans. *Diabetes* 48: 643–644.

Saar, K., Geller, F., Ruschendorf, F., Reis, A., Friedel, S., Schauble, N., Nurnberg, P., Siegfried, W., Goldschmidt, H.P., Schafer, H., Ziegler, A., Remschmidt, H., Hinney, A., and Hebebrand, J. (2003) Genome scan for childhood and adolescent obesity in German families. *Pediatrics* 111: 321–327.

Shihara, N., Yasuda, K., Moritani, T. et al. (2001) Synergic effect of polymorphisms of uncoupling protein1 and beta3-adrenergic receptor genes on autonomic nervous system activity. *Int. J. Obes. Relat. Metab. Disord.* 25(6): 761–766.

Slavotinek, A.M., Stone, E.M., Mykytyn, K. et al. (2000) Mutations in MKKS cause Bardet–Biedl syndrome. *Nat. Genet.* 26: 15–16.

Stone, S., Abkevich, V., Hunt, S.C. et al. (2002). A major predisposition locus for severe obesity, at 4p15-p14. *Am. J. Hum. Genet.* 70(6): 1459–1468.

Strobel, A., Issad, T., Camoin, L. et al. (1998) A leptin missense mutation associated with hypogonadism and morbid obesity. *Nat. Genet.* 18: 213–215.

Tavtiglian, S.V., Simard, J., Teng, D.H.F. et al. (2001) A candidate prostate cancer susceptibility gene at chromosome 17p. *Nat. Genet.* 27: 172–180.

Terwilliger, J.D. and Weiss, K.M. (1998) Linkage disequilibrium mapping of complex disease: fantasy or reality? *Curr. Opin. Biotechnol.* 9: 578–594.

Vaisse, C., Clement, K., Guy, G.B. et al. (1998) A frameshift mutation in human MC4R is associated with a dominant form of obesity. *Nat. Genet.* 20: 113–114.

Vaisse, C., Clement, K., Durand, E. et al. (2000) Melanocortin-4 receptor mutations are a frequent and heterogeneous cause of morbid obesity. *J. Clin. Invest.* 106: 253–262.

Vasseur, F., Helbecque, N., Dina, C., Lobbens, S., Delannoy, V., Gaget, S., Boutin, P., Vaxillaire, M., Lepretre, F., Dupont, S., Hara, K., Clement, K., Bihain, B., Kadowaki, T., and Froguel, P. (2002) Single-nucleotide polymorphism haplotypes in the both proximal promoter and exon 3 of the APM1 gene modulate adipocyte-secreted adiponectin hormone levels and contribute to the genetic risk for type 2 diabetes in French Caucasians. *Hum. Mol. Genet.* 11(21): 2607–2614.

Vionnet, N., Hani, E.H., Dupont, S. et al. (2000) Genomewide search for type 2 diabetes-susceptibility genes in French whites: evidence for a novel susceptibility locus for early-onset diabetes on chromosome 3q27-qter and independent replication of a type 2-diabetes locus on chromosome 1q21-q24. *Am. J. Hum. Genet.* 67: 1470–1480.

Walder, K., Norman, R., Hanson, R.L., et al. (1998) Association between uncoupling protein polymorphisms (UCP2-UCP3) and energy metabolism obesity in Pima Indians. *Hum. Mol. Genet.* 7: 1431–1435.

Walston, J., Silver, K., Bogardus, C. et al. (1995) Time of onset of non-insulin dependent diabetes mellitus and genetic variation in the beta3-adrenergic receptor gene. *N. Engl. J. Med.* 333: 343–348.

Widen, E., Lehto, M., Kanninen, T. et al. (1995) Association of a polymorphism in the beta3-adrenergic receptor gene with features of the insulin resistance syndrome in Finns. *N. Engl. J. Med.* 333: 348–352.

Woods, S.C., Seeley, R.J., Porte, D. et al. (1998) Signals that regulate food intake and energy homeostasis. *Science* 280: 1378–1383.

WHO (World Health Organization). Obesity: preventing and managing the global epidemic. Report of a WHO consultation on obesity. Geneva: WHO, 1997, June 3–5.

Yamauchi, T., Kamon, J., Waki, H. et al. (2001) The fat-derived hormone adiponectin reverses insulin resistance associated with both lipoatrophy and obesity. *Nat. Med.* 7(8): 941–946.

Yaswen, L., Diehl, N., Brennan, M.B. et al. (1999) Obesity in the mouse model of proopiomelanocortin deficiency responds to peripheral melanocortin. *Nat. Med.* 5: 1066–1070.

Yeo, G.S., Farooqi, I.S., Aminian, S. et al. (1998) A frameshift mutation in MC4R associated with dominantly inherited human obesity. *Nat. Genet.* 20(2): 111–112.

Zhang, C.Y., Baffy, G., Perret, P. et al. (2001) Uncoupling protein-2 negatively regulates insulin secretion and is a major link between obesity, beta cell dysfunction, and type 2 diabetes. *Cell* 15(6): 745–755.

Zhu, X., Cooper, R.S., Luke, A., Chen, G., Wu, X., Kan, D., Chakravarti, A., and Weder, A. (2002) A genome-wide scan for obesity in African–Americans. *Diabetes* 51(2): 541–544.

Zollner, S. and Von Haeseler, A. (2000) A coalescent approach to study linkage disequilibrium between single-nucleotide polymorphisms. *Am. J. Hum. Genet.* 66: 615–628.

4

Antipsychotic Drugs, Weight Gain, and Diabetes

Trino Baptista

CONTENTS

ABSTRACT   Numerous drugs induce hyperglycemia and may eventually lead to diabetes mellitus (DM). In current clinical practice, corticosteroids; thiazide diuretics; β-blockers; protease inhibitors; and atypical antipsychotic drugs (APDs) are the most widely pre-scribed agents associated with hyperglycemia. The propensity of APDs to induce hyper-glycemia (*de novo* or in previous diabetics) closely resembles their effect on body weight gain (BWG): (1) high for clozapine; olanzapine; thioridazine; and chlorpromazine; (2) moderate to low for risperidone; quetiapine; sertindole; and zotepin; and (3) very low for haloperidol; fluphenazine; pimozide; ziprasidone; and aripiprazole. The majority of type 2 DM reported cases received clozapine or olanzapine and some of them developed ketoacidosis. These results are preliminary and need confirmation with prospective and randomized studies.

The APDs do not primarily impair insulin production and release. Increased insulin resistance and insulin demand due to increased appetite may be determinant factors with or without BWG. Patients with schizophrenia and affective disorders may be genetically predisposed to glucose dysregulation. Preliminary studies reported a linkage between APD-induced BWG and a polymorphism in the 5-HT2C receptor gene allele, and between schizophrenia and enzymes involved in glycolysis. New data are expected in the near future. Thus, this is a remarkable example of interaction between genetic predisposition and an exogenous trigger. High-risk subjects should be detected before starting APD administration. Nutritional assistance, regular physical activity, blood glucose, and lipid monitoring are recommended. Small studies reported positive effects of amantadine; niza-tidine; topiramate; metformin; reboxetine; and orlistat to prevent APD-induced BWG. Treatment of overt DM in polymedicated psychiatric patients follows the same principles for nonpsychiatric populations, with the additional concern of potential adverse drug interaction and poor treatment compliance.

4.1   Introduction: Drugs, Obesity, and Diabetes Mellitus

Pharmacological agents may impair carbohydrate metabolism through excessive body weight gain (BWG) and obesity. The medical community's interest in this issue increased considerably after 1990, with the introduction of the atypical antipsychotic drugs (APDs) into clinical practice. Some atypical APDs often cause obesity and glucose dysregulation. After an overview of the general topic of drug-induced glucose dysregulation; the effects of APDs on body weight (BW); and the association of these agents with the development of DM, current treatment and research perspectives will be reviewed.

Converging evidence shows that obesity is a significant risk factor for development of diabetes mellitus (DM) type 2. The frequency of type 2 DM in men and women increases from 2.0 and 2.3%, respectively, in subjects with normal weight, to 10.7 and 19.9%, in people with class 3 obesity (Must et al., 1999). Obesity (particularly of the abdominal type) is also associated with increased risk of stroke; coronary heart disease; osteoarthritis; some types of cancer; complicated pregnancy; and infertility. The consensus is that abdominal obesity is particularly deleterious for carbohydrate and lipid metabolism (Kissebah and Krakover, 1994). The frequency of type 2 DM and obesity is increasing alarmingly in developed countries (Flegal et al., 2002; Harris et al., 1998). Thus, prevention or attenuation of these diseases is a critical concern in modern public health administration.

Obesity and type 2 DM are prototypical chronic diseases with multifactor etiology, including genetic predisposition, unhealthy dietary habits, and low physical activity among many other factors (Ravussin and Bouchard, 2000). The type 2 DM (formerly noninsulin-dependent type) comprises around 90% of all cases of DM, and insulin production is relatively preserved until intermediate phases of the disease. In contrast, type 1 DM (formerly insulin-dependent type) is generally related to immunologically based destruction of pancreatic β-cells, leading to absolute hypoinsulinemia (Lebovitz, 2002).

Pharmacological agents have also been causally implicated in excessive BWG and glucose intolerance. Clinically significant BWG may be observed during treatment with corticosteroids; antihistaminics; antidepressants such as tricyclic drugs and mirtazapine; lithium; anticonvulsants such as valproate; and some APDs (Luna and Feinglos, 2001; Zimmermann et al., 2003). An increased risk for glucose dysregulation was reported during treatment with an extensive list of drugs, including (Pandit, et al., 1993; Luna and Feinglos, 2001; Chan, 2002; Molazowski, 2002):

- APDs
- β-Blockers
- β-Adrenergic agonists
- Thiazide diuretics
- Corticosteroids
- Glucosamine
- Protease inhibitors
- Pyriminil
- Niacin
- Pentamidine
- Minoxidil
- Diazoxide

- Cyclosporine
- Oral contraceptives
- Growth hormones
- Sex and thyroid hormones

In current clinical practice, thiazide diuretics; β-blockers; protease inhibitors; corticosteroids; and atypical APDs are the most widely prescribed agents associated with hyperglycemia (Luna and Feinglos, 2001). Of all these agents, clinically significant BWG is mainly observed during corticosteroid and APD administration (Allison et al., 1999a, b; Taylor and McAskill, 2000; Baptista et al., 2002b; Lebovitz and McFarlane, 2001), and it may be causally associated with glucose dysregulation development.

The hyperglycemia observed with thiazides and β-blockers may be related to decreased insulin secretion. In the case of protease inhibitors, insulin resistance and a direct impairment in β-cell-function have been implicated (Luna and Feinglos, 2001; Lebovitz and McFarlane, 2001). The risk of hyperglycemia increases by up to 28% during prolonged treatment with β-blockers. This risk is lower during thiazide administration at the relatively low dose schedule currently used. Hyperglycemia with or without DM is reported in 3 to 17% of patients receiving active antiretroviral therapy (Luna and Feinglos, 2001).

The impairing effects of glucocorticoids on glucose metabolism were firmly established in 1940 by Long et al. and are observed in people with normal pretreatment glucose tolerance and in diabetic subjects (Pandit et al., 1993). Between 25 and 90% of nondiabetic people display abnormally high postprandial plasma glucose levels during prolonged treatment with glucocorticoids (Lebovitz and McFarlane, 2001). These agents induce glucose dysregulation by several mechanisms, such as enhanced gluconeogenesis; augmented insulin resistance at the insulin receptor and the signal transduction process; and increased glycogenolysis secondary to hyperglucagonemia (Pandit et al., 1993; Nyirenda et al., 1998). The effects of glucocorticoids on BW are complex: even though they induce redistribution of body fat in the abdomen, face, and upper back, they also induce protein catabolism, leading to thin extremities and thorax. Thus, total BW is not severely increased in many cases. Hormone withdrawal or dose reduction usually allows serum glucose level normalization or better control in well-established diabetics (Lebovitz and McFarlane, 2001).

Clinicians' concerns about drug-induced hyperglycemia increased considerably in the last 5 years after numerous case reports of DM during APD administration. These agents are classified as typical or atypical based on the propensity of the former group to induce neurological side effects and hyperprolactinemia (Reynolds, 1997). The APDs used between 1950 and 1990, e.g., chlorpromazine; thioridazine; haloperidol; fluphenazine; and pimozide, may be classified as typicals (conventional). The new atypical APDs belong to the so-called second (clozapine; olanzapine; risperidone; quetiapine; ziprasidone; sertindole; zotepin; amisulpiride) and third (aripiprazole) generation of APDs. Most APDs are antagonists of monoamine and acetylcholine receptors, with the exception of ziprasidone and aripiprazole, which display agonist properties on some $5HT_{1A}$ and D_2 receptors, respectively. Risperidone, ziprasidone, and chlorpromazine also show inverse agonist properties on $5\text{-}HT_{2C}$ receptors (Kroeze et al., 2003).

The atypical agents (notably clozapine) are more effective than the typicals in drug-resistant schizophrenia and in alleviating the negative symptoms of this disorder (Meltzer et al., 1990). In addition, atypical APDs are currently used in treatment of a diversity of mental disorders, such as bipolar; obsessive compulsive; resistant depression; anorexia nervosa; dementia; and conduct disorders, among many others. This review will focus on APD-induced glucose dysregulation, in which appetite increment and BWG may play a prominent role. Evidence will be presented that APDs display several effects that may induce DM. This is a remarkable example of a pathological condition arising from the interaction between genetic factors and an exogenous trigger, where preventive and therapeutic measures are available.

4.2   Antipsychotic Drugs and Obesity

Clinically significant BWG is an important side effect of prolonged treatment with some APDs. It is mainly observed with agents that interact in the brain with multiple neurotransmitter receptors such as dopamine; norepinephrine; serotonin; histamine; and acetylcholine, which are critically involved in appetite regulation (Ravussin and Bouchard, 2000; Baptista et al., 2002b). The differential propensity of the diverse APDs to induce excessive BWG in the short-term (10 to 15 weeks) is well established, as follows (Allison et al., 1999a; Taylor and McAskill, 2000; Weterling, 2001):

> clozapine > olanzapine > thioridazine > quetiapine > chlorpromazine >
> sertindole > risperidone = zotepine > amisulpiride > haloperidol >
> fluphenazine > ziprasidone > molindone

The effects of quetiapine may have been underestimated (Baptista et al., 2002b). The recently introduced atypical APD aripiprazole displays minimal effects on BW regulation (Kane et al., 2002). Increase of clinically relevant obesity is also observed after prolonged APD treatment, even with agents with low propensity to induce BWG in the short term (Baptista et al., 2001a).

Reliable predictors of APD-induced BWG are low body mass index (BMI) before treatment and good clinical outcome. Women are more susceptible to BWG during typical, but not during atypical, APD administration (Baptista et al., 2002b). The average BWG for some atypical APDs after a 10-week treatment is as follows (Allison et al., 1999a):

- Clozapine (4.45 kg)
- Olanzapine (4.15 kg)
- Thioridazine (3.19 kg)
- Sertindole (2.92 kg)
- Risperidone (2.1 kg)
- Ziprazidone (0.04 kg)

Massive BWG during treatment with risperidone (18 kg); olanzapine (38 kg); or clozapine (40 kg) has been observed after prolonged drug administration (reviewed in Baptista et al., 2002b). The BWG tends to reach a plateau after 39 weeks of olanzapine administration. For clozapine and risperidone, BWG was still observed after 46 and 24 weeks of treatment, respectively (Baptista et al., 2002b; Henderson, 2002). Between 58 and 73% of patients displayed abdominal obesity after prolonged APD administration (Stedman and Welhan, 1993; Allison et al., 1999b; Elsmlie et al., 2000). Body mass gain after APD administration is mainly due to fat accumulation in humans (Eder et al., 2001) and rats (Baptista et al., 2002c).

Mounting evidence points to direct appetite stimulation as a prominent mechanism underlying atypical APD-induced BWG (Baptista et al., 2002b). Hyperprolactinemia may enhance appetite through glucose metabolism impairment and gonadal steroid suppression (Baptista,

1999a, b; Baptista et al., 2001a). However, it appears to be a secondary mechanism because strong hyperprolactinemia is observed with APDs that induce little BWG. Moreover, clozapine and olanzapine administration, which induces considerable BWG, is associated with discrete prolactin elevation (Baptista, 1999a; Baptista et al., 2001a). Typical APD administration has an impact on gonadal steroid production (transient low estradiol and permanent low progesterone levels in women and low testosterone levels in men) (Baptista et al., 1999a, b, 2001b); this promotes abdominal fat deposition. Importantly, hyperandrogenicity in women (an important factor in insulin resistance) (Haffner, 2000), was not detected during treatment with conventional APDs (Baptista et al., 2001b). The atypical APs are not expected to affect the gonadal steroids because they tend to induce little hyperprolactinemia. However, scarce data on this subject have been published so far and the relationship between hormones and BW regulation has not been established (Canuso et al., 2002).

The interaction of the APDs with brain monoamines and acetylcholine plays a prominent role in appetite stimulation (Baptista et al., 2002b; Kroeze et al., 2003; Wirshing et al., 2002). For example, the author's research group conducted a theoretical study in which the APD-induced BWG in the short term positively correlated with a composed ratio of the affinity (potency) of each specific APD for neurotransmitter receptors involved in feeding regulation (Figure 4.1). The numerator comprised the affinity for those neurotransmitter receptors whose blockade increases appetite ($\alpha_1 + H_1 + $ muscarinic $ + 5HT_{2A-2C}$), whereas the denominator comprised those whose blockade decreases food intake ($\alpha_2 + D_2 + 5HT_{1A}$) (Baptista et al., 2002b).

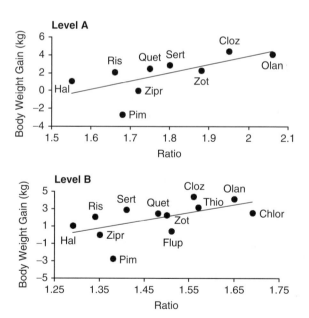

FIGURE 4.1

Correlation between weight gain (in kilograms) after 10 to 15 weeks of antipsychotic treatment (according to Allison et al., 1999a, and Taylor and McAskill, 2000) and a composed ratio of the log of the absolute drug affinities (potency) for receptors: $\alpha_1 + H_1 + $ muscarinic $ + 5HT_{2A-2C}/\alpha_2 + D_2 + 5HT_{1A}$; (according to Richelson, E. and Souder, T., *Life Sci.*, 68: 29–39, 2000, and E. Richelson, personal communication). (A) The affinities for all receptors were included — $r = 0.673$; $n = 9$; β coefficient $= 0.673$; $p = 0.047$. This analysis excludes chlorpromazine, thioridazine, and fluphenazine because the affinities for $5HT_{2C}$ receptors are not yet available. (B) The affinities for the $5HT_{2C}$ receptor were excluded — $r = 0.576$; $n = 12$; β coefficient $= 0.58$; $p = 0.05$. Chlor = chlorpromazine; Cloz = clozapine; Flup = fluphenazine; Hal = haloperidol; Olan = olanzapine; Pim = pimozide; Quet = quetiapine; Ris = risperidone; Sert = sertindole; Thio = thioridazine; Zipr = ziprasidone; Zot = zotepine. (From Baptista, T. et al., *Pharmacopsychiatry*, 35, 6–20, 2002. With permission.)

Although unsurprising mechanistically, the distribution of specific agents along the correlation line closely mirrors their propensity to induce glucose dysregulation, for example, high for clozapine and olanzapine; moderate or low for risperidone and quetiapine; and very low for haloperidol and ziprasidone (see next section). That result also reinforces the need for novel tools to quench the strong appetite stimulation often observed during APD treatment. In addition, it supports the search for clinically useful biological markers that might identify subjects at high risk of BWG. A notable example was recently provided by Reynolds et al. (2002), who showed that patients with the −759T variant allele of the 5-HT2C receptor gained little BW during APD administration, whereas those without that allele displayed significant BWG.

4.3 Antipsychotic Drugs and Diabetes Mellitus

Clinicians have traditionally been concerned with the apparently high frequency of DM observed in patients with some mental illnesses like schizophrenia and bipolar disorder (Cassidy et al., 1999; Dixon et al., 2000). In fact, indirect evidence of abnormal glucose metabolism (such as the requirement of extremely high insulin doses to induce hypoglycemic coma) had been observed in schizophrenics long before the introduction of APDs into clinical practice (reviewed in Baptista et al., 2002b; Henderson, 2002). Recent epidemiological studies have provided evidence to buttress this suspicion: between 9 and 14% of people with schizophrenia (mostly treated with typical APDs) have DM (Dixon et al., 2000). These values are significantly higher than the overall prevalence in the U.S. general population, which is around 2.6% (Harris et al., 1998).

In a recent study involving 243 inpatients, the following figures for DM in specific mental disorders were observed: schizoaffective (50%); bipolar I (26%); major depression (18%); and schizophrenia (13%) (Regenold et al., 2002). Importantly, first-degree relatives of schizophrenics also show a high prevalence of DM (Mukherjee et al., 1989). The nature of the genetic predisposition to DM in schizophrenia and affective disorders is currently under intense investigation. Notably, Stone et al. (2004) recently presented preliminary evidence showing linkage between regulatory enzymes in glycolysis and schizophrenia.

The APDs appear to add to genetic factors and life-style to promote type 2 DM in psychiatric patients. Several studies evaluated carbohydrate metabolism during treatment with the early, conventional APDs. For instance, Thonnard–Newman (1968) reported DM in 25% of a sample of 277 patients with schizophrenia receiving phenothiazines. Mukherjee et al. (1996) reported a global prevalence of DM of 15.8% in 95 subjects with schizophrenia. Keskiner (1973) also reported a differential propensity of typical APDs to be associated with glucose dysregulation. This author screened 249 subjects for DM with the 2-h glucose tolerance test and found blood glucose levels above 120 mg/dl in 11.5% of patients treated with thioridazine; 10.6% treated with chlorpromazine; 4.3% treated with fluphenazine; and 2.9% treated with haloperidol.

After the introduction of atypical agents in the early 1990s, clinicians' concerns with APD-induced DM increased considerably (Henderson, 2002; Wirshing et al., 2002). Koller et al. (2001) reviewed published cases and data from the Food and Drug Administration MedWatch surveillance program in the U.S. from 1990 to 2001 and identified 384 reports of DM among clozapine-treated patients. Numerous publications have summarized these and other case reports (Mir and Taylor, 2001; Liebzeit et al., 2001; McIntyre et al., 2001). Baptista (2002a) reviewed 56 published cases and found new-onset DM or disease exacerbation in 27 subjects on clozapine; 24 subjects on olanzapine; 2 on quetiapine; and 3 on risperidone. After 1999, new cases were reported almost at a monthly rate, with the notable absence of cases related to ziprasidone, sertindole, aripiprazole, or zotepine treatment. The great majority of cases belong to type 2 DM in adults (Mir and Taylor, 2001; Liebzeit et al., 2001; McIntyre et al., 2001), but there are reports of type 2 DM in adolescents (Saito and Kafantaris, 2002). Ketoacidosis was developed by 26 subjects (14 under olanzapine and 10 receiving clozapine), some of them after very short-term drug administration (Baptista, 2002a; Liebzeit et al., 2001; McIntyre et al., 2001; Mir and Taylor, 2001).

The differential propensity to induce glucose dysregulation *between* typical and atypical APDs and *within* the atypical group is currently under active investigation. Researchers have evaluated the frequency of already established DM (categorical studies) and carbohydrate metabolism (dimensional studies). Table 4.1 summarizes published categorical

TABLE 4.1

Frequency of Diabetes Mellitus during Typical and Atypical APDs Administration

Design	Findings	Ref.
Retrospective, case-control design; incidence rate for DM in 63 subjects under clozapine and 67 under typical APD administration	12% of clozapine-treated patients developed DM compared to 6% with DM during conventional depot APDs ($p = 0.06$)	Hagg et al., 1999
Naturalistic, retrospective; 82 clozapine-treated patients (55 with schizophrenia; 27 with schizoaffective disorder) followed for 5 years	30 Patients (36.6%) developed DM during the 5-year follow-up	Henderson et al., 2000
Medical and pharmacy claims; retrospective cohort design; incidence rate for DM in 552 clozapine-treated patients and 2461 patients receiving conventional APDs (haloperidol and/or chlorpromazine)	Similar overall incidence of DM in both groups; significant relative risk increase for subjects aged 20–34 years	Lund et al., 2001
Retrospective, claim data for psychotic patients; incidence rate for type 2 DM in 2.5 million individuals receiving risperidone, clozapine, olanzapine, high- or low-potency typical APDs compared to untreated patients after 12 months of exposure	Significantly high frequency in subjects treated with clozapine, olanzapine high- and low-potency typical APDs; similar frequency between risperidone and untreated subjects	Gianfrancesco et al., 2002
Retrospective, case-control study; odds ratio for APDs exposure (current: last 6 months; recent: 7–12 months) among 424 patients with DM and 1552 without DM	Significantly increased odds ratio of current exposure to conventional (1.7; 95% interval: 1.2–2.3) and atypical (4.7; 95% interval: 1.5–14.9) APDs among subjects with DM	Kornegay et al., 2002
Retrospective, nested case-control study; 19,637 subjects with schizophrenia treated with typical, atypical (olanzapine or risperidone) APDs or drug free; incident cases of DM matched with 2696 controls	Olanzapine, but not risperidone, increased risk of developing DM compared to patients receiving typical APDs or drug free	Koro et al., 2002
Retrospective, diagnosis of DM in outpatients with schizophrenia treated with atypical (n = 22,648) or typical (n = 15,984) APDs	In subjects aged <40 years, all atypical APDs increased frequency of DM; when age was controlled, clozapine, olanzapine, and quetiapine, but not risperidone, increased the prevalence	Sernyak et al., 2002
Retrospective, drug-claim, case-control study in a heterogeneous psychiatric population; comparison of APD treatment between 7227 new cases of DM and 6780 controls	Chlorpromazine, perphenazine, and prochlorperazine, but not clozapine, significantly increased risk of DM	Wang et al., 2002

studies with representative clinical samples. Numerous studies have also been presented as abstracts and await publication (reviewed in Henderson, 2002, and Baptista et al., 2002b). Contradictory results are evident, mostly with clozapine and, to a lesser extent, with typical APDs. One important issue is that categorical studies underestimate sub-threshold glucose dysregulation. This subject will only be clarified with prospective/randomized trials, including an exhaustive pretreatment evaluation.

Dimensional studies offer a more consistent picture. Baptista et al. (2001b) reported significantly higher basal glucose (p = 0.02) and 60-min insulin levels (p = 0.03) in 26 psychotic women treated with typical APDs compared to BMI-matched healthy controls. Kinon et al. (2001) found that at end point, nonfasting serum glucose levels were signifi-cantly higher in olanzapine-treated patients than in subjects treated with haloperidol (p = 0.001) or risperidone (p = 0.06). Henderson et al. (2002) used the Bergman's minimal model analysis to assess insulin sensitivity in 17 patients with schizophrenia treated with atypical APDs. Compared to risperidone, clozapine (p = 0.0017) and olanzapine (p = 0.0085) significantly decreased insulin sensitivity.

Newcomer et al. (2002) conducted a modified oral glucose tolerance test in schizo-phrenics receiving clozapine (n = 9); olanzapine (n = 12); risperidone (n = 10); typical APDs (n = 17); and untreated healthy controls (n = 31). At all time points (in the olanzapine group) and 75 min after load (clozapine group), glucose levels were significantly higher in the olanzapine group compared with the typical APD and control groups. The risperi-done group showed elevated fasting and postload glucose levels only in comparison to controls. No differences were observed between the risperidone and typical APD groups and between controls and the typical APD group. Hedenmalm et al. (2002) reviewed the WHO data base for reports of drug-induced glucose intolerance and found significant association for clozapine, olanzapine, and risperidone, but not for chlorpromazine and haloperidol.

Finally, Sowell et al. (2002) conducted a hyperglycemic clamp in healthy volunteers treated with olanzapine (n = 17); risperidone (n = 18); or placebo (n = 18) for 15 to 17 days. Both APDs significantly increased the insulin response to hyperglycemia, but only olan-zapine significantly decreased insulin sensitivity in the *within* group comparison. Both results were completely accounted for by the drug-induced BWG. This study shows that atypical APDs do not directly impair β-cell function and supports the role of appetite stimulation and BWG in APD-induced glucose dysregulation.

4.4   Mechanisms of Diabetes Mellitus Associated with Antipsychotics

Lebovitz (2002) summarized the following mechanisms by which a drug may promote DM:

1. Increase appetite and caloric intake
2. Change distribution of body fat
3. Decrease physical activity
4. Decrease oxidative metabolism in tissues
5. Interfere with action of insulin (synthesis, release, effects)
6. Increase counter-regulatory hormones
7. Increase free fatty acid release from adipose tissue

The first three mechanisms are well documented in humans and rats treated with APDs (Stedman and Welhan, 1993; Allison et al., 1999b; Eder et al., 2001; Theisen et al., 2001; Baptista et al., 2002b, c), but mechanisms 4 and 7 have not been explored in detail.

It was initially speculated that the APDs might decrease insulin synthesis and/or release, but this was not demonstrated in healthy people, as previously discussed (Sowell et al., 2002). An impairment of insulin sensitivity is expected, given the excessive BWG often observed during APD administration; this was preliminarily demonstrated by Sowell et al. (2002). Appetite stimulation (which may be intense enough to resemble a binge disorder) (Theisen et al., 2001) and hyperinsulinemia are expected to stimulate anti-insulin hormone levels, which further impair insulin sensitivity (Marmomier et al., 1999). These hormones have not been explored in detail during atypical APD administration (Newcomer et al., 2002). However, Baptista et al. (2001b) reported higher cortisol levels (in the afternoon and post dexamethasone suppression) in typical APD-treated women compared to BMI-matched healthy controls. It has been suggested that such an abnormal cortisol metabolism may be inherent to schizophrenia and some affective disorders (Tandom and Halbreich, 2003). Importantly, it could be a factor involved in the postulated drug-independent insulin resistance observed in this psychiatric population (Baptista et al., 2002b; Ryan et al., 2003).

The relationship between insulin response to hyperglycemia and insulin sensitivity describes a hyperbolic function (Kahn et al., 1993) (Figure 4.2). This important fact supports a heuristic proposal that may be tested at each level and has relevant applications for prevention and treatment (Baptista et al., 2002b). It is possible that many patients with schizophrenia and affective disorders have a clinically silent reduction in insulin sensitivity that is partially independent of drug treatment and BW (thus, they might be placed at level A of Figure 4.2). Administration of some typical APDs (haloperidol, pimozide, fluphenazine, trifluoperazine) could be neutral or induce an additional small deterioration of insulin sensitivity (Baptista et al., 2001b). However, atypical APDs (mainly clozapine and olanzapine) or typical APDs (notably chlorpromazine and thioridazine) increase anti-insulin hormones due to appetite stimulation, causing additional impairment of insulin sensitivity. The increased insulin demand may eventually lead to β-cell claudication.

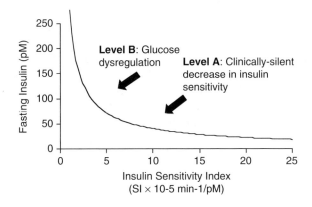

FIGURE 4.2
The relationship between insulin sensitivity ($S_I \times 10^{-5}$ min^{-1}/pM) and plasma fasting insulin level (pM) is hyperbolic. Thus, a moderate decrease in insulin sensitivity may be efficiently buffered without significant increase in insulin secretion (level A). Only after insulin sensitivity is severely impaired will overt changes take place in insulin (level B). Many psychiatric patients (untreated or receiving typical APDs) might be in level A. Treatment with some atypical APDs may pull them into the steep part of the curve, where glucose dysregulation will be noticeable (level B). (Adapted from Kahn, S.E. et al., *Diabetes*, 42: 1663–1672, 1993. With permission.)

Excessive BWG has additive deleterious effects on insulin sensitivity, but strong appetite stimulation, even without significant changes in BW, might be enough to pull some subjects into the steep part of the curve (Figure 4.2, level B), where overt glucose dysregulation may develop (Ramunkutty, 2002). Other mechanisms are under intense investigation, such as parent drug or metabolite effect on insulin dynamic (Hagg et al., 1999; Melkerson et al., 2000); on leptin and cytokines (Zimmermann et al., 2003); or on glucose transporters (Ardizzone et al., 2001). An unsolved issue that must be addressed is that antidepressants with potent appetite stimulating properties such as mirtzapine (Zimmermann et al., 2003) do not appear to be associated with DM. Besides differential pharmacological effects, a parsimonious explanation is that antidepressants are used in populations with lower risk for metabolic dysregulation.

Finally, there is no evidence that APDs have an independent effect on lipid metabolism. Therefore, while new data are presented, the numerous reports of atypical APD-related dyslipidemia (Meyer, 2001) may be prudently attributed to the insulin resistance syndrome (Baptista et al., 2002b). For example, in a large sample of olanzapine-treated patients, a positive correlation was observed between BWG and serum cholesterol (p = 0.001) (Kinon et al., 2001).

Animal research has provided limited information on the mechanisms of APD-induced glucose dysregulation. Significant hyperphagia has been induced after acute administration of risperidone, clozapine, or olanzapine in mice (Kaur and Kulkarni, 2002), and obesity has been induced in genetically intact rats by prolonged administration of sulpiride (a typical APD regarding its effects on serum prolactin), risperidone, and olanzapine (Baptista et al., 2002c; Goudie et al., 2002). However, the expected hyperinsulinemia accompanying obesity states was not observed during sulpiride or risperidone administration (Baptista et al., 2002c). In fact, sulpiride-treated rats consistently display lower serum glucose levels, with normal or lower insulin levels than vehicle-treated controls, suggesting increased insulin sensitivity (Baptista et al., 1999c; 2002c). Future studies should be conducted in genetically modified animals in which the human insulin resistance syndrome could be better modeled.

4.5 Treatment of Antipsychotic-Induced Metabolic Dysfunction

The atypical APDs represent a considerable advance in the treatment of mental disorders such as schizophrenia and bipolar disorders (Meltzer, 2001). It is unfortunate that mental illness treatment with very effective agents like clozapine and olanzapine has been associated with excessive BWG and glucose dysregulation; thus, a rigorous cost/benefit analysis will be necessary in many cases (Fontaine et al., 2001; Meltzer, 2001). For optimal drug selection, high-risk subjects should be ideally detected before atypical APD treatment. Baptista (2002a; 56 cases) and Jin et al. (2002; 45 cases) found the following risk factors in atypical APD-treated subjects with DM:

- Personal and family history of DM (18.5 and 24.1%, respectively)
- Overweight or obese before treatment (57.4%)
- BWG during APD treatment (38.9%)
- Male gender (87%)

Unfortunately, information about these factors was often not reported. For example, BW change was not described in 42.6% of cases. Koller et al. (2001) found an overrepresentation of African descendents among clozapine-treated subjects with DM. Diabetic ketoacidosis was presented in 42% of cases. After starting treatment, DM was detected within 3 or 6 months in 59 and 84% of cases respectively (Jin et al., 2002).

Once hyperglycemia or overt type 2 DM is detected, switching to another agent with low propensity to induce glucose dysregulation or combining agents is recommended (Reinstein et al., 1999). Intensive nutritional advice may effectively prevent olanzapine-induced glucose dysregulation in patients with schizophrenia (Rabin et al., manuscript in preparation). A realistic schedule of physical activity is also advisable. Several drugs have been tested in small studies to prevent or attenuate BWG, including amantadine; nizatidine; topiramate; reboxetine; metformin; and orlistat (Baptista et al., 2002b; Morrison et al., 2002; Puyurovsky et al., 2003; Werneke et al., 2002).

An understandable concern exists that anorectic agents acting through brain monoamines may worsen psychotic symptoms in some patients; thus, other avenues to quench appetite should be explored (Fernández–López et al., 2002). For example, high β-endorphin serum levels were detected in women receiving conventional APDs (Baptista et al., 2001b). Given the role of brain opiates in appetite regulation, the use of opiate antagonists such as naltrexone or naloxone might prove useful in selected patients. A promising strategy is the prophylactic use of insulin sensitizers such as metformin that may prevent excessive BWG and attenuate the development of insulin resistance without acting directly in the brain (Morrison et al., 2002).

As expected, psychiatric patients with DM have been successfully treated with oral antidiabetics (mainly metformin) and insulin. However, in current clinical practice, these patients often receive psychotropic drugs others than APDs, such as mood stabilizers; antidepressants; anxiolytics; and antiparkinsonians. Thus, treatment of DM and other aspects of the insulin resistance syndrome in this population is particularly difficult, given the risk of adverse drug interactions and poor treatment compliance (reviewed in Baptista et al., 2004).

4.6 Conclusions and Research Perspectives

Atypical APD administration (mainly of clozapine and olanzapine) is frequently associated with excessive BWG and glucose dysregulation in current clinical practice. Numerous cases of DM (mainly type 2) in APD-treated patients have been reported since 1994. Increased appetite (with or without significant BWG) may be a determinant factor causing DM, but other mechanisms are under active investigation. People with schizophrenia and some affective disorders are particularly prone to DM and may be more susceptible to the effects of APDs. Preliminary evidence demonstrates a linkage between schizophrenia and some regulatory enzymes involved in glycolysis, and between polymorphism at the 5-HT2C receptor gene allele and APD-induced BWG. Other aspects of carbohydrate metabolism such as insulin dynamics; insulin receptor and post-receptor functioning; and glucose transporters in psychiatric patients are central issues in current research. Novel agents that counteract APD-induced hyperphagia directly or through other mechanisms of BW regulation must also prove to be safe in patients with severe mental disorders. Prevention and treatment of DM and other aspects of the insulin resistance syndrome in these poly-medicated patients is a formidable challenge because of the risk of adverse drug interactions and poor treatment compliance. A close collaboration among psychiatrists, endocrinologists, and nutritionists is thus necessary to assist this particularly unstable clinical population.

Acknowledgments

The author thanks his colleagues Luis Hernández, Ximena Páez, N.M.K. Ng Ying Kin, and Serge Beaulieu who reviewed the manuscript and have been involved in collaborative research.

References

Allison, D.B. et al. (1999a) Antipsychotic-induced weight gain: a comprehensive research synthesis, *Am. J. Psychiatry*, 156: 1686–1696.

Allison, D.B. et al. (1999b) The distribution of body mass index among individuals with and without schizophrenia, *J. Clin. Psychiatry*, 60: 215–220.

Ardizzone, T.D. et al. (2001) Inhibition of glucose transport in PC12 cells by the atypical antipsychotic drugs risperidone and clozapine, and structural analogs of clozapine, *Brain Res.*, 923: 82–90.

Baptista, T. (1999a) Body weight gain induced by antipsychotic drugs: mechanisms and management, *Acta Psychiatrica Scand.*, 100: 3–16.

Baptista, T., Reyes, D. and Hernández, L. (1999b) Antipsychotic drugs and reproductive hormones: relationship to body weight regulation, *Pharmacol. Biochem. Behav.*, 62: 409–417.

Baptista, T. et al. (1999c) Glucose tolerance and serum insulin levels in an animal model of obesity induced by subacute or chronic administration of antipsychotic drugs, *Prog. Neuropsychopharmacol. Biol. Psychiatry*, 23: 277–287.

Baptista, T. et al. (2001a) Antipsychotic drugs and obesity: is prolactin involved? *Can. J. Psychiatry*, 46: 829–834.

Baptista, T. et al. (2001b) Endocrine and metabolic profile in the obesity associated to typical antipsychotic drug-administration, *Pharmacopsychiatry*, 34: 223–231.

Baptista, T. (2002a) Atypical antipsychotic drugs and glucose dysregulation, *Can. J. Psychiatry*, 47: 94–96.

Baptista, T. et al., (2002b) Obesity and related metabolic abnormalities during antipsychotic drug administration: mechanisms, management and research perspectives, *Pharmacopsychiatry*, 35, 6–20.

Baptista, T. et al. (2002c) Comparative effects of the antipsychotics sulpiride or risperidone in rats: I: bodyweight, food intake, body composition, hormones and glucose tolerance, *Brain Res.*, 957: 144–151.

Baptista, T., Ng Yin Kin, N.M.K. and Beaulieu, S. (2004) Treatment of the metabolic disturbances caused by antipsychotic drugs: focus on potential drug interactions, *Clin. Pharmacokinetics*, 43: 1–15.

Canuso, C.M. et al. (2002) Antipsychotic medication, prolactin elevation and ovarian function in women with schizophrenia and schizoaffective disorder, *Psychiatry Res.*, 111: 11–20.

Cassidy, F., Ahearn, E. and Carroll, B.J. (1999) Elevated frequency of diabetes mellitus in hospitalized manic-depressive patients, *Am. J. Psychiatry*, 156: 1417–1420.

Chan, N.M. et al. (2002) Drug-related hyperglycemia, *JAMA*, 287: 714.

Dixon, L. et al. (2000) Prevalence and correlates of diabetes in national schizophrenia samples, *Schizophr. Bull.*, 26: 903–912.

Eder, U. et al. (2001) Association of olanzapine-induced weight gain with an increase in body fat, *Am. J. Psychiatry*, 158: 1719–1722.

Elsmlie, J.L. et al. (2000) Prevalence of overweight and obesity in bipolar patients, *J. Clin. Psychiatry,* 61: 179–184.

Fernández–López, J.A. et al. (2002) Pharmacological approaches for the treatment of obesity, *Drugs,* 62: 915–944.

Flegal, K.M. et al. (2002) Prevalence and trends in obesity among U.S. adults, *JAMA,* 288: 1772–1773.

Fontaine, K.R. et al. (2001) Estimating the consequences of antipsychotic induced weight gain on health and mortality, *Psychiatry Res.,* 101: 277–280.

Gianfrancesco, F.D. et al. (2002) Differential effects of risperidone, olanzapine, clozapine, and conventional antipsychotics on type 2 diabetes: findings from a large health plan data base, *J. Clin. Psychiatry,* 63: 920–930.

Goudie, A.J., Smith, J.A. and Halford, J.C.G. (2002) Characterization of olanzapine-induced weight gain in rats, *J. Psychopharmacol.,* 16: 291–296.

Haffner, S.M. (2000) Sex hormones, obesity, fat distribution, type 2 diabetes and insulin resistance: epidemiological and clinical correlation, *Int. J. Obesity Relat. Metabolic Disorders,* 24 Suppl 2: S56–58.

Hagg, S. et al. (1999) Prevalence of diabetes and impaired glucose tolerance in patients treated with clozapine compared with patients treated with conventional depot neuroleptic medications, *J. Clin. Psychiatry,* 59: 294–299.

Harris, M.I. et al. (1998) Prevalence of diabetes, impaired fasting glucose, and impaired glucose tolerance in U.S. adults. The Third National Health and Nutrition Examination Survey, 1988–1994, *Diabetes Care,* 21: 518–524.

Hedenmalm, K. et al. (2002) Glucose intolerance with atypical antipsychotics, *Drug Saf.,* 25: 1107–1116.

Henderson, D.C. (2002) Atypical antipsychotic-induced diabetes mellitus: how strong is the evidence? *CNS Drugs,* 16: 77–89.

Jin, J., Meyer, J.M. and Jeste, D.V. (2002) Phenomenology of and risk factors for new-onset diabetes mellitus and diabetic ketoacidosis associated with atypical antipsychotics: an analysis of 45 published cases, *Ann. Clin. Psychiatry,* 14: 59–64.

Kahn, S.E. et al. (1993) Quantification of the relationship between insulin sensitivity and β-cell function in human subjects, *Diabetes,* 42:1663–1672.

Kane, J.M. et al. (2002) Efficay and safety of aripiprazole and haloperidol versus placebo in patients with schizophrenia and schizoaffective disorders, *J. Clin. Psychiatry,* 63: 763–771.

Kaur, G. and Kulkarni, S.K. (2002) Studies on modulation of feeding behavior by atypical antipsychotics in female mice, *Prog. Neuropsychopharmacol. Biol. Psychiatry,* 26: 277–285.

Keskiner, A., el-Toumi, A. and Bousquet, T. (1973) Psychotropic drugs and chronic mental patients, *Psychosomatics,* 14: 176–181.

Kinon, B.J. et al. (2001) Long-term olanzapine treatment: weight change and weight-related health factors in schizophrenia, *J. Clin. Psychiatry,* 62: 92–100.

Kissebah, A.H. and Krakower, G.R. (1994) Regional adiposity and morbidity, *Physiol. Rev.,* 74: 761–811.

Koller, E. et al. (2001) Clozapine-associated diabetes, *Am. J. Med.,* 111: 716–723.

Kornegay, C.J., Vasilakis–Scaramozza, C. and Jick, H. (2002) Incident diabetes associated with antipsychotic use in the United Kingdom general practice research database, *J. Clin. Psychiatry,* 63: 758–762.

Koro, C.E. et al. (2002) Assessment of independent effect of olanzapine and risperidone on risk of diabetes among patients with schizophrenia: population based nested case-control study, *Br. Med. J.,* 325: 243–249.

Kroeze, W.K. et al. (2003) H_1-histamine receptor affinity predicts short-term weight gain for typical and atypical antipsychotic drugs, *Neuropsychopharnacology,* 28: 519–526.

Lebovitz, H.E. (2002) Diagnosis, classification, and pathogenesis of diabetes mellitus, *J. Clin. Psychiatry,* 62 Suppl 27: 5–9.

Lebovitz, H.E. and McFarlane, S.I. (2001) Hyperglycemia secondary to nondiabetic conditions and therapies, in L.J. DeGroot and J.L. Jameson (Eds.) *Endocrinology,* Philadelphia: W.B. Saunders Company, pp. 959–967.

Liebzeit, K.A., Markowitz, J.S. and Caley, C.F. (2001) New onset diabetes and atypical antipsychotics, *Eur. Neuropsychopharmacol.,* 11: 25–32.

Long, C.N., Katzin, B. and Fry, E.G. (1940) The adrenal cortex and carbohydrate metabolism, *Endocrinology,* 26: 309–344.

Luna, B. and Feinglos, M.N. (2001) Drug-induced hyperglycemia, *JAMA,* 286: 1945–1948.

Lund, B.C. et al. (2001) Clozapine use in patients with schizophrenia and the risk of diabetes, hyperlipidemia, and hypertension: a claims-based approach, *Arch. Gen. Psychiatry,* 58: 1172–1176.

Marmomier, C., Chapelot, D. and Louis–Sylvestre, J. (1999) Metabolic and behavioral consequences of a snack consumed in a satiety state, *Am. J. Clin. Nutr.,* 70: 854–866.

McIntyre, R.S., McCann, S.M. and Kennedy, S.H. (2001) Antipsychotic metabolic effects: weight gain, diabetes mellitus, and lipid abnormalities, *Can. J. Psychiatry,* 46: 273–281.

Melkerson, K.I., Hulting, A.L. and Brismar, K.E. (2000) Elevated levels of insulin, leptin, and blood lipids in olanzapine-treated patients with schizophrenia or related psychoses, *J. Clin. Psychiatry,* 61: 742–749.

Meltzer, H.Y. et al. (1990) Effects of six months of clozapine treatment on the quality of life of chronic schizophrenic patients, *Hosp. Community Psychiatry,* 41: 892–897.

Meltzer, H.Y. (2001) Putting metabolic side effects into perspective: risks versus benefits of atypical antipsychotics, *J. Clin. Psychiatry,* 62 Suppl 27: 35–39.

Meyer, J.M. (2001) Novel antipsychotics and severe hyperlipidemia. *J. Clin. Psychopharmacol.,* 21: 369–374.

Mir, S. and Taylor, D. (2001) Atypical antipsychotics and hyperglycaemia, *Int. Clin. Psychopharmacol.,* 16: 63–73.

Molazowski, S. (2002) Drug-related hyperglycemia, *JAMA,* 287: 714.

Morrison, J.A., Cottingham, E.M. and Barton, B.A. (2002) Metformin for weight loss in pediatric patients taking psychotropic drugs, *Am. J. Psychiatry,* 159: 655–657.

Mukherjee, S., Schnur, D.B. and Reddy, R. (1989) Family history of type 2 diabetes in schizophrenic patients, *Lancet,* 1: 495.

Mukherjee, S. et al. (1996) Diabetes mellitus in schizophrenic patients, *Compr. Psychiatry,* 37: 68–73.

Must, A. et al. (1999) The disease burden associated with overweight and obesity, *JAMA,* 282: 1523–1529.

Newcomer, J.W. et al. (2002) Abnormalities in glucose regulation during antipsychotic treatment of schizophrenia, *Arch. Gen. Psychiatry,* 59: 337–345.

Nyirenda, M. et al. (1998) Glucocorticoid exposure in late gestation permanently programs rat hepatic phosphoenolpyruvate carboxykinase and glucocorticoid receptor expression and causes glucose intolerance in adult offspring, *J. Clin. Invest.,* 101: 2174–2181.

Pandit, M.K. et al. (1993) Drug-induced disorders of glucose tolerance, *Ann. Intern. Med.,* 118: 529–539.

Poyurovsky, M. et al. (2003) Attenuation of olanzapine-induced weight gain with reboxetine in patients with schizophrenia: a double-blind, placebo-controlled study, *Am. J. Psychiatry,* 160(2): 297–302.

Ramankutty, G. (2002) Olanzapine-induced destabilization of diabetes in the absence of weight gain, *Acta Psychiatrica Scand.,* 105: 235–236.

Ravussin, E. and Bouchard, C. (2000) Human genomics and obesity: finding appropriate drug targets, *Eur. J. Pharmacol.,* 410: 131–145.

Regenold, W.T. et al. (2002) Increased prevalence of type 2 diabetes mellitus among psychiatric patients with bipolar 1 affective and schizoaffective disorders independent of psychotropic drug use, *J. Affective Disorders,* 70: 19–26.

Reinstein, M.F., Sirotovskaya, L.A. and Jones, L.E. (1999) Effect of clozapine-quetiapine combination therapy on weight and glycaemic control, *Clin. Drug Invest.,* 18: 99–104.

Reynolds, G.P. (1997) What is an atypical antipsychotic?, *J. Psychopharmacol.,* 11: 195–199.

Reynolds, G.P., Zhang, Z.J. and Zhang, X.B. (2002) Association of antipsychotic drug-induced weight gain with a 5-HT2C receptor gene polymorphism, *Lancet,* 359: 2086–2087.

Richelson. E. and Souder, T. (2000) Binding of antipsychotic drugs to human brain receptors: focus on newer generation compounds, *Life Sci.,* 68: 29–39.

Ryan, M.C. et al. (2003) Impaired fasting glucose tolerance in first-episode, drug-naive patients with schizophrenia, *Am. J. Psychiatry,* 160(2): 284–289.

Saito, E. and Kafantaris, V. (2002) Can diabetes mellitus be induced by medication?, *J. Child Adolescent Psychopharmacol.*, 12: 231–236.

Sowell, M.O. et al. (2002) Hyperglycemic clamp assessment of insulin secretory responses in normal subjects treated with olanzapine, risperidone or placebo, *J. Clin. Endocrinol. Metab.*, 87: 2918–2923.

Stedman, T. and Welhan, J. (1993) The distribution of adipose tissue in female in-patients receiving psychotropic drugs, *Br. J. Psychiatry*, 162: 249–250.

Stone, W.S. et al. (2004) Evidence for linkage between regulatory enzymes in glycolysis and schizophrenia in a multiplex sample, *Neuropsychiatric Genet.*, (in press).

Tandom, R. and Halbreich, U. (2003) The second generation "atypical" antipsychotics: similar improved efficacy but different neuroendocrine effects, *Psychoneuroendocrinology*, supp 1: 1–7.

Taylor, D.M. and McAskill, R. (2000) Atypical antipsychotics and weight gain — a systematic review, *Acta Psychiatrica Scand.*, 101: 416–432.

Theisen, F.M. et al. (2001) Prevalence of obesity in adolescent and young adult patients with and without schizophrenia and in relationship to antipsychotic medication, *J. Psychiatric Res.*, 35: 339–345.

Sernyak, M.J. et al. (2002) Association of diabetes mellitus with use of atypical neuroleptics in the treatment of schizophrenia, *Am. J. Psychiatry*, 159: 561–566.

Thonnard–Neumann, E. (1968) Phenothiazines and diabetes in hospitalized women, *Am. J. Psychiatry*, 124: 978–982.

Wang, P.S. et al. (2002) Clozapine use and risk of diabetes mellitus, *J. Clin. Psychopharmacol.*, 22: 236–243.

Werneke, U., Taylor, D. and Sanders, T.A. (2002) Options for pharmacological management of obesity in patients treated with atypical antipsychotics, *Int. Clin. Psychopharmacol.*, 17: 145–160.

Wetterling, T. (2001) Bodyweight gain with atypical antipsychotics: a comparative review, *Drug Saf.*, 24: 59–73.

Wirshing, D.A. et al. (2002) The effects of novel antipsychotics on glucose and lipid levels, *J. Clin. Psychiatry*, 63: 856–865.

Zimmermann, U. et al. (2003) Implications and mechanisms underlying dug-induced weight gain in psychiatric patients, *J. Psychiatric Res.*, 37: 193–220.

Part II

General Therapeutic Aspects

5

Obesity and Associated Complications

Michael Hamilton and Frank Greenway

CONTENTS

5.1   Introduction

The broad goal of the clinician is to promote wellness, quality of life, and longevity. An increasingly common and difficult clinical challenge is that of weight gain leading to overweight and obesity, often complicated by a diversity of health problems, diminished quality of life, and premature death. Some whose weight is only moderately elevated are severely affected by weight-related health problems, while others who are significantly overweight are spared. Therefore, susceptibility to the complications of weight gain varies, based on differences in heredity, age, ethnicity, body fat distribution, gender, and life-style. Nevertheless, for any individual, being obese is a greater health risk compared to being normal weight.

Because of the increasing prevalence of obesity, clinicians will necessarily devote more time and thought to the treatment of patients with obesity and its complications. Also, as the prevalence of childhood and adolescent overweight increases, many of tomorrow's patients will be young adults with chronic diseases once considered to be diseases of aging. Therefore, clinicians will increasingly encounter the many and varied health consequences of overweight and obesity, from impairments in quality of life to the morbidities and mortality associated with weight gain.

Although life-style change will continue to be the mainstay of obesity treatment, the development of novel weight loss agents affecting one or more of the several pathways that influence food intake and energy expenditure will require that clinicians keep pace with a rapidly expanding body of information concerning the biology of weight regulation. They will need to be conversant with the effect of weight on mortality and morbidity, and the potential benefits of obesity treatment. Though little is known regarding the health benefits of long-term weight loss, the goal of this chapter is to describe the variety of clinical parameters that can be assessed in determining the benefits of emerging therapies.

TABLE 5.1

Classification of Adults according to BMI

Classification	BMI (kg/m²)	Risk of Co-Morbidities
Underweight	<18.5	Low (but risk of other problems increased)
Normal range	18.5–24.9	Average
Overweight	>25	
Preobese (overwt.)	25–29.9	Increased
Obese class I	30–34.9	Moderate
Obese class II	35–39.9	Severe
Obese class III	>40	Very severe

Source: Data from World Health Organization. Obesity: preventing and managing the global epidemic. Report of a WHO consultation on obesity. Geneva, 1998.

5.2 Effect of Overweight and Obesity on Mortality

The consensus that a positive relationship exists between obesity and mortality is based on studies involving large numbers of people followed over significant periods of time. Such studies were first initiated by the life insurance industry.[1] Other long-term studies involving large numbers of people have subsequently supported the findings of the life insurance studies.[2–4]

The severity and the duration of obesity influence mortality. According to the guidelines published by the World Health Organization, a body mass index (BMI) between 18.5 and 24.9 kg/m² is considered normal, i.e., associated with the least risk with respect to mortality (Table 5.1).[5] A modest increase in risk occurs as the BMI rises above 25 kg/m²; at a BMI of 30 kg/m², the increase in mortality risk begins to rise sharply (Table 5.2). In a study of morbidly obese men, mortality was as much as 12 times greater in persons 25 to 34 years of age and 6 times greater in those 35 to 44 years of age compared to persons in the BMI range of 18.5 to 24.9 kg/m².[6] It should be noted that a BMI of 30 kg/m² is associated with a 50% increase in relative mortality, equivalent to the increased mortality risk resulting from a blood pressure of 140/90 or a total cholesterol greater than 240 mg/dl.[7]

The long-term impact of excess weight, i.e., duration, is illustrated by a 55-year follow-up study of adolescents in which overweight in adolescence was a better predictor of coronary heart disease and other obesity co-morbidities than the onset of obesity in adulthood. The relative risk of death from coronary heart disease was 2.3 in men who had been overweight as adolescents compared to their normal-weight adolescent peers.[8] In addition to the severity and duration of obesity, the relationship between obesity and mortality is affected by a number of factors that include age; ethnicity; body composition; body fat distribution; stature; and fitness.

5.2.1 Age

In older persons, the optimal BMI with respect to mortality may be higher compared to those who are younger. For example, several studies suggest that the BMI associated with the lowest mortality in persons 55 to 74 years of age may be slightly above a BMI of 25 kg/m².[9–13] In terms of absolute mortality risk, older obese persons have higher rates of mortality for a given level of obesity than younger obese persons. However, between a BMI of 23.5 and 30 kg/m², the rise in relative risk of death that occurs with increasing

TABLE 5.2

Rates and Relative Risks of Death from all Causes among Subjects according to BMI by Age and Gender[a]

Group	Body Mass Index (kg/m²)						
	23.5–24.9[b]	25.0–26.4	26.5–27.9	28.0–29.9	30.0–31.9	32.0–34.9	>35
Men (30–64 yrs.)							
Rate/100,000 person yrs.[c]	250	301	296	367	432	557	659
Multivariate relative rate[d]	1.00	1.19	1.15	1.41	1.62	2.05	2.30
Men (65–74 yrs.)							
Rate/100,000 person yrs.[c]	898	941	1038	1270	1370	1798	2767
Multivariate relative rate[d]	1.00	1.04	1.12	1.34	1.42	1.85	2.75
Women (30–64 yrs.)							
Rate/100,000 person yrs.[c]	163	217	221	224	257	268	335
Multivariate relative rate[d]	1.00	1.31	1.33	1.33	1.51	1.53	1.86
Women (65–74 yrs.)							
Rate/100,000 person yrs.[c]	595	598	636	796	836	1111	1299
Multivariate relative rate[d]	1.00	0.99	1.04	1.28	1.32	1.71	1.99

[a] Subjects without history of cancer, heart disease, stroke, respiratory disease, current illness, or weight loss of at least 10 lb. in the previous year.
[b] Reference category = BMI 23.5 to 24.9 kg/m².
[c] Standardized for age within age and gender group.
[d] Adjusted for age, level of education, physical activity, alcohol use, marital status, aspirin use, fat and vegetable consumption, and use of estrogen replacement in women.

Source: Adapted from Calle, E.E. et al., *N. Engl. J. Med.*, 1999, 341: 1097–1105.

BMI is less in older persons compared to those who are younger. After a BMI of 32 kg/m², the relative risk of death in persons over 65 years approaches or exceeds that of younger persons (Table 5.2).[14,15]

5.2.2 Race and Ethnicity

Many industrialized nations have assimilated large numbers of immigrants from developing countries. In the U.S., the annual number of immigrants is approximately 800,000, predominantly from Asian, Latin American, Caribbean, and African countries.[16] These immigrants, in addition to second-generation immigrants and their descendents, reflect the diversity of cultures and ethnicities that must be considered in assessing the effect of weight on health.

To the nonepidemiologist, studies of the effect of race/ethnicity on the relationship between BMI and mortality have been conflicting if not confusing.[17] The Cancer Prevention Study II, a study with a large cohort including Caucasian and African Americans followed for up to 14 years, showed that obesity had less impact on mortality in African Americans, particularly women, compared to Caucasians.[14] In other words, the relative increase in mortality risk with increasing BMI was less in African Americans compared to Caucasians. However, analogous to the effect of aging on the mortality risk associated with obesity, absolute mortality risk in African Americans is higher than in Caucasians for an equivalent BMI. In another example of the influence of ethnicity on weight and health, BMI cut-off points for obesity in Asian populations may need to be lower than in Caucasians; studies indicate that Asian populations have a higher percent body fat for a given BMI,[18,19] suggesting that Asian populations may experience the negative health effects of adiposity at a lower BMI than Caucasians.[20]

5.2.3   Body Composition

Population studies generally show a curvilinear, J-shaped relationship between weight and mortality, i.e., slightly increased mortality at the lower end of the weight continuum and significantly greater mortality at higher weights. The common explanation for this observation has been that such studies included smokers as well as persons with chronic diseases, both of whom tend to have lower BMIs but higher and earlier mortality.[21] One technique for dealing with this confounding factor has been to exclude those who die within the first 5 years of the study. However, in the large population study of Calle et al.,[14] the J-shaped curve persisted even when smokers and those with a history of disease were excluded from the analysis. In a meta-analysis of additional studies reporting on the relationship of BMI and mortality, Allison and Saunders found that the elimination of early deaths had very little effect.[22] Because BMI is really a surrogate measure of body fat, Allison has suggested that greater accuracy in the measurement of body fat will lead to a truer understanding of the relationship between adiposity and mortality.[23] Advancing technologies that allow greater accuracy and ease in the measurement of body composition in large population samples will lead to a clearer picture of the relationship between body fat and mortality risk.

5.2.4   Body Fat Distribution and Stature

Body fat distribution has been shown to influence mortality, with central obesity playing a greater role than body mass index on mortality risk.[24,25] On the other hand, lower body obesity may offer relative protection against cardiovascular risk factors.[26] In a population-based study of 38- to 64-year-old women,[27] hip circumference was inversely related to the 24-year incidence of myocardial infarction, combined cardiovascular diseases, and diabetes even after adjusting for age, smoking, and BMI and waist circumference. The effect of height also needs to be considered; for example, decreasing height with age leads to higher calculated BMI values in older persons leading to an "artifactual" increase in BMI[28] and possible systematic bias in the relationship between BMI and mortality. In addition, height may affect health risk: some studies have shown that short stature increases the risk of coronary heart disease,[29,30] while tall stature increases cancer risk.[31]

5.2.5   Fitness

Physical fitness also appears to influence the impact of weight on mortality. Blair and colleagues have found that, in obese men and women, a high level of fitness as determined by a maximal exercise stress test is associated with a reduction in mortality to levels comparable to normal-weight subjects, albeit with low levels of fitness.[32-34] A study by Stevens et al.,[35] however, found that fitness did not completely "neutralize" the mortality risk of obesity.

5.2.6   Intrauterine Environment

Birth weight, a reflection of intrauterine environment, may also influence adult weight. A study based on 1850 interviews with women, ages 50 to 79, reported that women with lower or higher birth weights were more likely to have a BMI > 30 kg/m² compared to women with mid-range birth weights.[36] Despite the many factors that influence the relationship between body weight and mortality, the fact remains that the WHO BMI guidelines (Table 5.1) offer a practical tool to evaluate the mortality risk of excess weight. Even within distinctly differing populations, a BMI of 30 kg/m² carries a greater risk than a BMI of 25 kg/m², and BMI levels above 30 kg/m² are predictive of a higher risk for disease and mortality, no matter the age, gender, ethnicity, or physical abilities of the individual.

5.2.7 Causes of Death in Overweight and Obese Persons

The causes of mortality in overweight and obese persons are heavily weighted towards cardiovascular diseases and cerebrovascular accidents. Predisposing factors to these final events include 1) hypertension; 2) the components of the metabolic syndrome, i.e., diabetes, dyslipidemia, and the production of proinflammatory and prothrombotic cytokines by adipose tissues; and 3) the mechanical effects of excessive adiposity on the respiratory and circulatory systems. Because of incomplete and often inaccurate information listed on death certificates, it is difficult to know the precise cause of death in most overweight/obese persons. However, based on morbidity data, it is not unreasonable to conclude that certain morbidities associated with overweight and obesity are major contributors to cardiovascular risk and death, i.e., diabetes, hypertension, and dyslipidemia. For example, Wolf[37] estimated that in the U.S., 61% of type 2 diabetes; 17% of hypertension; and 17% of coronary heart disease could be attributed to obesity. Although, the adverse health effects of obesity are largely manifested through its co-morbidities, the effect of obesity alone on cardiovascular risk is illustrated by a study of 310 women in whom carotid artery wall thickness was related to BMI and waist-to-hip ratio independently of blood pressure, lipid abnormalities, and fasting insulin.[38]

Obesity predisposes to venous stasis/thrombosis in the lower extremities and therefore may be a significant factor in obesity-related deaths due to pulmonary emboli, many of which may be erroneously attributed to coronary artery disease and stroke. It is interesting that, in a small series of patients who died following gastric bypass surgery, autopsies showed that 80% had pulmonary emboli although only 20% were clinically suspected of having pulmonary emboli before death.[39] Another autopsy study compared the BMI of patients who died of acute pulmonary embolism with a control group who died suddenly without evidence of pulmonary embolism; patients who died of pulmonary embolism had an average BMI of 34.1 kg/m² compared with a BMI of 25.9 kg/m² in the control group.[40] Sleep apnea leading to hypoxia, pulmonary hypertension, heart failure, and fatal cardiac arrhythmias[41–44] may be related to sudden death in those whose sleep apnea was undetected and therefore untreated.

Surprisingly, autopsy studies of severely obese persons have shown relatively little coronary arteriosclerotic disease, although cardiac hypertrophy and cardiomyopathy have been noted.[45,46] In Kortelainen's study, subcutaneous fat thickness in women was negatively associated with the severity of atherosclerosis. In men, a higher BMI was associated with greater dilatation of myocardial arterioles. One explanation given for such findings is that severely obese persons, because of an enhanced ability to store fat within adipose cells, are able to limit the deposition of fat in "ectopic" tissues such as muscle and liver. The deposition of fat in these ectopic tissues is associated with insulin resistance and therefore an increased risk for the metabolic syndrome and its vascular complications.[47]

Obesity is also associated with a greater risk for certain cancers.[1] However, obesity is probably underreported as a contributor to cancer-related deaths because, in all likelihood, these deaths are attributed to the primary neoplasm with frequent omission of obesity as a contributing factor.

5.2.8 Effect of Weight Loss on Mortality

Intuitively, weight loss should lead to greater longevity because of the significant health risks associated with weight gain. However, the beneficial impact of weight loss on mortality has been difficult to demonstrate. Epidemiological/observational studies of weight loss and mortality must deal with a difficult methodologic problem: how to determine the cause of weight loss correctly in those who have lost weight i.e., whether by intention or alternatively, unintentionally, due to overt or subclinical disease that increases the potential for early death. Therefore, studies that include subjects who have lost weight unintentionally will bias the results toward the conclusion that weight loss increases mortality.

Thus, studies that have combined subjects who intentionally as well as unintentionally lost weight have generally increased mortality with weight loss. A meta-analysis of 11 population studies by Andres et al.[48] in 1993 indicated that the highest mortality rates occurred in those who lost weight or in those who gained significant weight. The lowest mortality rates were seen in those who gained a modest amount of weight. Several other studies have also found weight loss to be associated with increased mortality.[49–51] Williamson and colleagues examined the effect of intentional vs. unintentional weight loss and found that intentional weight loss was associated with decreased mortality, particularly from diabetes.[52–54] On the other hand, unintentional weight loss was associated with increased mortality.[55]

As mentioned, body weight and BMI are surrogate measures of body fat and may obscure the relationship between fat loss and mortality. In a 13- to 15-year mortality follow-up of 10,169 subjects participating in the first and second National Health and Nutrition Examination Survey (NHANES), Allison showed a monotonic decrease in mortality with decreasing amounts of fat tissue and an increase in mortality with decreasing amounts of lean tissue.[56] Although fatness and leanness were determined by relatively crude methods (skin fold thickness and arm circumferences), the number of subjects and the length of follow-up give this study special significance. Body composition measurement by DEXA scanning in the current and future cycles of the NHANES should introduce greater accuracy in answering this important question: does fat loss prolong life and loss of lean tissue shorten it?

5.3 Morbidity

5.3.1 Mechanisms by which Obesity Affects Health

Overweight and obesity impact health in several ways: 1) by the physical effects of excess weight, 2) through the development of insulin resistance and hyperinsulinemia associated with central obesity, the secretory products of adipose cells, and, the deposition of fat in non-adipose cells such as those of liver and muscle, and 3) by increased blood pressure associated with weight gain. In this chapter we shall focus on the consequences of the physical enlargement of adipose tissues as well as several morbidities that do not fit exactly into the above categories.

5.3.2   Complications Resulting from the Physical Effects of Excess Weight

Certain obesity co-morbidities seem clearly related to the physical effects of excess adipose tissue and increased weight. For example, osteoarthritis of the weight bearing joints due to increased body weight and sleep apnea associated with upper airway obstruction related to increased adiposity of the pharyngeal tissues are easily understood examples of the aversive physical effects of obesity. Other comorbidities may not, at first glance, appear to be related to the physical effects of adiposity. However, evidence from the surgical field offers a new perspective on the physical effects of excess weight.

Trauma surgeons have long appreciated the acute abdominal compartment syndrome (a condition in which intra-abdominal pressure increases) as a life-threatening complication of abdominal trauma. When intra-abdominal pressure increases to more than 20 cm of water, as reflected by urinary bladder pressure, venous return is compromised. Under these circumstances, the release of intra-abdominal pressure by laparotomy can be life-saving. Some of the same symptoms seen in the acute abdominal compartment syndrome — decreased venous return with lower leg edema; decreased renal venous return with hypertension; and decreased venous return to the thoracic cavity with increased intracranial pressure and seizures — are characteristic of the hypertensive syndromes of pregnancy. Preliminary evidence suggests that reduction in intra-abdominal pressure during the hypertensive syndromes of pregnancy reverses toxemia or eclampsia.[57]

With abdominal trauma, intra-abdominal pressure (as reflected by internal bladder pressure) may increase acutely due to the rapid accumulation of blood and fluid in the peritoneal cavity. In the hypertensive syndromes of pregnancy, the rise in intra-abdominal pressure is subacute in nature and results from the enlarging uterus within the peritoneal cavity. Increased intra-abdominal pressure has also been found to be associated with central adiposity; however, in obesity, the increase in intra-abdominal pressure is chronic in nature because of the gradual accumulation of intra-abdominal fat. Therefore, the bladder pressures in obesity can be much greater than those in acute trauma due to the length of time available for adaptation to take place. Animal study results support the relationship between intra-abdominal pressure and several of the complications of obesity.

Studies infusing nonabsorbed fluids into the abdominal cavity of pigs have been shown to produce increases in pleural pressure; cardiac filling pressure; femoral venous pressure; renal venous pressure; aldosterone and renin; systemic blood pressure and vascular resistance; and intracranial pressure.[57] Thus, increased intra-abdominal pressure associated with severe obesity may play a role in development of several very different clinical manifestations of excess weight; congestive heart failure; hypoventilation; venous stasis ulcers; venous thrombosis and pulmonary embolism; proteinuria; hypertension; and pseudotumor cerebri, as well as urinary incontinence and gastroesophageal reflux (Figure 5.1).

Finally, even in the absence of medical complications, obesity can have a profound effect on quality of life.[58] Obese persons are also more likely to experience bias and discrimination, even from health providers from whom they seek care.[59]

5.3.3   Cardiovascular Physiology and Increased Body Mass

In reviewing the cardiovascular complications of obesity, much of the medical literature focuses on coronary artery disease and risk factors that predispose to atherosclerosis and coronary occlusion, i.e., hypertension and the components of the metabolic syndrome. However, the purely physical consequences of weight gain, particularly severe weight gain, are also important and result in significant circulatory, hemodynamic, and electrophysiological changes that affect cardiovascular morbidity and mortality.

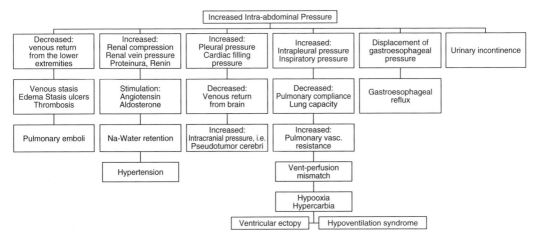

FIGURE 5.1
Proposed mechanisms for the clinical manifestations of central obesity.

Obesity is associated with an increase in blood volume to which the heart responds by increasing cardiac output through an increase in diastolic filling and stroke volume. Increased left ventricular filling leads to dilatation of the left ventricle, followed by hypertrophy as the ventricle responds to the stress of ejecting an ever greater volume of blood with increasing obesity. This sequence of events leads to a form of hypertrophy characteristic of obesity — eccentric left ventricular hypertrophy — in which dilatation of the left ventricle is proportional to the increase in left ventricular wall mass.[60,61]

Cardiac hypertrophy is directly related to the degree of obesity. Although cardiac hypertrophy is a structural adaptation to maintain cardiac output, it increases the risk for congestive heart failure and sudden death.[62] Thus, with increasing obesity and volume overload, left ventricular dilatation may increase to such an extent that left ventricular contractility is impaired, leading to systolic dysfunction, clinically measured as a decrease in the ejection fraction. Progressive dilatation of the left ventricle also leads to a decrease in the compliance of the left ventricle and therefore diastolic dysfunction. Systolic and diastolic dysfunction separately or combined can lead to congestive failure.

5.3.4   Congestive Heart Failure

A recent study of 5881 participants followed for a mean of 14 years in the Framingham Heart Study reported that, for each unit increase in body mass index, risk of heart failure increased 5% for men and 7% for women, even after adjusting for traditional risk factors.[63] Compared to normal-weight persons, obese persons were two times more likely to develop congestive heart failure. Paradoxically, in a study of 1203 patients with advanced heart failure, obesity was not associated with increased mortality, but instead with a slightly better prognosis.[64]

5.3.5   Ventricular Ectopy

It is difficult to estimate how frequently ventricular arrhythmias are a cause of death in obese persons. However, it is known that ventricular ectopic beats are more frequently observed in obese compared to normal-weight persons.[65,66] It is also known that obesity is associated with left ventricular hypertrophy and prolongation of the QT interval, both of which are risk factors for development of ventricular arrhythmias and sudden death.[67] The mechanism by which such arrhythmias arise is not known, but may relate to obesity-related structural changes in the conduction pathways of the heart; Bharati and Lev found significant fat and fibrous tissue around and within the conducting pathways of seven young obese people who died suddenly.[68]

5.3.6   Venous Stasis, Ulcers, Venous Thrombosis and Pulmonary Embolism

Severe obesity increases the risk of lower extremity venous stasis, presumably related to increased intra-abdominal pressure with impedance of venous return from the legs. Venous stasis is often accompanied by a bronze-like skin discoloration, secondary to extravasation of blood and residual heme pigmentation beneath the skin. Edema, skin ulceration and secondary cellulitis are also seen with severe obesity and a central deposition of body fat. Weight loss leads to improvements in these complications of obesity,[69] except for skin discoloration.

Venous thrombosis is a serious complication of increased intra-abdominal pressure because of its association with pulmonary embolism and sudden death. A prospective study of 19,293 men and women followed for a median time of 8 years showed a clear relationship of thromboembolism to severe obesity, with a relative risk of 2.7 in those with a BMI of 40 kg/m² or more compared to the reference group with a BMI less than 25 kg/m².[70] Diabetes was also associated with increased risk, possibly related to the fact that diabetes is associated with central obesity. Risk was also increased in men vs. women, black vs. white, and older vs. younger — groups more likely to have increased intra-abdominal fat.

Interestingly, thromboembolism was not associated with other traditional cardiovascular risk factors: cigarette smoking; hypertension; dyslipidemia; or physical inactivity. Other risk factors for thromboembolism exist, of course.[71] One of these is linked to a relatively new hazard of modern living: air travel. A recent study found that the risk of pulmonary embolism was 0.01 cases per million passengers traveling less than 5000 km; 1.5 cases per million passengers traveling more than 5000 km; and 4.8 cases per million for those traveling more than 10,000 km.[72] Because many people who fly today undoubtedly have established risk factors for thromboembolism, for example, obesity, diabetes, or advanced age, the incidence of thromboembolism may increase significantly in the future.

5.3.7   Effect of Weight Loss on Cardiovascular Health

Weight loss leads to a decrease in left ventricular hypertrophy. A 21-week trial of obese hypertensive subjects showed greater decreases in blood pressure and left ventricular mass with dietary weight loss than with metoprolol.[73] Weight loss has also been shown to improve left ventricular function in severely obese patients treated by gastric surgery, as demonstrated by reductions in left ventricular dilatation and hypertrophy, and increases in left ventricular work.[74,75]

Weight loss may also decrease the risk of sudden death in patients with left ventricular hypertrophy and QT prolongation; a 7-day weight loss regimen resulted in a significant reduction in the QT interval duration.[76] One exception to the observation that the risks of cardiac arrhythmias are reduced by weight loss may be very low calorie diets. Sours and colleagues reported sudden cardiac death in young women without arteriosclerotic cardiovascular disease who had been on very low calorie diets for more than 8 weeks.[77] These women had prolonged QT intervals, low QRS voltage, and findings on autopsy that were consistent with starvation. Pringle et al. demonstrated that QRS voltage on the electrocardiogram decreased after 7 weeks of fasting and that, after 8 weeks, the QT interval was prolonged, placing subjects at risk for malignant arrhythmias.[78] Greenway demonstrated that the QRS complex voltage decreased with diets of less than 600 kcal/d regardless of protein levels that varied from 45 to 70 g per day.[79] Modern very low calorie diets rarely consist of less than 800 kcal/d and have been shown to produce weight losses not different from diets containing 420 kcal/d.[80]

Weight loss also leads to improvements in the complications of increased venous pressure in the lower extremities. In one report of 37 patients with pretibial venous stasis ulcers who reduced their BMI from 62 to 40 kg/m[2] through gastric surgery, all but three had resolution of their venous stasis ulcers.[57]

5.3.8 Respiratory Physiology and Increased Body Mass

Severe obesity, particularly obesity involving the chest wall, has detrimental effects on the mechanics and physiology of breathing. Thus, obesity can lead to a decrease in chest wall and lung compliance, resulting in an increase in the work of breathing; hypoventilation; hypercarbia; and hypoxia. Pulmonary function tests may show a restrictive breathing pattern with decreases in total lung volume, functional reserve, and expiratory reserve volumes. Ventilation–perfusion mismatching may also be present, especially in the supine position as the abdominal contents displace the diaphragm upward resulting in atelectasis in the lung bases. Those with reduced sensitivity of CO_2 chemoreceptors may be severely affected by these abnormalities and go on to develop the obesity-hypoventilation syndrome. Not surprisingly, significantly obese persons complain of dyspnea at rest and/or with exertion.

5.3.8.1 Sleep Apnea

The prevalence of sleep apnea has been estimated to be between 1.3 and 4% in middle-aged adults;[81,82] men are more often affected than women in a ratio of 3.3:1.[83] The prevalence of sleep apnea is greater in postmenopausal women, although significantly less in those on hormone replacement therapy.[83] Obesity is the major predictor of the severity of the disorder, which is determined by the apnea–hypopnea index, which is the number of apneas and hypopneas lasting 10 sec or more per hour (hypopnea is a reduction in breathing amplitude/airflow, while apnea is a period of complete breathing cessation). A common threshold for the diagnosis of sleep apnea is the presence of more than 10 apnea–hypopnea incidents per hour or more than 30 during an overnight observation.

Although narrowing of the upper airway passages due to adiposity is one element in the pathogenesis of sleep apnea, the physiological consequences of increased intra-abdominal pressure (IAP) secondary to central obesity set the stage for the development of significant decrements in respiratory function. Thus, in persons with sleep apnea and central obesity, IAP can lead to increased pleural pressure; high inspiratory pressures; hypoventilation; hypoxia; and hypercarbia.[57] These in turn increase the risk of diurnal hypertension; nocturnal dysrhythmias;[84,85] pulmonary hypertension; right and left ventricular failure; myocardial infarction; and stroke.[86] Vgontzas et al. found visceral fat to be related positively to the severity of sleep apnea, but in contrast to other studies, not to BMI.[87] In addition to the medical consequences of sleep apnea, daytime sleepiness resulting from disrupted sleep impairs quality of life and work performance, as well as increasing the rate of motor vehicle accidents,[88] reportedly seven times higher in persons with sleep apnea compared to the general public.[89]

Dietary weight loss alone has a beneficial effect on sleep apnea,[90,91] but surgical weight loss interventions result in larger weight losses and greater decreases in the apnea–hypopnea index, i.e., reductions of –33 to –75% vs. –89 to –98%, respectively.[92] In the absence of significant weight loss or insufficient improvement with a given loss of weight, the use of continuous positive airway pressure (CPAP) is effective in those who tolerate wearing this device at night. Although no effective pharmacological interventions are available for sleep apnea, it is important to avoid using certain drugs, such as alcohol and hypnotic agents, that reduce muscle tone and therefore increase the tendency of the upper airway passages to collapse as intra-airway pressure decreases during inspiration.

5.3.9   Gastrointestinal Disorders Resulting from Effects of Increased Weight

The gastrointestinal consequences of obesity are surprisingly underrepresented considering the number of health consequences associated with overweight and obesity. Gallbladder disease and gastroesophageal reflux disease (GERD) are the most prominent of the gastrointestinal problems, along with a variety of common symptoms (bloating, gas, etc.) that are generally not the focus of clinical research because of their relatively benign effect on overall health. GERD is related, in part, to the physical effects of increased intra-abdominal pressure. Gallbladder disease is not related to increased intra-abdominal pressure to our knowledge and will therefore be addressed in another section of this chapter. Steatosis, or "fatty liver" manifested by elevated liver enzymes is a common finding in obese persons.

5.3.9.1   *Gastroesophageal Reflux Disease*

Gastroesophageal reflux disease (GERD) occurs more commonly in obese persons compared to those who are lean. Among 1524 randomly selected subjects, ages 25 to 74, a BMI greater than 30 kg/m² was associated with an odds ratio of 2.8 for the presence of reflux symptoms. Smoking, consuming more than seven drinks per week, and a family history of esophageal or stomach disease were other significant risk factors.[93] The latter was demonstrated in a study of mono- and dizygotic twins, which showed a significantly greater intraclass correlation for the symptoms of reflux symptoms in mono- compared to dizygotic twins. The increased incidence of esophageal disease with obesity was also shown in an 18.5 year follow-up of 12,349 subjects in the First National Health and Nutrition Examination Survey; the risk of hospitalization for esophagitis or hiatal hernia was 22% higher for every increase in BMI of 5 kg/m².[94]

Conditions associated with increased intra-abdominal pressure, for example, pregnancy, laparoscopic pneumoperitoneum, and ascites, are accompanied by esophageal reflux. It is therefore reasonable to conjecture that increased intra-abdominal pressure associated with central obesity is an additional mechanism that may predispose to esophageal reflux disease.[57] Barak has suggested that increased intra-abdominal pressure displaces the lower esophageal pressure upwards and also affects the gastroesophageal pressure gradient; together, these are conducive to reflux. In addition, obesity is associated with hiatal hernia, which promotes reflux by impairing the integrity of the lower esophageal sphincter.[95]

The incidence of esophageal adenocarcinoma has increased by more than 350% since the 1970s in the U.S.[96] Because GERD is a risk factor for Barrett's esophagus, which is a precancerous lesion, the increasing prevalence of obesity and therefore GERD may portend future increases in the prevalence of esophageal cancer.[97]

Weight loss improves the symptoms of esophageal reflux; changes in diet associated with weight loss may be a major contributor to the improvement (a personal observation is that GERD in severely obese persons almost always improves within 2 days of a calorie-restricted, low-fat diet). Gastric bypass surgery appears to produce better relief of GERD than restrictive procedures, possibly because of greater ease of outflow of gastric contents with bypass procedures.[98]

5.3.10 Skeletal Consequences of Increased Weight

Arthritis is more common in those who are obese. In a study of 195,000 people participating in the Behavioral Risk Factor Surveillance System in 2001, the risk of arthritis in persons with a BMI of 40 kg/m² increased fourfold compared to those with a normal BMI.[99] The two types of arthritis that affect obese persons most commonly are osteoarthritis and gout. The mechanical stress of excess weight is related to the development of osteoarthritis, particularly in the knee and to a lesser extent in the hip, while the arthritis of gout results primarily from metabolic factors that influence excretion of uric acid. Both forms of arthritis are more symptomatic with increasing weight.

5.3.10.1 Osteoarthritis

Osteoarthritis is more common in those who are overweight or obese. Although for many years it was uncertain which preceded the other, a consensus has emerged that obesity increases the risk of osteoarthritis.[100,101] A study of 1180 males at age 23 followed at intervals for a median time of 36 years[102] found that the incidence of osteoarthritis at age 65 was three times greater in the group that was heaviest at baseline (BMI 24.7 to 37.6 kg/m²) compared to the leanest group (BMI 15.6 to 22.8 kg/m²): 12.8 vs. 4.0%, respectively. Furthermore, a dose–response effect was suggested: increased body mass index at age 20 to 29 was more predictive of subsequent osteoarthritis than an elevated BMI between ages 30 and 50. The relationship between obesity and osteoarthritis is thought to result from the destructive effect of excess weight on joint structure and function, particularly in the knees. For example, it has been estimated that for every 1-lb increase in weight, pressure across the knee during impact increases by 2 to 3 lb.[103]

Systemic factors may also influence the development of osteoarthritis but are less well understood. Several observations support this view:

- Non weight-bearing joints are involved, i.e., hand osteoarthritis.
- Gender differences exist in the prevalence of osteoarthritis; females are affected more commonly than males.[104]
- Some studies have found an inverse association between osteoarthritis and osteoporosis.[105,106]

Systemic factors that have been suggested include adipose-derived inflammatory proteins and growth factors; oxygen radicals coupled with an insufficient intake of antioxidant nutrients; and gonadal hormones.[107–109] Although gout and rheumatoid arthritis are attributable to systemic factors, the severity of their symptoms is greatly influenced by the mechanical stress of excessive weight. Therefore, the physical effect of weight also affects these clearly systemic forms of arthritis.

The relationship of overweight and obesity to hip osteoarthritis is less strong than the relationship of overweight and obesity to knee osteoarthritis. In Gelber and colleagues' study,[102] weight at age 23 did not predict the subsequent development of hip osteoarthritis. Another report reviewing studies of hip osteoarthritis published through 2000 concluded that the influence of obesity on the development of hip osteoarthritis is moderate.[110]

Like that of hip osteoarthritis, the relationship between overweight/obesity and hand osteoarthritis has been difficult to prove. Several case control studies have reported negative as well as positive associations between obesity and hand osteoarthritis. A 23-year follow-up of 1276 participants in the Tecumseh Community Health Study showed that higher baseline relative weight was associated with an increased incidence and severity of subsequent hand osteoarthritis.[111] In contrast, a 13-year radiological follow-up of participants in the Baltimore Longitudinal Study of Aging found no association between baseline BMI and hand osteoarthritis.[112]

Weight loss leads to improvement in the symptoms of knee osteoarthritis.[113] In a much earlier study of phentermine for weight reduction, improvement in symptoms of knee and hip arthritis occurred after an average loss of 5 kg.[114]

5.3.11 Neurological Consequences of Central Obesity

5.3.11.1 *Pseudotumor Cerebri*

Pseudotumor cerebri, also known as idiopathic intracranial hypertension, is characterized by elevated intracranial pressure in the absence of an explanatory structural lesion, such as hydrocephalus. Clinically, it is recognized by headaches, visual symptoms, dizziness, and nausea. Pseudotumor cerebri can also lead to visual loss; however, frequently no symptoms are present and the diagnosis is suspected only after the finding of papilledema. The condition is often associated with severe obesity, and recently it has been proposed that intra-abdominal obesity, i.e., increased intra-abdominal pressure, is a significant factor in the pathogenesis of this disorder.[115] This hypothesis is supported by the following facts:

- Pseudotumor cerebri is a complication of late-term pregnancy.
- Symptoms of pseudotumor cerebri are relieved by application of a device to the abdomen that provides continuous negative pressure, much like a suction cup.[115]
- Clinical features of the disorder disappear with weight loss — through diet or through gastric surgery.[115,116]

The finding that pseudotumor cerebri occurs more commonly in females than males[117] suggests that additional factors beyond increased intra-abdominal pressure may play a role in the etiology of the disease (men might be expected to have an equal or greater incidence of pseudotumor cerebri because of their tendency toward central obesity).

Sleep apnea frequently accompanies pseudotumor cerebri.[118] One study involving four patients with papilledema and sleep apnea syndrome found normal daytime cerebrospinal pressures in all four patients. Nocturnal monitoring in one patient, however, showed repeated episodes of increased cerebrospinal pressure associated with apnea and arterial oxygen desaturation. The author proposed that repeated apneas with hypoxia and hypercarbia could lead to cerebral vasodilatation and papilledema.[119]

As mentioned, weight loss resolves the symptoms and clinical signs of pseudotumor cerebri in most patients. Considering that persistence of papilledema can lead to significant visual impairment, and that the only treatment for many years was to relieve intracerebral pressure by repeated lumbar punctures or shunt procedures, aggressive, relatively safe weight loss therapies should be strongly considered in the definitive management of these patients.

5.3.11.2 *Meralgia Paresthetica*

Meralgia paresthetica is caused by entrapment of the lateral femoral cutaneous nerve as it passes beyond the inguinal ligament into the leg. The symptoms are not dangerous but are disagreeable and nagging: paresthesias with numbness and tingling and sometimes pain, usually localized to the lateral thigh. Although rarely mentioned as a complication of obesity in the medical literature, clinicians who treat severe obesity frequently encounter this syndrome.

5.3.12   Dermatological Disorders

Skin problems associated with obesity fall into two categories: those that result from the physical effects of excess weight and those associated with hormonal changes that often accompany obesity (discussed later in the chapter).

5.3.12.1   *Striae*

Striae distensae, commonly known as stretch marks, are often seen in obese persons.[120] They appear as smooth atrophic bands of skin, generally seen over the abdomen, buttocks, and thighs, and are perpendicular to the natural cleavage lines of the skin. Initially, they appear red/purple but with time fade to a color paler than the surrounding skin. Woman following childbirth often develop striae, as do many adolescents who gain significant weight. Although weight gain, and therefore the physical effect of "stretching" the skin, is the common antecedent of striae, not all significantly obese persons develop them, suggesting an additional etiologic factor. The similarity between the striae seen in patients with hypercorticoidism and those with obesity has prompted many a beginning clinician to search fruitlessly for a cortisol-secreting tumor. In fact, it appears that the steroid excretion of obese patients with striae is higher compared with equally obese patients without striae.[121] Defective development of the integument has also been suggested to play a role.

5.3.12.2   *Intertrigo*

In severely obese patients, redundant folds of fat predispose to persistent moisture, maceration, and development of fungal or bacterial infections. The areas most usually affected are the intertriginous areas. A common initial presentation of patients with diabetes is a Candida albicans infection of the skin.

5.3.12.3   *Lymphedema*

Increased intra-abdominal pressure impedes lymphatic return from the legs and may cause edema, sometimes even resistant to diuretics. Chronic edema complicated by the development of one or more skin ulcers can lead to a dramatic and copious seepage of clear fluid, a complication difficult to ignore that generally prompts early consultation with a clinician.

5.3.12.4   *Venous Insufficiency Bronzing and Stasis Ulcers*

As with lymphedema, increased intra-abdominal pressure plays a role in the development of venous insufficiency, causing obstruction to venous return from the legs, and therefore increased pressure and dilation of the veins. With dilation, the venous valves become incompetent, allowing greater pressures to be transmitted to downstream capillaries. Extravasation of fluid and blood from capillaries leads to tissue edema and deposition of hemoglobin pigment in the subcutaneous tissues, manifested by so-called bronzing edema. If this process continues, ulceration of the skin and cellulitis may occur. Weight loss can resolve the edema, the ulcerative changes, and infection. However, bronzing generally persists due to the deposition of pigment beneath the skin.

5.3.12.5   *Cellulite*

Cellulite is the cobblestone appearance of the skin caused by the tethering of fibrous elements of the superficial fascia to the dermis coupled with bulging of fat contained within the honeycomb-like structure of the superficial fascia. Cellulite may occur in obese and normal-weight persons. Women are at greater risk than men. Although weight loss is possibly helpful, the topical application of aminophylline cream has been shown to help by stimulating lipolysis of superficial fat cells.[122]

5.3.12.6   *Hyperkeratoses at Pressure Points in the Feet*

Excess weight leads to abnormal alignment of foot structures with walking and hyperkeratosis at points of increased pressure. A horseshoe-shaped hyperkeratosis of the posterior rim of the sole has been found to be related to the degree of obesity.[120]

5.4   Disorders Unrelated to Physical Effects of Adiposity

5.4.1   Gallbladder Disease

Manifested primarily by gallstones, gallbladder disease and its complications, biliary colic, cholecystitis, and pancreatitis, is more common in people who are overweight and obese compared to those who are lean. A 10-year follow-up of women in the Nurses Health Study and men in the Health Professionals Follow-up Study found an almost twofold increase in the risk of developing gallstones in those with a BMI between 25 and 30 kg/m² compared to those who were leaner.[123] Another study using the Nurses Health Study cohort found that women with a BMI greater than 45 kg/m² had a sevenfold increase in the risk of symptomatic gallstone disease compared to women with a BMI less than 24 kg/m². In some studies central obesity has been associated with an increased prevalence of gallstones.[124]

Factors other than weight also influence the risk of developing gallstones. Advancing age is associated with a greater incidence of gallstones. Also, compared to men, women have a higher prevalence of gallstones, possibly related to their higher estrogen levels.[125] The incidence of gallstones also varies among ethnic groups,[126] and it has been suggested that genetic factors may account for as much as 30% of the variability in risk for gallstones.[127] Although gallstones are a risk factor for cholecystitis, two thirds of patients with gallstones are asymptomatic.[128]

Weight loss is also a risk factor for the development of gallstones and occurs primarily with the use of diets that are extremely low in fat. Such diets have been found to diminish gallbladder contractility thereby leading to bile stasis and gallstone formation. Not surprisingly then, weight cycling has been found to be positively related to cholecystectomy rates, with greater weight losses and regains during cycles associated with higher rates of cholecystectomy.[129] In a study by Syngal in which weight maintainers were used as a control group, the relative risk of cholecystectomy was 20% higher in those who lost and gained 5 to 9 lbs; 31% higher in those who lost and gained 10 to 19 lbs; and 68% higher in those who lost and gained >20 lbs. Surgical treatment of obesity with rapid and large weight losses would also be expected to increase the risk of gallstone formation; among 81 patients who did not have gallstones prior to gastric bypass surgery, 36% developed gallstones, and of these 40% developed symptoms and 28% underwent elective cholecystectomy.[130] For this reason, most patients who have gastric bypass undergo cholecystectomy at the time of surgery.

The pathogenesis of gallstone formation is complex but depends on three conditions, which together predispose to the development of gallstones:

- *Supersaturation of bile with cholesterol* — In obesity, cholesterol supersaturation of bile results from a higher than normal production of cholesterol by the liver, leading to an increase in the cholesterol/bile acid ratio. During weight loss, cholesterol is mobilized from fat stores and bile cholesterol supersaturation increases in proportion to the rapidity of weight loss.[131] During maintenance of lower weight cholesterol, supersaturation of bile is less and the risk of stone formation decreases.

- *Nucleation of cholesterol crystals in bile* — Nucleation of cholesterol results from higher than normal concentrations of cholesterol in the gallbladder, and from increasing bile concentration resulting from the absorption of water across the gallbladder mucosa. Mucins and glycoproteins secreted by the gallbladder mucosa may also stimulate stone development.

- *Decreased motility of the gallbladder* — If gallbladder motility and therefore emptying are diminished, i.e., during prolonged low-calorie and low-fat diets, bile stasis, yet another predisposing factor for gallstone formation, will occur.[128] Hormonal and neural stimuli following food intake affect gallbladder function. Thus, cholecystokinin increases gallbladder contractility, as does vagal stimulation. The maximal contraction of the gallbladder occurs after meals and is significantly influenced by meal composition. The observation that diets with little or no fat were associated with a high incidence of gallstones led to recognition of the importance of fat in maintaining normal contractility and therefore normal emptying of the gallbladder. Based on several studies, it is now recommended that weight-reducing diets include an intake of at least 10 g of fat with one meal[132,133] and that the rate of weight loss not exceed 1.5 kg per week.[134]

5.4.2 Cancer

Overweight or obesity increases the risk for several types of cancer. The most common obesity related cancers include those affecting the breast; endometrium; colon; prostate; and gallbladder.[1] In varying degrees, these cancers are related to hormonal changes that are affected by age, menstrual status, weight, and body fat distribution.

A relatively new concept in carcinogenesis ties hyperinsulinemia to the development and promotion of tumor growth. A "modern lifestyle" characterized by minimal physical activity and greater consumption of saturated fats, refined and simple carbohydrates leads to weight gain, central obesity, insulin resistance, and compensatory hyperinsulinemia. Hyperinsulinemia persists for as long as the pancreas is able to meet the heightened tissue needs for insulin due to insulin resistance. During this period, which may last many years, a number of hormonally sensitive tissues/organs are exposed to higher than normal insulin levels. In those who are genetically at risk and who have been exposed to additional environmental factors that increase carcinogenesis, hyperinsulinemia alone or in combination with these factors, may contribute to the development of cancer.

Hyperinsulinemia promotes tumor growth in several ways. Hyperinsulinemia increases the synthesis of insulin-like growth factor 1 (IGF-1), and also enhances its actions by decreasing binding proteins for IGF-1, thus increasing free IGF-1 and its bioavailability. Insulin and IGF-1 stimulate cell proliferation and inhibit apoptosis (cell death). In addition, insulin decreases the production of sex hormone-binding globulins, which increases the bioavailability of circulating sex steroids and therefore their potential to stimulate tumor growth. Also, IGF-1 increases production of endothelial growth factor, thus enhancing

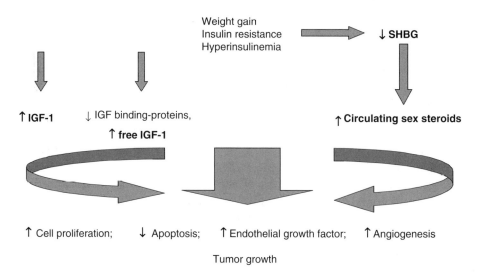

FIGURE 5.2
Obesity and cancer.

angiogenesis — a process that favors the growth of tumor cells and increases their metastatic potential[135] (Figure 5.2). These effects of insulin and IGF-1 are believed to be involved in the development of colon, breast, endometrial, and possibly prostate cancers. With the exception of the colon, these tissues are also sensitive to the actions of sex steroids, which will be discussed briefly later.

5.4.2.1   Colon Cancer

A positive relation exists between increased relative weight and colon cancer;[1] central adiposity is also important. In a study of 47,723 male health professionals with a follow-up of 5 years, waist circumference was found to be strongly associated with colon cancer.[136,137] This is consistent with the hypothesis that hyperinsulinemia plays a role in the development of colon cancer because central adiposity is associated with insulin resistance and hyperinsulinemia. The following findings support the role of hyperinsulinemia and IGF-1 in the development of colon cancer:

- Insulin promotes the growth of tumors in rats.[138]
- Acromegalic patients produce excessive amounts of growth hormone and IGF-1 and have a greater risk of developing colon cancer.[135,139]
- Insulin resistance and hyperinsulinemia are characteristic of the central adiposity positively associated with colon cancer.
- Studies report an increased risk of colon cancer in those with type 2 diabetes, a condition in which hyperinsulinemia exists during the first several years of the disorder.[135]
- Baseline levels of IGF-1 have been found to be higher in those who subsequently developed colon cancer or adenomas.[140,141]
- Hyperinsulinemia is associated with skin tags that, in turn, are associated with colon polyps.[142]
- Postprandial insulin levels increase the risk of subsequently developing colon cancer.[143]

- Physical activity, which increases insulin sensitivity, reduces the risk of colon cancer.[144]
- Increased stature, a result of different factors that include higher levels of growth hormone and IGF-1, is associated with an increased risk of colon cancer.[137]
- Diets that negatively affect insulin sensitivity, and therefore increase insulin levels, may increase the risk of colon cancer.[145]

5.4.2.2 Breast Cancer

Breast cancer is one of the most common cancers in women, accounting for 17% of all cancer deaths in women in the U.S.[146] Overweight and obese women are at greater risk from breast cancer than lean women, and overweight/obesity after menopause may be a greater risk although this has been an issue of some debate. Hormonal factors are important in the development of breast cancer. Endogenous estrogens may play a significant role (because breast cancer is rare in males) as well as hyperinsulinemia.

Several types of evidence support the role of estrogen in the risk of breast cancer. Epidemiological data indicate an increased risk of breast cancer in those who have had greater exposure to endogenous estrogen. Thus, early menarche; late menopause; late first pregnancy; low parity; or infertility are risk factors, while removal of the ovaries at an early age is protective.[147] Women with higher bone density, a reflection of higher exposure to estrogen, are at increased risk for breast cancer.[148] A prospective case control study of women 65 years and older reported that women who developed breast cancer 3 years after a baseline measurement of estradiol had higher levels of free estradiol (and free testosterone) compared to a control group without breast cancer.[149]

The ovaries are the major source of estrogens before menopause. After menopause, fat tissue becomes a major source through the conversion of endogenous androgens to estrogens by fat tissues. Although still a subject of debate, the lower risk of premenopausal breast cancer in obese compared to lean women may be due to higher levels of leptin noted with obesity, and a possible relationship to the *in vitro* finding that leptin inhibits insulin's action to increase estradiol production by cultured ovarian granulosa cells.[150]

After menopause, the increased risk of breast cancer in obese compared to lean women may reflect not only higher estrogen levels due to conversion of androgens to estrogens but also changes in insulin metabolism associated with weight gain and the development of central obesity so often seen after menopause. The tumor-enhancing actions of hyperinsulinemia; increased levels of IGF-1; and the greater bioavailability of estrogens and testosterone due to decreases in SHBG were previously discussed. These actions are thought to influence the risk of breast cancer as well as the other sex hormone-related cancers.

5.4.2.3 Endometrial Cancer

Endometrial cancer is the most common cancer of the female reproductive system in the U.S.[151] The incidence of endometrial cancer is highest in North America and Western Europe, with lower rates in Eastern Europe, Latin America, Asia, and Africa.[152] Obesity is one of several risk factors for endometrial cancer, and the geographic variation in the incidence of endometrial cancer may reflect differences in the prevalence of obesity throughout the world. Most cases of endometrial cancer occur after the age of 50, which is also a period in a woman's life when weight peaks and the distribution of body fat changes to the more central pattern associated with a hormonal profile conducive to the development of endometrial cancer.

Hormonal factors, including sex hormones and possibly insulin, are believed to play an important role in the development of endometrial cancer. The dominant hypothesis explaining this development posits that estrogen increases the mitotic activity of endometrial cells, leading to endometrial hyperplasia and malignancy. Thus, early menarche, late menopause, and nulliparity are associated with an increased risk of endometrial cancer. A complete or relative deficiency of progesterone further increases the risk, possibly related to a hypothesized inhibition of mitotic activity by progesterone.[153] Thus, "unopposed" estrogen replacement therapy after menopause increases endometrial hyperplasia and the risk of endometrial cancer, while the addition of progesterone decreases and/or neutralizes that risk.[154]

At first glance, the greater incidence of endometrial cancer in obese women before menopause is inconsistent with the "unopposed estrogen" theory. However, in premenopausal women, obesity is associated with a greater number of anovulatory cycles[155] and therefore less progestational exposure during the luteal phase of the menstrual cycle. After menopause and cessation of ovarian function, obese women are still exposed to higher estrogen levels because fat cells are able to aromatize androstenedione to estrone, the major estrogen after menopause. In addition, obesity is associated with increased adrenal production of androstenedione, thus providing greater amounts of substrate for the aromatization process. As mentioned, obesity is also associated with a decrease in the production of SHBG by the liver, resulting in greater bioavailability of estrone and other estrogenic compounds.[156–158]

The levels of insulin and IGF-1 are increased in obesity, and for reasons described earlier, may add to the risk of endometrial cancer, particularly in those with central obesity. The finding that the incidence of endometrial cancer is increased in type 2 diabetes, which is characterized by central obesity, insulin resistance, and hyperinsulinemia, but not in type 1 diabetes supports the role of insulin and IGF-1 in the development of endometrial cancer.[159] Hyperinsulinemia also stimulates ovarian androgen production and enhances the peripheral conversion of androstenedione to estrogens.[160,161]

Thus, the hormonal changes associated with obesity and a central distribution of body fat offer a plausible explanation for the increased risk of endometrial cancer in premenopausal and postmenopausal women.

5.4.2.4   Ovarian Cancer

The relationship between obesity and ovarian cancer is unclear. Studies have shown an increase in the relative risk of ovarian cancer with increasing weight;[162] no increase in risk with adult weight gain;[163] or a decrease in risk with increasing weight.[164] Risk factors that have been consistently observed include nulliparity, early menarche, late menopause, and a family history of ovarian cancer. Multiparity and the use of oral contraceptives are protective, suggesting that a higher number of ovulations during a woman's life is a risk factor.[165–167] It is interesting that increased height may be positively related to the risk of ovarian cancer.

5.4.2.5   Prostate Cancer

Although obesity is widely reported to increase the risk of prostate cancer, not all studies support this relationship. One study of 8922 men (mean age 67 years) followed for 5 years, from 1988 to 1993, found that the incidence of prostate cancer was not related to BMI at age 18.[168] A case control study of 238 cases and 471 controls conducted in China showed no relation between usual adult BMI and prostate cancer, although increasing waist/hip ratio was significantly related to the risk of prostate cancer: men in the highest quartile of waist/hip ratio had a threefold increase in risk compared to men in the lowest quartile.[169] Two large long-term follow up studies conducted by the American Cancer Society, Cancer

Prevention Study (CPS) I and II (381,638 and 434,630 men followed for 13 and 14 years, respectively), reported a significant association between obesity and mortality from prostate cancer. In CPS-I (but not CPS-II), an inverse association between height and prostate cancer risk was found.[170] Another large, long-term follow-up study (135,006 construction workers followed for 20 years) found a relative risk of 1.40 in men in the highest compared to the lowest BMI categories.[171] The risk was also slightly greater in the tallest men. Of clinical importance, obesity may be associated with more advanced disease; one study reported that obese patients with prostatic cancer were more likely to be younger and to have more advanced disease at the time of diagnosis.[172]

The mechanisms leading to the initiation of prostate cancer are unclear. The etiologic role of testosterone, once thought to be a key factor, has been disputed but not entirely discarded. A relatively recent hypothesis posits that hyperinsulinemia may play an important role by stimulating the synthesis of IGF-1 while decreasing the synthesis of IGF-1-binding proteins, thus increasing the bioavailability of IGF-1. As mentioned earlier, IGF-1 stimulates cell division and inhibits apoptosis, thereby enhancing tumor growth.[173] This hypothesis is consistent with studies reporting that obesity and a central distribution of body fat increase the risk for prostate cancer.

5.4.3 Menstrual Irregularity and Infertility; Polycystic Ovary Syndrome

Menstrual irregularity and infertility are more common in obese women. The hormonal changes associated with obesity are complex and often lead to anovulatory cycles, leading to menstrual irregularity and diminished fertility. Obesity with hyperinsulinemia stimulates the production of androgens by the ovary and adrenals. Hyperinsulinemia also decreases the liver's production of sex hormone-binding globulin, resulting in higher blood levels of free androgens available for conversion to estrone by fat cells. Elevated estrone levels interfere with the normal hypothalamohypophysial feedback system, resulting in a rise in the secretion of gonadotropins, manifested clinically by hirsutism and infertility.

Poorly understood, polycystic ovary syndrome is characterized by a more severe form of the preceding constellation of findings; abnormal gonadotropin secretion; an elevated LH/FSH ratio; anovulation; hyperandrogenism; insulin resistance; amenorrhea; and infertility. Following weight loss and increases in insulin sensitivity, women with menstrual irregularity, infertility, and polycystic ovary syndrome may in some cases re-establish menstrual regularity and fertility.[174,175]

5.4.4 Skin Problems Resulting from Hormonal Changes Associated with Obesity

5.4.4.1 *Acanthosis Nigricans and Skin Tags*

Obesity, insulin resistance, and hyperinsulinemia are at the heart of the pathophysiological mechanisms leading to acanthosis and skin tags.[120] High levels of insulin increase the production of IGF-1, which has a stimulative effect on the growth of keratinocytes and fibroblasts. The severity of acanthosis and skin tags appears to be related to the degree of obesity; insulin levels in patients with these skin lesions are higher than in those without acanthosis or skin tags.

5.4.4.2 *Hirsutism*

Hyperinsulinemia stimulates the production of androgens by the adrenal and inhibits the production of sex hormone-binding globulin by the liver, thereby increasing the bioavailability of free testosterone. Women who are obese, especially those who have central obesity, have higher levels of free testosterone, which leads to the typical features of hirsutism with increased facial hair. Reduction of insulin levels through weight loss or the use of insulin-sensitizing agents such as metformin may relieve this manifestation of obesity.

5.5   Quality of Life; Social and Psychological Consequences of Weight Gain

Given the many health problems described previously, it is not surprising that studies indicate that obese persons often perceive themselves as having a diminished quality of life.[58] Even those without health problems may consider their lives to be less than full.

Although size does not reflect intelligence, character, or personality, society does form judgments about people based solely on appearance.[59] Thus, obese adults and children are more likely to face discrimination and bias than their peers of normal weight.[176] Compared to those who are normal weight, obese persons are less likely to be hired, and if hired, are more likely to receive less pay, fewer promotions, and to be terminated from their jobs.[177] Basic opportunities to which most persons aspire are less available to those who are heavy; one study of adult women showed that those who were overweight or obese as adolescents were less likely to marry and more likely to complete fewer years of schooling and to have lower household incomes than their normal-weight adolescent peers, independent of aptitude test scores and socioeconomic status at baseline.[178] Obese people also experience greater bias when they seek medical care.[179,180] Perhaps for this reason, overweight and obese women, in spite of an increased risk for cancers of the reproductive system, are less likely to seek yearly screening for these cancers compared to normal-weight women.[181]

Not surprisingly, weight reduction appears to lessen the negativity that obese people encounter: severely obese persons who had previously experienced overwhelming prejudice and discrimination reported little or no discrimination following a body weight reduction of 100 lbs. through gastric surgery.[182] Weight loss is also associated with a perceived improvement in quality of life.[183] Although obese persons had been thought to have no greater psychopathology than normal-weight persons, recent studies report an increased risk of depression and preoccupation with suicide in obese persons.[184] Obesity is also associated with lower self-esteem, centering primarily on negative feelings and attitudes concerning body image.

5.6   Economic Costs of Obesity

The healthcare costs of obesity and its morbidities constitute a significant portion of all healthcare costs. A study conducted by Wolf and Colditz found that, for the U.S., the total costs attributable to obesity, including direct medical costs and indirect costs (excess lost work days, restricted activity, etc.), were almost 100 billion dollars in 1995, of which approximately 52 billion dollars were expended for direct medical costs, representing 5.7% of total health care expenditure.[37] In a Kaiser Permanente System study, the total healthcare costs of persons with a BMI of 25 to 30 kg/m^2 were 10% higher than those of persons with a BMI between 20 and 25 kg/m^2.[185] In both studies, a significant proportion of the total costs were attributed to the cost of treating diabetes, one of the most common medical complications of obesity and one that is expected to become more common with the increasing prevalence of obesity in adults and children.

5.7 Summary

Weight gain leading to overweight and obesity is complicated by a diversity of health problems, diminished quality of life, and premature death. The increasing prevalence of overweight and obesity will require clinicians to be well versed in the consequences of excess weight as well as current and emerging pharmacological treatments for obesity and its complications.

Common complications of obesity are diabetes; dyslipidemia; hypertension; and cardio-vascular disease. The pathophysiological mechanisms leading to these complications are related to insulin resistance and are usually discussed in the context of changes in body fat distribution and fat cell size referred to as the metabolic syndrome. The physical effects of adiposity are less often considered. This chapter concentrated on the physical effects of excess adiposity on the cardiovascular; respiratory; gastrointestinal; musculoskeletal; and neurological systems. Thus, clinical complications of obesity as different as congestive failure; sleep apnea; venous stasis ulcers and gastroesophageal reflux; arthritis; and pseudotumor cerebri are related to the physical effects of adiposity.

Although insulin resistance and hyperinsulinemia are known to be important in the development of the metabolic syndrome and cardiovascular disease, the association of insulin and insulin-like growth factors with the development of obesity-related cancers, i.e., colon, breast, and endometrium, is a newly appreciated relationship that reinforces the importance of weight as a determinant of health.

Additional obesity-related complications affecting quality of life, emotional well-being, and self-image complete the picture of a problem that deserves to be treated scientifically and compassionately.

References

1. Lew, E.A. and Garfinkel, L. Variations in mortality by weight among 750,000 men and women. *J. Chronic Dis.* 1979, 32: 563–576.
2. Hubert, H.B., Feinleib, M., McNamara, P.M., and Castelli, W.P. Obesity as an independent risk factor for cardiovascular disease: a 26-year follow-up of participants in the Framingham Heart Study. *Circulation* 1983, 67: 968–977.
3. Hoffmans, M.D., Kromhout, D., and de Lezenne Coulander, C. The impact of body mass index of 78,612 18-year old Dutch men on 32-year mortality from all causes. *J. Clin. Epidemiol.* 1988, 41: 749–756.
4. Manson, J.E., Colditz, G.A., and Stampfer, M.J. et al. A prospective study of obesity and risk of coronary heart disease in women. *N. Engl. J. Med.* 1990, 322: 882–889.
5. World Health Organization. Obesity: preventing and managing the global epidemic. Report of a WHO consultation on obesity. Geneva, 1998.
6. Drenick, E.J., Bale, G.S., Seltzer, F., and Johnson, D.G. Excessive mortality and causes of death in morbidly obese men. *JAMA* 1980, 243: 443–445.

7. Bray, G.A. Coherent, preventive and management strategies for obesity. *Ciba Found. Symp.* 1996, 201: 228–246, discussion 246–254.

8. Must, A., Jacques, P.F., Dallal, G.E., Bajema, C.J., and Dietz, W.H. Long-term morbidity and mortality of overweight adolescents. A follow-up of the Harvard Growth Study of 1922 to 1935. *N. Engl. J. Med.* 1992, 327: 1350–1355.

9. Andres, R., Elahi, D., Tobin, J.D., Muller, D.C., and Brant, L. Impact of age on weight goals. *Ann. Intern. Med.* 1985, 103: 1030–1033.

10. Durazo–Arvizu, R.A., McGee, D.L., Cooper, R.S., Liao, Y., and Luke, A. Mortality and optimal body mass index in a sample of the U.S. population. *Am. J. Epidemiol.* 1998, 147: 739–749.

11. Grabowski, D.C. and Ellis, J.E. High body mass index does not predict mortality in older people: analysis of the longitudinal study of aging. *J. Am. Geriatr. Soc.* 2001, 49: 968–979.

12. Heiat, A., Vaccarino, V., and Krumholz, H.M. An evidence-based assessment of federal guidelines for overweight and obesity as they apply to elderly persons. *Arch. Intern. Med.* 2001, 161: 1194–1203.

13. Sorkin, J.D., Muller, D., and Andres, R. Body mass index and mortality in Seventh-Day Adventist men. A critique and reanalysis. *Int. J. Obes. Relat. Metab. Disord.* 1994, 18: 752–754.

14. Calle, E.E., Thun, M.J., Petrelli, J.M., Rodriguez, C., and Heath, C.W., Jr. Body-mass index and mortality in a prospective cohort of U.S. adults. *N. Engl. J. Med.* 1999, 341: 1097–1105.

15. Stevens, J., Cai, J., Pamuk, E.R., Williamson, D.F., Thun, M.J., and Wood, J.L. The effect of age on the association between body-mass index and mortality. *N. Engl. J. Med.* 1998, 338: 1–7.

16. Singh, G.K. and Siahpush, M. Ethnic-immigrant differentials in health behaviors, morbidity, and cause-specific mortality in the United States: an analysis of two national data bases. *Hum. Biol.* 2002, 74: 83–109.

17. Stevens, J. Obesity and mortality in Africans–Americans. *Nutr. Rev.* 2000, 58: 346–353.

18. Deurenberg, P., Yap, M., and van Staveren, W.A. Body mass index and percent body fat: a meta analysis among different ethnic groups. *Int. J. Obes. Relat. Metab. Disord.* 1998, 22: 1164–1171.

19. Ko, G.T., Tang, J., Chan, J.C. et al. Lower BMI cut-off value to define obesity in Hong Kong Chinese: an analysis based on body fat assessment by bioelectrical impedance. *Br. J. Nutr.* 2001, 85: 239–242.

20. Deurenberg, P. Universal cut-off BMI points for obesity are not appropriate. *Br. J. Nutr.* 2001, 85: 135–136.

21. Andres, R. Beautiful hypotheses and ugly facts: the BMI-mortality association. *Obes. Res.* 1999, 7: 417–419.

22. Allison, D.B., Faith, M.S., Heo, M., Townsend–Butterworth, D., and Williamson, D.F. Meta-analysis of the effect of excluding early deaths on the estimated relationship between body mass index and mortality. *Obes. Res.* 1999, 7: 342–354.

23. Allison, D.B. and Saunders, S.E. Obesity in North America. An overview. *Med. Clin. North Am.* 2000, 84: 305–332, v.

24. Folsom, A.R., Kushi, L.H., Anderson, K.E. et al. Associations of general and abdominal obesity with multiple health outcomes in older women: the Iowa Women's Health Study. *Arch. Intern. Med.* 2000, 160: 2117–2128.

25. Lapidus, L., Bengtsson, C., Larsson, B., Pennert, K., Rybo, E., and Sjostrom, L. Distribution of adipose tissue and risk of cardiovascular disease and death: a 12 year follow up of participants in the population study of women in Gothenburg, Sweden. *Br. Med. J.* (Clin. Res. Ed.) 1984, 289: 1257–1261.

26. Snijder, M.B., Dekker, J.M., Visser, M. et al. Larger thigh and hip circumferences are associated with better glucose tolerance: the Hoorn study. *Obes. Res.* 2003, 11: 104–111.

27. Lissner, L., Bjorkelund, C., Heitmann, B.L., Seidell, J.C., and Bengtsson, C. Larger hip circumference independently predicts health and longevity in a Swedish female cohort. *Obes. Res.* 2001, 9: 644–646.

28. Sorkin, J.D., Muller, D.C., and Andres, R. Longitudinal change in the heights of men and women: consequential effects on body mass index. *Epidemiol. Rev.* 1999, 21: 247–260.

29. Forsen, T., Eriksson, J., Qiao, Q., Tervahauta, M., Nissinen, A., and Tuomilehto, J. Short stature and coronary heart disease: a 35-year follow-up of the Finnish cohorts of the seven countries study. *J. Intern. Med.* 2000, 248: 326–332.

30. Nwasokwa, O.N., Weiss, M., Gladstone, C., and Bodenheimer, M.M. Higher prevalence and greater severity of coronary disease in short versus tall men referred for coronary arteriography. *Am. Heart J.* 1997, 133: 147–152.

31. Albanes, D., Jones, D.Y., Schatzkin, A., Micozzi, M.S., and Taylor, P.R. Adult stature and risk of cancer. *Cancer Res.* 1988, 48: 1658–1662.

32. Blair, S.N., Kohl, H.W., III, Paffenbarger, R.S., Jr., Clark, D.G., Cooper, K.H., and Gibbons, L.W. Physical fitness and all-cause mortality. A prospective study of healthy men and women. *JAMA* 1989, 262: 2395–2401.

33. Blair, S.N., Kampert, J.B., Kohl, H.W., III et al. Influences of cardiorespiratory fitness and other precursors on cardiovascular disease and all-cause mortality in men and women. *JAMA* 1996, 276: 205–210.

34. Farrell, S.W., Braun, L., Barlow, C.E., Cheng, Y.J., and Blair, S.N. The relation of body mass index, cardiorespiratory fitness, and all-cause mortality in women. *Obes. Res.* 2002, 10: 417–423.

35. Stevens, J., Cai, J., Evenson, K.R., and Thomas, R. Fitness and fatness as predictors of mortality from all causes and from cardiovascular disease in men and women in the lipid research clinics study. *Am. J. Epidemiol.* 2002, 156: 832–841.

36. Leong, N.M., Mignone, L.I., Newcomb, P.A. et al. Early life risk factors in cancer: the relation of birth weight to adult obesity. *Int. J. Cancer* 2003, 103: 789–791.

37. Wolf, A.M. and Colditz, G.A. Current estimates of the economic cost of obesity in the United States. *Obes. Res.* 1998, 6: 97–106.

38. De Michele, M., Panico, S., Iannuzzi, A. et al. Association of obesity and central fat distribution with carotid artery wall thickening in middle-aged women. *Stroke* 2002, 33: 2923–2928.

39. Melinek, J., Livingston, E., Cortina, G., and Fishbein, M.C. Autopsy findings following gastric bypass surgery for morbid obesity. *Arch. Pathol. Lab. Med.* 2002, 126: 1091–1095.

40. Blaszyk, H., Wollan, P.C., Witkiewicz, A.K., and Bjornsson, J. Death from pulmonary thromboembolism in severe obesity: lack of association with established genetic and clinical risk factors. *Virchows Arch.* 1999, 434: 529–532.

41. Bananian, S., Lehrman, S.G., and Maguire, G.P. Cardiovascular consequences of sleep-related breathing disorders. *Heart Dis.* 2002, 4: 296–305.

42. Fletcher, E.C. Obstructive sleep apnea and cardiovascular morbidity. *Monaldi Arch. Chest Dis.* 1996, 51: 77–80.

43. Becker, H., Brandenburg, U., Peter, J.H., and Von Wichert, P. Reversal of sinus arrest and atrioventricular conduction block in patients with sleep apnea during nasal continuous positive airway pressure. *Am. J. Respir. Crit. Care Med.* 1995, 151: 215–218.

44. Shepard, J.W., Jr., Garrison, M.W., Grither, D.A., and Dolan, G.F. Relationship of ventricular ectopy to oxyhemoglobin desaturation in patients with obstructive sleep apnea. *Chest* 1985, 88: 335–340.

45. Drenick, E.J. and Fisler, J.S. Myocardial mass in morbidly obese patients and changes with weight reduction. *Obes. Surg.* 1992, 2: 19–27.

46. Kortelainen, M.L. Myocardial infarction and coronary pathology in severely obese people examined at autopsy. *Int. J. Obes. Relat. Metab. Disord.* 2002, 26: 73–79.

47. Kelley, D.E., Goodpaster, B.H., and Storlien, L. Muscle triglyceride and insulin resistance. *Annu. Rev. Nutr.* 2002, 22: 325–346.

48. Andres, R., Muller, D.C., and Sorkin, J.D. Long-term effects of change in body weight on all-cause mortality. A review. *Ann. Intern. Med.* 1993, 119: 737–743.

49. Pamuk, E.R., Williamson, D.F., Madans, J., Serdula, M.K., Kleinman, J.C., and Byers, T. Weight loss and mortality in a national cohort of adults, 1971–1987. *Am. J. Epidemiol.* 1992, 136: 686–697.

50. Wedick, N.M., Barrett–Connor, E., Knoke, J.D., and Wingard, D.L. The relationship between weight loss and all-cause mortality in older men and women with and without diabetes mellitus: the Rancho Bernardo Study. *J. Am. Geriatr. Soc.* 2002, 50: 1810–1815.

51. Nilsson, P.M., Nilsson, J.A., Hedblad, B., Berglund, G., and Lindgarde, F. The enigma of increased non-cancer mortality after weight loss in healthy men who are overweight or obese. *J. Intern. Med.* 2002, 252: 70–78.

52. Williamson, D.F., Pamuk, E., Thun, M., Flanders, D., Byers, T., and Heath, C. Prospective study of intentional weight loss and mortality in never-smoking overweight U.S. white women aged 40–64 years. *Am. J. Epidemiol.* 1995, 141: 1128–1141.

53. Williamson, D.F., Pamuk E., Thun, M., Flanders, D., Byers, T., and Heath, C. Prospective study of intentional weight loss and mortality in overweight white men aged 40–64 years. *Am. J. Epidemiol.* 1999, 149: 491–503.

54. Williamson, D.F., Thompson, T.J., Thun, M., Flanders, D., Pamuk, E., and Byers, T. Intentional weight loss and mortality among overweight individuals with diabetes. *Diabetes Care* 2000, 23: 1499–1504.

55. French, S.A., Folsom, A.R., Jeffery, R.W., and Williamson, D.F. Prospective study of intentionality of weight loss and mortality in older women: the Iowa Women's Health Study. *Am. J. Epidemiol.* 1999, 149: 504–514.

56. Allison, D.B., Zhu, S.K., Plankey, M., Faith, M.S., and Heo, M. Differential associations of body mass index and adiposity with all-cause mortality among men in the first and second National Health and Nutrition Examination Surveys (NHANES I and NHANES II) follow-up studies. *Int. J. Obes. Relat. Metab. Disord.* 2002, 26: 410–416.

57. Sugerman, H.J. Effects of increased intra-abdominal pressure in severe obesity. *Surg. Clin. North. Am.* 2001, 81: 1063–1075, vi.

58. Kolotkin, R.L., Meter, K., and Williams, G.R. Quality of life and obesity. *Obes. Rev.* 2001, 2: 219–229.

59. Puhl, R. and Brownell, K.D. Bias, discrimination, and obesity. *Obes. Res.* 2001, 9: 788–805.

60. Saltzman, E. and Benotti, P. The effects of obesity on the cardiovascular system. In: Bray, G.A., Bouchard, C., and James, W.P., Eds. *Handbook of Obesity.* New York: Marcel Decker, 1997: 637–649.

61. Lauer, M.S., Anderson, K.M., Kannel, W.B., and Levy, D. The impact of obesity on left ventricular mass and geometry: the Framingham Heart Study. *JAMA* 1991, 266: 231–236.

62. Lavie, C.J., Ventura, H.O., and Messerli, F.H. Left ventricular hypertrophy. Its relationship to obesity and hypertension. *Postgrad. Med.* 1992, 91: 131–132, 135–138, 141–143.

63. Kenchaiah, S., Evans, J.C., Levy, D. et al. Obesity and the risk of heart failure. *N. Engl. J. Med.* 2002, 347: 305–313.

64. Horwich, T.B., Fonarow, G.C., Hamilton, M.A., MacLellan, W.R., Woo, M.A., and Tillisch, J.H. The relationship between obesity and mortality in patients with heart failure. *J. Am. Coll. Cardiol.* 2001, 38: 789–795.

65. Messerli, F.H., Nunez, B.D., Ventura, H.O., and Snyder, D.W. Overweight and sudden death. Increased ventricular ectopy in cardiopathy of obesity. *Arch. Intern. Med.* 1987, 147: 1725–1728.

66. Zemva, A. and Zemva, Z. Ventricular ectopic activity, left ventricular mass, hyperinsulinemia, and intracellular magnesium in normotensive patients with obesity. *Angiology* 2000, 51: 101–106.

67. Messerli, F.H. and Soria, F. Ventricular dysrhythmias, left ventricular hypertrophy, and sudden death. *Cardiovasc. Drugs Ther.* 1994, 8 Suppl 3: 557–563.

68. Bharati, S. and Lev, M. Cardiac conduction system involvement in sudden death of obese young people. *Am. Heart J.* 1995, 129: 273–281.

69. Sugerman, H.J., Sugerman, E.L., Wolfe, L., Kellum, J.M., Jr., Schweitzer, M.A., and DeMaria, E.J. Risks and benefits of gastric bypass in morbidly obese patients with severe venous stasis disease. *Ann. Surg.* 2001, 234: 41–46.

70. Tsai, A.W., Cushman, M., Rosamond, W.D., Heckbert, S.R., Polak, J.F., and Folsom, A.R. Cardiovascular risk factors and venous thromboembolism incidence: the longitudinal investigation of thromboembolism etiology. *Arch. Intern. Med.* 2002, 162: 1182–1189.

71. Heit, J.A. Venous thromboembolism epidemiology: implications for prevention and management. *Semin. Thromb. Hemost.* 2002, 28 Suppl 2: 3–13.

72. Lapostolle, F., Surget, V., Borron, S.W. et al. Severe pulmonary embolism associated with air travel. *N. Engl. J. Med.* 2001, 345: 779–783.

73. MacMahon, S.W., Wilcken, D.E., and Macdonald, G.J. The effect of weight reduction on left ventricular mass. A randomized controlled trial in young, overweight hypertensive patients. *N. Engl. J. Med.* 1986, 314: 334–339.

74. Alaud-din, A., Meterissian, S., Lisbona, R., MacLean, L.D., and Forse, R.A. Assessment of cardiac function in patients who were morbidly obese. *Surgery* 1990, 108: 809–818, discussion 818–820.

75. Karason, K., Wallentin, I., Larsson, B., and Sjostrom, L. Effects of obesity and weight loss on cardiac function and valvular performance. *Obes. Res.* 1998, 6: 422–429.

76. Pietrobelli, A., Rothacker, D., Gallagher, D., and Heymsfield, S.B. Electrocardiographic QTC interval: short-term weight loss effects. *Int. J. Obes. Relat. Metab. Disord.* 1997, 21: 110–114.

77. Sours, H.E., Frattali, V.P., Brand, C.D. et al. Sudden death associated with very low calorie weight reduction regimens. *Am. J. Clin. Nutr.* 1981, 34: 453–461.

78. Pringle, T.H., Scobie, I.N., Murray, R.G., Kesson, C.M., and Maccuish, A.C. Prolongation of the QT interval during therapeutic starvation: a substrate for malignant arrhythmias. *Int. J. Obes.* 1983, 7: 253–261.

79. Greenway, F. Higher calorie content preserves myocardial electrical activity during very-low-calorie dieting. *Obes. Res.* 1994, 2: 95–99.

80. Foster, G.D., Wadden, T.A., Peterson, F.J., Letizia, K.A., Bartlett, S.J., and Conill, A.M. A controlled comparison of three very-low-calorie diets: effects on weight, body composition, and symptoms. *Am. J. Clin. Nutr.* 1992, 55: 811–817.

81. Gislason, T., Almqvist, M., Eriksson, G., Taube, A., and Boman, G. Prevalence of sleep apnea syndrome among Swedish men — an epidemiological study. *J. Clin. Epidemiol.* 1988, 41: 571–576.

82. Young, T., Palta, M., Dempsey, J., Skatrud, J., Weber, S., and Badr, S. The occurrence of sleep-disordered breathing among middle-aged adults. *N. Engl. J. Med.* 1993, 328: 1230–1235.

83. Bixler, E.O., Vgontzas, A.N., Lin, H.M. et al. Prevalence of sleep-disordered breathing in women: effects of gender. *Am. J. Respir. Crit. Care Med.* 2001, 163: 608–613.

84. Harbison, J., O'Reilly, P., and McNicholas, W.T. Cardiac rhythm disturbances in the obstructive sleep apnea syndrome: effects of nasal continuous positive airway pressure therapy. *Chest* 2000, 118: 591–595.

85. Javaheri, S. Effects of continuous positive airway pressure on sleep apnea and ventricular irritability in patients with heart failure. *Circulation* 2000, 101: 392–397.

86. Yamashiro, Y. and Kryger, M.H. Review: sleep in heart failure. *Sleep* 1993, 16: 513–523.

87. Vgontzas, A.N., Papanicolaou, D.A., Bixler, E.O. et al. Sleep apnea and daytime sleepiness and fatigue: relation to visceral obesity, insulin resistance, and hypercytokinemia. *J. Clin. Endocrinol. Metab.* 2000, 85: 1151–1158.

88. Young, T., Blustein, J., Finn, L., and Palta, M. Sleep-disordered breathing and motor vehicle accidents in a population-based sample of employed adults. *Sleep* 1997, 20: 608–613.

89. He, J., Kryger, M.H., Zorick, F.J., Conway, W., and Roth, T. Mortality and apnea index in obstructive sleep apnea. Experience in 385 male patients. *Chest* 1988, 94: 9–14.

90. Schwartz, A.R., Gold, A.R., Schubert, N. et al. Effect of weight loss on upper airway collapsibility in obstructive sleep apnea. *Am. Rev. Respir. Dis.* 1991, 144: 494–498.

91. Smith, P.L., Gold, A.R., Meyers, D.A., Haponik, E.F., and Bleecker, E.R. Weight loss in mildly to moderately obese patients with obstructive sleep apnea. *Ann. Intern. Med.* 1985, 103: 850–855.

92. Strohl, K.P., Strobel, R.J., and Parisi, F.A. Obesity and pulmonary function. In: Bray, G.A., Bouchard, C., and James, W.P., Eds. *Handbook of Obesity.* New York: Marcel Deckker, 1979: 725–739.

93. Locke, G.R., III, Talley, N.J., Fett, S.L., Zinsmeister, A.R., and Melton, L.J., III. Risk factors associated with symptoms of gastroesophageal reflux. *Am. J. Med.* 1999, 106: 642–649.

94. Ruhl, C.E. and Everhart, J.E. Overweight, but not high dietary fat intake, increases risk of gastroesophageal reflux disease hospitalization: the NHANES I epidemiologic followup study. First national health and nutrition examination survey. *Ann. Epidemiol.* 1999, 9: 424–435.

95. Barak, N., Ehrenpreis, E.D., Harrison, J.R., and Sitrin, M.D. Gastro-oesophageal reflux disease in obesity: pathophysiological and therapeutic considerations. *Obes. Rev.* 2002, 3: 9–15.

96. Devesa, S.S., Blot, W.J., and Fraumeni, J.F., Jr. Changing patterns in the incidence of esophageal and gastric carcinoma in the United States. *Cancer* 1998, 83: 2049–2053.
97. Mayne, S.T. and Navarro, S.A. Diet, obesity and reflux in the etiology of adenocarcinomas of the esophagus and gastric cardia in humans. *J. Nutr.* 2002, 132: 3467S–3470S.
98. Schauer, P., Hamad, G., and Ikramuddin, S. Surgical management of gastroesophageal reflux disease in obese patients. *Semin. Laparosc. Surg.* 2001, 8: 256–264.
99. Mokdad, A.H., Ford, E.S., Bowman, B.A. et al. Prevalence of obesity, diabetes, and obesity-related health risk factors, 2001. *JAMA* 2003, 289: 76–79.
100. Dougados, M., Gueguen, A., Nguyen, M. et al. Longitudinal radiologic evaluation of osteoarthritis of the knee. *J. Rheumatol.* 1992, 19: 378–384.
101. Schouten, J.S., van den Ouweland, F.A., and Valkenburg, H.A. A 12 year follow up study in the general population on prognostic factors of cartilage loss in osteoarthritis of the knee. *Ann. Rheum. Dis.* 1992, 51: 932–937.
102. Gelber, A.C., Hochberg, M.C., Mead, L.A., Wang, N.Y., Wigley, F.M., and Klag, M.J. Body mass index in young men and the risk of subsequent knee and hip osteoarthritis. *Am. J. Med.* 1999, 107: 542–548.
103. Felson, D.T., Lawrence, R.C., Dieppe, P.A. et al. Osteoarthritis: new insights. Part 1: the disease and its risk factors. *Ann. Intern. Med.* 2000, 133: 635–646.
104. Felson, D.T., Anderson, J.J., Naimark, A., Walker, A.M., and Meenan, R.F. Obesity and knee osteoarthritis: the Framingham Study. *Ann. Intern. Med.* 1988, 109: 18–24.
105. Hart, D.J., Mootoosamy, I., Doyle, D.V., and Spector, T.D. The relationship between osteoarthritis and osteoporosis in the general population: the Chingford Study. *Ann. Rheum. Dis.* 1994, 53: 158–162.
106. Dequeker, J. and Johnell, O. Osteoarthritis protects against femoral neck fracture: the MEDOS study experience. *Bone* 1993, 14 Suppl 1: S51–6.
107. Sowers, M. Epidemiology of risk factors for osteoarthritis: systemic factors. *Curr. Opinion Rheumatol.* 2001, 13: 447–451.
108. Clark, A.G., Jordan, J.M., Vilim, V. et al. Serum cartilage oligomeric matrix protein reflects osteoarthritis presence and severity: the Johnston County Osteoarthritis Project. *Arthritis Rheum.* 1999, 42: 2356–2364.
109. Haynes, M.K., Hume, E.L., and Smith, J.B. Phenotypic characterization of inflammatory cells from osteoarthritic synovium and synovial fluids. *Clin. Immunol.* 2002, 105: 315–325.
110. Lievense, A.M., Bierma–Zeinstra, S.M., Verhagen, A.P., van Baar, M.E., Verhaar, J.A., and Koes, B.W. Influence of obesity on the development of osteoarthritis of the hip: a systematic review. *Rheumatology* (Oxford) 2002, 41: 1155–1162.
111. Carman, W.J., Sowers, M., Hawthorne, V.M., and Weissfeld, L.A. Obesity as a risk factor for osteoarthritis of the hand and wrist: a prospective study. *Am. J. Epidemiol.* 1994, 139: 119–29.
112. Hochberg, M.C., Lethbridge–Cejku, M., Scott, W.W., Jr., Plato, C.C., and Tobin, J.D. Obesity and osteoarthritis of the hands in women. *Osteoarthritis Cartilage* 1993, 1: 129–135.
113. Felson, D.T., Zhang, Y., Anthony, J.M., Naimark, A., and Anderson, J.J. Weight loss reduces the risk for symptomatic knee osteoarthritis in women: the Framingham Study. *Ann. Intern. Med.* 1992, 116: 535–539.
114. Williams, R. and Foulsham, B. Weight reduction in osteoarthritis using phentermine. *Practitioner* 1981, 225: 231–232.
115. Sugerman, H.J., Felton, W.L.R., Sismanis, A., Kellum, J.M., DeMaria, E.J., and Sugerman, E.L. Gastric surgery for pseudotumor cerebri associated with severe obesity. *Ann. Surg.* 1999, 229: 634–640, discussion 640–642.
116. Newborg, B. Pseudotumor cerebri treated by rice reduction diet. *Arch. Intern. Med.* 1974, 133: 802–807.
117. Durcan, F.J., Corbett, J.J., and Wall, M. The incidence of pseudotumor cerebri. Population studies in Iowa and Louisiana. *Arch. Neurol.* 1988, 45: 875–877.
118. Marcus, D.M., Lynn, J., Miller, J.J., Chaudhary, O., Thomas, D., and Chaudhary, B. Sleep disorders: a risk factor for pseudotumor cerebri? *J. Neuroophthalmol.* 2001, 21: 121–123.
119. Purvin, V.A., Kawasaki, A., and Yee, R.D. Papilledema and obstructive sleep apnea syndrome. *Arch. Ophthalmol.* 2000, 118: 1626–3160.

120. Garcia–Hidalgo, L., Orozco–Topete, R., Gonzalez–Barranco, J., Villa, A.R., Dalman, J.J., and Ortiz–Pedroza, G. Dermatoses in 156 obese adults. *Obes. Res.* 1999, 7: 299–302.

121. Simkin, B. and Arce, R. Steroid excretion in obese patients with colored abdominal striae. *N. Engl. J. Med.* 1962, 266: 1031–1035.

122. Greenway, F.L., Bray, G.A., and Heber, D. Topical fat reduction. *Obes. Res.* 1995, 3 Suppl 4: 561S–568S.

123. Field, A.E., Coakley, E.H., Must, A. et al. Impact of overweight on the risk of developing common chronic diseases during a 10-year period. *Arch. Intern. Med.* 2001, 161: 1581–1586.

124. Ruhl, C.E. and Everhart, J.E. Relationship of serum leptin concentration and other measures of adiposity with gallbladder disease. *Hepatology* 2001, 34: 877–883.

125. Henriksson, P., Einarsson, K., Eriksson, A., Kelter, U., and Angelin, B. Estrogen-induced gallstone formation in males. Relation to changes in serum and biliary lipids during hormonal treatment of prostatic carcinoma. *J. Clin. Invest.* 1989, 84: 811–816.

126. Everhart, J.E. Gallstones and ethnicity in the Americas. *J. Assoc. Acad. Minor Phys.* 2001, 12: 137–143.

127. Nakeeb, A., Comuzzie, A.G., Martin, L. et al. Gallstones: genetics versus environment. *Ann. Surg.* 2002, 235: 842–849.

128. Ko, C.W. and Lee, S.P. Obesity and gallbladder disease. In: Bray, G.A., Bouchard, C., and James, W.P., Eds. *Handbook of Obesity.* New York: Marcel Dekker, 1997: 709–724.

129. Syngal, S., Coakley, E.H., Willett, W.C., Byers, T., Williamson, D.F., and Colditz, G.A. Long-term weight patterns and risk for cholecystectomy in women. *Ann. Intern. Med.* 1999, 130: 471–477.

130. Shiffman, M.L., Sugerman, H.J., Kellum, J.M., Brewer, W.H., and Moore, E.W. Gallstone formation after rapid weight loss: a prospective study in patients undergoing gastric bypass surgery for treatment of morbid obesity. *Am. J. Gastroenterol.* 1991, 86: 1000–1005.

131. Grundy, S.M. and Kern, F., Jr. Workshop on regulation of hepatic cholesterol and bile acid metabolism. *J. Lipid Res.* 1980, 21: 496–500.

132. Stone, B.G., Ansel, H.J., Peterson, F.J., and Gebhard, R.L. Gallbladder emptying stimuli in obese and normal-weight subjects. *Hepatology* 1992, 15: 795–798.

133. Hoy, M.K., Heshka, S., Allison, D.B. et al. Reduced risk of liver-function-test abnormalities and new gallstone formation with weight loss on 3350-kJ (800-kcal) formula diets. *Am. J. Clin. Nutr.* 1994, 60: 249–254.

134. Weinsier, R.L., Wilson, L.J., and Lee, J. Medically safe rate of weight loss for the treatment of obesity: a guideline based on risk of gallstone formation. *Am. J. Med.* 1995, 98: 115–117.

135. Giovannucci, E. Insulin, insulin-like growth factors and colon cancer: a review of the evidence. *J. Nutr.* 2001, 131: 3109S–3120S.

136. Giovannucci, E., Ascherio, A., Rimm, E.B., Colditz, G.A., Stampfer, M.J., and Willett, W.C. Physical activity, obesity, and risk for colon cancer and adenoma in men. *Ann. Intern. Med.* 1995, 122: 327–334.

137. Giovannucci, E. Insulin and colon cancer. *Cancer Causes Control* 1995, 6: 164–79.

138. Tran, T.T., Medline, A., and Bruce, W.R. Insulin promotion of colon tumors in rats. *Cancer Epidemiol. Biomarkers Prev.* 1996, 5: 1013–1015.

139. Jenkins, P.J. Acromegaly and colon cancer. *Growth Horm. IGF Res.* 2000, 10 Suppl A: S35–36.

140. Ma, J., Pollak, M.N., Giovannucci, E. et al. Prospective study of colorectal cancer risk in men and plasma levels of insulin-like growth factor (IGF)-I and IGF-binding protein-3. *J. Natl. Cancer Inst.* 1999, 91: 620–625.

141. Giovannucci, E., Pollak, M.N., Platz, E.A. et al. A prospective study of plasma insulin-like growth factor-1 and binding protein-3 and risk of colorectal neoplasia in women. *Cancer Epidemiol. Biomarkers Prev.* 2000, 9: 345–349.

142. Leavitt, J., Klein, I., Kendricks, F., Gavaler, J., and VanThiel, D.H. Skin tags: a cutaneous marker for colonic polyps. *Ann. Intern. Med.* 1983, 98: 928–930.

143. Schoen, R.E., Tangen, C.M., Kuller, L.H. et al. Increased blood glucose and insulin, body size, and incident colorectal cancer. *J. Natl. Cancer Inst.* 1999, 91: 1147–1154.

144. Colditz, G.A., Cannuscio, C.C., and Frazier, A.L. Physical activity and reduced risk of colon cancer: implications for prevention. *Cancer Causes Control* 1997, 8: 649–667.

145. Slattery, M.L., Boucher, K.M., Caan, B.J., Potter, J.D., and Ma, K.N. Eating patterns and risk of colon cancer. *Am. J. Epidemiol.* 1998, 148: 4–16.

146. Parker, S.L., Tong, T., Bolden, S., and Wingo, P.A. Cancer statistics, 1997. *CA Cancer J. Clin.* 1997, 47: 5–27.

147. Kelsey, J.L. and Bernstein, L. Epidemiology and prevention of breast cancer. *Annu. Rev. Public Health* 1996, 17: 47–67.

148. Zhang, Y., Kiel, D.P., Kreger, B.E. et al. Bone mass and the risk of breast cancer among postmenopausal women. *N. Engl. J. Med.* 1997, 336: 611–617.

149. Cauley, J.A., Lucas, F.L., Kuller, L.H., Stone, K., Browner, W., and Cummings, S.R. Elevated serum estradiol and testosterone concentrations are associated with a high risk for breast cancer. Study of osteoporotic fractures research group. *Ann. Intern. Med.* 1999, 130: 270–277.

150. Spicer, L.J. and Francisco, C.C. The adipose obese gene product, leptin: evidence of a direct inhibitory role in ovarian function. *Endocrinology* 1997, 138: 3374–3379.

151. Cancer facts and figures. Atlanta, GA: American Cancer Society, 2000.

152. Parkin, D.M. and Muir, C.S. Cancer incidence in five continents. Comparability and quality of data. *IARC Sci. Publ.* 1992: 45–173.

153. Key, T.J. and Pike, M.C. The dose-effect relationship between 'unopposed' oestrogens and endometrial mitotic rate: its central role in explaining and predicting endometrial cancer risk. *Br. J. Cancer* 1988, 57: 205–212.

154. Gelfand, M.M. and Ferenczy, A. A prospective 1-year study of estrogen and progestin in postmenopausal women: effects on the endometrium. *Obstet. Gynecol.* 1989, 74: 398–402.

155. Rogers, J. and Mitchell, G. The relation of obesity to menstrual disturbances. *N. Engl. J. Med.* 1952, 247: 55–57.

156. Austin, H., Austin, J.M., Jr., Partridge, E.E., Hatch, K.D., and Shingleton, H.M. Endometrial cancer, obesity, and body fat distribution. *Cancer Res.* 1991, 51: 568–572.

157. Potischman, N., Hoover, R.N., Brinton, L.A. et al. Case-control study of endogenous steroid hormones and endometrial cancer. *J. Natl. Cancer Inst.* 1996, 88: 1127–1135.

158. Zeleniuch–Jacquotte, A., Akhmedkhanov, A., Kato, I. et al. Postmenopausal endogenous oestrogens and risk of endometrial cancer: results of a prospective study. *Br. J. Cancer* 2001, 84: 975–981.

159. Parazzini, F., La Vecchia, C., Negri, E. et al. Diabetes and endometrial cancer: an Italian case-control study. *Int. J. Cancer* 1999, 81: 539–542.

160. Poretsky, L. and Kalin, M.F. The gonadotropic function of insulin. *Endocr. Rev.* 1987, 8: 132–141.

161. Garzo, V.G. and Dorrington, J.H. Aromatase activity in human granulosa cells during follicular development and the modulation by follicle-stimulating hormone and insulin. *Am. J. Obstet. Gynecol.* 1984, 148: 657–662.

162. Rodriguez, C., Calle, E.E., Fakhrabadi–Shokoohi, D., Jacobs, E.J., and Thun, M.J. Body mass index, height, and the risk of ovarian cancer mortality in a prospective cohort of postmenopausal women. *Cancer Epidemiol. Biomarkers Prev.* 2002, 11: 822–828.

163. Fairfield, K.M., Willett, W.C., Rosner, B.A., Manson, J.E., Speizer, F.E., and Hankinson, S.E. Obesity, weight gain, and ovarian cancer. *Obstet. Gynecol.* 2002, 100: 288–296.

164. Lukanova, A., Toniolo, P., Lundin, E. et al. Body mass index in relation to ovarian cancer: a multi-centre nested case-control study. *Int. J. Cancer* 2002, 99: 603–608.

165. Key, T.J., Allen, N.E., Verkasalo, P.K., and Banks, E. Energy balance and cancer: the role of sex hormones. *Proc. Nutr. Soc.* 2001, 60: 81–89.

166. Key, T.J. Hormones and cancer in humans. *Mutat. Res.* 1995, 333: 59–67.

167. Mink, P.J., Folsom, A.R., Sellers, T.A., and Kushi, L.H. Physical activity, waist-to-hip ratio, and other risk factors for ovarian cancer: a follow-up study of older women. *Epidemiology* 1996, 7: 38–45.

168. Lee, I.M., Sesso, H.D., and Paffenbarger, R.S., Jr. A prospective cohort study of physical activity and body size in relation to prostate cancer risk (United States). *Cancer Causes Control* 2001, 12: 187–193.

169. Hsing, A.W., Deng, J., Sesterhenn, I.A. et al. Body size and prostate cancer: a population-based case-control study in China. *Cancer Epidemiol. Biomarkers Prev.* 2000, 9: 1335–1341.

170. Rodriguez, C., Patel, A.V., Calle, E.E., Jacobs, E.J., Chao, A., and Thun, M.J. Body mass index, height, and prostate cancer mortality in two large cohorts of adult men in the United States. *Cancer Epidemiol. Biomarkers Prev.* 2001, 10: 345–353.
171. Andersson, S.O., Wolk, A., Bergstrom, R. et al. Body size and prostate cancer: a 20-year follow-up study among 135006 Swedish construction workers. *J. Natl. Cancer Inst.* 1997, 89: 385–389.
172. Amling, C.L., Kane, C.J., Riffenburgh, R.H. et al. Relationship between obesity and race in predicting adverse pathologic variables in patients undergoing radical prostatectomy. *Urology* 2001, 58: 723–728.
173. Kaaks, R. and Lukanova, A. Energy balance and cancer: the role of insulin and insulin-like growth factor-I. *Proc. Nutr. Soc.* 2001, 60: 91–106.
174. Hollmann, M., Runnebaum, B., and Gerhard, I. Effects of weight loss on the hormonal profile in obese, infertile women. *Hum. Reprod.* 1996, 11: 1884–1891.
175. Clark, A.M., Ledger, W., Galletly, C. et al. Weight loss results in significant improvement in pregnancy and ovulation rates in anovulatory obese women. *Hum. Reprod.* 1995, 10: 2705–2712.
176. Hill, A.J. and Silver, E.K. Fat, friendless and unhealthy: 9-year old children's perception of body shape stereotypes. *Int. J. Obes. Relat. Metab. Disord.* 1995, 19: 423–430.
177. Loh, E. The economic effects of physical appearance. *Soc. Sci. Q.* 1993, 74: 420–437.
178. Gortmaker, S.L., Must, A., Perrin, J.M., Sobol, A.M., and Dietz, W.H. Social and economic consequences of overweight in adolescence and young adulthood. *N. Engl. J. Med.* 1993, 329: 1008–1012.
179. Klein, D., Najman, J., Kohrman, A.F., and Munro, C. Patient characteristics that elicit negative responses from family physicians. *J. Fam. Pract.* 1982, 14: 881–888.
180. Price, J.H., Desmond, S.M., Krol, R.A., Snyder, F.F., and O'Connell, J.K. Family practice physicians' beliefs, attitudes, and practices regarding obesity. *Am. J. Prev. Med.* 1987, 3: 339–345.
181. Fontaine, K.R., Heo, M., and Allison, D.B. Body weight and cancer screening among women. *J. Womens Health Gend. Based Med.* 2001, 10: 463–470.
182. Rand, C.S. and Macgregor, A.M. Morbidly obese patients' perceptions of social discrimination before and after surgery for obesity. *South Med. J.* 1990, 83: 1390–1395.
183. Kolotkin, R.L., Crosby, R.D., Williams, G.R., Hartley, G.G., and Nicol, S. The relationship between health-related quality of life and weight loss. *Obes. Res.* 2001, 9: 564–571.
184. Carpenter, K.M., Hasin, D.S., Allison, D.B., and Faith, M.S. Relationships between obesity and DSM-IV major depressive disorder, suicide ideation, and suicide attempts: results from a general population study. *Am. J. Public Health* 2000, 90: 251–257.
185. Thompson, D., Brown, J.B., Nichols, G.A., Elmer, P.J., and Oster, G. Body mass index and future healthcare costs: a retrospective cohort study. *Obes. Res.* 2001, 9: 210–218.

6

Psychosocial Aspects of Obesity

Esther Biedert and Jürgen Margraf

CONTENTS

SUMMARY   Obesity is generally a life-long problem with numerous weight-related medical complications. The relationship between body weight and risk of developing a significant disease, as well as total mortality and morbidity, has been examined in many epidemiological studies. Such studies provide insight into biological relationships. In addition to negative physical effects, obesity may also have deleterious psychological and social effects on the individuals concerned. It is not obesity as a physical state that creates a psychological burden for many obese individuals, but rather the people or society who create this burden and suffering. Discrimination and prejudice may have adverse effects on the psychological well-being of a subgroup of obese persons. The psychosocial consequences of obesity will be described in this chapter. Furthermore the possible specific psychopathology of obese individuals in clinical settings, e.g., binge eating disorder and body dissatisfaction, will be discussed. The second part of this chapter addresses treatment possibilities for obesity. Additional associated characteristics such as increasing physical activity, enhancing self-esteem, binge eating disorder, and body dissatisfaction are discussed.

0-415-30321-4/04/$0.00+$1.50
© 2004 by CRC Press LLC

6.1 Introduction

The World Health Organization described obesity as a "global epidemic" (World Health Organization [WHO], 1997) and a major health problem. In Western societies, the rates for childhood and adult obesity are rising (Flegal et al., 1998; Seidell and Rissanen, 1998). An increasing number of obese people will suffer from many weight-related medical complications, including cardiovascular disease; type 2 diabetes; certain cancers; musculoskeletal disorders; and sleep apnea (Bray et al., 1998; Visscher and Seidell, 2001; Field et al., 2002). In addition, they will be at an increased risk of adverse psychological and social consequences of obesity (Gortmaker et al., 1993; Stunkard and Sobal, 1995). In other words obesity is not only a physical problem but also, to a considerable extent, a psychosocial one.

This problem is compounded by the failure of many attempts to reduce weight and the fact that, viewed from a long-term perspective, most people regain their lost weight even after a specialized treatment program. Obesity is generally a life-long problem against which short-term treatment strategies offer no success. Even with behavioral state-of-the-art programs, the long-term results are more than sobering because the lost weight is almost always regained within 5 years (Garner and Wooley, 1991; Goodrick et al., 1991). For obese people, this often means a life-long psychological burden.

In contrast to physical ill effects, the psychosocial consequences of obesity are not inevitable but derive from culture-bound values by which people view body fat as unhealthy and ugly. This derogation of obesity is most frequent in Western society as a function of social attitudes specific to particular times and places (Wilfley and Rodin, 1995). Stereotypes about obesity abound and particularly subscribe to the psychological characteristics attributed to obese persons.

6.2 Prejudice, Discrimination, and Psychological Consequences of Obesity

6.2.1 Prejudice and Discrimination

Although in former times and in other parts of the world corpulence was and still is regarded as a valued symbol of affluence, being overweight nowadays has a negative connotation, especially in the industrialized Western world (Sobal, 1995). The ideal of slimness first became dominant in the 1960s and 1970s. Photomodels (e.g., "Twiggy") and actresses (e.g., Marilyn Monroe or Jane Fonda) became ever thinner, as shown in the oft-quoted study by Garner et al., (1980) which found that, between 1959 and 1979, the average weight of contestants in the Miss America contest fell just as strikingly as did that of the centerfold models of *Playboy* magazine. At the same time, attitudes toward obese people became increasingly negative; the percentage of Germans prepared to accept an overweight person as a friend fell from 40% in 1971 to only 3% in 1979.

Discrimination starts during childhood, as evidenced by findings that show that, even before puberty, children dislike obese bodies; 6-year-old children associate adjectives such as lazy, dirty, stupid, and unattractive significantly more often with the silhouette of an obese child than with that of a nonobese child (Staffieri, 1967). When shown black and white line drawings of an obese child and of children with various severe handicaps, including missing hands and facial disfigurement, children and adults rated the obese child as the least likeable (Maddox et al., 1968). Sadly, obese persons manifest precisely the same kind of prejudice.

Prejudice against obese individuals is associated with discrimination in virtually every domain of life. An exemplary study by Gortmaker et al. (1993) followed a community sample of adolescents ($N = 10,309$) for 7 years and found that, compared with normal-weight women of comparable intellectual aptitude, overweight females completed significantly fewer months of school; were less likely to be married; and had lower household incomes. Overweight males were also less likely to be married than were their normal-weight peers. This applied even after all other differentiating characteristics were controlled. By contrast, people with other chronic conditions (e.g., cerebral palsy, asthma, rheumatoid arthritis) did not differ from normal-weight participants in any of these outcome variables.

Discrimination also exists in education and employment. Thus, overweight high-school students were found to be less likely to win a place at prestigious colleges than were normal-weight students, despite comparable scholastic performance between the two groups (Pargaman, 1969). Laboratory studies that experimentally manipulated job applicants' perceived weights showed a strong bias against obese individuals in almost every stage of employment, e.g., selection, placement, compensation, promotion, discipline, and discharge (Frieze et al., 1994; Roehling, 1999). This effect seems to be more pronounced for women than for men. Further evidence of discrimination against overweight individuals in the workplace is given by another study. Pingitore et al. (1994) asked participants to rate videotaped job interviews of actors who appeared to be normal-weight or were made up to look overweight. The applicants' apparent weight was the strongest determinant of the hiring decision. The same applicant, when made to look overweight, was selected significantly less often than when the appearance was of normal-weight. Again, this finding was stronger against overweight-appearing women than against such men.

The preceding negative attitudes toward obese people prevail even in medical institutions. Health care insurance does not grant obesity the status of an illness because it is regarded as self-inflicted (Rand and Macgregor, 1990). This view is shared by most of the normal-weight population, which generally regards being overweight as a consequence of a freely chosen self-indulgent life-style. Furthermore, 78% of obese persons reported that doctors often treat them with a lack of respect because of their weight and doctors generally categorize their overweight patients as weak-willed, inept, and ugly (Rand and Macgregor, 1990). Such negative attitudes on the part of medical professionals may partly explain why obese people are reluctant to seek medical help for their problem. The previously mentioned negative attitudes even have effects on concrete treatment strategies of obese individuals: overweight patients were found to be considerably less likely to be prescribed lipid-lowering drugs than were other categories of patients (e.g., smokers). Moreover, the general practitioners concerned openly acknowledged that their prescribing habits were skewed in this way (Rand and Macgregor, 1990).

Studies clearly demonstrate that obese people bear overt prejudice and discrimination in today's Western society. Given this burden, one can assume that these individuals suffer from greater psychological distress than normal-weight individuals. This clearly appears to be the case with obese patients who seek weight reduction. The assumed psychological distress is probably one of the factors leading them to seek weight loss. Surprisingly, the results of several studies have shown that, in standard psychological tests, the scores of obese persons differ little if at all from those of nonobese persons. In the face of the reviewed prejudices and discriminations, this finding is truly surprising; according to Stunkard and Sobal (1995), it is a tribute to the resilience of the human spirit. As the following section shows, however, the stigma attached to obese individuals because of their overweight does take its toll on the emotional health of some obese people.

6.2.2 Psychological Consequences of Obesity

Discussion of the psychological consequences of obesity must be done separately for general and clinical populations (i.e., obese individuals who do not seek treatment vs. those who do).

6.2.2.1 General Population

The psychological consequences of the previously described experiences include a generally low self-esteem and severe mental distress, as well as psychological disturbances that can be so severe as to rank as mental illness, particularly in young women. In a representative study of 2063 young women in Germany, Soeder et al. (1999) found the lifetime prevalence of mental disorders (assessed with clinical structured interviews) in women with a body mass index (BMI) of 30 kg/m² or more to be over 50%. In detail, anxiety disorders and depression were predominant, whereas the number of other mental disorders was not significant. The dependence of prevalence rates on weight category is especially clear in the case of anxiety disorders. Though weaker, this pattern is also apparent in the second most common group of mental illness, namely, affective disorders.

Several studies suggest (e.g., Istvan et al., 1992; Carpenter et al., 2000) that obesity has different psychosocial consequences in males and females (in the general population). Women and teenage girls, especially, appear to be particularly vulnerable to low self-esteem and depression when they do not fit the slim body ideal seen everywhere. However, it would be incorrect to assume that a majority of obese women (or men) suffers from depression or anxiety. It seems to be a subgroup of obese individuals in the general population that shows more of these mental disorders (Stunkard et al., 1992; Friedman and Brownell, 1995).

Quality of life seems to be obesity's most significant adverse psychosocial effect. Health-related impairments in quality of life include limitations and suffering at work and in social functioning associated with illness. Health-related quality of life is most commonly measured by the Short-Form Health Survey (SF-36; Ware and Sherbourne, 1992). The SF-36 contains 36 questions that measure the following eight areas:

- Physical functioning
- Role limitations due to physical health problems
- Social functioning
- Physical pain
- General mental health
- Role limitations due to emotional problems
- Vitality
- General health perceptions

Several studies of obese individuals in the general population as well as in the clinical one show significantly more complaints of pain (low back pain); reduced vitality; shortness of breath when walking up hill; and impairment in social or occupational roles compared with nonobese controls (e.g., Barofsky et al., 1998; LePen et al., 1998; Lean et al., 1999). An increasing BMI is associated with increased physical comorbidities and with more reports of poorer physical health (Doll et al., 2000). These results suggest that many obese individuals in the general population suffer from undesired physical or social consequences due to their overweight and that this suffering reduces quality of life. Typically, the emotional consequences do not require any professional help, but they influence the individual well-being nonetheless. To give the best treatment possibilities, those who are at high risk of developing a mental disorder must be detected as soon as possible.

6.2.2.2 Clinical Populations

Earlier studies of obese individuals in clinical settings show significant psychopathology in contrast to population studies, as Wadden and Stunkard (1985) and Friedman and Brownell (1995) report in their reviews. These authors conclude that the shortcoming of these early investigations is the lack of appropriate control groups. Increased anxiety and depression are very often observed in persons who seek medical care, regardless of body weight, and are therefore not specific or unique to obese individuals. However, one very well-conducted and controlled study of psychopathology indicated that obese individuals who seek treatment are likely to have higher rates of psychopathology (emotional distress, i.e., symptoms of anxiety or depression) than obese people in the general population and nonobese persons (Fitzgibbon et al., 1993). In addition to mood disorders, obese individuals in clinical settings are more likely to suffer from body dissatisfaction and a specific eating disorder, namely, binge eating disorder (BED).

6.2.2.2.1 Body Image

Regarding the widespread prevalence of weight-related prejudice, one might expect all obese persons to suffer from their physical appearance and disparagement of the body image. However, such is not the case, although body image dissatisfaction is more common in obese persons than is binge eating (Cargill et al., 1999). The disturbance of the body image most often occurs in young women of middle and upper middle socioeconomic status (Stunkard and Sobal, 1995). The disturbance is generally confined to persons who have suffered from obesity since childhood; adolescence appears to be the highest risk period for developing these problems. Although obese women appear to experience significantly greater body image dissatisfaction than normal-weight controls, a great majority does not suffer under clinically significant distress. However a small minority of obese individuals who seek treatment do suffer from severe body image dissatisfaction related to clinically significant depression or related complications (Sarwer et al., 1998). Further studies are needed to investigate the possible factors contributing to the development of severe body image dissatisfaction. Some primary findings indicate that a childhood history of weight-related teasing by peers (Grilo et al., 1994) and the presence of binge eating disorder are risk factors for the specific etiology (Mussell et al., 1996; French et al., 1999).

6.2.2.2.2 Binge Eating Disorder

A second psychological disorder that occurs with increased frequency among obese individuals is binge eating. This disorder is so far not an officially recognized eating disorder; rather, it is one example within the EDNOS (eating disorder not otherwise specified) category of DSM-IV-TR (American Psychiatric Association [APA], 2000). A set of diagnostic criteria has been provided for further study. These criteria include frequent and regular binges (an objectively large amount of food with an associated sense of loss of control over eating) without the regular, inappropriate compensatory behaviors characteristic of bulimia nervosa and significant distress and discomfort about and during binge eating. For the full criteria for binge eating disorder, see Table 6.1.

TABLE 6.1

Research Criteria for Binge Eating Disorder

A.	*Recurrent episodes of binge eating. An episode of binge eating is characterized by both of the following:* In a discrete period of time (e.g., within any 2-hour period), eating an amount of food definitely larger than most people would eat in a similar period of time under similar circumstances. A sense of lack of control over eating during the episodes (e.g., a feeling that one cannot stop eating or control what or how much one is eating).
B.	*Binge-eating episodes are associated with three (or more) of the following:* Eating much more rapidly than normal Eating until feeling uncomfortably full Eating large amounts of food when not feeling physically hungry Eating alone because of being embarrassed by how much one is eating Feeling disgusted with oneself, depressed, or very guilty after overeating
C.	*Marked distress regarding binge eating is present.*
D.	*Binge eating occurs, on average, at least 2 days a week for 6 months.* The method of determining frequency differs from that used for bulimia nervosa; future research should address whether the preferred method of setting a frequency threshold is counting the number of days on which binges occur or counting the number of episodes of binge eating.
E.	*Binge eating is not associated with the regular use of inappropriate compensatory behaviors (e.g., purging, fasting, excessive exercise) and does not occur exclusively during the course of anorexia nervosa or bulimia nervosa.*

Source: American Psychiatric Association (APA). *Diagnostic and Statistical Manual of Mental Disorders*, 4th ed., text revision. Washington, D.C.: American Psychiatric Association, 2000.

The prevalence of binge eating disorder shows widely varying estimates. Studies based upon self-report questionnaires (e.g., Spitzer et al., 1992) showed that about 30% of obese people seeking treatment for their obesity had binge eating disorder, with the disorder about 1.5 times more common in overweight women than in overweight men. In contrast, interview-based studies of treatment-seeking obese individuals found a lower prevalence of about 10% (e.g., Stunkard et al., 1996) and in the general population the prevalence was about 2% (Bruce and Agras, 1992; Spitzer et al., 1992).

With increasing degrees of overweight, the prevalence of binge eating disorder is increasing (Telch et al., 1988). Persons with binge eating disorder have an earlier onset of overweight and dieting (Marcus et al., 1992; Yanovski, 1993) and show a greater psychopathology (especially affective and anxiety disorders) than those obese people without binge eating (Mitchell and Mussell, 1995; Marcus et al., 1996). The possibilities for the treatment of binge eating disorder are described in one of the following sections.

6.2.2.2.3 *Psychosocial Status of Extremely Obese Individuals*

What is happening to the psychological status of extremely obese individuals? Concerning the medical consequences; the likelihood of adverse health consequences increases with greater BMI, i.e., obese people with a BMI × 40 kg/m² have at least a twofold greater risk of fatal and nonfatal myocardial infarction than those with a BMI of 27 to 29 kg/m² and at least a fourfold greater risk than individuals with a BMI of 19 to 22 kg/m² (Manson et al., 1995). One can assume that morbidly obese individuals are at greater risk for adverse psychological consequences of their obesity because of the greater prejudice and discrimination to which they are probably subjected. This assumption is confirmed by a study of Sullivan et al. (1993), in which extremely obese people reported significantly poorer mental well-being than moderately obese individuals.

In addition to this decreased general well-being, obese individuals with a BMI ≥ 40 kg/m² have significantly more symptoms of depression and a lower self-esteem than obese patients with a BMI ≤ 40 kg/m² (Wadden et al., 2002). A study by Rand and Macgregor (1991) showed the enormous perceived liability of severely obese persons: in this study these perceptions were quantified by an imaginative method — "owing one's disability." In this method, patients are asked a series of forced-choice questions about whether they would prefer their current disability to a variety of other handicaps. In previous tests of this method, 62 to 95% of respondents selected their own disability when it was randomly paired with other severe disabilities. Obesity was a striking exception; when severely obese persons who had successfully maintained a 45-kg weight loss for more than 3 years were investigated, not a single patient preferred his or her obesity to being deaf, dyslexic, diabetic, or having heart disease. Leg amputation was preferred by 91.5% and legal blindness by 89.4%. When asked to choose between being normal weight or a severely obese multimillionaire, all patients said that they would prefer to be normal weight.

The previous section showed that a great majority of obese persons appear to have essentially normal psychological functioning, despite their daily exposure to weight-related prejudice and discrimination in a Western society that attributes beauty, attractiveness, health, and success only to thinness. However, among obese persons who show up in the clinical setting, approximately 10 to 20% suffer from clinically relevant symptoms of depression; negative body image; binge eating disorder; or decreased health-related quality of life. Those with extreme obesity are at a higher risk of suffering even more from these possible negative consequences of obesity.

From this point of view, obesity seems to be a risk factor for the occurrence of mental disorders. For the conclusion of this causal link, it must be demonstrated that being overweight precedes the mental disturbance and is causally related to it. The findings of Soeder et al. (1999) that obese women did not show an increased prevalence of mental disorders during their childhood and adolescence could be important to underscore the assumed causal link. If obesity is a consequence of an increased susceptibility to mental disorders, the prevalence of mental illness during childhood must be increased in obese individuals. The fact that this is not the case suggests that the increased frequency of mental illness reported in obese people is a consequence rather than a cause of obesity.

6.3 What to Do against Negative Psychosocial Consequences of Obesity?

The negative psychosocial consequences of obesity could be an indication for intervention, depending on the degree to which they contribute to individual suffering. For example, measures could be taken to break down prejudices against obesity and to counter the prevailing ideal of slimness. These objectives could be pursued via social interaction. Of course, establishing a new and healthier ideal of body weight and changing people's negative attitudes towards obesity takes a long time and is probably no immediate help for the obese individual. Developing more resilience against prevailing prejudices by changing their judgments of their obesity and its associated dysfunctional cognitions about their body and themselves could be more helpful to obese individuals.

Of course the treatment of obesity is valuable because it is characterized by the negative medical and psychosocial consequences. The following section will focus on treatment possibilities for obesity and their possible associated negative consequences. The treatment of obesity thus can also include aspects of social skills training (e.g., refusing to have negative attitudes toward obese people); changing dysfunctional cognitions about one's person and body; enhancing self-esteem; changing eating psychopathology (e.g., binge eating disorder); or modifying body image dissatisfaction.

6.3.1 Treatment of Obesity

A substantial body of evidence supports the use of behavior therapy in treatment of obesity (Wing, 1998). It reliably results in an average weight reduction of about 10% of the initial weight (among completers). A weight loss thought to result in clinically significant health benefits, this means even a slight reduction of 5 to 10% leads to a definite and medically relevant improvement in the major risk factors associated with overweight (Tremblay et al., 1999). However, the lost weight is just as likely to be regained over the following 3 years (Perri, 1998).

Behavior treatment of obesity is usually delivered in group settings, presented as a series of preplanned lessons and involving weekly meetings for 16 to 24 weeks with a series of less frequent meetings thereafter. The principal components of such program usually include self-monitoring of eating; stimulus control; problem solving; cognitive restructuring; social support; nutrition education; physical activity; and use of reinforcement contingencies (Wing, 1998; Brownell, 2000; Wadden and Foster, 2000). The effectiveness of such program is well documented, not only in the clinical setting but also in general practice (Munsch et al., 2003). Many of the behavioral programs for obesity are presented by a team of specialists (e.g., behavior therapist, nutritionist, exercise physiologist). Behavioral treatment is very goal-oriented; participants are given homework assignments specified in terms easily put into operation and measured (Wadden et al., 2002).

The internationally accepted definition of successful weight loss of about 10% is practically always contrary to the patient's wishes. It is critically important, therefore, that even slight weight loss be maintained over the long term. Leading obesity researchers suggest that, in order to reach this higher-level aim, after an achieved weight reduction of 10 to 15%, patients should actively be discouraged from losing more weight and focus on strategies to maintain the weight loss in the future (Cooper and Fairburn, 2001). This treatment approach is designed to minimize the weight regain that generally follows weight loss. Cooper and Fairburn (2001) describe three main issues to be addressed: the treatment must

- Help patients accept and value the weight reduction that they have achieved
- Encourage the adoption of weight maintenance and not weight loss as a goal
- Help patients acquire and then use the behavioral skills and cognitive responses required for successful long-term weight control

For the objective of long-term weight control, obese individuals must accept first that obesity is a chronic problem and that only strategies and measures that minimize restrictions on the enjoyment of food and life in general will help to deal with this problem. In other words, long-term weight control cannot be achieved with strategies of renunciation, abnegation, self-control, and suffering. Instead, it is important that obese individuals are able to enjoy their lives, including eating and drinking. It is clear that weight reduction and weight maintenance are not the same, but rather require different mechanisms; different modes of behavior; and different strategies. In order to achieve the goal of weight maintenance, adequate motivation of the patients is essential. How is this to be done?

Typically, most obese individuals have a long history of failed attempts to lose weight, which implies frequent weight loss and weight regain — the so called weight cycling — and they have unrealistic goals for their weight reduction. These goals are not harmless because they lead to disparagement of realistically achievable progress and to a negation of achieved successes that are judged inadequate or unsuccessful. A recent study by Teixeira et al. (2002) shows that individuals who indicated larger weight loss as "acceptable" or "happy" weight (i.e., subjects who evaluated smaller weight loss as less satisfying)

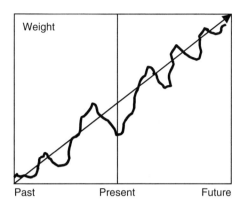

FIGURE 6.1
Normal course of weight change in a typical obese patient.

lost significantly less weight by the end of a weight reduction program than subjects with less stringent evaluations. These results were independent of baseline body weight. Therefore, a very important feature of successful treatment is the motivation of the patient to achieve realistic goals. Goals of weight loss must be realistic in terms of weight loss and in terms of the time required to achieve the specific weight loss (e.g., losing 6 kg in 6 months instead of 20 kg in 6 months).

To set realistic goals, individual patterns of weight changes must first be assessed. Plotting the time course and fluctuations of the patient's weight on a graph can do this. After entering the time course of the patient's weight to the current date, the probable future pattern of weight development without treatment can be entered on the graph. Figure 6.1 shows a typical time course of weight for an obese person. Based on this individual graph, reasons and causes for the course of the weight can be discussed and false assumptions can be corrected.

In a next step, the patient's wishes concerning the terms of a successful treatment should be discussed. Once again, the desired course of weight can be plotted on a graph, upon which any unrealistic expectations or wishes show up. Figure 6.2 is a typical wish that obese patients hope to achieve during the course of obesity treatment. Of course, all unrealistic expectations must be discussed before going on to the next step. During the discussion of realistic and probable goals of weight loss, it must be explained to the patient that even a 5% reduction of weight attributes to a medically worthwhile degree of success. With suitable

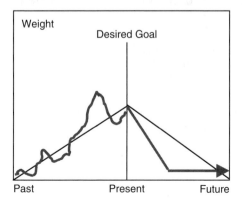

FIGURE 6.2
Results that obese patients typically hope to achieve during obesity therapy.

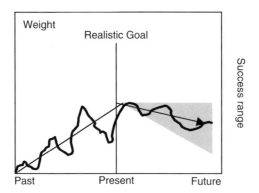

FIGURE 6.3
Results that obesity treatment can realistically be expected to produce.

strategies, as much as 10 to 15% weight reduction can be achieved. The graphical representation shown in Figure 6.3 can be useful to underline the importance of long-term success instead of rapid short-term weight loss (which would be regained even faster).

Before the action phase with all the preceding therapeutic implements can start, the information on the origin, causality, and maintenance of obesity should be repeated and summarized. Part of this discussion should be the fact that

- A genetic predisposition to fat storage exists.
- This genetic predisposition is revealed only in the presence of high-fat nutrition and a sedentary life-style.
- If fat stores are to be broken down, fat intake must be reduced.
- Exercise increases the body's energy consumption, i.e., the total metabolic rate.
- A lasting reduction in body weight can be achieved only slowly and in small steps.

Next steps in the treatment of obesity can be started when this first phase of motivation and goal setting is concluded. If long-term success is to be achieved, traditional ideas on weight reduction must be changed. First, genetic predisposition must be taken into account. The individual attitude to one's obesity is important in this respect: the patient learns to accept his or her overweight as a condition determined by fate in which any unnecessary and surplus food consumption is used to build up energy reserves, i.e., fat. This does not mean that the patient is powerless or without any possibilities to change body weight; instead, he or she can influence this fate by adequate behavioral strategies rather than by modifying the genetic predisposition.

The core element of modern behavioral treatment programs for obesity is a flexible control of eating. This control contradicts well-known crash diets based upon a rigid control that require no food or only certain foods be eaten over a certain period of time. Flexible control over eating makes it possible to change eating habits and behavior as open-ended, long-term strategies with possibilities for compensation. All types of food may be eaten; the only restriction is that fat consumption should be normalized or reduced. With this type of eating, the typical craving for favored, but forbidden, food rarely arises.

6.3.1.1   *Increasing Physical Activity*

In addition to fat reduction, the increase of physical activity is important for the reduction of weight and maintenance of the achieved weight loss. Many studies and recent guidelines show that physical activity plays a role in the etiology and treatment of overweight and obesity (Bouchard and Blair, 1999). It is very difficult for people to lose large amounts of weight, or at least to lose weight quickly by exercise alone. Even though physical activity is not the most effective method of losing weight, it appears to be crucial for maintaining weight loss (McGuire et al., 1998).

Although the immediate effects of exercise are limited, the long-term cumulative effect of small changes in the activity level can be beneficial. Increased physical activity and cardiorespiratory fitness have significant benefits for obese and overweight individuals that extend far beyond the contributions of exercise to weight loss and maintenance. Fit men in each fatness stratum have a substantially lower risk of cardiovascular disease and all-cause mortality than unfit men in the same fatness stratum, i.e., fit but obese men have a lower mortality risk than lean men who are unfit (Blair and Leermakers, 2002). Unfortunately, up till now this positive effect has only been proven for men and not for women.

An increase in physical activity does not mean participating in competitive sports, but rather increasing (daily) life-style physical activity. Various public health recommendations can be summarized to create a consensus public health recommendation for physical activity (Blair and Leermakers, 2002): all sedentary adults should accumulate at least 30 minutes of at least moderate-intensity physical activity over the course of most, preferably all, days of the week. These recommendations include the concept of intermittent activity (e.g., activity does not need to be done all in one setting), and a focus on moderate-intensity activities. The advantage of these recommendations is that it allows for innumerable possibilities for increasing physical activities. Incorporating physical activity into everyday life is already beneficial for health and weight maintenance; in other words, sedentary individuals can be encouraged to increase their physical activities in their daily lives.

The benefits of regular physical activity are well known but, although this knowledge exists, increasing physical activity represents a big obstacle for many individuals (regardless of body weight). Overweight and obese persons face a combination of physical and psychosocial burdens when they begin to exercise. For one reason, the excess weight makes exercising understandably more difficult and another often mentioned reason is negative feelings about exercise due to past experiences. Many obese individuals report having been teased as children or selected last for teams; they may be embarrassed by their lack of cardiovascular fitness or coordination, or their appearance when dressed for exercising. All the possible obstacles must be kept in mind when advising obese people to increase their physical activity and the recommendation alone may not be sufficient for a successful exercise adherence. It may be necessary to work with the person to overcome these barriers in order to improve exercise adherence. How is this to be done?

Several studies have investigated the effectiveness of interventions of physical activity. For example, studies by Andersen et al. (1999) and Perri et al. (1997) addressed the question of whether a supervised group exercise program, conducted at a designated location, was more or less effective than a home-based or life-style approach to physical activity. The group setting could be favored because of greater social support from peers and more guidance and reinforcement from the group leader. However, the extra time spent in traveling to the exercise location, as well as the fact that exercise lessons are held at a designated time, could limit the long-term appeal of this approach. The results of these studies suggest that a home-based life-style approach or a supervised group exercise program can be used in the initial phase of treatment for obesity; however, the home-based condition in the Perri et al. (1997) study stands out as the best long-term outcome across these two studies (regarding exercise adherence and weight loss).

In a study by Jeffery et al. (1998), the use of personal trainers and financial incentives was evaluated as strategies to improve exercise adherence and long-term weight loss. Personal trainers went walking with the obese individuals and made phone calls to remind them to exercise. Financial incentives ranged from $1 to $3 per bout of walking. Although these strategies increased attendance at supervised exercise lessons, neither strategy improved weight loss. Consistent with the finding from Perri et al. (1997), the control group, which received a home-based exercise regimen, showed better maintenance of weight loss at follow-up than the other conditions.

When trying to maximize exercise adherence in obese individuals, the following recommendations can be very helpful (for the full set of recommendations, see Grilo et al., 1993):

- General principles
  - Sensitivity to psychological and physical barriers
  - Emphasis on consistency and enjoyment (not amount and type)
  - Beginning at a person's individual level of fitness
  - Defining routine daily activities as "exercise"
- Specific interventions
  - Providing information about importance of physical activity, including psychological benefits and possible barriers
  - Maximizing daily activities such as walking, using stairs instead of escalators
  - Introducing self-monitoring, feedback, and goal-setting techniques
  - Identifying important targets other than weight loss, including physical changes, increased endurance, lowered resting heart rate
  - For maintenance and relapse prevention, identifying possible high-risk situations for skipping exercise (e.g., stressful times, busy schedule), developing plans to cope with such high-risk situations, and knowing that one day lapsed is not failure

6.3.1.2   Enhancing Self-Esteem

The previously mentioned prejudices and discriminations against obese people stem from beliefs that are usually inaccurate or simply wrong. Not only are obese people regarded or judged as physically unattractive, but they are also assumed to be weak of character. Independently of the wrongness of these negative assumptions, they can have a worse effect on the self-esteem of obese individuals. Being judged only on the basis of one's weight and size leads not surprisingly to a severely wounded self-esteem — but how to pump up the self-esteem of obese people? As Johnson (2002) describes, this is not an easy task because many obese individuals believe that the only way to repair their self-esteem is by losing a great amount of weight (not just a modest amount). They have been conditioned by Western society to believe that they are not entitled to self-esteem without being thin or, at least, normal weight. This might be the most unfortunate aspect of all because most obese people will never be thin in a healthy way.

So far little scientific research has been conducted on how to improve the self-esteem of obese individuals. The ideal solution would be to eliminate size and weight prejudices. Of course, the culture must change so that being overweight is no longer a stigma, but as Quinn and Crocker (1998) conclude, a move by culture in that direction is not evidenced. In other words, overweight individuals must take responsibility for their self-esteem and research findings exist that can differentiate specific characteristics distinguishing overweight persons with good self-esteem from those with poor self-esteem.

The interesting question concerns what makes some overweight individuals more "resilient" to psychological distress caused by the stigma of being overweight. Overweight persons with this resilience do not view other overweight individuals with disgust or dislike, and they do not base their self-regard on others' approval; in this way, they can build a more solid and stable self-esteem on self-appraisal. Resilient overweight persons realize that not all outcomes are deserved and not all things (including size and weight) are under full personal control. This viewpoint allows people to realize that, despite their very best efforts, the desired outcome may not be achievable and that this is not due to their personal failure and is not their fault (Crandall, 1994). A further characteristic of this subset of overweight individuals concerns the ability to reject or ignore society's dictates about ideal and acceptable body weight and to focus on other factors besides body weight and size, such as personal style and presentation, when evaluating their attractiveness (Heatherton et al., 1995; Parker et al., 1995).

These research findings undermine the importance of self-image and give many hints about possibilities for individual cognitive restructuring of dysfunctional beliefs. Johnson (2002) summarizes 20 suggestions given to overweight individuals on how to help heal their self-esteem. For example, she suggests stopping comparing oneself to others, especially comparisons that destroy self-esteem concerning body image. If comparing is inevitable, the comparison must be done with real people and not media images because, by looking at everyday people, the different shapes and sizes that nature creates can be observed.

Another suggestion is to focus on positive attributes and to contrast the small part of appearance plays in total individuality. When focusing only on weight and shape, the individual strengths, talents, and accomplishments are forgotten. Another frequent dysfunctional opinion of overweight persons is to put anything on hold while waiting to lose weight. Postponing personally relevant activities and life challenges to the time of possible slimness raises the chance of never achieving many personal goals and aspirations. Most of the time, there is no valid reason not to pursue goals and activities at one's actual weight. These are only a few possible dysfunctional beliefs and attitudes that can decrease self-esteem. For further reading, see Johnson (2001, 2002).

6.3.2 Treatment of Binge Eating Disorder

As mentioned previously, a minority of obese individuals suffer from clinically significant binge eating problems — the frequent and regular intake of an objectively large amount of food with an associated sense of loss of control over eating without inappropriate compensatory behaviors. Obesity and disordered eating are associated with significant morbidity; therefore, effective treatment for obese binge eating patients is needed. Treatment approaches for this disorder have often followed the precedent of treatments for bulimia nervosa (Fairburn et al. 1993). The most distinctive have involved the use of cognitive–behavior therapy. The best evaluated treatment approaches are cognitive–behavior therapy; interpersonal therapy; dialectical behavior therapy; and behavioral weight reduction programs.

6.3.2.1 *Cognitive–Behavior Therapy (CBT)*

The CBT treatment approach of binge eating disorder focuses on the eating disturbance and the associated problematic cognitions and attitudes toward eating, body shape, and weight. Food intake should be neither over- nor under-restrictive and physical activity should be increased during treatment. Several studies have shown the effectiveness of CBT for significantly reducing binge eating (Wilfley and Cohen, 1997). The primary goal in CBT is the control of binge eating, which for many researchers is necessary before obese persons can lose weight. That is, efforts to reduce weight should be postponed until binge eating is controlled.

6.3.2.2   Interpersonal Therapy (IPT)

Wilfley et al. (1993) modified the interpersonal therapy for the treatment of binge eating disorder following the precedent of bulimia nervosa. Interpersonal therapy has been examined as an alternative treatment to target binge eating by directly addressing the social and interpersonal deficits observed among these individuals. This treatment approach also produces a clinically significant reduction in binge eating (Wilfley et al., 1993, 2000).

A randomized comparison of group cognitive–behavioral therapy and group interpersonal therapy for the treatment of overweight individuals with binge eating disorder showed that IPT is a viable alternative to CBT in reducing binge eating. Both treatments showed initial and long-term efficacy for the core and related symptoms of binge eating disorder (Wilfley et al., 2002). Despite the effective reduction in binge eating, neither CBT nor IPT produced significant weight loss. How can this be explained, considering that the binges are successfully reduced and thus energy intake should be decreased? One possible explanation is that energy intake during binges may be distributed to the non binge-eating caloric intake. The other assumption is that the energy intake of the binges is not as excessive as expected and therefore has only a small or even no influence on body weight.

6.3.2.3   Dialectical Behavior Therapy (DBT)

Telch et al. (2001) adopted dialectical behavior therapy for binge eating disorder. This treatment model postulates that binge eating serves to regulate affect. A considerable amount of research evidence supporting the affect regulation model of binge eating exists (for review, see Polivy and Herman, 1993). DBT, a treatment found to be effective for borderline personality disorder (Linehan et al. 1991), specifically targets emotion regulation by teaching adaptive skills to enhance emotion regulation capabilities. Compared to no treatment, the group DBT is better in eliminating binge eating (Telch et al., 2001), but unfortunately the comparison to any other treatment condition is so far outstanding.

6.3.2.4   Behavioral Weight Loss Programs

Interestingly, behavioral weight reduction programs are also effective in reducing binges in binge eating disorder patients (e.g., Agras et al., 1994; Marcus et al., 1995; Gladis et al., 1998). This effectiveness is surprising, considering that such programs do not focus on the core symptom of binge eating disorder, namely, the binges. These results are encouraging because with this treatment approach two goals in the treatment of obese binge eating disorder patients can be achieved: reduction of binges and of body weight. The crucial point so far is the question about the long-term results of behavioral weight loss programs for binge eating disorder individuals. The long-term course of reduced weight is well known, but the long-term effects of behavioral weight loss programs on binge eating are not known.

From a clinical viewpoint, it appears that cognitive–behavioral therapy; interpersonal therapy; dialectical behavior therapy; and behavioral weight reduction programs may have the same effect on individuals with binge eating disorder. These findings show the possibility for a treatment of binge eating disorder that does not especially and directly focus on eating behaviors. Given the marked differences among all these treatment approaches, it seems likely that differential predictors of outcome might be identified; this would allow more precise triage of individuals into one or the other treatment. Further studies must be conducted to answer this clinically important question.

6.3.3 Treatment of Body Dissatisfaction

Cognitive-behavioral treatment approaches to obesity such as the one from Cooper and Fairburn (2001, 2002) have integrated special lessons concerning body image. The goal is to identify individual concerns of body image and to change possible inappropriate cognitions or behavior. Possible dissatisfaction with shape or appearance that is not a problem for the individual is very common; it becomes clinically relevant when it affects general self-evaluation and functioning in everyday life. Compared to normal-weight individuals, obese persons overestimate or distort their body size more; are more dissatisfied and preoccupied with their appearance; and avoid more social situations due to their appearance (Cash, 1990). As Rosen et al. (1995) summarize, all three components of body image — perception, cognition/affect, and behavior — can be more troublesome for obese individuals.

Rosen (1997) developed techniques and strategies for addressing problems with body image. Such strategies include an overview of body image and the social aspects of being overweight in a weight-conscious society. People learn that body image is a psychological construct and that the two variables, physical appearance and body image, can be independent; in other words, body image can be changed without changing physical appearance. A further goal is to recognize and question society's weight and shape ideal and learn to protect and to distance from this social pressure to be thin. Another topic to address is possible avoidance and body-checking behavior: the goal is to learn to tolerate distress during exposure of one's physical appearance and to reduce and eliminate checking behavior that promotes preoccupation with the appearance (e.g., decreasing weighing, inspecting the body in the mirror). A further goal in the treatment of body dissatisfaction is to identify and restructure maladaptive assumptions about body shape. This way of thinking plays an important role in maintaining a poor body image because, despite its excessively critical, and therefore in most cases false, nature, it tends to be accepted as true.

The administration of such strategies and techniques is effective for treating negative body image (Rosen et al., 1995). Although helping obese individuals to feel less negative about their shape and body weight is strongly emphasized, the goal is also to encourage positive acceptance of appearance. This is important regarding the life-long character of obesity and the moderate weight reduction possibilities in most cases.

6.4 Summary and Conclusions

As Brownell (1991) summarizes, modern society searches for the perfect body. Today's aesthetic ideal is extremely thin and, superimposed on this, is the need to be physically fit. People see this ideal because of expected health benefits and because of what the ideal symbolizes in Western society especially: acceptance, self-control, and success. Overweight and obese individuals do not fit this aesthetic ideal, which can have possible negative consequences. The psychosocial status of overweight and obese individuals is quite heterogeneous. The great majority of these persons appear to have essentially normal psychological functioning, despite their daily exposure to weight-related prejudice and discrimination in a society that glorifies thinness.

Several studies indicate that overweight and obesity during adolescence and young adulthood have important social and economic consequences that are more severe for women than for men and greater than those associated with a variety of other chronic conditions during adolescence. These results remain the same, even after adjustments for socioeconomic origins, ability, or socioeconomic attainment. Despite widespread weight-related prejudice and discrimination, the majority of obese and overweight individuals are resilient to negative consequences. However, among persons encountered in clinical settings, approximately 10 to 20% are likely to suffer from clinically significant symptoms of depression, negative body image, or impaired health-related quality of life. These problems are most likely to occur in individuals with extreme obesity (BMI > 40 kg/m^2); in women; and in those suffering from binge eating disorder.

In addition to a great majority of obese and overweight individuals with an enormous amount of resilience, a clinical subgroup exists that is suffering significantly from the stigma associated with obesity and the poor fit to the aesthetic ideal of Western society. Unfortunately, two crucial assumptions are associated with body weight and shape: (1) the body is infinitely malleable with only the right combination of weight reduction programs, exercises, and eating plans; and (2) vast rewards await persons who reach this goal, i.e., when one becomes slimmer, fitter, and more attractive, life will improve dramatically in all areas.

Moreover, being overweight differs from other chronic conditions in its visibility. Unlike other attributes such as skin color or sex, body weight is regarded as under voluntary personal control; obese and overweight individuals are held responsible for their body weight and possible changes. However, research on the etiology of obesity and overweight has shown that, besides behavioral variables, biological variables, particularly genetics, have great influence on body weight and shape; in other words, how much a person can change body weight and shape has its limits. This fact places the aesthetic ideal in conflict with physiology and contributes to stigmatization of obese and overweight individuals.

The actual possibilities for treatment of obesity are promising regarding the positive consequences on physical health, even though no miraculous treatments will make obese individuals thin and deliver them from stigma. Thus, in addition to the effort to reduce body weight in a healthy and reasonable way, the stigma itself must be attacked — on the one hand, helping obese individuals to cope with the stigmatization of obesity and to establish reasonable weight and shape goals, and on the other, educating the public to the etiology of obesity, based on biological and psychological realities rather than cultural ideals or pressure.

References

Agras, W.S., Telch, C.F., Arnow, B., Eldredge, K., Wilfley, D.E., Raeburn, E.D., Henderson, J. and Marnell, M. (1994). Weight loss, cognitive, behavioral and desipramine treatments in binge eating disorder: an additive design. *Behav. Ther.*, 25, 225–238.

American Psychiatric Association (APA) (2000). Diagnostic and Statistical Manual of Mental Disorders, 4th ed., text revision, Washington, D.C.: American Psychiatric Association.

Andersen, R.E., Wadden, T.A., Bartlett, S.J., Zemel, B., Verde, T.J. and Franckowiak, S.C. (1999). Effects of lifestyle activity vs. structured aerobic exercise in obese women: a randomized trial. *JAMA*, 281(4), 335–340.

Barofsky, I., Fontaine, K.R. and Cheskin, L.J. (1998). Pain in the obese: impact on health-related quality-of-life. *Ann. Behav. Med.*, 19(4), 408–410.

Blair, S.N. and Leermakers, E.A. (2002). Exercise and weight management. In T.A. Wadden and A.J. Stunkard (Eds.), *Handbook of Obesity Treatment* (pp. 283–300). New York: Guilford Press.

Bouchard, C. and Blair, S.N. (1999). Roundtable introduction: introductory comments for the consensus on physical activity and obesity. *Med. Sci. Sports Exercise*, 31(11 Suppl.), S498–S501.

Bray, G.A., Bouchard, C. and James, W.P.T. (1998). *Handbook of Obesity*. New York: Marcel Dekker.

Brownell, K.D. (1991). Dieting and the search for the perfect body: where physiology and culture collide. *Behav. Ther.*, 22, 1–12.

Brownell, K.D. (2000). *The LEARN Program for Weight Management* 2000. Dallas: American Health.

Bruce, B. and Agras, W.S. (1992). Binge eating in females: a population-based investigation. *Int. J. Eating Disorders*, 12, 365–373.

Cargill, B.R., Clark, M.M., Pera, V., Niaura, R.S. and Abrams, D.B. (1999). Binge eating, body image, depression, and self-efficacy in an obese clinical population. *Obes. Res.*, 7(4), 379–386.

Carpenter, K.M., Hasin, D.S., Allison, D.B. and Faith, M.S. (2000). Relationships between obesity and DSM-IV major depressive disorder, suicide ideation, and suicide attempts: results from a general population study. *Am. J. Public Health*, 90(2), 251–257.

Cash, T.F. (1990). The psychology of physical appearance: aesthetics, attributes and images. In T.F. Cash and T. Pruzinsky (Eds.), *Body Images: Development, Deviance, and Change* (pp. 51–79). New York: Guilford Press.

Cooper, Z. and Fairburn, C.G. (2001). A new cognitive behavioral approach to the treatment of obesity. *Behav. Res. Ther.*, 39(5), 499–511.

Cooper, Z. and Fairburn, C.G. (2002). Cognitive-behavioral treatment of obesity. In A.J. Stunkard and T.A. Wadden (Eds.), Handbook of obesity and treatment (pp. 465–479). New York: Guilford Press.

Crandall, C.S. (1994). Prejudice against fat people: ideology and self-interest. *J. Pers. Soc. Psychol.*, 66(5), 882–894.

Doll, H.A., Petersen, S.E. and Stewart–Brown, S.L. (2000). Obesity and physical and emotional well-being: associations between body mass index, chronic illness, and the physical and mental components of the SF-36 questionnaire. *Obes. Res.*, 8(2), 160–170.

Fairburn, C.G., Marcus, M.D. and Wilson, G.T. (1993). Cognitive-behavioral therapy for binge eating and bulimia nervosa: a comprehensive treatment manual. In C.G. Fairburn and G.T. Wilson (Eds.), *Binge Eating: Nature, Assessment, and Treatment* (pp. 361–404). New York: Guilford Press.

Field, A.E., Barnoya, J. and Colditz, G.A. (2002). Epidemiology and health and economic consequences of obesity. In T.A. Wadden and A.J. Stunkard (Eds.), *Handbook of Obesity Treatment*. pp. 3–18. New York: Guilford Press.

Fitzgibbon, M.L., Stolley, M.R. and Kirschenbaum, D.S. (1993). Obese people who seek treatment have different characteristics than those who do not seek treatment. *Health Psychol.*, 12(5), 342–345.

Flegal, K.M., Carroll, M.D., Kuczmarski, R.J. and Johnson, C.L. (1998). Overweight and obesity in the United States: prevalence and trends, 1960–1994. *Int. J. Obesity Relat. Metab. Disorders*, 22, 39–47.

French, S.A., Jeffery, R.W., Sherwood, N.E. and Neumark–Sztainer, D. (1999). Prevalence and correlates of binge eating in a nonclinical sample of women enrolled in a weight gain prevention program. *Int. J. Obes. Relat. Metab. Disord.*, 23(6), 576–585.

Friedman, M.A. and Brownell, K.D. (1995). Psychological correlates of obesity: moving to the next research generation. *Psychol. Bull.*, 117(1), 3–20.

Frieze, I.H., Olson, J.E. and Good, D.C. (1994). Perceived and actual discrimination in the salaries of male and female managers. *J. Appl. Social Psychol.*, 20, 46–67.

Garner, D.M. and Wooley, S.C. (1991). Confronting the failure of behavioral and dietary treatments for obesity. *Clin. Psychol. Rev.*, 11, 729–780.

Garner, D.M., Garfinkel, P.E., Schwartz, D. and Thompson, M. (1980). Cultural expectations of thinness in women. *Psychol. Rep.*, 47(2), 483–491.

Gladis, M.M., Wadden, T.A., Vogt, R., Foster, G., Kuehnel, R.H. and Bartlett, S.J. (1998). Behavioral treatment of obese binge eaters: do they need different care? *J. Psychosom. Res.*, 44(3–4), 375–384.

Goodrick, G.K. and Foreyt, J.P. (1991). Why treatments for obesity don't last. *J. Am. Diet. Assoc.*, 91(10), 1243–1247.

Gortmaker, S.L., Mist, A., Perrin, J.M., Sobol, A.M. and Dietz, W.H. (1993). Social and economic consequences of overweight in adolescence and young adulthood. *N. Engl. J. Med.*, 329, 1008–1012.

Grilo, C.M., Brownell, K.D. and Stunkard, A.J. (1993). The metabolic and psychological importance of exercise in weight control. In A.J. Stunkard and T.A. Wadden (Eds.), *Obesity: Theory and Therapy* (pp. 253–273). New York: Raven Press.

Grilo, C.M., Wilfley, D.E., Brownell, K.D. and Rodin, J. (1994). Teasing, body image, and self-esteem in a clinical sample of obese women. *Addict. Behav.*, 19(4), 443–450.

Heatherton, T.F., Kiwan, D. and Hebl, M.R. (1995). The stigma of obesity in women: the difference is black and white. Paper presented at the annual meeting of the American Psychological Association, New York.

Istvan, J., Zavela, K. and Weidner, G. (1992). Body weight and psychological distress in NHANES I. *Int. J. Obes. Relat. Metab. Disord.*, 16(12), 999–1003.

Jeffery, R.W., Wing, R.R., Thorson, C. and Burton, L.R. (1998). Use of personal trainers and financial incentives to increase exercise in a behavioral weight-loss program. *J. Consult. Clin. Psychol.*, 66(5), 777–783.

Johnson, C. (2002). Obesity, weight management, and self-esteem. In T.A. Wadden and A.J. Stunkard (Eds.), *Handbook of Obesity and Treatment* (pp. 480–493). New York: Guilford Press.

Johnson, C.A. (2001). Self-esteem comes in all sizes: how to be happy and healthy at your natural weight. Carlsbad, CA: Gürze Books.

Lean, M.E., Han, T.S. and Seidell, J.C. (1999). Impairment of health and quality of life using new U.S. federal guidelines for the identification of obesity. *Arch. Intern. Med.*, 159(8), 837–843.

LePen, C., Levy, E., Loos, F., Banzet, M.N. and Basdevant, A. (1998). "Specific" scale compared with "generic" scale: a double measurement of the quality of life in a French community sample of obese subjects. *J. Epidemiol. Community Health*, 52, 445–450.

Linehan, M.M., Armstrong, H.E., Suarez, A., Allmon, D. and Heard, H.L. (1991). Cognitive-behavioral treatment of chronically parasuicidal borderline patients. *Arch. Gen. Psychiatry*, 48(12), 1060–1064.

Maddox, G.L., Back, K.W. and Liederman, W.R. (1968). Overweight as social deviance and disability. *J. Health Soc. Behav.*, 9(4), 287–298.

Manson, J.E., Willett, W.C., Stampfer, M.J., Colditz, G.A., Hunter, D.J., Hankinson, S.E., Hennekens, C.H. and Speizer, F.E. (1995). Body weight and mortality among women. *N. Engl. J. Med.*, 333(11), 677–685.

Marcus, M.D., Amith, D., Santelli, R. and Kaye, W. (1992). Characterization of eating disordered behavior in obese binge eaters. *Int. J. Eating Disorders*, 12, 249–255.

Marcus, M.D., Wing, R.R., Ewing, L., Kern, E., Gooding, W. and McDermott, M. (1996). Psychiatric disorders among obese binge eaters. *Int. J. Eating Disorders*, 9, 69–77.

Marcus, M.D., Wing, R.R. and Fairburn, C.G. (1995). Cognitive behavioral treatment of binge eating vs. behavioral weight control on the treatment of binge eating disorder. *Ann. Behav. Med.*, 17, S090.

McGuire, M.T., Wing, R.R., Klem, M.L., Seagle, H.M. and Hill, J.O. (1998). Long-term maintenance of weight loss: do people who lose weight through various weight loss methods use different behaviors to maintain their weight? *Int. J. Obes. Relat. Metab. Disord.*, 22(6), 572–577.

Mitchell, J.E. and Mussell, M.P. (1995). Comorbidity and binge eating disorder. *Addict. Behav.*, 20(6), 725–732.

Munsch, S., Biedert, E. and Keller, U. (2003). Evaluation of a lifestyle change programme for the treatment of obesity in general practice. *Swiss Med. Wkly.*, 133, 148–154.

Mussell, M.P., Peterson, C.B., Weller, C.L., Crosby, R.D., de Zwaan, M. and Mitchell, J.E. (1996). Differences in body image and depression among obese women with and without binge eating disorder. *Obes. Res.*, 4(5), 431–439.

Pargaman, D. (1969). The incidence of obesity among college students. *J. Sch. Health*, 29, 621–625.

Parker, S., Nichter, M., Vuckovic, N., Sims, C. and Rittenbaugh, C. (1995). Body image and weight concerns among African–American and white adoslescent females: differences that make a difference. *Hum. Organ.*, 54, 103–114.

Perri, M.G. (1998). The maintenance of treatment effects in the long-term management of obesity. *Clin. Psychol.: Sci. Pract.*, 5, 526–543.

Perri, M.G., Martin, A.D., Leermakers, E.A., Sears, S.F. and Notelovitz, M. (1997). Effects of group- vs. home-based exercise in the treatment of obesity. *J. Consulting Clin. Psychol.*, 65, 278–285.

Pingitore, R., Dugoni, B.L., Tindale, R.S. and Spring, B. (1994). Bias against overweight job applicants in a simulated employment interview. *J. Appl. Psychol.*, 79(6), 909–917.

Polivy, J. and Herman, C.P. (1993). Etiology of binge eating: psychological mechanisms. In C.G. Fairburn and G.T. Wilson (Eds.), *Binge Eating: Nature, Assessment and Treatment*. New York: Guilford Press.

Quinn, D. and Crocker, J. (1998). Vulnerability to the Affective Consequences of the Stigma of Overweight. San Diego, CA: Academic Press.

Rand, C.S. and Macgregor, A.M. (1990). Morbidly obese patients' perceptions of social discrimination before and after surgery for obesity. *South Med. J.*, 83(12), 1390–1395.

Rand, C.S. and Macgregor, A.M. (1991). Successful weight loss following obesity surgery and the perceived liability of morbid obesity. *Int. J. Obes.*, 15(9), 577–579.

Roehling, M.V. (1999). Weight-based discrimination in employment: psychological and legal aspects. *Personnel Psychol.*, 52, 969–1016.

Rosen, J.C. (1997). Cognitive-behavioral body image therapy. In D.M. Garner and P.E. Garfinkel (Eds.), *Handbook of Treatment for Eating Disorders* (pp. 188–201). New York: Guilford Press.

Rosen, J.C., Orsan, P. and Reiter, J. (1995). Cognitive behavior therapy for negative body image in obese women. *Behav. Ther.*, 26, 25–42.

Sarwer, D.B., Wadden, T.A. and Foster, G.D. (1998). Assessment of body image dissatisfaction in obese women: specificity, severity, and clinical significance. *J. Consult. Clin. Psychol.*, 66(4), 651–654.

Seidell, J.C. and Rissanen, A.M. (1998). Time tends in the worldwide prevalence of obesity. In C. Bouchard, G.A. Bray and W.P.T. James (Eds.), *Handbook of Obesity.* (pp. 79–91). New York: Marcel Dekker.

Sobal, J. (1995). Social influences on body weight. In K.D. Brownell and C.G. Fairburn (Eds.), *Eating Disorders and Obesity — a Comprehensive Handbook* (pp. 73–77). New York: Guilford Press.

Soeder, U., Margraf, J. and Becker, E. (1999). Adipositas ist oft von psychischen Störungen begleitet: Adipositas Brief.

Spitzer, R.L., Devlin, M., Walsh, B.T., Hasin, D., Wing, R., Marcus, M., Stunkard, A.J., Wadden, T.A., Yanovski, S., Agras, S., Mitchell, J. and Nonas, C. (1992). Binge eating disorder: a multisite field trial of the diagnostic criteria. *Int. J. Eating Disorders*, 11, 191–203.

Staffieri, J.R. (1967). A study of social stereotype of body image in children. *J. Pers. Soc. Psychol.*, 7(1), 101–104.

Stunkard, A.J., Berkowitz, R., Wadden, T.A., Tanrikut, C., Reiss, E. and Young, L. (1996). Binge eating disorder and night eating syndrome. *Int. J. Obesity*, 20, 1–6.

Stunkard, A.J. and Sobal, J. (1995). Psychosocial consequences of obestiy. In K.D. Brownell and C.G. Fairburn (Eds.), *Eating Disorders and Obesity.* New York: Guilford Press.

Stunkard, A.J. and Wadden, T.A. (1992). Psychological aspects of severe obesity. *Am. J. Clin. Nutr.*, 55(2 Suppl), 524S–532S.

Sullivan, M., Karlsson, J., Sjostrom, L., Backman, L., Bengtsson, C., Bouchard, C., Dahlgren, S., Jonsson, E., Larsson, B., Lindstedt, S. et al. (1993). Swedish obese subjects (SOS) — an intervention study of obesity. Baseline evaluation of health and psychosocial functioning in the first 1743 subjects examined. *Int. J. Obes. Relat. Metab. Disord.*, 17(9), 503–512.

Teixeira, P.J., Going, S.B., Houtkooper, L.B., Cussler, E.C., Martin, C.J., Metcalfe, L.L., Finkenthal, N.R., Blew, R.M., Sardinha, L.B. and Lohman, T.G. (2002). Weight loss readiness in middle-aged women: psychosocial predictors of success for behavioral weight reduction. *J. Behav. Med.*, 25(6), 499–523.

Telch, C.F., Agras, W.S. and Linehan, M.M. (2001). Dialectical behavior therapy for binge eating disorder. *J. Consult. Clin. Psychol.*, 69(6), 1061–1065.

Telch, C.F., Agras, W.S. and Rossiter, F.M. (1988). Binge eating increases with increasing adiposity. *Int. J. Eating Disorders*, 7, 115–119.

Tremblay, A., Doucet, E., Imbeault, P., Mauriege, P., Despres, J.P. and Richard, D. (1999). Metabolic fitness in active reduced-obese individuals. *Obes. Res.*, 7(6), 556–563.

Visscher, T.L. and Seidell, J.C. (2001). The public health impact of obesity. *Annu. Rev. Public Health*, 22, 355–375.

Wadden, T.A. and Foster, G.D. (2000). Behavior therapy of obesity. *Med. Clin. North Am.*, 84, 441–461.

Wadden, T.A. and Osei, S. (2002). The treatment of obesity: an overview. In T.A. Wadden and A.J. Stunkard (Eds.), *Handbook of Obesity and Treatment* (pp. 229–248). New York: Guilford Press.

Wadden, T.A., Womble, L.G., Stunkard, A.J. and Anderson, D.A. (2002). Psychosocial consequences of obesity and weight loss. In T.A. Wadden and A.J. Stunkard (Eds.), *Handbook of Obesity Treatment*. New York: Guilford Press.

Ware, J.E., Jr. and Sherbourne, C.D. (1992). The MOS 36-item short-form health survey (SF-36). I. Conceptual framework and item selection. *Med. Care*, 30(6), 473–483.

Wilfley, D. and Rodin, J. (1995). Cultural influences on eating disorders. In K.D. Brownell and C.G. Fairburn (Eds.), *Eating Disorders and Obesity*. New York: Guilford Press.

Wilfley, D.E., Agras, W.S., Telch, C.F., Rossiter, E.M., Schneider, J.A., Cole, A.G., Sifford, L.A. and Raeburn, S.D. (1993). Group cognitive-behavioral therapy and group interpersonal psycho-therapy for the nonpurging bulimic individual: a controlled comparison. *J. Consult. Clin. Psychol.*, 61(2), 296–305.

Wilfley, D.E. and Cohen, L.R. (1997). Psychological treatment of bulimia nervosa and binge eating disorder. *Psychopharmacol. Bull.*, 33(3), 437–454.

Wilfley, D.E., Schwartz, M.B., Spurrell, E.B. and Fairburn, C.G. (2000). Using the eating disorder examination to identify the specific psychopathology of binge eating disorder. *Int. J. Eat. Disord.*, 27(3), 259–269.

Wilfley, D.E., Welch, R.R., Stein, R.I., Spurrell, E.B., Cohen, L.R., Saelens, B.E., Dounchis, J.Z., Frank, M.A., Wiseman, C.V. and Matt, G.E. (2002). A randomized comparison of group cognitive-behavioral therapy and group interpersonal psychotherapy for the treatment of overweight individuals with binge-eating disorder. *Arch. Gen. Psychiatry*, 59(8), 713–721.

Wing, R.R. (1998). Behavioral approaches to the treatment of obesity. In G.A. Bray, C. Bouchard and W.P.T. James (Eds.), *Handbook of Obesity* (pp. 855–873). New York: Marcel Dekker.

World Health Organization (WHO). (1997). Obesity: preventing and managing the global epidemic. Geneva: World Health Organization.

Yanovski, S.Z. (1993). Binge eating disorder: current knowledge. *Obesity Res.*, 1, 306–324.

7

Basic Considerations and Guidelines for Treatment

Michael E. J. Lean

CONTENTS

SUMMARY   Modern weight management has four components that need to be assessed and addressed separately:

- Prevention of weight gain/regain (life-long) (proposed target to restrict <0.5 kg/year)
- Induction of weight loss (target 5 to 10 kg in 3 to 6 months)
- Treatment of obesity-related symptoms
- Reduction of coexisting coronary risk factors

Drug therapy may be considered for all these components, although obesity-related symptoms and risk factors may be adequately controlled by weight loss and maintenance. A treatment that checks the disease process of weight gain (effectively cures obesity) should not be expected to produce continued or indefinite weight loss. The reduction of coexisting coronary risk factors commonly requires other specific drugs. Obese patients are a high-risk group, particularly for long-term risks of coronary heart disease, but also for many other disabling consequences. The primary role of drugs for weight management is to contribute to symptomatic improvement and well-being. If they also contribute to reduced cardiovascular disease, then this will be a bonus. Long-term data on safety will be welcomed, given the need for long-term treatment in increasing numbers of younger patients, but on current evidence, clinical guidelines assess the benefit/hazard balance of existing drugs to be positive.

7.1 Uses of Drugs

Drugs are used in medicine to treat or to prevent disease. Sometimes they can be used alone, sometimes in conjunction with nonpharmacological measures. The vast majority of drugs have been developed to relieve symptoms or distress — to help people feel better; it is easy to assess their value to an individual patient, often immediately. A small number of available drugs are intended to modify the course of disease progression, to reduce or delay pathology. Very few drugs indeed have the capacity to effect a cure; even antibiotics only serve to tip the balance in favor of host defense systems — although certain chemotherapeutic agents can radically stop specific cancers in their tracks. The value of these drugs to an individual must be made early on clinical evidence of a response so that, if they fail, other alternatives can be tried. In most cases with drugs effective in changing the course of a disease progression, a symptomatic improvement also takes place.

More recently, increasing numbers of drugs have been designed for purely preventive purposes. They are not intended to help people feel better, but to modify or block a pathogenetic process at an early stage with a goal of delaying disease development. The best known are drugs to delay the clinical appearance of coronary heart disease (CHD) by improving risk factors. It is possible to identify nonresponders (e.g., patients whose blood pressure does not fall with a specific antihypertensive drug); however, the value of these drugs cannot be assessed fully in individual cases because the processes of pathogenesis are multifactorial. For example, the value of a lipid-lowering drug to an individual will depend on how important lipids are to heart disease development in that patient (in relation to blood pressure, insulin sensitivity, and a host of other genetic behavioral and circumstantial factors). The decision to treat, and to continue treatment, is guided by statistically secure evidence in large trials, comforted by measurable signs of an effect on a risk factor in the individual.

As a rule, drugs intended to treat symptoms or to modify disease progression are indicated for as long as the patient has symptoms or evidence of active disease. Drugs intended for prevention are usually continued indefinitely. Although it seems self-evident to doctors, the concept that a drug's effect stops when the drug is stopped may not be obvious to some patients, who commonly believe that a course of treatment will have a permanent effect on disease progression.

7.2 Prescribing

For all drugs, clinical decisions about treatment must be made based on an evaluation of the benefit of treatment to that patient and balanced against actual or potential hazards associated with the treatment. It is in this context that the use of drugs in weight management must be considered and guidelines developed. In many ways obesity (ICD-10 Code E.66) is an unusual disease, and previous guidance about drug treatments has not always been informed by doctors who are expert in their use. As an example, the anti-obesity drugs phentermine and diethylpropion have had their licensing decisions in Europe reversed twice in the last 3 years. In 2002, the European Court of First Instance finally established that repeated decisions to revoke the licenses were based on prejudice and ignorance.

Clinical management guidelines come in several forms. Some treatment protocols are more or less mandatory (e.g., penicillin for meningitis); others, like treatments for obesity, recognize the complexity of interaction between diet and life-style advice and drug actions, variability between patients, and relative skills and enthusiasm of therapists, and thus are presented in the form of a blueprint from which specific protocols can be developed locally.

7.3   What Is Obesity?

Obesity is the disease process of excess fat accumulation, with multiple pathological consequences affecting almost every organ system. The word *obesity* (Latin *ob-, esum*) identifies the problem as having eaten too much (stating the obvious rather unhelpfully). Several definitions are available for different purposes. For epidemiology, the WHO has provided criteria based on body mass index (BMI, weight/height^2) to adjust weight for differences in height. BMI > 30 kg/m^2 = (grade II obesity); BMI > 25 kg/m^2 = (grade I obesity).

For health promotion, the waist circumference has found greater favor than BMI. It identifies those at risk through excess total fat and also from the more serious intra-abdominal fat (even when total body fat is relatively low). Waist is measured using fixed boney landmarks — between the iliac crest and the lowest rib. It does not vary much with height, so does not need adjustment. Waist > 80 cm (women)/94 cm (men) identifies people with increasing risks who should take positive steps to avoid weight gain. Waist > 88 cm (women)/102 cm (men) generates high risks. At this level, people should seek professional help to achieve and maintain 10% weight loss.

However, an understanding of the disease process and its demands a more clinically relevant definition. This is the disease process of excess fat accumulation, which generates over time a catalogue of organ-specific pathological manifestations affecting virtually every body system. All its effects are age related and often misattributed. Obesity results from polygenic–environmental interactions, such that its development and consequences vary among individuals.

For epidemiological classifications and for certain clinical purposes, the WHO body mass index (BMI) criteria are used to identify people with obesity. However, it is important to recognize that BMI is a rather crude guide to body fat content. Variations in muscle (which is heavier than fat) mean that not every person with BMI > 30 kg/m^2 is fat. Some, such as rugby players, are in fact very thin — with body fat < 10%! Conversely, some individuals with BMI well below 30 kg/m^2 severely obese (i.e., high body fat content) but have very little muscle. Obesity and its serious metabolic consequences may be manifested and need treatment at BMI below 30 kg/m^2, particularly in most Asian and Chinese people (WHO, IASO and IOTF report, 2000). A better index of total body fat is the waist circumference (Lean et al., 1996). Waist circumference is also influenced by (intra-) abdominal fat preponderance; however, this is an advantage because people with large waists tend to have particularly increased health risks as a close association, probably as a consequence of excess intra-abdominal fat (Han et al., 1995).

TABLE 7.1

Medical Consequences of Overweight and Obesity Account for 4 to 8% of Total Health Care Costs

Physical Symptoms	Metabolic Problems	Social Problems	Anaesthetic/ Surgical	Endocrine Problems	Psychological Problems
Tiredness	Hypertension	Isolation	Sleep apnea	Hirsutism	Low self-esteem
Breathlessness	Impaired glucose tolerance, type 2 diabetes	Agoraphobia	Chest infections	Oligomenorrhea/ infertility	Self-deception
Varicose veins		Unemployment	Wound dehiscence	Metromenorrhagia	Cognitive disturbance
Back pain	Hepatic steatosis	Family/marital stress	Hernia	Estrogen dependent	Distorted body image
Arthritis	Hyperlipidemia	Discrimination	Venous thrombosis	Cancers: breast, uterus, prostate	Depression
Edema/cellulitis	Hypercoagulation	Financial			
Sweating/ intertrigo	Coronary heart disease and stroke				
Stress incontinence					

Obesity is a disabling, symptomatic disease. Its clinical impact varies, manifested through a long list of symptoms (Table 7.1). These are common, age-related, multifactorial symptoms that occur earlier and with greater severity in more overweight people. The relevance of underlying obesity is often recognized in principle, but the true impact of obesity is often underestimated until a full history is taken, and it becomes clear that the patient has many different coexisting symptoms. These easily become disabling and contribute to a sense of helplessness, coupled with discrimination, low self-esteem, and social isolation. Obese people commonly complain of "depression." This obesity-related symptom does not have the same roots as endogenous depression and responds poorly to antidepressants. Obesity has important social consequences, for example, in absenteeism and the need for social support (Rissanen, 1996).

Obesity is also a major contributor to a range of serious metabolic and physical disorders (Table 7.1). The best recognized is its influence in revealing the phenotypic expression of "metabolic syndrome." Over half of all people will, if they become overweight, develop clear evidence of the triad of interrelated major risk factors (hypertension, dyslipidaemia, type 2 diabetes) that herald premature heart disease or stroke. These disorders are rare in people who manage to remain at or near "ideal body weight" (BMI 21 to 22 kg/m^2) throughout adult life, but become more common as BMI increases from 23 to 25 kg/m^2. Half of all type 2 diabetes develops below BMI 28 kg/m^2, and the main risk of heart disease is already established with impaired glucose tolerance (IGT), at BMI 23 to 27 kg/m^2.

All the clinical problems mentioned (and many more, see Table 7.1) increase or accelerate as the BMI grows higher, although the exact BMI at which problems develop, and the sequence of their appearance, varies among individuals.

Because obesity is a disease *process*, (Figure 7.1), weight gain tends to continue (commonly about 2 kg/year among people heading into clinical problems) and so, once started, the burden of ill health on an individual tends to increase with time. The *average* weight gain through adult life for the whole population is about 15 kg (0.5 kg/year). For people developing obesity, the average rate of weight gain is 1 to 2 kg per year.

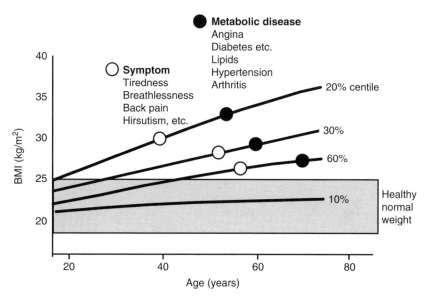

FIGURE 7.1
Centiles of weight gain in adults.

7.4   What Should Be the Aims of Weight Management?

In the past, in terms of weight loss, "obesity treatment" was viewed simplistically as synonymous with slimming, with cosmetic overtones. A greater understanding of the disease process and its clinical impact has led to the more comprehensive, clinically oriented term "weight management."

7.4.1   Symptomatic Treatment

In general it may still be helpful to treat individual symptoms. However, when obesity is a major factor, symptomatic approaches to pain; tiredness; breathlessness; indigestion; depression; etc. are often rather incomplete and unrewarding. The symptoms listed in Table 7.2 commonly coexist, so patients often end up on many drugs. This table lists the 10 most common symptoms of newly presenting type 2 diabetic patients in UKPDS. Most are in fact related to BMI (which was 28 kg/m^2). If weight continues to increase over time, these symptoms will get worse.

Obesity does not often contribute symptoms below the age of 40, by which time BMI is often very high. The assumption is often made that major weight loss must be necessary for improvement. For symptoms that have been studied, it is clear that quite modest weight loss (5 to 10 kg) can bring major improvements. This being the case, it is perhaps surprising that patients usually express dissatisfaction with this degree of weight loss. Part of the explanation lies in the dominance for obese people of discrimination, or perceived discrimination, felt from other people in every walk of life. Weight loss of 5 to 10 kg is often not noticed by others, and most patients remain "obese" even after this treatment.

TABLE 7.2

Symptoms in 430 Newly Diagnosed Type 2 Diabetes[a]

Symptom	Prevalence	Independent Association	
		FPG[a]	BMI[a]
Dry mouth	66%	<0.001	
Thirst	66%	<0.01	
Nocturia	75%		<0.01
Stomach pain	21%	0.02	<0.01
Shortness of breath	34%		<0.01
Swollen ankles	21%		<0.01
Headache	53%		<0.01
Heartburn	20%		<0.01
Excess sweating	37%		<0.01
Wheezing	20%		<0.01
Diarrhea	12%		<0.01

[a] Mean fasting plasma glucose (FPG) 9 mmol/L; BMI 29 kg/m².

It is also a problem that conventional "treatment" to produce a 5- to 10-kg weight loss and improvement in symptoms usually leads to a situation in which indefinite, life-long restrained eating is still required. For many people with obesity, an elevated appetite, left unsatisfied, is an intolerable new symptom.

7.4.2 Treatment of the Disease Process

Theoretically, it should be possible to produce a total cure for obesity, i.e., abolition of the process of excess fat accumulation. Ideally, this could be instituted *before* any excess fat has accumulated. Seen from another perspective, this could be viewed as primary prevention of the "state" of obesity (e.g., to keep BMI <25 kg/m²; <28 kg/m²; or <30 kg/m², depending on how much secondary disease is to be prevented). This possibility has actually arisen in the extremely rare cases of babies who can now have genetic leptin deficiency diagnosed at birth. Exogenous leptin treatment would be started at once; without it obesity is guaranteed.

Usually, however, the diagnosis of obesity is only made when the patient has clearly become seriously overweight. The earlier such patients can be helped to prevent further gain, the better, but the usually obvious benefits from weight loss take immediate clinical precedence. Tragically, in the past the need for active, life-long measures to check the disease process (i.e., to prevent weight regain) has often been neglected. Enlightened guidelines recognize this as the most important component of weight management. A practical target of reducing weight gain to the average in the population (<0.5 kg/year in Europe) is reasonable. Zero gain is improbable.

It is only very recently that obesity treatments have begun to be evaluated for their role in prevention of weight gain (or regain). Most treatments that produce weight loss (which is usually complete in 3 to 6 months) are effective for long-term weight maintenance, but there is no intrinsic reason why specific treatments should be used for both. Certain drugs may be appropriate for weight loss (3- to 6-month course), while others may be more suitable for long-term weight maintenance. The writers of guidelines and regulatory bodies are beginning to understand that *weight loss* and *weight maintenance* are two distinct components of weight management and should be studied separately in clinical trials.

A practical problem that faces doctors in using drugs (or even offering dietary advice) for weight maintenance is that the patient has no identifiable benefit, and it is not sensible to use a therapeutic trial of treatment withdrawal because of the multiple long-term negative effects of weight regain. Patients virtually always identify weight maintenance as their greatest problem (not weight loss — most of them can lose weight), but they are very apt to stop drug treatment once the initial weight loss phase is complete and then express surprise when weight regain occurs. Some reinforcement is possible if the weight management is instituted in order to treat a monitorable metabolic disorder, e.g., type 2 diabetes or hyperlipidaemia. However, overweight is only one of many contributing, and fluctuating, factors, so monitoring in an individual can produce misleading short-term changes.

7.4.3 Treatment of Obesity-Related Risk Factors and Prevention of Secondary "Hard" End Points

The Cartesian principle of doubt leads to the correct observation that associations between obesity or BMI and coronary risk factors are definite associations, but not necessarily indications of a causal relationship between obesity and heart disease or stroke. The causal link is strengthened greatly by the evidence that (in young people at least) obesity is strongly associated with myocardial infarction, coronary death, and stroke. Moreover, in the Nurses Health Study, a powerful interaction has been shown between high BMI, as it rises from 25 to 29 kg/m^2 or above, to increase the risk of myocardial infarction up to 12-fold if conventional risk factors are also present (Figure 7.2) (Manson et al., 1990).

The evidence to justify weight loss on the basis of reduced coronary risk factors is very strong and consistent across various study designs. Nevertheless, doubters need evidence from long-term randomized controlled trials to prove that the known improvement in risk factors with weight loss will translate into reduced (i.e., delayed) myocardial infarction, stroke, and deaths. Such studies are being undertaken and can be completed relatively quickly (e.g., 4 to 5 years) because obese patients are at high risk; untreated they will suffer frequent cardiac problems. Most of the evidence from comparable studies on risk factors in high-risk groups (e.g., lipid lowering, or antihypertensive drugs) has shown modest reductions in the "hard" end points, so a betting doctor would predict similar improvement from antiobesity drugs. It is already known that the incidence of type 2 diabetes can be reduced by 30% with orlistat, which adds an extra 4 years with a mean weight loss of 3 kg.

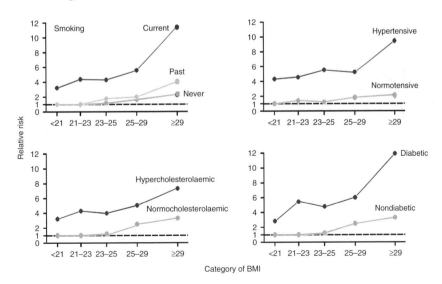

FIGURE 7.2
Relative risks of myocardial infarction (Manson et al., 1990).

An important issue, however, for those conducting long-term "hard end point" trials of antiobesity drugs is that cardiovascular disease is only one of many clinical consequences of obesity, and it is a fairly distant consequence of which obesity is only one of many contributors. It will therefore be of some value to prove a reduction in myocardial infarction from long-term weight management, as well as reassuring if the benefit/hazard balance is positive for antiobesity drugs in this respect. However, the main values of antiobesity drugs remain for symptomatic treatment and for checking the disease process. More potent drugs are available to reduce blood pressure, and lipids, and blood glucose. Antiobesity drugs are not licensed for these purposes, although weight loss brings some improvement in all of them.

7.5   Antiobesity Drugs, Mechanisms, Benefits, and Risks

A drug can contribute to medical weight management if it helps to *reduce* energy (calorie) intake and absorption or to increase energy expenditure. Patients will lose weight as long as this balance is negative. If a drug continued indefinitely to generate a negative balance in the energy balance equation (Figure 7.3), then it would continue to produce further weight loss. This would of course ultimately become dangerous. In practice, all of the many drugs used over the years for weight management gave a more or less fixed effect size, such that a step change in energy intake or expenditure results in a set amount of weight loss followed by re-establishment of energy balance at a lower weight. That amount of weight loss varies among individuals and of course takes time to complete.

The different drugs used over the years have a remarkable variety of mechanisms (Table 7.3), which illustrate the complexity of physiological regulation of appetite and energy balance. However, these drugs have remarkably similar effect sizes on average. Clearly, some individual patients can do much better than others, but on average antiobesity drugs will generate an imbalance of energy balance of about 300 kcal/day. Patients are usually able to adhere to weight loss (dieting) programs for about 3 to 4 months, with support. A deficit of 300 kcal/day for 100 days produces a total deficit of 30,000 kcal. Adipose tissue contains about 7000 kcal/kg (stored lipid is 9000 kcal/kg, but vascular and sup-

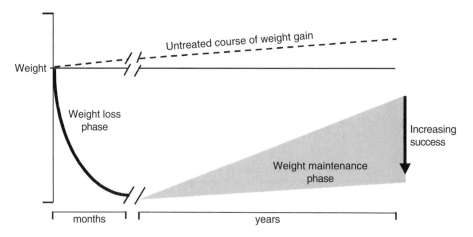

FIGURE 7.3
Phases of success in weight management.

TABLE 7.3

Drugs Used or Developed for Weight Management

Amphetamines
Diethylpropion
Phentermine
Mazindol
Fenfluramines
Methyl cellulose
Caffeine + ephedrine
Orlistat (lipase inhibitor)
Sibutramine
Leptin
Topiramate
Cannabinoid receptor antag. (rimonabant)

porting structure is also in adipose tissue); thus, the pharmacological effect will in theory be able to reduce weight about 4 kg more than diet and life-style alone. This is almost exactly what is found in randomized clinical trials, compared to placebo.

However, with the help of trained, experienced, supportive health professionals, and on an antiobesity drug without the uncertainty of possible placebo allocation, patients are commonly able to lose 10 to 15 kg. This has been shown in several large studies with different agents. The problem then is weight maintenance, and this is probably when antiobesity drugs have the greatest clinical benefit and application. A drug-induced deficit of 300 kcal/day, when applied to a weight-maintenance situation, means that weight stability will be achieved at body weight 12 to 13 kg lower, on average. Again, this theoretical effect is exactly what is seen in weight maintenance studies — for example, among patients who respond to orlistat (Rissanen et al., 2003) or with sibutramine after open intervention with conventional diet and exercise in the STORM Trial (James et al., 2000) or after initial weight loss achieved by very low calorie diet (Apfelbaum et al., 1999).

It is important to recognize that a drug that reduces food intake will only affect body weight if compensation from reduced energy expenditure is incomplete, and vice versa. With most drugs that affect appetite or satiety by noradrenergic or serotoninergic mechanisms (e.g., fenfluramines, sibutramine, phentermine), there is some evidence for modest "thermogenic" actions to attenuate the expected decline in metabolic rate with weight loss. Similarly, most of the experimental thermogenic drugs (e.g., β-3 stimulants) can be shown in animals to prevent any compensatory increase in appetite and food intake.

With active weight loss (i.e., usually in the first 3 to 6 months of treatment), substantial symptomatic improvements commonly occur, as well as disproportionately large improvements in obesity-related risk factors. The effect of weight loss on blood pressure, lipids, and glucose tolerance can be overestimated if studied when a negative energy balance still exists. When energy balance is re-established at a lower maintenance weight, the acutely suppressed HDL-cholesterol usually rises, but the other cardiac risk factors also tend to revert to a position more proportionate to the lower weight (possibly including effects from improved exercise capacity).

That said, the metabolic improvements from quite modest weight loss (5 to 10 kg) and their maintenance are much greater than most doctors appreciate. The XENDOS study found a 30% reduction in new cases of type 2 diabetes from a mean 3-kg weight loss with orlistat for 4 years. Table 7.4 shows the 2-year improvements in patients treated with orlistat who clearly responded to treatment (5 kg weight loss at 12 weeks). These results are comparable to those seen with multiple drug therapies directed at the risk factors individually.

TABLE 7.4

Percent Body Weight Loss of Orlistat "Responders"[a]

	Diet Lead-In Loss < 2.5 kg	Diet Lead-In Loss > 2.5 kg	All Responders
1 year	−12.0 (0.9)	−15.7 (0.7)	−14.5 (0.6)
2 years	−11.3 (1.1)	−12.2 (1.0)	−11.9 (0.8)
N (% of total)	33 (15%)	71 (32%)	104 (47%)

[a] Those who lost >5% body weight at 12 weeks and so would qualify for continued, long-term treatment according to EU prescribing guidelines.

Note: Results are little different between those who succeeded or failed to achieve 2.5 kg loss in a diet-alone lead-in period of 4 weeks. Mean (SEM).

Source: Risannen, A. et al., *Int. J. Obes.* 27(1), 103–109, 2003.

It is important to consider also possible adverse effects from antiobesity drug treatment. Historically, this was an issue because the first drugs to be introduced, the amphetamines, turned out to be addictive and to have a range of destructive side effects. Clinical trials with subsequent agents (centrally and peripherally acting) have described large numbers of adverse effects, but with placebo as well as active treatments.

Orlistat is essentially not absorbed and so has no systemic effects. Its only adverse effect, to produce steatorrhea, is in fact the result of continuing to eat too much fat (above about 20 g/meal). The noradrenergic and serotoninergic agents have the capacity to produce central side effects, but they tend to be uncommon, minor, and transient. Undoubtedly, noradrenergic agents have an effect on pulse and blood pressure, but this action tends to be neutralized by the opposite effect from weight loss. Monitoring is important in order to withdraw treatments that do not lead to weight loss and to identify new hypertension. Of course, new hypertension is common in people with obesity, so the multiple risks of withdrawing effective antiobesity treatment need to be weighed against possible benefits in relation to blood pressure.

In some situations, specific antiobesity drugs have additional clinical benefits beyond the effect on body weight. For example, by blocking fat absorption as its mechanism in generating weight loss, orlistat has an extra effect on hyperlipidaemia that is maintained in the long term.

7.6   Guidelines for Antiobesity Drug Use

A number of national bodies have produced guidelines for antiobesity drug use, with different perspectives. The first evidence-based guideline (SIGN, 1996) broke new ground in stating first that drugs could not be recommended without evidence for long-term safety and efficacy, but then tacitly recognizing that lack of such evidence does not mean that the drugs are unsafe or ineffective. To have understood this would have spared regulatory authorities some embarrassment. The Scottish Intercollegiate Guidelines Network (SIGN) guidelines and the National Institutes of Health (NIH, 1998) guidelines (which actually list the 700 references used) observe that the needs for weight loss and for weight maintenance may be different and should be assessed separately. Both guidelines agreed that 5 to 10 kg weight loss should be considered clinically valuable; subsequent national guidelines have concurred (Table 7.5).

Other guidelines from professional bodies have focused on the need for doctors treating obesity to assess weight and its management in the context of the overall health of the

TABLE 7.5

Benefits of 5- to 10-kg Weight Loss

Mortality	Diabetes	Blood Pressure	Lipids
Fall of >20% total mortality	Fall of 50% fasting plasma glucose (newly diagnosed)	Fall of 10 mm Hg systolic	Fall of 10% total cholesterol
Fall of >30% diabetes-related		Fall of 20 mm Hg diastolic	Fall of 15% LDL cholesterol
Fall of >40% obesity-related cancers			Fall of 30% triglycerides
			Rise of 8% HDL cholesterol

Note: Some subsequent systematic reviews indicate lesser reductions in blood pressure in normotensive individuals, although it must be remembered that conventional randomized controlled trials include long-term treatment of nonresponders. The benefits to responders are greater.

Sources: SIGN, No 8. (http://www.sign.ac.uk), 1996. After Goldstein, D.J. *Int. J. Obes.* 16, 1992, 397–415; Lean, M.E.J. et al., *Diab. Med.* 7, 228–233, 1990; Williamson, D.R. et al., *Am. J. Epidemiol.* 141, 1128–1141, 1995.

TABLE 7.6

Drugs That Promote Weight Gain

Drug Class	Main Disease Treated
Insulin	Diabetes[a]
Sulphonylureas	Diabetes[a]
Thiazolidinediones	Diabetes[a]
Corticosteroids	Inflammatory diseases
Some contraceptives	Contraception
β-Adrenergic blockers	Hypertension, angina[a]
Cyproheptadine	Allergy, hay fever
Pizotifen	Vasomotor headache
Sodium valproate	Epilepsy
Lithium	Bipolar disease[a]
Some antidepressants	Depression[a]
Most antipsychotics	Schizophrenia

[a] Diseases likely to be aggravated by weight gain.

whole patient, with responsibilities to document findings, management decisions, and clinical monitoring (Royal College of Physicians, 2003). A better understanding of the principles of human nutrition and an awareness of the obesity-promoting capacity of several major drugs classes is important (Table 7.6). The National Institute for Clinical Excellence takes the lead in the U.K. for evaluating treatments and their cost/benefit balance.

7.7   Antiobesity Drug Licensing Restrictions

The issue of license indications and restrictions is unusual for obesity and weight management. These include a lower limit of BMI 30 kg/m^2, but different lower limits for different drugs and variations of BMI 27 or 28 kg/m^2 to permit earlier treatment of patients with obesity-related "comorbidities" (i.e., secondary or compounding disorders). A lower age limit of 18 is usual. Most doctors, in most clinical situations, would only very rarely have reasons to consider prescribing outside these limits. Exceptions might occur, e.g., an Asian with multiple risk factors and BMI 26 kg/m^2, or uncontrollable obesity and type 2 diabetes in a 17-year-old. Antiobesity drugs should be stopped, of course, if they do not work, e.g., fail to produce weight loss of 5% at 12 weeks or 2 kg at 4 weeks.

More problematic is the new habit of placing a duration limit of 1 or 2 years on treatment on the grounds that few clinical trials have extended beyond 2 years. This seems to be a pure expression of prejudice against obesity and weight management because clinical trials of antiobesity drugs have been much longer than trials of other drugs for life-long conditions such as hyperlipidaemia, hypertension, or diabetes, which carry no duration limit.

From clinical trials, as well as common sense, it is not in patients' best interests to stop effective treatment for a progressive, disabling, and expensive disease simply because few clinical trials have extended beyond 2 years. No worrying problems have been met in clinical trials up to 4 years, and the evidence for clinical benefit continues to accumulate. The notion that patients with obesity should be able to "pull themselves together" and do without drugs after 1 or 2 years is extraordinarily naïve and destructive. It is to be hoped that regulatory authorities will take more advice from doctors experienced in obesity and weight management and from their patients.

7.8   Health Economic Assessment

The health burden of obesity is difficult to estimate because data for appropriate attributable risk calculation are sparse. Analyses in the U.S. (Wolf and Colditz, 1998); Netherlands (Seidell, 1995); and U.K. (Hughes et al., 1999) concur that it is a very expensive disease, with health care costs of the order 4 to 8% of total health care spending. This is greater than the costs of other diseases such as diabetes, epilepsy, or major cancers. These enormous costs, plus the social burden of obesity, are growing; they justify substantial investment in effecting diet and life-style programs; preventing modifications of the total food supply; and optimal use of all medical approaches for management.

Some guidelines (e.g., National Institute for Clinical Excellence [NICE]) have attempted to evaluate the cost/benefit ratio of antiobesity drugs in terms of quality adjusted life years. This is an appropriate aim, but the calculations (which suggested extraordinarily high costs of treatment) were based on long-term randomized-controlled trial evidence and the assumption that all patients started on the drugs would continue indefinitely. In clinical practice, however, as directed elsewhere in the guidelines, the drug will always be stopped in nonresponders, who can comprise 50% or more, depending on how effective the primary diet and life-style interventions are. To continue ineffective treatment in long-term clinical trials is unethical if such patients can be identified at an early stage.

References

Apfelbaum, M., P. Vague, O. Ziegler, C. Hanotin, F. Thomas, and E. Leutenegger, Long-term maintenance of weight loss after a very-low calorie diet: a randomized blinded trial of the efficacy and tolerability of sibutramine. *Am. J. Clin. Nutr.* 106, 1999, 179–184.

Goldstein, D.J., Beneficial health effects of modest weight loss, *Int. J. Obes.* 16, 1992, 397–415.

Han, T.S., E.M. van Leer, J.C. Seidell, and M.E.J. Lean, Waist circumference action levels in the identification of cardiovascular risk factors: prevalence study in a random sample, *Br. Med. J.* 311, 1995, 1041–1045.

Hughes, D., A. McGuire, H. Elliot, N. Finer, M.E.J. Lean, A.M. Prentice, and L. Ritchie, The cost of obesity in the United Kingdom, *J. Drug Assess.* 2, 1999, 327–396.

James, W.P., A. Astrup, N. Finer, J. Hilsted, P. Kopelman, S. Rossner, W. Saris, and L.F. Van Gaal, Effect of sibutramine on weight maintenance after weight loss: a randomized trial. STORM Study Group. *Lancet* 356, 2000, 2119–2125.

Lean, M.E.J., J.K. Powrie, A.S. Anderson, and P.H. Garthwaite, Obesity, weight loss and prognosis in type 2 diabetes, *Diab. Med.* 7, 1990, 228–233.

Lean, M.E.J., T.S. Han, and P. Duerenberg, Predicting body composition by densitometry from simple anthropometric measurements, *Am. J. Clin. Nutr.* 63, 1996, 4–14.

Lean, M.E.J., T.S. Han, and J.C. Seidell, Impairment of health and quality of life in people with large waist circumference, *Lancet* 351, 1998, 853–856.

Manson, J.E., G.A. Colditz, M.J. Stampfer, W.C. Willett, B. Rossner, R.R. Monson, F.F. Speizer, and C.H. Hennekens, A prospective study of obesity and risk of coronary heart disease in women, *New Engl. J. Med.* 332, 1990, 882–889.

National Institute for Clinical Excellence (NICE), Guidance on the use of orlistat for the treatment of obesity in adults (March 2001) (http://www.nice.org.uk).

National Institute for Clinical Excellence (NICE), Guidance on the use of sibutramine for the treatment of obesity in adults (October 2001) (http://www.nice.org.uk).

National Institutes of Health (NIH), National Heart Lung and Blood Institute (NLLBI), Clinical guidelines on the identification, evaluation and treatment of overweight and obesity: the evidence report. U.S. Government Press, Washington, D.C., 1998. (http://www.nhlbi.nih.gov).

Rissanen, A.M., The economic and psychosocial consequences of obesity, *Ciba Found. Symp.* 201, 1996, 194–201.

Rissanen, A., M.E.J. Lean, S. Rossner, K.R. Segal, and L. Sjostroum, Predictive value of early weight loss in obesity management with orlistat: an evidence-based assessment of prescribing guidelines, *Int. J. Obes.* 27(1), 2003, 103–109.

Royal College of Physicians of London, A report of the Nutrition Committee of the RCP. Anti-obesity drugs — guidance on appropriate prescribing and management, 2003.

SIGN (Scottish Intercollegiate Guidelines Network), Obesity in Scotland: integrating prevention with weight management. No 8. SIGN 1996. (http://www.sign.ac.uk).

Seidell, J.C., What is the cost of obesity? *Int. J. Obes.* 19, 1995, S, 513–516.

U.K. Prospective Diabetes Study 7: response of fasting plasma glucose to diet therapy in newly presenting type II diabetic patients, UKPDS Group, *Metabolism*, 39(9), 1990, 905–912.

WHO, Steering Committee of the WHO Western Pacific Region, IASO and IOTF, The Asia-Pacific perspective: redefining obesity and its treatment, 2000.

Williamson, D.R., E. Pamuk, M. Thun, D. Flanders, T. Byers, and C. Heath, Prospective study of intentional weight loss and mortality in never-smoking overweight U.S. white women aged 40–64 years, *Am. J. Epidemiol.* 141, 1995, 1128–1141.

Wolf, A.M. and G.A. Colditz, Current estimates of the economic cost of obesity in the United States, *Obes. Res.* 6(2), 1998, 97–106.

Part III

Benefits of Weight Loss

8

Weight Loss and Cardiovascular Risk Factors

Tobias Pischon, James D. Douketis, and Arya M. Sharma

CONTENTS

8.1   Introduction

The association between obesity, cardiovascular risk factors, and cardiovascular disease is well established.[1] Compared to normal-weight subjects, obese individuals (BMI ≥ 30 kg/m^2) have an about 3.5-fold increased risk for type 2 diabetes and hypertension, a 2-fold increased risk for hypercholesterolemia, and a 50% increased risk for cardiovascular disease.[2,3] Consequently, numerous studies have investigated weight reduction interventions for people with obesity, and epidemiologic studies have estimated the potential benefits that may be expected from preventive measures.[1]

Obesity, in most cases, is a chronic condition in which a life-long management strategy is required; therefore, weight reduction and maintenance requires a long-term approach.[4–6] Most weight reduction trials, however, are limited by a short follow-up duration of 6 months or less because they are designed to show a maximal treatment benefit in terms of weight reduction over a short time period. Furthermore, most intervention trials focus on body weight reduction as the primary outcome, rather than on health consequences such as cardiovascular risk factors or clinical endpoints. Therefore, the long-term health consequences and effectiveness of weight reduction interventions are less clear. In most (of the few) long-term weight reduction intervention trials, weight regain is typically observed after an initial 6- to 12-month period of weight loss.[7] This weight regain can occur while the subjects are still receiving a weight reduction intervention, and often exacerbates once the treatment has ended. Consequently, patients may regain most, or in some cases all, of the weight lost.

Despite the apparent difficulty in sustaining esthetically pleasing major weight reduction, modest weight loss, consisting of 5 to 10% of body weight, is associated with improvements in lipid levels, glycemic control, and blood pressure control.[1] Consequently, current guidelines recommend modest weight reduction and weight maintenance that can be sustained over the long term, anticipating that this strategy may have profound beneficial effects on the incidence of clinically important outcomes such as type 2 diabetes, myocardial infarction, and death.[1] These issues, again, cannot be addressed with short-term studies.

Although the pharmacological and nonpharmacological treatment of obesity and its capability in terms of weight reduction are addressed in other sections of this book, the objective of this chapter is to review long-term studies that have investigated the effectiveness of weight loss on diseases associated with obesity. However, because few studies have investigated clinical endpoints such as coronary artery disease or death, this chapter is limited to studies reporting the effect of weight loss on surrogate markers of cardiovascular disease, consisting of blood lipid levels, glycemic status, and blood pressure control. Studies focusing on nonpharmacological weight reduction lasting at least 2 years or pharmacological weight reduction with at least 1-year duration were included.

Furthermore, it is important to note that the vast majority of studies have been conducted in the "healthy" obese, i.e., obese individuals with little or no metabolic or cardiovascular abnormalities associated with obesity. Thus, the rather modest results of most studies on these parameters most likely represent a substantial underestimation of the beneficial effects that can be achieved in a less healthy population. Additionally, in almost all of the studies reviewed here, changes in metabolic parameters were reported as secondary outcomes only.

8.2   Hypertension

Overweight and obesity have long been recognized as important determinants of elevated blood pressure in African–American and Caucasian hypertensive and normotensive individuals.[8] The same appears true for Asian populations.[9] It is well established that weight gain is consistently associated with increased blood pressure, and that weight loss decreases blood pressure independent of changes in sodium intake. Nevertheless, the mechanisms underlying this relationship remain poorly understood. Several mechanisms, including increased sympathetic activity; sodium and volume retention; renal abnormalities; insulin resistance; and, more recently, hyperleptinemia, have been implicated in the development of obesity-related hypertension.[10]

The Clinical Guidelines on the Identification, Evaluation, and Treatment of Overweight and Obesity in Adults[1] recently assessed 76 clinical trials (including short-term studies) investigating the effect of life-style and pharmacological weight loss interventions on blood pressure. The authors concluded that strong evidence indicated that weight loss by life-style modifications reduced blood pressure levels. Furthermore, evidence suggested that weight loss produced by most weight loss medications in combination with life-style modifications will be accompanied by reductions in blood pressure. Importantly, a modest weight loss of 5 to 10% of initial weight is associated with blood pressure reduction and normalization, and decreased requirements for antihypertensive medications.

8.2.1   Nonpharmacological Treatment (Table 8.1)

Few studies have investigated the long-term efficacy of dietary interventions on blood pressure control. These studies can be divided into those that specifically focused on the effect of dietary intervention on blood pressure control and those focusing on other outcomes.

8.2.1.1   Studies not Focusing on Hypertension

A study by Eriksson and Lindgarde[11] tested the feasibility of a long-term intervention, consisting of dietary advice and increase of physical activity, in 41 subjects with type 2 diabetes (12% on antihypertensive medication) and 181 subjects with impaired glucose tolerance (IGT) (15% on antihypertensive medication) compared to no specific intervention in 79 subjects with IGT (18% on antihypertensive medication) and 114 healthy controls (1% on antihypertensive medication), over 5 years. In the intervention group, BMI decreased by 3.7% in subjects with type 2 diabetes ($p < .001$) and by 2.3% in those with IGT ($p < .001$). In the comparison groups, however, BMI increased by 0.5% in subjects with IGT ($p = NS$), and by 1.7% in controls ($p < .001$).

Weight changes were significantly different between the intervention and control groups. In the intervention group, systolic blood pressure (SBP) was reduced by 7.2% ($p < .01$) in patients with type 2 diabetes and by 6.4% ($p < .001$) in subjects with IGT. In the comparison groups, SBP decreased by 6.2% ($p < .05$) in subjects with IGT and by 3.0% ($p < .01$) in the control group. Reductions in diastolic blood pressure (DBP) in the intervention group were 6.3% ($p < .01$) in subjects with type 2 diabetes and 5.4% ($p < .001$) in subjects with IGT, whereas in the comparison group it was 7.2% ($p < .001$) in subjects with IGT and 1.3% ($p = NS$) in controls.

It should be noted that in the intervention group, use of antihypertensive medication increased in subjects with type 2 diabetes to 20.6%, but decreased to 7.4% in subjects with IGT. In the comparison group, usage increased to 23.9% in subjects with IGT, but decreased to 0% in controls. Although this analysis shows that diet and physical activity were somewhat successful in terms of weight reduction, its analysis with regard to blood pressure control is limited. Furthermore, comparing the effects of different interventions on blood pressure control across four groups with different baseline co-morbidity is problematic.

A study by Flechtner–Mors et al.[12] investigated the effect of snack replacements for weight maintenance over 4 years in 100 subjects (79 women). Subjects received a diet

TABLE 8.1

Effects of Nonpharmacologic Weight Reduction on Physiological and Biochemical Markers of Cardiovascular Disease

Study (Ref.)	Study Design	Follow-Up (Months)	Patients	Intervention	Baseline Weight (kg)	Weight (kg)	Change from Baseline in Markers of Cardiovascular Disease[a]						
							SBP (mmHg)	DBP (mmHg)	LDL (mmol/L)	HDL (mmol/L)	TG (mmol/L)	FBG (mmol/L)	2-h BG (mmol/L)
Stevens, 2001	RCT	36	2382 with nonmedicated hypertension	Diet counselling	93.4	-0.2	(-0.8)	(-3.2)	n/a	n/a	n/a	n/a	n/a
				Na+ restriction	94.0	-1.7	(-0.7)	(-3.0)	n/a	n/a	n/a	n/a	n/a
				Diet + Na+ restriction	93.6	-0.3	(-0.5)	(-2.9)	n/a	n/a	n/a	n/a	n/a
				Usual care	93.6	-1.8	(+0.6)	(-2.4)	n/a	n/a	n/a	n/a	n/a
Whelton, 1998	RCT	3.2	585 (age 60–80) with treated hypertension	Reduced Na+ intake			-3.4	-1.9	n/a	n/a	n/a	n/a	n/a
				Diet regimen			-4.0	-1.1	n/a	n/a	n/a	n/a	n/a
				Reduced Na+ intake + diet			-5.3	-3.4	n/a	n/a	n/a	n/a	n/a
				Usual care			-0.8	-0.8	n/a	n/a	n/a	n/a	n/a
Eriksson and Lindgarde, 1991		60	41 with T2D	Diet counselling + exercise	87.0	-2.0	(-7.2)	(-6.3)	(-3.8)	n/a	(-8.2)	n/a	-0.1
			181 with IGT	Diet counselling + exercise	82.0	-3.3	(-6.4)	(-5.4)	(+0.9)	n/a	(-8.6)	n/a	-1.1
			79 with IGT	Usual care	84.0	-0.2	(-6.2)	(-7.2)	(-0.3)	n/a	(+22.5)	n/a	n/a
			114 without IGT	Usual care	114.0	-2.0	(-3.0)	(-1.3)	(+1.0)	n/a	(+24.6)	n/a	n/a
Flechtner–Mors et al., 2000	RCT	48	50	Low-calorie diet	92.7	-4.1	-1.0	-3.0	n/a	-0.06	-0.69	-0.7	n/a
			50	Snack replacements	92.6	-9.5	-13.0	-4.0	n/a	-0.05	-0.94	-0.6	n/a
Tuomilheto, 2001	RCT	48	265 with IGT	Diet counselling	n/a	-3.5	-5.0	-5.0	n/a	+0.05	-0.2	-0.2	n/a
			257 with IGT	Usual care	n/a	-0.8	-1.0	-3.0	n/a	+0.03	-0.01	+0.05	n/a
Stamler, 1987	RCT	48	78 with treated hypertension	Stop antihypertensive + diet counselling	80.7	n/a	+5.2	+10.8	n/a	n/a	n/a	n/a	n/a
			78 with treated hypertension	Stop antihypertensive + usual care	77.7	n/a	+6.7	+11.4	n/a	n/a	n/a	n/a	n/a
			20 with treated hypertension	Continue antihypertensive + usual care	78.6	n/a	+1.0	+2.5	n/a	n/a	n/a	n/a	n/a

[a] Values in parentheses reflect percent changes because absolute values were not available from some papers.

Notes: ref. = Reference; RCT = randomized controlled trial; T2D = type 2 diabetes; IGT = impaired glucose tolerance; LDL = low–density lipoprotein cholesterol; HDL = high–density lipoprotein cholesterol; TG = triglycerides; FBG = fasting blood glucose; 2-h BG = 2-h postglucose load; SBP = systolic blood pressure; DBP = diastolic blood pressure; n/a = not available.

providing 1200 to 1500 kcal/d (19 to 21% of energy as protein; 48 to 54% as carbohydrate; and 25 to 34% as fat; three meals and 2 snacks a day) and were randomized to a meal replacement group (two of the three main meals were replaced with milk shakes, soups, or hot chocolate) or a control group and followed for 3 months. After that period, all subjects were instructed to replace one meal and one snack with the energy-controlled, nutrient-dense meal and snack replacements. The control group (group A) and the meal-replacement group (group B) lost weight; however, although both groups received the same energy intake, group B lost significantly more weight during the first 3 months of the trial.

Thereafter, additional weight loss was observed up to 27 months, followed by a slight weight regain until the end of the follow-up period. These weight changes were not substantially different between the two treatment regimens. After 4 years, body weight had decreased significantly ($p < .01$) by 4.1 kg in group A and 9.5 kg in group B. Reductions ($p < .01$) in systolic and diastolic blood pressure in groups A and B were also significant. This study indicates that meal replacements may be of additional benefit to an energy-restricted diet to promote weight loss and control blood pressure.

The Finnish Diabetes Prevention Study[13] investigated the feasibility and effects of a lifestyle modification program designed to prevent or delay the onset of type 2 diabetes in a randomized trial that involved 523 subjects (350 women) with IGT over a mean follow-up period of 3.2 years. Subjects in the control group received oral and written information about diet and exercise at baseline and at subsequent annual visits, whereas those in the intervention group received detailed advice about how to achieve the intervention goals (i.e., reduction in weight of 5% or more; reduction of fat intake and intake of saturated fat to less than 30 and 10% of energy, respectively; increase in fiber intake to at least 15 g per 1000 kcal; and moderate exercise for at least 30 min per day). This group also had regular sessions with a nutritionist and supervised exercise programs were offered.

The mean weight loss between baseline and the end of year 1 (year 2) was 4.2 kg (3.5 kg) in the intervention group and 0.8 kg (0.8 kg) in the control group ($p < .001$). Over a mean follow-up of 3.2 years, the risk of type 2 diabetes was reduced by 58% in the intervention group ($p < .001$). After 1 year and 2 years, SBP and DBP were significantly lower in the intervention group compared to the control group. This study indicates that changes in lifestyle can lower blood pressure levels in high-risk patients. However, it also suggests that a structured, individualized program is necessary to achieve this goal.

8.2.1.2 Studies Focusing on Hypertension

The Trials of Hypertension Prevention II[14] was a 36-month randomized trial of weight loss vs. usual care in 1191 overweight adults (mean BMI ~ 31 kg/m^2) with nonmedicated diastolic blood pressure of 83 to 89 mm Hg and systolic blood pressure less than 140 mm Hg. Participants who lost at least 4.5 kg at 6 months and maintained this weight reduction for the next 30 months had a 65% decreased risk of developing hypertension (hazard ratio [HR] = 0.35; 95% CI: 0.20, 0.59); however, this group comprised only 13% of the participants in the weight-loss arm. Sadly, over the 36 months, body weight returned to –0.2 kg below baseline in the weight loss group and increased by 1.8 kg in the control group. Thus, this study illustrates the limited success of achieving and maintaining weight loss by lifestyle measures even over a relatively short time period.

The trial of nonpharmacological interventions in the elderly (TONE)[15] included 585 obese men and women aged 60 to 80 years with systolic blood pressure lower than 145 mm Hg and diastolic blood pressure lower than 85 mm Hg on antihypertensive mono-therapy (withdrawn after 1 month). Participants were randomized to reduced sodium intake, weight loss, both, or usual care for 29 months. Compared to usual care, there was a significant reduction in risk for the combined outcome measure (diagnosis of hypertension, antihypertensive drug therapy, or a cardiovascular event) with reduced sodium intake alone (HR = 0.60; 95% CI: 0.45, 0.80); weight loss alone (HR = 0.64; 95% CI: 0.49, 0.85); and combined reduced sodium intake and weight loss (HR = 0.47; 95% CI: 0.35, 0.64).

The Hypertension Control Program[16] investigated whether people with medicated hypertension could discontinue drug therapy and remain normotensive by following a nutritional intervention program. Patients were randomized to nutritional intervention throughout the trial plus withdrawal of antihypertensive medication (group 1); withdrawal of antihypertensive medication without nutritional intervention (group 2); or continued antihypertensive therapy without nutritional intervention (group 3). The intervention consisted of weight reduction in overweight subjects and reduced sodium and alcohol intake. Over a 4-year period, body weight decreased by 1.8 kg in group 1, but increased by 2 kg in groups 2 and 3 ($p < .001$). SBP and DBP increased in all three groups; however, after 4 years, 39% in group 1 remained normotensive without drug therapy compared with 5% in group 2 ($p < .001$). This study indicates that a substantial proportion of hypertensive individuals may benefit from nutritional therapy and could consequently avoid antihypertensive medication.

8.2.2 Pharmacological Treatment

8.2.2.1 Orlistat (Table 8.2)

Several randomized, double-blind, placebo-controlled trials report the effect of weight loss due to treatment with orlistat, a gastrointestinal lipase inhibitor, on blood pressure levels. However, many of these studies excluded hypertensive subjects, and most trials focused on weight loss as their primary objective. Consequently, changes in blood pressure levels under treatment are usually only reported as secondary outcomes. It is important to keep in mind that the blood pressure-lowering effect of any potential antihypertensive treatment is more pronounced in hypertensive subjects. For example, although the antihypertensive effects of the widely used ACE inhibitor ramipril are well documented in hypertensive subjects, it had little effect on the mean blood pressure level in a large cohort of high-risk patients with overall normotensive blood pressure.[17] Only a few studies focused on the antihypertensive effects of orlistat treatment in hypertensive subjects.

In general, the following studies included obese subjects who were otherwise healthy or had well-controlled chronic diseases. If hypertensive subjects were included, blood pressure was usually well controlled in these trials and mean blood pressure levels of these study populations were generally normal or borderline.

- Sjöström et al.[18] found a weight loss of 10.2% in 350 obese patients who received orlistat, 120 mg three times a day, for 1 year compared with a weight loss of 6.1% in 350 placebo-treated patients ($p < .05$). Orlistat-treated patients experienced a greater decrease in blood pressure than did placebo-treated patients ($p < .05$). In addition to orlistat therapy, both groups received a hypocaloric diet containing roughly 30% of energy as fat.

- In a 2-year study by Davidson et al.,[19] 892 obese patients received a hypocaloric diet for 1 year; they were randomly allocated to receive orlistat or placebo for the first year and rerandomized to receive orlistat or placebo during the second year. After 1 year of follow-up, patients who received orlistat had an 8.8% weight loss associated with decreased blood pressure levels compared to a weight loss of 5.8% in placebo-treated subjects that was associated with an increase in blood pressure.

TABLE 8.2

Effects of Orlistat Therapy on Physiological and Biochemical Markers of Cardiovascular Disease

Study (Ref.)	Study Design	Follow-Up (Months)	Patients	Intervention	Baseline Weight (kg)	Change from Baseline in Markers of Cardiovascular Disease							
						Weight (kg)	SBP (mmHg)	DBP (mmHg)	LDL (mmol/L)	HDL (mmol/L)	TG (mmol/L)	FBG (mmol/L)	HbA1c (%)
Sjostrom, 1998	RCT	12	686	Placebo	99.8	-6.1	-2.0	-1.2	+0.02	+0.04	+0.08	+0.04	n/a
				orlistat, 120 mg TID	99.1	-10.0	-4.0	-2.1	-0.36	+0.05	-0.18	-0.1	n/a
Davidson et al., 1999	RCT	24	880	Placebo	100.6	-4.5	-1.0	-1.3	-0.22	+0.03	+0.03	+0.20	n/a
				orlistat, 120 mg TID	100.7	-7.6	-0.8	-1.0	-0.24	-0.01	-0.12	+0.05	n/a
Lindgarde, 2000	RCT	12	376 patients at risk for CAD	Placebo	95.9	-4.3	-4.1	-2.9	-0.07	-0.02	-0.15	+0.1	-0.05
				orlistat, 120 mg TID	96.1	-5.6	-4.9	-2.5	-0.25	0.0	0	-0.5	-0.25
Rossner et al., 2000	RCT	24	718	Placebo	97.7	-4.3	-5.1	-2.7	+0.03	+0.08	-0.17	-0.14	n/a
				orlistat, 120 mg TID	96.7	-7.4	-6.1	-2.6	-0.17	+0.04	-0.28	-0.07	n/a
Hauptman et al., 2000	RCT	24	422	Placebo	101.8	-1.7	+5.0	+4.0	+0.17	0.0	+0.01	+0.24	n/a
				orlistat, 120 mg TID	100.5	-5.0	+4.0	+1.0	-0.15	0.0	+0.11	+0.07	n/a
Finer et al., 2000	RCT	12	228	Placebo	98.4	1.3	n/a	n/a	+0.21	+0.16	n/a	n/a	n/a
				orlistat, 120 mg TID	97.9	3.3	n/a	n/a	-0.11	+0.15	n/a	n/a	n/a
Hollander et al., 1998	RCT	12	391 with type 2 diabetes	Placebo	99.7	-4.3	n/a	n/a	+0.22	+0.08	+0.21	+0.54	+0.18
				orlistat, 120 mg TID	99.6	-6.2	n/a	n/a	-0.13	+0.06	-0.1	-0.2	-0.28
Kelley et al., 2002	RCT	12	535 with type 2 diabetes	Placebo	101.8	-1.3	-0.9	-2.9	-0.1	+0.1	+0.31	-1.08	-0.27
				orlistat, 120 mg TID	102.0	-3.9	-1.1	-2.3	-0.38	0.0	+0.18	-1.63	-0.62
Miles et al., 2002	RCT	12	503 with type 2 diabetes	Placebo	101.1	-1.8	-0.3	n/a	-0.05	+1.0	+0.03	-0.7	-0.41
				orlistat, 120 mg TID	102.1	-4.7	-2.1	n/a	-0.25	+0.9	-0.25	-2.0	-0.75

Note: ref. = reference; RCT = randomized controlled trial; IGT = impaired glucose tolerance; LDL = low-density lipoprotein cholesterol; HDL = high-density lipoprotein cholesterol; TG = triglycerides; FBG = fasting blood glucose; HbA1c = hemoglobin-A1C; SBP = systolic blood pressure; DBP = diastolic blood pressure; n/a = not available; CAD = coronary artery disease; T2D = type 2 diabetes; TID = three times a day.

These differences between orlistat and placebo were statistically significant. No data were available on blood pressure levels in the second year of follow-up.

- A study by Rössner et al.[20] found no differences in the effect of orlistat or placebo, three times daily, on systolic or diastolic blood pressure levels after 2 years of treatment in 718 obese patients. In this study, weight loss after 1 year (2 years) was 6.6% (4.5%) and 9.7% (7.6%) in patients who received placebo or orlistat 120 mg, respectively (differences between orlistat and placebo were statistically significant). Overall, orlistat therapy was not associated with a significant decrease in blood pressure, except in DBP after 1 year of treatment.

- A study by Hauptman et al.[21] compared the effect of orlistat with placebo treatment in 635 obese patients over a period of 2 years (first year: hypocaloric diet; second year: eucaloric diet). In this study, patients on orlistat treatment lost significantly more weight after 1 year (7.94 kg) and 2 years (5.02 kg) than those treated with placebo (4.14 kg after 1 year and 1.65 kg after 2 years). However, the changes in blood pressure levels were not significantly different after 1 or 2 years.

- Kelley et al.[22] compared the effect of 120 mg orlistat with placebo, three times daily, over a 1-year period in 535 obese patients with type 2 diabetes and suboptimal glycemic control. In this study, patients who received orlistat therapy lost 3.76% of baseline body weight, compared to 1.22% in the placebo group ($p < .001$). However, changes in blood pressure levels were not significantly different between orlistat and placebo-treated patients.

- Finally, Miles et al.[23] compared the effect of orlistat with placebo over a 1-year period in 503 obese patients with suboptimal control of type 2 diabetes who were receiving metformin alone or in combination with sulfonylurea therapy. In this study, patients who received orlistat lost significantly more of their baseline weight than those in the placebo group (4.6 vs. 1.7%; $p < .001$). Compared to placebo, orlistat therapy was associated with a significant reduction in systolic but not diastolic blood pressure.

As mentioned earlier, all studies summarized here included obese subjects who were otherwise healthy or had well-controlled chronic diseases. Consequently, baseline blood pressure levels in the studies were generally not hypertensive. The only long-term study that reported results of a population with hypertensive mean blood pressure levels (145/88) was a study by Lindgärde,[24] which investigated orlistat therapy, 120 mg three times daily, in 376 obese patients at high risk for coronary artery disease. This study found no significant difference to placebo therapy on systolic or diastolic blood pressure levels. Although mean weight loss was greater with orlistat compared to placebo (5.9 vs. 4.6%; $p < .05$), changes in blood pressure levels were not significantly different between the orlistat and placebo groups.

Taken together, these studies indicate that weight loss that occurs with orlistat therapy is not consistently associated with reductions in blood pressure levels. These discrepant findings might be due to differences in baseline patient characteristics. Normotensive obese patients, who comprised the majority of patients in these studies, might not demonstrate significant reduction in blood pressure with orlistat-associated weight loss compared to hypertensive obese patients. However, in the only study that included subjects whose mean BP levels were hypertensive,[24] the effect of orlistat on blood pressure was not significantly different from placebo.

8.2.2.2   Sibutramine (Table 8.3)

Four randomized, double-blind, placebo-controlled trials have investigated the effect of sibutramine, a serotonin and noradrenaline reuptake inhibitor that induces satiety and

TABLE 8.3

Effects of Sibutramine Therapy on Physiological and Biochemical Markers of Cardiovascular Disease

Study (Ref.)	Study Design	Follow-Up (Months)	Patients	Intervention	Baseline Weight (kg)	Change from Baseline in Markers of Cardiovascular Disease							
						Weight (kg)	SBP (mmHg)	DBP (mmHg)	LDL (mmol/L)	HDL (mmol/L)	TG (mmol/L)	FBG (mmol/L)	HbA1c (%)
James et al., 2000	RCT	24	467	Placebo	102.1	-4.9	-4.7	-1.6	+0.08	+0.11	-0.11	+0.06	-0.09
				Sibutramine, 10 mg OD	102.3	-8.9	+0.1	+2.3	+0.01	+0.24	-0.47	-0.1	-0.30
Smith and Goulder, 2001	RCT	24	485	Placebo	87.0	-1.6	-0.5	-0.9	n/a	n/a	-1.3	-0.2	n/a
				Sibutramine, 10 mg OD	87.0	-4.4	+1.0	+1.6	n/a	n/a	-6.1	-0.9	n/a
				Sibutramine, 20 mg OD	87.0	-6.4	+0.3	-0.1	n/a	n/a	-9.8	-1.7	n/a
McMahon et al., 2000	RCT	12	224 with treated hypertension	Placebo	95.5	-0.5	+1.5	-1.3	-0.11	+0.06	-0.01	+0.31	n/a
				Sibutramine, 20 mg OD	97.0	-4.4	+2.7	+2.0	-0.10	+1.4	-0.19	+0.23	n/a
McMahon et al., 2002	RCT	12	220 with treated hypertension	Placebo	99.0	-0.4	+1.1	-0.1	-0.10	+0.03	-0.08	n/a	n/a
				Sibutramine, 20 mg OD	96.7	-4.5	+3.8	+3.0	-0.10	+0.10	-0.30	n/a	n/a

Note: Ref. = reference; RCT = randomized controlled trial; IGT = impaired glucose tolerance; LDL = low–density lipoprotein cholesterol; HDL = high-density lipoprotein cholesterol; TG = triglycerides; FBG = fasting blood glucose; HbA1c = hemoglobin-A1C; SBP = systolic blood pressure; DBP = diastolic blood pressure; n/a = not available; OD = once daily.

increases basal energy expenditure, on blood pressure levels.[25] In general, sibutramine use in obese hypertensive patients has been limited by the potential for drug-related increases in blood pressure and resting heart rate.[26] Consequently, the following studies limited the inclusion of hypertensive subjects to those with well-controlled blood pressure.

8.2.2.3   Studies not Focusing on Hypertensive Subjects

James et al.[27] reported the effect of 10 mg sibutramine daily on weight loss and maintenance during a 2-year period in 467 obese patients. After 2 years, weight loss was 10.2 kg in the sibutramine group and 4.7 kg in the placebo group. However, systolic and diastolic blood pressure and heart rate increased in the sibutramine group, but decreased in the placebo group. Smith and Goulder[28] compared the effect of 10 and 15 mg sibutramine per day with placebo over a 1-year period in 485 obese subjects. Weight loss in patients who received 10 or 15 mg sibutramine or a placebo had a mean weight loss of 6.4, 4.4, and 1.6 kg, respectively. Sibutramine was associated with a nonsignificant increase in systolic and diastolic blood pressure; heart rate increased by 1.8 beats/min on 10 mg and 3.5 beats/min on 15 mg ($p < .1$ vs. placebo).

8.2.2.4   Studies Focusing on Hypertensive Subjects

McMahon et al.[26] investigated treatment with 20 mg sibutramine daily over a 1-year period in 224 obese subjects with controlled hypertension. Patients who received sibutramine lost 4.7% of body weight compared to 0.7% in the placebo group ($p < .05$). Concomitantly, systolic blood pressure was associated with an increase in systolic and diastolic pressure and an increased heart rate of 4.9 beats/min, the latter significantly higher than after placebo ($p < .05$). In a similar study, McMahon et al.[29] investigated the effect of 20 mg sibutramine daily during a 1-year period in 220 obese hypertensive patients whose blood pressure was controlled with an angiotensin-converting enzyme inhibitor with or without a coadministered thiazide diuretic. Although sibutramine therapy was associated with a significantly greater weight reduction than placebo (4.5 vs. 0.4 kg; $p < .05$), sibutramine-treated patients had higher levels of systolic and diastolic blood pressure compared to placebo. Furthermore, resting heart rate increased by 5.7 beats/min in the sibutramine group and decreased by 0.3 beats/min in the placebo group. Overall, these studies indicate that despite significantly greater weight reduction with sibutramine therapy compared to placebo, this effect does not confer favorable effects on blood pressure. In fact, sibutramine therapy may be associated with modest increases in blood pressure and heart rate.

8.3   Dyslipidemia

8.3.1   Nonpharmacological Treatment (Table 8.1)

Few data are available on the long-term efficacy of dietary intervention to improve blood lipids, consisting of low-density lipoprotein (LDL) cholesterol; high-density lipoprotein (HDL) cholesterol; and triglyceride (TG) levels, which are markers of cardiovascular disease risk.[30] None of the following studies specifically focused on subjects with hyper- or dyslipidemia.

- In the aforementioned study by Eriksson and Lindgarde,[11] cholesterol levels decreased significantly by 3.8% in the intervention group (consisting of dietary advice and increased physical activity) in subjects with type 2 diabetes, but increased by 0.9% in subjects with IGT (p = NS). In the comparison groups, cholesterol levels decreased by 0.3% in subjects with IGT, but increased by 1.0% in controls (both p = NS). Changes in cholesterol levels were not significantly different between the groups. In the intervention groups, triglyceride levels decreased by 8.2% (p = NS) in subjects with type 2 diabetes and by 8.6% (p < .05) in those with IGT. In the comparison groups, levels increased by 22.5% (p = NS) in participants with IGT, but decreased by 24.6% (p < .001) in controls. The increase in subjects with IGT in the comparison group was significantly different from the decrease in those with IGT in the intervention group and from controls.

- The study by Flechtner–Mors et al.[12] found that HDL cholesterol levels did not significantly change over time and were not significantly different between the meal replacement group and the control group. In contrast, subjects who had replaced two of three meals with shakes, soups, or hot chocolate in the first 3 months had significantly lower TG levels compared to baseline and to the control group. After 4 years, TG levels were decreased from 2.23 to 1.29 mmol/L in the meal replacement group (p < .01), and from 2.13 to 1.44 mmol/L (p > .05) in the control group.

- Similarly, in the Finnish Diabetes Prevention Study[13] in subjects with IGT, HDL cholesterol levels were not significantly different after 1 or 2 years between subjects in the intervention group and controls. However, TG levels were significantly lower in the intervention group (p < .001). After 1 year, TG levels had decreased by 18 mg/dL in the intervention group compared to 1 mg/dL in controls. Taken together and based on limited data, these results indicate that dietary and behavioral interventions have no long-term effect on HDL cholesterol levels, but may decrease TG levels.

8.3.2 Pharmacological Treatment

8.3.2.1 *Orlistat (Table 8.2)*

In the study by Sjöström et al.,[18] orlistat therapy resulted in significant reductions in LDL cholesterol levels after 2 years compared to placebo, whereas changes in HDL cholesterol and TG levels were comparable between the two groups. LDL cholesterol levels decreased from 3.82 to 3.46 mmol/L (orlistat), and from 3.72 to 3.68 mmol/L (placebo). HDL cholesterol levels did not change on orlistat treatment (1.25 mmol/L), and increased from 1.24 to 1.26 mmol/L on placebo. Triglyceride concentrations fell from 1.66 to 1.53 mmol/L (orlistat), and from 1.72 to 1.59 mmol/L (placebo). Interestingly, LDL cholesterol levels fell in the orlistat group further than would have been expected from weight loss alone.

Similarly, Davidson et al.[19] found that total and LDL cholesterol were significantly more reduced with orlistat treatment than with placebo, whereas HDL cholesterol and TG levels changed similarly between the two groups. After 2 years, LDL cholesterol levels fell from 3.38 to 3.14 mmol/L (orlistat), and from 3.44 to 3.22 mmol/L (placebo). A study by Rössner et al.[20] revealed that after the first year of orlistat therapy, LDL cholesterol levels were significantly lower with orlistat therapy than with placebo, whereas HDL cholesterol and TG levels did not differ significantly between the two groups. After the second year of treatment, total and LDL cholesterol levels increased with orlistat and placebo therapy above the initial level before randomization, but still below the levels at the beginning of the 4-week placebo lead-in period (except for LDL cholesterol that, on placebo, was even higher after 2 years than at the beginning of the trial). This increase was significantly less on orlistat compared to placebo. LDL cholesterol fell from 3.80 (lead-in) to 3.55 (randomization) to 3.49 mmol/L (year 1), and increased to 3.83 mmol/L (year 2) on placebo; dropped from 3.69 (lead-in) to 3.49 (randomization) to 3.18 (year 1), and increased to 3.42 (year 2) on 60 mg orlistat; and fell from 3.65 (lead-in) to 3.44 (randomization) to 3.11 mmol/L (year 1), and increased to 3.48 mmol/L (year 2) on orlistat 120 mg.

The significant effect of orlistat therapy compared to placebo on LDL cholesterol levels and the lack of effect on HDL and TG levels were also observed by Hauptman et al.[21] In this study, the most pronounced changes in lipid levels occurred during the lead-in period. During the first year, LDL cholesterol levels increased on placebo, but decreased slightly more with orlistat therapy. During the second year, levels increased in all groups, but were still lower than compared with the levels at the beginning of the trial in the orlistat group, whereas levels were even higher in the placebo group.

Similarly, Finer et al.[31] investigated the efficacy and tolerability of orlistat in producing and maintaining weight loss over a 12-month period in 228 obese patients with a mean BMI of 36.8 kg/m^2. LDL cholesterol levels decreased in orlistat-treated patients, but increased in the placebo group. The difference in changes over 1 year was 8.98% lower LDL cholesterol ($p < .001$) in orlistat-treated patients compared to placebo; the change in HDL cholesterol was not significantly different between the groups. In this study, patients on orlistat had lost 3.29 kg compared to 1.31 kg in those on placebo (p for difference = .016).

Hollander et al.[32] investigated the role of orlistat in the treatment of 391 obese patients with type 2 diabetes over 1 year. Over the course of the study, patients on orlistat lost 6.2% of initial body weight compared to 4.3% in those on placebo (p for difference < .001). Total cholesterol (LDL cholesterol) decreased by 0.08 mmol/L (0.13 mmol/L) in patients on orlistat but increased by 0.39 mmol/L (0.22 mmol/L) in those on placebo ($p < .001$ for both total and LDL cholesterol). Triglycerides decreased by 0.01 mmol/L on orlistat and increased by 0.21 mmol/L on placebo ($p = .036$). Changes in HDL levels were not significantly different between orlistat and placebo.

Kelley et al.[22] found a similar pattern in subjects with type 2 diabetes: total and LDL cholesterol levels were significantly more reduced in subjects treated with 120 mg orlistat over 1 year compared to placebo, but HDL,[24] cholesterol, and triglyceride levels changed similarly between the two groups. Lindgärde's study included patients at high risk for cardiovascular disease; it was found that LDL cholesterol was significantly lower with orlistat therapy than with placebo, whereas HDL cholesterol and TG levels were not significantly different between the two groups. LDL cholesterol fell by 0.25 mmol/L in orlistat-treated patients, compared to 0.07 mmol/L in those on placebo.

Taken together, these studies suggest that in the long term, treatment with orlistat is more effective in achieving a reduction in LDL cholesterol levels than placebo, but has no benefit with regard to HDL cholesterol or TG levels. The largest reductions in LDL cholesterol levels are usually observed during the placebo lead-in periods of the trials, where the sharpest weight loss occurs. Nevertheless, orlistat therapy resulted in a further decrease in body weight and LDL cholesterol levels compared to placebo and, over the long term, helped to achieve reduced body weight and lipid levels.

8.3.2.2   Sibutramine (Table 8.3)

The study by James et al.[27] found substantial decreases in concentrations of TG levels proportional to weight loss with sibutramine or placebo; however, these decreases were not significantly different between the two groups. LDL cholesterol levels did not substantially change in each group. In contrast, HDL cholesterol levels increased in both groups and, after 2 years, this effect was significantly greater in subjects treated with sibutramine compared to placebo.

Smith and Goulder[28] found significant changes in TG levels after 6 months of treatment with sibutramine compared with placebo; however, after 1 year of treatment, sibutramine and placebo did not differ significantly with regard to TG or cholesterol levels. In the study by McMahon et al.,[26] HDL cholesterol levels increased significantly more in hypertensive subjects taking sibutramine compared to placebo, whereas changes in LDL cholesterol and TG levels were not significantly different between the two groups. In another study by McMahon et al.,[29] subjects taking sibutramine had significantly greater reductions in TG levels and significant increases in HDL cholesterol concentrations compared to placebo. Changes in LDL cholesterol, however, were not significantly different between the two groups. Overall, these findings suggest that sibutramine does not confer consistent improvements in blood lipid levels.

8.4 Diabetes and Impaired Glucose Tolerance (IGT)

8.4.1 Nonpharmacological Treatment (Table 8.1)

The study by Flechtner–Mors et al.[12] investigated the effect of snack replacements on weight maintenance and found no difference in fasting blood glucose levels between the intervention and the control groups. However, this study did not focus on diabetic subjects.

The aforementioned study by Eriksson and Lindgarde[11] tested the feasibility of a long-term intervention, consisting of dietary advice and increased physical activity, in subjects with type 2 diabetes and IGT, compared to no specific intervention in subjects with IGT and healthy controls, over 5 years. In the intervention group, subjects with type 2 diabetes and IGT showed improvements in glucose tolerance during the first 2 years of the study. This improvement was maintained throughout the study in patients with IGT; their 2-h glucose levels decreased from 8.2 to 7.1 mmol/L ($p < .001$). In diabetics, 2-hour glucose levels following a glucose load were essentially unchanged (from 10.0 to 9.9 mmol/L). In the comparison groups, glucose tolerance deteriorated significantly in subjects with IGT and did not substantially change in controls. In the intervention group, glycemic control was improved in 53.8% of subjects with type 2 diabetes and 75.8% of subjects with IGT, of whom only 10.6% progressed to type 2 diabetes. In subjects with IGT who received no intervention, glycemic control worsened in 67.1% of cases; 28.6% developed type 2 diabetes. None of the healthy control subjects developed diabetes. Thus, the lifestyle modification was associated with a 63% reduction in the risk for diabetes (HR = 0.37; 95% CI: 0.20, 0.68).

The Finnish Diabetes Prevention Study[13] was designed to investigate the feasibility and effects of a program of changes in lifestyle to prevent or delay the onset of type 2 diabetes in a randomized trial among subjects with IGT. Over a mean follow-up of 3.2 years, diabetes developed in 32 cases per 1000 person-years in the intervention group, and in 78 per 1000 person-years in the control group. Thus, the risk of developing type 2 diabetes was 58% lower in the intervention group than in the control group ($p < .001$). Fasting plasma glucose levels decreased by 4 mg/dL in the intervention group, and increased by 1 mg/dL in controls ($p < .001$). Two-hour post glucose load and insulin concentrations also improved significantly.

The Diabetes Prevention Program Research Group[33] randomly assigned 3234 nondiabetic persons with elevated fasting and postglucose load plasma glucose concentrations to placebo, metformin (850 mg twice daily), or a life-stlye modification program with the goals of at least 7% weight loss and at least 150 min of physical activity per week. Patients in the placebo and the metformin groups were provided with written information and an annual 20- to 30-min individual session that emphasized the importance of a healthy lifestyle. Participants were also encouraged to follow the food guide pyramid and the equivalent of a National Cholesterol Education Program step 1 diet to reduce their weight, and to increase their physical activity. In the intervention group, a 16-lesson curriculum covering diet, exercise, and behavior modification was designed. The curriculum was taught by case managers on a one-to-one basis and was flexible, culturally sensitive, and individualized. The mean BMI of the subjects was 34 kg/m^2.

Over a mean follow-up period of 2.8 years, the incidence of type 2 diabetes was decreased by 58% (95% CI: 48 to 66) in the lifestyle intervention group, and by 31% (95% CI: 17 to 43) in the metformin group, compared to the placebo group. It is noteworthy that the lifestyle intervention was associated with a 39% lower incidence of diabetes than was metformin therapy. The average weight loss was 5.6 kg in the lifestyle intervention group; 2.1 kg in the metformin group; and 0.1 kg in the placebo group. Thus, this study provides strong evidence that changes in lifestyle can effectively lead to long-term weight loss and reduce the incidence of type 2 diabetes. Furthermore, it also demonstrates that a structured, long-term multidisciplinary program involving physicians, nurses, dieticians, nutritionists, and exercise physiologists is needed to achieve sustained weight reduction. Taken together, these findings indicate that nonpharmacological weight reduction and metformin therapy confer significant benefits on glycemic control and prevention of type 2 diabetes.

8.4.2 Pharmacological Treatment: Orlistat (Table 8.2)

8.4.2.1 *Studies not Focusing on Diabetic Subjects*

In the study by Sjöström et al.,[18] orlistat therapy was associated with a significantly better glycemic control after 2 years of treatment compared to placebo therapy. Fasting blood glucose increased by 2.3% in the placebo group and decreased by 0.92% in the orlistat group ($p < .05$). Davidson et al.[19] found that fasting glucose levels were significantly higher in the placebo group compared to the orlistat group. In the study by Rössner et al.,[20] treatment with 120 mg orlistat was associated with significant reductions in fasting blood glucose after 1 year.

8.4.2.2 *Studies Focusing on Subjects with Diabetes or Impaired Glucose Tolerance*

In the study by Lindgärde[24] that investigated the effect of orlistat in obese patients at high risk for coronary artery disease, fasting glucose and HbA1c levels showed significantly greater improvements in patients treated with orlistat compared to placebo. Fasting glucose and HbA1c dropped significantly in the orlistat group compared to the placebo group. Similar improvements were also seen with orlistat in the subgroup of patients with type 2 diabetes. In the orlistat group, 23.3% of type 2 diabetics were able to stop or reduce oral hypoglycemic requirements compared to 18.2% in the placebo group.

Kelley et al.[22] compared the effect of 120 mg orlistat with placebo three times a day in obese patients with type 2 diabetes (treated with insulin alone or combined with oral agents, but with suboptimal metabolic control) over a period of 1 year. In this study, the orlistat group experienced a greater decrease in fasting glucose and HbA1c levels than did the placebo group. Furthermore, more patients in the orlistat group decreased or discontinued at least one oral diabetes medication during the study, compared to the placebo group (41.3 vs. 30.9%).

A similar study by Miles et al.[23] compared the effect of 120 mg orlistat with placebo, three times daily, over a 1-year period in obese patients with suboptimal control of type

2 diabetes who were treated with metformin only or in combination with sulfonylurea therapy. In this study, orlistat therapy was associated with significantly greater reductions in metformin and sulfonylurea requirements than placebo. Compared to the placebo group, subjects in the orlistat group had significant reductions in HbA1c and fasting glucose levels.

Finally, in the study by Hollander et al.[32] that had investigated the role of orlistat in obese patients with type 2 diabetes, treatment with orlistat was associated with significant improvements in HbA1c levels, fasting plasma glucose levels, and oral hypoglycemic requirements. Overall, orlistat therapy appears to confer modest benefits in glycemic control, but this effect is most favorable in patients with type 2 diabetes or IGT. Importantly, orlistat therapy also reduced oral hypoglycemic drug requirements in such patients.

8.4.2.3   *Sibutramine (Table 8.3)*

The study by James et al.[27] showed no significant difference in fasting glucose levels between the sibutramine- and placebo-treated groups. Smith et al.[28] also found no significant differences in fasting glucose levels among placebo, 10 mg sibutramine, or 15 mg sibutramine. Similarly, the study by McMahon et al.[26] found no significant differences in fasting glucose levels between all patients treated with sibutramine or placebo, although some differences were found when the analysis was limited to sibutramine-treated subjects who lost 5 or 10% of body weight. These finding were confirmed in another study by McMahon et al.[29] Thus, sibutramine therapy does not appear to confer a consistently favorable effect on glycemic control, although the benefits may be contingent on attaining a target weight loss. Furthermore, this agent has not been adequately investigated in patients with type 2 diabetes or IGT, in whom the potential benefits may be more pronounced.

8.5   Conclusions and Perspectives

Two main conclusions follow from this analysis of weight reduction intervention studies that investigated the effects of weight loss on blood pressure control, lipid levels, and blood glucose control. First, nonpharmacological and pharmacological obesity therapies have the potential to lessen the health burden associated with obesity through a decreased need for comedication (e.g., antihypertensive drugs); symptom improvement (e.g., blood glucose control); improved cardiovascular risks (e.g., decreased LDL cholesterol and blood pressure); and preventing disease progression in patients with borderline hypertension and impaired glucose tolerance.

Second, the beneficial effects of weight reduction on blood pressure control, lipid levels, and glycemic control appear to depend, to some degree, on the weight reduction intervention. Thus, nonpharmacological and orlistat therapy had beneficial effects on blood pressure control and the need for antihypertensive drug therapy, whereas sibutramine therapy was associated with a modest, but statistically significant, increase in blood pressure. In addition, nonpharmacological therapy reduced cholesterol and TG levels, orlistat therapy decreased LDL levels only, and sibutramine therapy increased HDL levels without any significant effects on other lipid parameters. Finally, nonpharmacological and orlistat therapy improved glycemic status and decreased disease progression and oral hypoglycemic requirements, whereas sibutramine had no consistent effects on glycemic status.

The review in this chapter has potential limitations:

- No study in this review correlated changes in markers of cardiovascular risk with hard clinical outcomes such as myocardial ischemia or stroke, thereby precluding an assessment of the clinical significance of these weight loss-associated biochemical and physiologic effects.

- Because of heterogeneity of weight loss interventions, study follow-up, and outcome reporting across studies, quantitative meta-analyses of findings were precluded.

- Except in two studies (McMahon et al.[26,29]), outcome data were not presented according to whether patients attained a target weight loss such as 5 or 10% of initial weight. Consequently, these findings might have underestimated the potential health benefits of weight reduction interventions if analyses had been reported separately in patients who achieved a prespecified weight loss target.

In summary, weight reduction with nonpharmacological methods and treatment with orlistat and sibutramine confer improvements in biochemical and physiological markers of cardiovascular risk. Additional studies are required to determine if such effects confer reductions in cardiovascular morbidity and mortality.

References

1. Expert Panel. Executive summary of the clinical guidelines on the identification, evaluation, and treatment of overweight and obesity in adults. *Arch. Intern. Med.* 1998; 158:1855–1867.
2. Mokdad, A.H., Ford, E.S., Bowman, B.A., Dietz, W.H., Vinicor, F., Bales, V.S., and Marks, J.S. Prevalence of obesity, diabetes, and obesity-related health risk factors, 2001. *JAMA* 2003; 289:76–79.
3. Wilson, P.W., D'Agostino, R.B., Sullivan, L., Parise, H., and Kannel, W.B. Overweight and obesity as determinants of cardiovascular risk: the Framingham experience. *Arch. Intern. Med.* 2002; 162:1867–1872.
4. Rossner, S. Long-term intervention strategies in obesity treatment. *Int. J. Obes. Relat. Metab. Disord.* 1995; 19 Suppl 7:S29-S33; discussion S34–S35.
5. Jeffcoate, W. Obesity is a disease: food for thought. *Lancet* 1998; 351:903–904.
6. Rippe, J.M., Crossley, S., and Ringer, R. Obesity as a chronic disease: modern medical and lifestyle management. *J. Am. Diet. Assoc.* 1998; 98:S9–15.
7. Douketis, J.D., Feightner, J.W., Attia, J., and Feldman, W.F. Periodic health examination, 1999 update: 1. Detection, prevention and treatment of obesity. Canadian Task Force on Preventive Health Care. *CMAJ* 1999; 160:513–525.
8. Must, A., Spadano, J., Coakley, E.H., Field, A.E., Colditz, G., and Dietz, W.H. The disease burden associated with overweight and obesity. *JAMA* 1999; 282:1523–1529.
9. James, W.P., Chunming, C., Inoue, S. Appropriate Asian body mass indices? *Obes. Rev.* 2002; 3:139.
10. Kolanowski, J. Obesity and hypertension: from pathophysiology to treatment. *Int. J. Obes. Relat. Metab. Disord.* 1999; 23 Suppl 1:42–46.
11. Eriksson, K.F. and Lindgarde, F. Prevention of type 2 (non-insulin-dependent) diabetes mellitus by diet and physical exercise. The 6-year Malmo feasibility study. *Diabetologia* 1991; 34:891–898.
12. Flechtner–Mors, M., Ditschuneit, H.H., Johnson, T.D., Suchard, M.A., and Adler, G. Metabolic and weight loss effects of long-term dietary intervention in obese patients: four-year results. *Obes. Res.* 2000; 8:399–402.
13. Tuomilheto, J., Lindstrom, J., Eriksson, J.G., Valle, T.T., Hamalainen, H., Ilanne-Parikka, P., Keinanen–Kiukaanniemi, S., Laakso, M., Louheranta, A., Rastas, M., Salminen, V., and Uusitupa, M. Prevention of type 2 diabetes mellitus by changes in lifestyle among subjects with impaired glucose tolerance. *N. Engl. J. Med.* 2001; 344:1343–1350.

14. Stevens, V.J., Obarzanek, E., Cook, N.R., Lee, I.M., Appel, L.J., Smith West, D., Milas, N.C., Mattfeldt–Beman, M., Belden, L., Bragg, C., Millstone, M., Raczynski, J., Brewer, A., Singh, B., and Cohen, J. Long-term weight loss and changes in blood pressure: results of the trials of hypertension prevention, phase II. *Ann. Intern. Med.* 2001; 134:1–11.

15. Whelton, P.K., Appel, L.J., Espeland, M.A., Applegate, W.B., Ettinger, W.H., Jr., Kostis, J.B., Kumanyika, S., Lacy, C.R., Johnson, K.C., Folmar, S., and Cutler, J.A. Sodium reduction and weight loss in the treatment of hypertension in older persons: a randomized controlled trial of nonpharmacologic interventions in the elderly (TONE). TONE Collaborative Research Group. *JAMA* 1998; 279:839–846.

16. Stamler, R., Stamler, J., Grimm, R., Gosch, F.C., Elmer, P., Dyer, A., Berman, R., Fishman, J., Van Heel, N., Civinelli, J. et al. Nutritional therapy for high blood pressure. Final report of a four-year randomized controlled trial — the hypertension control program. *JAMA* 1987; 257:1484–1491.

17. Yusuf, S., Sleight, P., Pogue, J., Bosch, J., Davies, R., and Dagenais, G.. Effects of an angiotensin-converting-enzyme inhibitor, ramipril, on cardiovascular events in high-risk patients. The Heart Outcomes Prevention Evaluation Study Investigators. *N. Engl. J. Med.* 2000; 342:145–153.

18. Sjostrom, L., Rissanen, A., Andersen, T., Boldrin, M., Golay, A., Koppeschaar, H.P., and Krempf, M. Randomised placebo-controlled trial of orlistat for weight loss and prevention of weight regain in obese patients. European Multicentre Orlistat Study Group. *Lancet* 1998; 352:167–172.

19. Davidson, M.H., Hauptman, J., DiGirolamo, M., Foreyt, J.P., Halsted, C.H., Heber, D., Heimburger, D.C., Lucas, C.P., Robbins, D.C., Chung, J., and Heymsfield, S.B. Weight control and risk factor reduction in obese subjects treated for 2 years with orlistat: a randomized controlled trial. *JAMA* 1999; 281:235–242.

20. Rossner, S., Sjostrom, L., Noack, R., Meinders, A.E., and Noseda, G. Weight loss, weight maintenance, and improved cardiovascular risk factors after 2 years treatment with orlistat for obesity. European Orlistat Obesity Study Group. *Obes. Res.* 2000; 8:49–61.

21. Hauptman, J., Lucas, C., Boldrin, M.N., Collins, H., and Segal, K.R. Orlistat in the long-term treatment of obesity in primary care settings. *Arch. Fam. Med.* 2000; 9:160–167.

22. Kelley, D.E., Bray, G.A., Pi–Sunyer, F.X., Klein, S., Hill, J., Miles, J., and Hollander, P. Clinical efficacy of orlistat therapy in overweight and obese patients with insulin-treated type 2 diabetes: A 1-year randomized controlled trial. *Diabetes Care* 2002; 25:1033–1041.

23. Miles, J.M., Leiter, L., Hollander, P., Wadden, T., Anderson, J.W., Doyle, M., Foreyt, J., Aronne, L., and Klein, S. Effect of orlistat in overweight and obese patients with type 2 diabetes treated with metformin. *Diabetes Care* 2002; 25:1123–1128.

24. Lindgarde F. The effect of orlistat on body weight and coronary heart disease risk profile in obese patients: the Swedish Multimorbidity Study. *J. Intern. Med.* 2000; 248:245–254.

25. Bray, G.A., Blackburn, G.L., Ferguson, J.M., Greenway, .FL., Jain, A.K., Mendel, C.M., Mendels, J., Ryan, D.H., Schwartz, S.L., Scheinbaum, M.L., and Seaton, T.B. Sibutramine produces dose-related weight loss. *Obes. Res.* 1999; 7:189–198.

26. McMahon, F.G., Fujioka, K., Singh, B.N., Mendel, C.M., Rowe, E., Rolston, K., Johnson, F., and Mooradian, A.D. Efficacy and safety of sibutramine in obese white and African American patients with hypertension: a 1-year, double-blind, placebo-controlled, multicenter trial. *Arch. Intern. Med.* 2000; 160:2185–2191.

27. James, W.P., Astrup, A., Finer, N., Hilsted, J., Kopelman, P., Rossner, S., Saris, W.H., and Van Gaal, L.F. Effect of sibutramine on weight maintenance after weight loss: a randomised trial. STORM Study Group. Sibutramine Trial of Obesity Reduction and Maintenance. *Lancet* 2000; 356:2119–2125.

28. Smith, I.G. and Goulder, M.A. Randomized placebo-controlled trial of long-term treatment with sibutramine in mild to moderate obesity. *J. Fam. Pract.* 2001; 50:505–512.

29. McMahon, F.G., Weinstein, S.P., Rowe, E., Ernst, K.R., Johnson, F., and Fujioka, K. Sibutramine is safe and effective for weight loss in obese patients whose hypertension is well controlled with angiotensin-converting enzyme inhibitors. *J. Hum. Hypertens.* 2002; 16:5–11.

30. Third Report of the National Cholesterol Education Program (NCEP) Expert Panel on Detection, Evaluation, and Treatment of High Blood Cholesterol in Adults (Adult Treatment Panel III) final report. *Circulation* 2002; 106:3143–3421.

31. Finer, N., James, W.P., Kopelman, P.G., Lean, M.E., and Williams, G. One-year treatment of obesity: a randomized, double-blind, placebo- controlled, multicentre study of orlistat, a gastrointestinal lipase inhibitor. *Int. J. Obes. Relat. Metab. Disord.* 2000; 24:306–313.

32. Hollander, P.A., Elbein, S.C., Hirsch, I.B., Kelley, D., McGill, J., Taylor, T., Weiss, S.R., Crockett, S.E., Kaplan, R.A., Comstock, J., Lucas, C.P., Lodewick, P.A., Canovatchel, W., Chung, J., and Hauptman, J. Role of orlistat in the treatment of obese patients with type 2 diabetes. A 1-year randomized double-blind study. *Diabetes Care* 1998; 21:1288–1294.

33. Knowler, W.C., Barrett–Connor, E., Fowler, S.E., Hamman, R.F., Lachin, J.M., Walker, E.A., and Nathan, D.M. Reduction in the incidence of type 2 diabetes with lifestyle intervention or metformin. *N. Engl. J. Med.* 2002; 346:393–403.

9

Weight Loss and Associated Diseases

Paolo M. Suter

CONTENTS

9.1   Introduction

Overweight and obesity are increasing worldwide in all age groups (Flegal et al. 2002; Kuczmarski et al. 1994; McLellan 2002; Vorster 2002; Walker et al. 2001), especially in children and young adults (Ebbeling et al. 2002). Due to alterations in life-style (mainly nutrition and patterns of physical activity), overweight and obesity are also emerging problems in Third World countries. Large differences in the mean body mass index (BMI) as well as the prevalence rates of obesity are found between rural and urban areas — a clear indication of the pathophysiological importance of environmental and life-style factors. Presently, two in three U.S. adults are overweight or obese (Flegal et al. 2002). An increased body weight is associated with an increased risk of death and shortening of life expectancy (Lee et al. 2001; Peeters et al. 2003).

Overweight and obesity represent the most important risk factors and risk modulators for most if not all chronic diseases, i.e., coronary artery disease; type 2 diabetes mellitus; hypertension; dyslipidemia; or the metabolic syndrome (Ford et al. 2002; Mokdad et al. 2003). Weight loss leads to a reduced risk for these conditions (Knowler et al. 2002; Will et al. 2002). Nevertheless, the relationship among body weight, weight loss, morbidity and mortality remains controversial (Lee et al. 2001). In the present epidemiological transition in chronic disease risk factors, overweight and obesity will soon bypass smoking as the most important preventable cause of death. Thus, strategies for prevention of and therapy for overweight and obesity at the individual as well as the population level should be implemented and developed as a top priority in health care. In this chapter, the relationship among body weight, weight loss, and chronic disease risk, especially risk of developing the metabolic syndrome, will be reviewed in the context of individual and population levels. In addition, evidence regarding control of weight at the population level will be reviewed briefly.

9.2 Body Weight Changes and Disease Risk

The increased incidence and prevalence of overweight and obesity represent the most dramatic epidemiologic shift worldwide. In the 1960s, one in four U.S. adults was overweight or obese; presently this ratio is two in three (Flegal et al. 2002; Kuczmarski et al. 1994; Mokdad et al. 1999, 2003). In a recent study using data from the Framingham Heart Study (follow-up from 1948 to 1990), Peeters et al. (2003) reported a decrease in life expectancy due to overweight and obesity that is similar to smoking. According to this study, an obese adult at age 40 had a 6- to 7-year shorter life span than a normal-weight adult. The combination of smoking and overweight had even more deleterious effects. Smoking increased the shortening of the life-span by 13 to 14 years in obese adults. Although the study by Peeters et al. (2003) did not identify the exact cause of the premature mortality, it is known from many other studies that body weight affects virtually all cellular, metabolic, and organ systems negatively. All risk factors for chronic diseases and all chronic disease conditions (except osteoporosis; see Albala et al. 1996) are affected by body weight.

9.3 Body Weight Changes and Diabetes Risk

More than 70% of people with diabetes type 2 are obese. Individuals with a BMI > 27 have at least a 70% chance of having an obesity induced co-morbid condition (Wolf 1998). Weight gain is strongly linked to the development of diabetes type 2 in men and in women (Chan et al. 1994; Colditz et al. 1990; Looker et al. 2001). In the Nurses Health Study, the risk for diabetes type 2 increased with increasing BMI even within the normal range (Colditz et al. 1995). Women showing a weight gain of 5.0 to 7.9 kg had a relative risk for diabetes mellitus of 1.9 (95% CI 1.5 to 2.3) compared to those showing a weight change of less than 5.0 kg (Colditz et al. 1995). The relative risk of diabetes for women gaining 8.0 to 10.9 kg was 2.7 (95% CI 2.1. to 3.3). However, women losing ≥5.0 kg had a reduction of the risk of diabetes by ≥50% (91% CI 0.4 to 1.0) (Colditz et al. 1995).

A similar increase in risk of diabetes type 2 with changes in body weight was observed in the National Health and Examination Survey Epidemiologic Follow-up Study (Ford et al. 1997). The latter study calculated a population-attributable risk of 27% for weight increases of 5 kg or more. It is important to note that the observed effects of body weight on the risk of diabetes type 2 were independent of the family history of diabetes, age, sex, or race (Colditz et al. 1995; Ford et al. 1997). These as well as other data support the importance of weight maintenance throughout adulthood. In view of the increase in the prevalence of obesity as well as the very profound effects of already small changes in body weight, the increases in diabetes rates are not surprising (Mokdad et al. 2003; Skyler and Oddo 2002).

Another often neglected aspect of these studies is the observation that an increase of body weight within the limits of "normality" (i.e., body mass index (BMI) < 25 kg/m²) will lead to an increase in disease risk. Present data clearly show the great impact of weight stability (absence of weight increase; see the next section) during adulthood on the risk of developing chronic diseases. Nevertheless, most guidelines promote weight loss and do not promote weight stability.

9.3.1 The Importance of Weight Maintenance

Insulin resistance and hyperinsulinemia are of central pathophysiological importance in the development of diabetes type 2 and the metabolic syndrome (Reusch 2002). However, whether obesity precedes or follows hyperinsulinemia is still controversial. In prospective data from the Kuopio Ischaemic Heart Disease Risk Factor Study, weight gain increased the risk of developing hyperinsulinemia in nondiabetic middle-aged men (Lakka et al. 2002). A BMI of > 26.7 kg/m² was associated with an incidence of hyperinsulinemia six times higher than for a BMI < 24.4 kg/m². Weight gain of ≥4 kg at middle age during a 4-year period was associated with a sixfold increase in the incidence of hyperinsulinemia compared to the incidence for men with stable weight and/or weight loss (Lakka et al. 2002).

The pathophysiological importance of overweight and obesity in the modulation of diabetes risk is well established; additionally, the study by Lakka et al. shows that relatively small changes in body weight have a very large impact. However, it should be remembered that overweight and obese subjects can reduce their risk considerably by avoiding further weight gain. In a recent prospective study, the age-adjusted incidence for diabetes increased from 9.6% in subjects with a BMI < 29 kg/m² to 26% in subjects with a BMI of ≥ 37 kg/m² (Resnick et al. 2000). In this prospective cohort study, for overweight subjects, each kilogram of weight gained annually resulted in a 49% increase in the risk for developing diabetes in the 10 subsequent years compared to the risk for overweight individuals with stable body weight (Resnick et al. 2000). Losing 1 kg of body weight in these overweight individuals led to 33% reduction of the diabetes risk in the subsequent 10 years. These data support the concept that body weight should at least be maintained independently from the actual body weight.

Most people lose and regain weight. However, to modulate disease risk, a sustained weight loss is important. An analysis from the Framingham Study showed the importance of a sustained weight loss in overweight subjects (BMI ≥ 27 kg/m²) (Moore et al. 2000). Weight cycling may even be associated with adverse metabolic effects and a higher chronic disease risk (Olson et al. 2000; Roessner 1989; Sea et al. 2000). Compared to subjects with stable weight, a sustained weight loss led to a 37% reduction in the risk of diabetes; the risk reduction was significantly stronger for more obese subjects (i.e., BMI $\geq$ 29 kg/m^2), who showed a relative risk of 0.38 (95% CI 0.18 to 0.81) (Moore et al. 2000). In addition, the study reported a clear correlation with a higher risk reduction with increasing weight loss. However, those regaining their weight did not experience any risk reduction for diabetes (Moore et al. 2000).

For daily practice, this means any weight loss will affect risk as long as the loss can be maintained at lower levels. If weight loss cannot be sustained, all efforts should focus on weight stability. (In this chapter, weight stability corresponds to weight maintenance.) It is well known that in the setting of weight maintenance at a higher than normal body weight, the risk of type 2 diabetes remains increased; however, it will be lower than in a setting in which body weight is continuously increasing. In addition, weight maintenance represents an important initial step toward body weight loss.

It seems that weight stability (i.e., avoidance of weight gain) during adulthood is of prime importance in preventing hyperinsulinemia (Lakka et al. 2002) and type 2 diabetes (Colditz et al. 1995; Ford et al. 1997). Weight stability is also associated with a lower mortality risk (Peeters et al. 2003; Somes et al. 2002).

9.3.2   Effects of Weight Loss on Mortality and Morbidity

In view of the pathophysiological effects of weight gain on the risk of diabetes, hyperinsulinemia, and other chronic diseases, it can be assumed that weight loss will unequivocally have favorable health effects. Despite the powerful association between weight gain and disease risk and mortality (Peeters et al. 2003), weight loss does not always lead to reduced mortality, especially when weight loss episodes are associated with weight regain ("weight cycling") (Lee et al. 2001; Wannamethee et al. 2002; Yaari and Goldbourt 1998). Some of the controversial results can be readily explained by methodological issues (such as lack of separation between intentional and unintentional weight loss or length of follow-up). In 1942, Newburgh reported that weight reduction improved glycemic control in obese subjects. It has been shown in many studies that a moderate weight loss (5 to 10% weight reduction) is associated with highly significant improvement of most cardiovascular risk factors, as well as certain end points (e.g., diabetes) (Dixon and O'Brien 2002a; Eriksson and Lindgarde 1991; Pasanisi et al. 2001; Vidal 2002).

No single prospective therapeutic long-term study has examined the effect of sustained weight loss on overall morbidity and mortality. Nevertheless, the evidence from large prospective cohort studies reporting a strong association between obesity and an increased mortality is convincing (Rhoads and Kagan 1983; van Italie 1985). In diabetic subjects, weight loss leads to improved fasting blood glucose levels as well as improved postprandial glucose levels (UKPDS Group 1990) and a reduction of antidiabetic or antihypertensive medication dosage and use (Amatruda et al. 1988; Dixon and O'Brien 2002b). The dramatic effect of weight loss on glucose homeostasis and diabetes risk can be nicely illustrated in patients after bariatric surgery with a comparatively large weight loss within a short time. The incidence of diabetes in a group of patients with a follow-up of more than 3000 patient-years after bariatric surgery was zero (Dixon and O'Brien 2002b).

Similarly, with a comparably small weight loss in combination with other life-style strategies, the incidence of diabetes was dramatically reduced for participants in several diabetes prevention studies (Eriksson and Lindgarde 1991; Knowler et al. 2002; Long et al. 1994; Tuomilehto et al. 2001). In the Diabetes Prevention Program Research Group study (Knowler et al. 2002), the incidence of diabetes could be reduced to a larger degree by the implementation of selected life-style interventions as compared to a drug therapy with metformin. During the 2.8-year-long intervention, the incidence of diabetes type 2 declined in the life-style intervention group by 58% (CI 48 to 66%) and in the metformin group by 31% (CI 17 to 43%) (Knowler et al. 2002).

The life-style intervention consisted of a weight reduction of at least 7% of the initial weight achieved by a hypocaloric fat-reduced diet and increased physical activity (at least 150 min of physical activity per week) (Knowler et al. 2002). In addition, the life-style group was required to attend 16 educational sessions about healthy nutrition, eating behavior, and physical activity. The metformin group received only a quick-fix educational session of 20 to 30 min. Although the life-style group could reduce body weight by 7% during the first half year, in the further course of the study it regained up to 40 to 50% of the initial weight loss. It seems that the increased physical activity could be maintained rather well during the whole study period. Accordingly, whether the hypocaloric diet and the small weight loss or the increased level of physical activity alone or in combination with a small weight loss is of greater therapeutic importance must be considered (Astrand and Rodahl 1986; Gwinup 1975; Levine et al. 1999; Ravnikar 1993).

Another recent diabetes prevention study is from the Finnish Diabetes Prevention Study Group (Tuomilehto et al. 2001), which reported a similar diabetes risk reduction by a life-style intervention in high-risk patients, i.e., individuals with a positive family history of diabetes and overweight individuals. The intervention consisted of a weight reduction of ≥5% of the baseline weight; reduced dietary fat intake (<30% energy from fat; <10% saturated fat); and increased dietary fiber intake (> 15 g/1000 kcal). In addition, it was recommended to increase the consumption of reduced-fat dairy products, lean meat, fruits and vegetables, and soft margarine, as well as to increase intake of plant-based oils and monounsaturated fat. These strategies were combined with the recommendation to increase the duration of physical activity to at least 30 min per day (Tuomilehto et al. 2001).

These life-style changes led to a reduction of the incidence of diabetes. The cumulative incidence of diabetes type 2 during a 2-year follow-up period was 11% (95% CI 6 to 15) in the intervention group and 23% (95% CI 17 to 29) in the control group. Again, the weight loss at the end of the 2-year period was comparatively small in the intervention group (3.5 ± 5.5 kg vs. 0.8 ± 4.4 in the control group, $p < .001$) (Tuomilehto et al. 2001). The results of this study are impressive; however, one cannot ignore the importance of factors other than weight loss (i.e., physical activity and nutritional factors). It seems that the combination of a moderate weight loss *and* exercise is more effective in reducing disease risk than weight loss alone. In view of the metabolic effects of exercise, this is not surprising (Jeukendrup 2002). In addition, regular physical activity is of crucial importance for weight stability (Weinsier et al. 2002); however, the level of activity in that study seemed to be rather high, and it is unclear whether this high level (regarding duration and intensity) of physical activity can be implemented in the long term.

Because of the relation between the percent of weight loss and the likelihood of remission and/or progression of type 2 diabetes, a larger weight loss would be preferable. Bariatric surgery is promoted with several arguments, e.g., that even a moderate weight loss is difficult to achieve; that weight loss could generally not be maintained; and that a large weight loss is needed to affect the incidence of the chronic diseases (e.g., diabetes) (Dixon and O'Brien 2002). To the contrary, present evidence shows that a comparatively small weight loss in combination with life-style modification (especially physical activity) has a large impact on the risk of developing diabetes (Knowler et al. 2002; Tuomilehto et al. 2001). In daily practice, any weight loss — independently from the amount — should be acknowledged and promoted as long as the loss will be maintained.

TABLE 9.1

Clinical Definition and Identification of the Metabolic Syndrome

Risk Factor	Defining Level
Abdominal obesity (waist circumference)	Men > 102 cm (>40 in.); women > 88 cm (>35 in.)
Triglyceride	≥1.69 mmol/L (≥150 mg/dl)
HDL cholesterol	Men ≤ 1.0 mmol/L (≤40 mg/dl); women ≤ 1.29 mmol/L (≤50 mg/dl)
Blood pressure	≥130/≥85 mmHg
Fasting glucose	≥6.0 mmol/L (≥110 mg/dl)

Source: From Expert Panel on Detection and Treatment of High Cholesterol in Adults, *JAMA*, 285: 2486–2497, 2001.

9.4 Effect of Weight Loss on Selected Components of the Metabolic Syndrome

According to the National Cholesterol Education Program (NCEP) Adult Treatment Panel III (ATP III) (Expert Panel 2001), the metabolic syndrome is a secondary target of therapy and is diagnosed based upon a clinical identification of selected conditions (Table 9.1). Besides the clinical features summarized in Table 9.1, other symptoms and signs cluster in the setting of the metabolic syndrome (Hauner 2002; Ukkola and Bouchard 2001) (e.g., albuminuria; proteinuria; inflammation and proinflammatory state; disorders of coagulation; and fibrinolysis and elevated uric acid). Weight loss affects all components of the metabolic syndrome. In this section, selected aspects of the effect of body weight and weight loss on the components of the metabolic syndrome are briefly addressed.

9.4.1 Abdominal Obesity

One important component of the metabolic syndrome is visceral (abdominal) obesity (Bosello and Zamboni 2000; Busetto 2001; Despres 2001; Wajchenberg 2000). Independently from body weight, visceral obesity is associated with an increased risk for hypertension; dyslipidemia; hypercoagulability; diabetes; inflammation; and the corresponding clinical end points (Nguyen–Duy et al. in press; Wajchenberg 2000). A moderate weight loss will also result in a reduction of visceral obesity as assessed with the measurement of the waist circumference or using modern imaging techniques, which correlate directly with the visceral fat mass (Despres 2001; Smith and Zachwieja 1999; Wajchenberg 2000). In addition to a positive energy balance, several risk factors for the abdominal accumulation of fat have been identified (Wajchenberg 2000). These risk factors are:

- Physical inactivity (Despres 1997)
- Smoking (Shimokata et al. 1989)
- Psychological stress (e.g., depression) (Bjoerntorp 1991)
- Weight cycling
- Alcohol consumption (Suter and Vetter 1995, 1997; Suter et al. 1997b)
- Genetics (hormonal changes) (Wajchenberg 2000).

With the exception of the genetic predisposition, all of these risk factors can be modulated favorably by nonpharmacological means.

9.4.2 Glucose Homeostasis

Body weight represents the most important determinant of diabetes risk (see other sections of this chapter and other chapters of this book) (Moore et al. 2000; Resnick et al. 2000). Not only absolute body weight or absolute fat mass determines the risk for an impaired glucose homeostasis, but also body fat distribution affects this risk (Goodpaster et al. 2003). Visceral abdominal fat is usually higher in subjects with type 2 diabetes and subjects with impaired glucose tolerance (IGT) than in subjects with normal glucose tolerance (NGT) (Goodpaster et al. 2003). Prospective data showed that only subjects with abdominal deposition of fat developed an impaired glucose tolerance (Despres 1997, 2001; Despres et al. 2000; Lamarche et al. 1999). The prevention of obesity is of top priority and, even more so, abdominal obesity (Bosello and Zamboni 2000). Individuals gaining only moderate amounts of weight with mainly abdominal deposition will have a considerably higher diabetes risk compared to individuals gaining the same amount of weight (or fat mass) but storing the fat in more peripheral tissues (e.g., subcutaneous adipose tissue). The most important modifiable risk factors for abdominal obesity have been mentioned earlier.

9.4.3 Hypertension

Body weight is one of the most important modulators of the level of blood pressure and overall cardiovascular risk (Poirier 2002). The exact mechanism by which an increased body weight augments blood pressure is not exactly known; however, certain factors are pathophysiologically relevant, such as (Frohlich 2002; Hall et al. 2002; Parati 2002; Suter et al. 1997a; Thakur et al. 2001):

- Hyperinsulinemia
- Insulin resistance
- Volume expansion
- Chronic renal damage
- Alterations in the renin–angiotensin–aldosterone system
- Increased salt sensitivity
- Leptin and other fat-derived hormonal factors
- Activation of sympathetic activity

In view of the complex pathogenesis and interrelationship of risk factors, the pharmacological therapy for obesity-related hypertension is difficult and often suboptimal. Whether β-blocking agents are associated with a higher risk of weight gain is controversial (Pischon and Sharma 2002; Sharma et al. 2001). Clinical practice suggests that β-blocker-related weight increase if only of minor importance — if at all. Other weight-promoting factors are of greater importance in hypertensive patients than the potential side effects on body weight by β-blocking agents (Suter and Vetter 1995). In view of the favorable effects of β-blocking agents in general and especially also in obese individuals, these drugs should not be withheld but patients should be monitored more closely. Basically, all effects of β-blocking agents on lipid and glucose metabolism can be controlled and prevented by the optimal implementation of nonpharmacological strategies.

Weight loss is often associated with a decrease in blood pressure (MacMahon et al. 1987); however, it should be mentioned that weight reduction does not reduce blood pressure in all patients and that the response shows a rather large variability. Based upon a meta-analysis, a 1-kg weight loss is associated with a decline in systolic and diastolic blood pressure by 0.68 and 0.34 mmHg, respectively (MacMahon et al. 1987). A systematic review in the Cochrane Database reported that a 4 to 9% weight reduction leads to a systolic and/or diastolic blood pressure reduction of roughly 3 mmHg (Mulrow et al. 2000).

As with most other disease conditions, however, a weight rebound will lead to a return of blood pressure to the preweight-loss level. The blood pressure-lowering effects of weight loss seem to be small compared to the pharmacological treatment of blood pressure, although, in the analysis by Mulrow et al. (2000), the therapeutic combination of weight-reducing diet and drugs led to a reduced requirement (dosage) of antihypertensive drugs. Again, it is important to remember that a modest weight loss without achieving ideal body weight will reduce blood pressure and thus cardiovascular risk in many patients.

Of special concern is the increase in the prevalence of childhood obesity (Ebbeling et al. 2002). Obesity in children is associated with an increase in blood pressure and frank hypertension that tracks into adulthood (Sorof and Daniels 2002). The antihypertensive benefit of weight loss for blood pressure control has also been shown in children (Belsha 2002; Sorof and Daniels 2002).

9.4.4 Dyslipidemia

High plasma triglycerides and low HDL cholesterol levels are the characteristic dyslipidemia of the metabolic syndrome (Expert Panel on Detection 2001). It is important to remember that the definition criteria do not include LDL cholesterol, which means that a metabolic syndrome could be present despite normal LDL cholesterol; many patients and also physicians are still focused exclusively on LDL cholesterol. With increasing body weight, total cholesterol and triglyceride plasma levels increase in a nearly linear manner and HDL cholesterol plasma levels decline (Hubert et al. 1983; Wilson et al. 1994)

Based upon data from a recent meta-analysis that included 70 trials, Dattilo and Kris–Etherton (1992) reported that, per kilogram of body weight lost, total cholesterol was reduced by 0.05 mmol/L; LDL cholesterol by 0.02 mmol/L; and plasma triglyceride levels by 0.015 mmol/L. Conversely, a weight loss of 1 kg (after stabilization of the weight on the new lower level) was associated with a 0.009-mmol/L increase of HDL cholesterol (Dattilo and Kris–Etherton 1992). What do these changes mean in the context of cardiovascular risk? Reducing LDL cholesterol by 0.025 mmol/L would imply a 1% coronary artery disease (CAD) risk reduction; however a change of HDL cholesterol by 0.025 mmol/L would be associated with a change in CAD-risk by 3%. The HDL cholesterol levels should be as high as possible and several important modulators of this level have been identified (obesity, smoking, physical activity, oral contraceptive agents, alcohol) (Wilson et al. 1994).

Different metabolic factors influence HDL cholesterol; however, hypertriglyceridemia seems to be of major importance (Gotto 2002; Hokanson 2002). Elevated plasma triglyceride (TG) levels are regarded as a coronary artery risk factor (Austin 1989, 1999). Hypertriglyceridemia has important metabolic consequences and represents one important component of the metabolic syndrome. The correction of the dyslipidemia is important because several of the metabolic abnormalities are induced and maintained by the hypertriglyceridemia. An inverse relationship exists between the fasting or postprandial plasma triglyceride concentration and the HDL cholesterol concentration (Gotto 2002). HDL cholesterol will only increase in the setting of a reduction of plasma triglyceride concentration.

In the Copenhagen Male Study, an increased fasting plasma triglyceride and low plasma HDL cholesterol concentration were associated with a twofold higher prevalence and incidence of ischemic heart disease (Jeppesen et al. 1997). In a recent study, the same authors reported that, in men free of clinical symptoms of ischemic heart disease (IHD), ischemic ECG changes were significantly more predictive of fatal IHD in men with high TG–low HDL cholesterol compared to men with low TG–high HDL cholesterol (Jeppesen et al. 2003).

Obesity (especially abdominal obesity) is one important determinant of the plasma HDL concentration and a higher body weight is associated with a lower HDL concentration (Gotto 2002). The low HDL concentration is usually a characteristic feature of abdominal obesity (Despres 2000, 2001). In this situation, HDL-raising strategies such as weight loss and a healthy diet in combination with regular physical activity seem to be of primary importance (Despres 2000). Evidence is now sufficient to support any strategy to correct the characteristic dyslipidemia of the metabolic syndrome. Weight loss and weight control in general (stabilization) are important (Noakes and Clifton 2000). Again, it is important to mention that a small weight loss of around 10% of the initial weight will have favorable effects on the plasma triglyceride concentration (Jones 2000).

Regular physical activity (with or without weight loss) is associated with favorable lipid effects (Durstine et al. 2001). There is a correlation between the volume of exercise training (i.e., energy expenditure) and the blood lipid changes (Durstine et al. 2001). As a function of duration and intensity of aerobic exercise, an improvement of plasma lipid levels can be achieved (Halbert et al. 1999) that may be additive to the effects of weight loss. The exercise effects on plasma lipids occur independently from body weight loss (Despres 1997; Durstine et al. 2001; Halbert et al. 1999). The lipid constellation of low HDL cholesterol and high plasma triglyceride levels seems to be more responsive to weight loss and/ or exercise than other lipid abnormalities.

Clearly, many factors lead to the dyslipidemia in the setting of the metabolic syndrome. It seems that an increased and prolonged postprandial lipemia is of considerable importance in atherosclerosis and the development of other chronic diseases. Many years ago Zilversmit (1979) postulated that atherosclerosis is a postprandial phenomenon; in the meantime, evidence has accumulated that this hypothesis may be correct (Parks 2001). An inverse relationship exists between the fasting or postprandial triglyceride concentration and the HDL cholesterol plasma concentration (Despres 2000, 2001; Lamarche et al. 1999). Several strategies, such as decreased fat intake, reduction of the meal frequency, or weight loss, would lead to an improvement of the postprandial lipemia (Suter 2001) (and thus also increase of HDL cholesterol). Postprandial lipemia is considerably lower in individuals pursuing regular physical activity and a preprandial exercise session leads to a reduction of the postprandial lipemia (Suter 2001).

In severe cases of hypertriglyceridemia, the gastrointestinal lipase inhibitor tetrahydrolipstatin (orlistat) may represent an additional important pharmacological agent (Wierzbicki et al. 2002). Furthermore, it was showed recently that orlistat may favorably affect postprandial lipemia as well as lipoprotein particle distribution pattern during the postprandial phase (Suter et al. manuscript submitted).

9.5 Body Weight and Other Components of the Metabolic Syndrome

In addition to the basic components of the metabolic syndrome (see Table 9.1), other clinical conditions and signs may occur; accordingly, the metabolic syndrome is also defined as a metabolic risk factor clustering. The effect of weight loss on some of these additional risk factor clusters will be briefly discussed in this section.

9.5.1   Albuminuria and Proteinuria

Another component of the metabolic syndrome is albuminuria as a surrogate marker for endothelial dysfunction in diabetics and in the general population (Liese et al. 2001; Naidoo 2002). Microalbuminuria is a strong predictor for future cardiovascular risk and is now generally accepted as a cardiovascular risk factor. Several studies report that microalbuminuria is an early sign of endothelial dysfunction and that microalbuminuria is independent from hypertension or diabetes associated with obesity and/or central adiposity (De-Jong et al. 2002; Kim et al. 2001; Liese et al. 2001; Mulyadi et al. 2001; Reid et al. 1998). Obesity may damage the kidney independently from other factors and associated conditions (e.g., hypertension, dyslipidemia, diabetes) and evidence suggests that the obesity-associated renal damage is similar to the damage induced by diabetes (De-Jong et al. 2002). A recent study reported that, in subjects with identical percent fat mass, the age-adjusted relative risk of albuminuria was 18 times greater in centrally obese subjects compared with controls, while only 4 times greater in peripherally obese subjects (Mulyadi et al. 2001).

Some studies failed to identify an independent relationship between obesity and increased albumin excretion (Hoffmann et al. 2001), which can be explained in part by different patient characteristics. Body weight reduction improves microalbuminuria and albuminuria (Ohashi et al. 2001). In addition to weight loss, nutritional factors (e.g., lipid intake regarding quality and quantity) may contribute to an increased urinary albumin excretion rate (Valensi et al. 1996). Experimental animal data reported a reduction in proteinuria during calorie restriction (Van-Liew et al. 1992).

9.5.2   Inflammation

During the last few years inflammation and inflammatory processes have been identified as central pathophysiological phenomena in the induction and maintenance of chronic diseases, including the metabolic syndrome and atherosclerosis (Ridker et al. 2003). Several factors have been suggested to promote or induce the onset of the metabolic syndrome, including genetic factors and dietary factors, hyperinsulinemia, and inflammation (Das 2002). Low-grade systemic inflammation, as associated with overweight and obesity, modulates insulin action. In nondiabetic and diabetic individuals, obesity, especially visceral obesity, correlates with the C-reactive protein (CRP), which is a sensitive marker of inflammation (Leinonen et al. 2003). Weight loss is associated with a reduction of the CRP, which may accordingly (independently from body weight) improve the metabolic syndrome as well as the overall cardiovascular risk (McLaughlin et al. 2000; Ziccardi et al. 2002).

In a recent Italian study, a 10% weight reduction in obese subjects (mean BMI 37 kg/ m^2) induced a down-regulation of the inflammatory state (Ziccardi et al. 2002). In view of the potentially great importance of inflammation in the pathogenesis of the metabolic syndrome and atherogenesis, the observation of the highly significant effect of weight loss on inflammation seems to be of great importance because moderate weight loss is a realistic goal achievable at realistic cost. An independent relationship exists between the most important cardiovascular risk factors (BMI; smoking; blood pressure; diabetes; alcohol use; age; HDL cholesterol) and the CRP (Bermudez et al. 2002). All of these risk factors can be controlled by nonpharmacological strategies.

Another cornerstone of weight control is exercise, which would represent another cheap and effective strategy to reduce low-grade inflammation (Bermudez et al. 2002; Pedersen and Bruunsgaard 2003). The effect of moderate body weight reduction and exercise on inflammation underlines the importance of nonpharmacological therapeutic strategies in the obese patient. The effects of the different nonpharmacological and pharmacological strategies on inflammation are probably additive.

9.5.3 Uric Acid

Elevated uric acid or frank hyperuricemia is one of the risk factors often found in the setting of the metabolic syndrome. Insulin resistance and hyperuricemia are often associated, and it has been suggested that renal effects due to insulin resistance may lead to hyperuricemia (Ter-Maaten et al. 1997). Elevated uric acid is associated with an increased incidence of cardiovascular morbidity and mortality (Alderman et al. 1999). Overweight and obesity lead independently from other factors to elevated plasma uric acid levels. In a large hyperuricemia-free cohort of 1312 male office workers (with no medication and no hypertension), obesity and alcohol were identified as independent predictors for the development of hyperuricemia over an 8-year period (Nakanishi et al. 2001). Due to the metabolic changes during weight loss, a short-term increase in uric acid may occur during the first days of weight loss and may even lead to symptomatic gout (Heyden 1978). However, in the long term, weight loss is associated with a reduction of the plasma uric acid concentration (Heyden 1978; Tsunoda et al. 2002).

9.5.4 Coagulation and Fibrinolysis

The increased risk of thrombosis and emboli (venous and/or arterial) in obesity is well known (De-Pergola et al. 2002). In a recent autopsy study of bariatric patients, a very high rate of clinically silent pulmonary emboli was observed (Melinek et al. 2002). Due to direct and indirect mechanisms, overweight and obesity as well as the clinical entity of the metabolic syndrome are associated with a reduced fibrinolysis and an activation of the coagulation system (Kohler 2002). These disturbances in the coagulation system are even more pronounced in the presence of other risk factors (e.g., hypertension, smoking, or age) (Franz et al. 2002). Insulin resistance leads to a clustering of thrombogenic factors such as suppression of fibrinolysis as a consequence of high plasma PAI-1 (plasminogen activator inhibitor 1) concentration or an increase in factor VII, factor VIII, factor IX, fibrinogen or the von Willebrand factor (Kohler 2002). These alterations lead to an increase in atherothrombotic risk.

Weight loss is associated with an improved coagulability and fibrinolysis (Rissanen et al. 2001); however, this improvement is only observed as long as the body weight remains at the lower level. In the latter study, weight loss paralleled the decline in the PAI-1 and factor VII activity. The effect of body weight on hemostasis is already seen in children (Sudi et al. 2001). Although different metabolic factors may affect hemostasis, body mass and age remain of primary importance (Vambergue et al. 2001). Again, the abdominal fat distribution pattern was associated with more pronounced abnormalities in hemostasis and fibrinolysis (Mertens and Van-Gaal 2002).

9.5.5 Age and Aging

The prevalence of the metabolic syndrome increases with aging in men and women (Ford et al. 2002). Body weight represents the most important risk modulator of the prevalence independently from age. Aging is associated with characteristic changes in body composition, especially an increase in fat mass and reduction in muscle mass; in fact, most individuals consider weight gain with aging a normal phenomenon. As in other countries, in Switzerland body weight increases with age and after the fifth decade of life approximately 50% of the population shows a BMI > 25 kg/m² (Egger et al. 2001). More than 40 years ago, McGandy et al. reported in the Baltimore Longitudinal Study on Aging that the majority of the age-related increase in body weight is due to a decline in physical activity and the associated decline in lean body mass (McGandy et al. 1966).

Accumulating evidence indicates that the age-related change in body composition and increase in fat mass is one of the major pathophysiological stimuli for the development of insulin resistance and diabetes mellitus, as well as other chronic diseases including the metabolic syndrome. However, this increase in body weight over age is largely avoidable (Dennis et al. 2000; Klesges and Klesges 1988; Lahmann et al. 2000; McGandy et al. 1966; Rissanen et al. 1991; Swinburn et al. 1991; Williamson et al. 1991). The reduction of weight gain with aging would have a great impact on prevalence and incidence of the metabolic syndrome.

9.6   Weight Loss Interventions: The Problem of Weight Maintenance

Long-term success rates of weight loss vary considerably; in a recent review the long term success rate were set at only 15% (Ayyad and Andersen 2000). Weight rebound is usually independent from the strategy of weight loss (Bray et al. 1998); however, interventions aiming at permanent life-style changes (including eating behavior and patterns of physical activity) seem to be more promising in the long term (Ayyad and Andersen 2000). In view of the generally not very encouraging long-term outcomes, the major strategies should focus on the maintenance of body weight.

Despite the great public health importance, it is surprising that hardly any interventional studies are targeting body weight control at the population level. Short-term intervention studies for the control of cardiovascular risk factors (including body weight) such as the well known life-style trial by Ornish et al. (1990) have been very successful, but only in a selected small population. The approach of the life-style trial is very intense and costly and not feasible at the population level. The success of this study is probably due to the fact that multidimensional types of interventions, including nutrition; physical activity; behavior; meditation; and stress-control in a highly motivated group, are not representative of the population at large. Nevertheless, these studies point to the type of intervention and the potentially ideal components of intervention.

Using similar strategies, two recent studies (Knowler et al. 2002; Tuomilehto et al. 2001) about the prevention of diabetes by life-style strategies gained a lot of attention. In most studies, weight loss was at least partially regained despite an intense multidisciplinary approach (Guy–Grand et al. 1989; Knowler et al. 2002; Shepard et al. 2000; Sjöström et al. 1998; Stevens et al. 1993; Tuomilehto et al. 2001; Weintraub 1992). Also, the addition of very low calorie diets (VLCD) as well as behavioral therapies did not prevent weight gain (Holden et al. 1992; Wing 1995). The maintenance of physical activity seemed to be more promising. Normal-weight individuals maintaining their body weight over time are (1) physically very active and/or (2) show an energy intake according to their requirements based upon a very consciously controlled eating behavior (Bray et al. 1998; Filozof and Gonzalez 2000; Rissanen et al. 1991).

9.7 Weight Control at the Community Level: Realistic and Feasible?

In view of the present pandemic expansion of overweight and obesity, prevention of these conditions at the community level is a public health priority. It is surprising that hardly any long-term community-based studies are aimed at body weight reduction or body weight control in healthy ambulant individuals (Farquhar et al. 1985; Jeffery 1993; Jeffery et al. 1993; Taylor et al. 1991). Most studies about body weight control are of much shorter duration than studies about other chronic diseases, such as diabetes, hypertension, dyslipidemia, or coronary artery disease, which usually span an observational period of several years.

One of the first community-based studies aiming at weight control was the Healthy Worker Project study in Minnesota (Jeffery et al. 1993). More than 2000 individuals from 32 worksites participated in this randomized intervention study for a duration of 2 years. From each worksite, a random sample was recruited and evaluated at the baseline level. Then the study participants were randomized to receive no treatment or to receive an intervention with health education sessions and an incentive system. With the aim of keeping or gaining control of their body weight, 1567 individuals (corresponding to 16% of all potentially eligible individuals respectively corresponding to 36% of overweight individuals) participated.

After 6 months, the mean weight loss was 2.2 kg (Jeffery et al. 1993); after 2 years, no significant difference was found in the change of body weight in the intervention group compared to the control group. The observed weight loss was a function of the participation rate in the worksite, which probably reflects the importance of the motivation between the individuals of a specific worksite and supports a broad approach at the population level. Despite the rather disappointing result of the Minnesota study regarding body weight loss, this study shows the feasibility of interventions targeted at the level of single worksites or communities.

An interesting community-based approach was chosen in the Minnesota Direct Mail Intervention trial (Jeffery et al. 1993). In the Invest in Your Health Weight Loss Correspondence Program, a fee-for-service program with a $5 registration fee or a free-program requiring a $60 deposit was offered. More than 1300 individuals participated over a 6-month period, resulting in a 2-kg weight loss in the fee-for-service program and a weight loss of 4 kg in the free program (Jeffery et al. 1993). The participants received a self-help weight loss manual and monthly information in the form of newsletters. In addition, the participants monitored their body weight, diet, and physical activity (Jeffery et al. 1993). This study shows that a significant weight loss can be achieved at the community or population level within a short time frame.

Another community-based study about weight control is the Stanford Five-City Project, a program with the primary goal of cardiovascular health (Farquhar et al. 1985). The project aimed to evaluate community-wide health education on cardiovascular risk factors, including body weight. The education of the target population was based upon communication with the help of mass media channels and interpersonal education, as well as local community organizations. A cohort and cross-sectional sample were studied. The effects of the intervention in the treatment cities were compared to two control cities (without any intervention). The duration of the Stanford Five-City Project was 6 years and the strategies for weight control were initiated in year 4 only (Taylor et al. 1991). During this year of the intervention program, a potential participant was exposed 27.3 times to any educational aspect related to weight loss (e.g., by mailing, TV, radio, newspaper). During the two remaining years, the exposure frequency was between 0.4 and 5 times. In the intervention, communities' weight gains over the 6-year period were lower than in the control communities (0.57 vs. 1.25 kg, $p < .05$).

It is interesting that the knowledge regarding cardiovascular risk factors (other than body weight) improved considerably; however, the knowledge regarding overweight and obesity as a risk factor did not change significantly! Despite the increase in body weight, the study participants became more self-confident of their ability to keep control over their body weight. This apparent paradox is difficult to explain but illustrates the difficulties of understanding and controlling for the different factors and components of the energy balance and the complex interplay of exogenous and endogenous factors in weight control.

At the end of the study, no significant difference existed between the control and intervention groups; the prevalence of obesity increased in both groups. Nevertheless, the Stanford Five-City Project showed that a large-scale educational intervention is feasible. The study results also clearly show that any strategy for weight control (avoiding weight gain or even attaining weight reduction) at the population level should be long term (for years if not permanent), with regular "refresher" activities. It seems that implementing weight control at the population/community level is more difficult than implementing strategies for the control of hypercholesterolemia or hypertension. Furthermore, the data from the cohort study suggest that the amount of weight gain over time could be reduced, which would already represent a considerable success.

9.8   Conclusion and Recommendation

The increasing prevalence of overweight and obesity represents the most important public health problem. Independently of age, the body weight of the population is increasing and so is the incidence of most chronic diseases such as diabetes mellitus, hypertension, dyslipidemia, and the metabolic syndrome. Interventional studies reported at the level of individual patients and patient groups that a multidimensional therapeutic approach can lead to a reduction of body weight and thus influence single risk factors (e.g., hypertension, dyslipidemia) as well as clusters of risk factors (e.g., the metabolic syndrome) and the corresponding end points (e.g., diabetes). Small studies have tested potentially successful strategies for weight control; however, cost-efficient means and strategies for weight control at the level of the whole population have yet to be established. The development of comprehensive strategies to promote physical activity and energy intake according to one's requirement are urgently needed. In view of the increasing prevalence of obesity in childhood and the tracking of childhood obesity into adulthood, special concerns should be focused on this age group.

References

Albala, C., Yanez, M., Devoto, E., Sostin, C., Zeballos, L. and Santos, J.L. (1996) Obesity as a protective factor for postmenopausal osteoporosis, *Int. J. Obes. Relat. Metab. Disord.*, 20: 1027–1032.

Alderman, M.H., Cohen, H., Madhavan, S. and Kivlighn, S. (1999) Serum uric acid and vardiovascular events in successfully treated hypertensive patients, *Hypertension*, 34: 144–150.

Amatruda, J.M., Richeson, J.F., Welle, S.L., Brodows, R.G. and Lockwood, D.H. (1988) The safety and efficacy of a controlled low-energy ("very-low-calorie") diet in the treatment of non-insulin-dependent diabetes and obesity, *Arch. Intern. Med.*, 148: 873–877.

Astrand, P.O. and Rodahl, K. (1986) *Textbook of Work Physiology. Physiological Bases of Exercise* 3rd ed., New York: McGraw–Hill Book Company, pp. 756.

Austin, A.M. (1989) Plasma triglyceride as a risk factor for coronary heart disease, *Am. J. Epidemiol.*, 129: 249–259.

Austin, M.A. (1999) Epidemiology of hypertriglyceridemia and cardiovacular disease, *Am. J. Cardiol.*, 13: 13F–16F.

Ayyad, C. and Andersen, T. (2000) Long-term efficacy of dietary treatment of obesity: a systematic review of studies published between 1931 and 1999, *Obes. Rev.*, 1: 113–119.

Belsha, C.W. (2002) Systemic hypertension: management in children and adolescents, *Curr. Treat. Options Cardiovasc. Med.*, 4: 351–360.

Bermudez, E.A., Rifai, N., Buring, J., Manson, J.E. and Ridker, P.M. (2002) Interrelationships among circulating interleukin-6, C-reactive protein, and traditional cardiovascular risk factors in women, *Arterioscler. Thromb. Vasc. Biol.*, 22: 1668–1673.

Bjoerntorp, P. (1991) Visceral fat accumulation: the missing link between psychosocial factors and cardiovascular disease? *J. Int. Med.*, 230: 195–201.

Bosello, O. and Zamboni, M. (2000) Visceral obesity and metabolic syndrome, *Obes. Rev.*, 1: 47–56.

Bray, G.A., Bouchard, C. and James, W.P.T. (Eds.) (1998) *Handbook of Obesity*, New York: Marcel Dekker Inc., pp. 1–1012.

Busetto, L. (2001) Visceral obesity and the metabolic syndrome: effects of weight loss, *Nutr. Metab. Cardiovasc. Dis.*, 11: 195–204.

Chan, J.M., Rimm, R.B., Colditz, G.A., Stampfer, M.J. and Willett, W.C. (1994) Obesity, fat distribution, and weight gain as risk factors for clilnical diabetes in men, *Diabetes Care*, 17: 961–969.

Colditz, G.A., Willett, W.C., Rotnitzky, A. and Manson, J.E. (1995) Weight gain as a risk factor for clinical diabetes in women, *Ann. Intern. Med.*, 122: 481–486.

Colditz, G.A., Willett, W.C., Stampfer, M.J., Manson, J.E., Hennekens, C.H., Arky, R.A. and Speizer, F.E. (1990) Weight as a risk factor for clinical diabetes in women, *Am. J. Epidemiol.*, 132: 501–513.

Das, U.N. (2002) Is metabolic syndrome X an inflammatory condition? *Exp. Biol. Med.*, 227: 989–997.

Dattilo, A.M. and Kris–Etherton, P.M. (1992) Effects of weight reduction on blood lipids and lipo-proteins: a meta-analysis, *Am. J. CLin. Nutr.*, 56: 320–328.

De-Jong, P.E., Verhave, J.C., Pinto–Sietsma, S.J. and Hillege, H.L. (2002) Obesity and target organ damage: the kidney, *Int. J. Obes. Relat. Metab. Disord.*, 26 (Suppl. 4): S21–S24.

Dennis, B.H., Pajak, A., Pardo, B., Davis, C.E., Williams, O.D. and Piotrowski, W. (2000) Weight gain and its correlates in Poland between 1983 and 1993, *Int. J. Obes. Relat. Metab. Disord.*, 24: 1507–1513.

De-Pergola, G. and Pannacciulli, N. (2002) Coagulation and fibrinolysis abnormalities in obesity, *J. Endocrinol. Invest.*, 25: 899–904.

Despres, J.P. (1997) Visceral obesity, insulin resistance, and dyslipidemia: contribution of endurance exercise training to the treatment of the plurimetabolic syndrome, *Exerc. Sport Sci. Rev.*, 25: 271–300.

Despres, J.P. (2001) Health consequences of visceral obesity, *Ann. Med.*, 33: 534–541.

Despres, J.P., Lemieux, I., Dagenais, G.R., Cantin, B. and Lamarche, B. (2000) HDL-cholesterol as a marker of coronary heart disease risk: the Quebec cardiovascular study, *Atherosclerosis*, 153: 263–272.

Dixon, J.B. and O'Brien, P.E. (2002a) Changes in comorbidities and improvement in quality of life after LAP-Band placement, *Am. J. Surg.*, 184: 51S–54S.

Dixon, J.B. and O'Brien, P.E. (2002b) Health outcomes of severly obese type 2 diabetic subjects 1 year after laparoscopic adjustable gastric banding, *Diabetes Care*, 25: 358–363.

Durstine, J.L., Grandjean, P.W., Davis, P.G., Ferguson, M.A., Alderson, N.L. and DuBose, K.D. (2001) Blood lipid and lipoprotein adaptations to exercise: a quantitative analysis, *Sports Med.*, 31: 1033–1062.

Ebbeling, C.B., Pawlak, D.B. and Ludwig, D.S. (2002) Childhood obesity: public-health crisis, common sense cure, *Lancet*, 360: 473–482.

Egger, S., Wieland, R., Ludin, M., Brändli, O., Vetter, W. and Suter, P. (2001) Übergewicht und Adipositas im Kanton Zürich: Eine LuftiBus Studie, PRAXIS (Schweizerische Rundschau für Medizin), 90: 531–538.

Eriksson, K.F. and Lindgarde, F. (1991) Prevention of type 2 (non-insulin-dependent) diabetes mellitus by diet and physical exercise: the 6-year Malmo feasibility study, *Diabetologica*, 34: 891–898.

Expert Panel on Detection and Treatment of High Cholesterol in Adults. (2001) Executive summary of the third report of the National Cholestrerol Education Program (NCEP) expert panel on detection, evaluation, and treatment of high blood cholesterol in adults (Adult Treatment Panel III), *JAMA*, 285: 2486–2497.

Farquhar, J.W., Fortmann, S.P., Maccoby, N., Haskell, W.L., Williams, P.T., Flora, J.A., Taylor, C.B., Brown, B.W., Solomon, D.S. and Hulley, S.B. (1985) The Stanford Five-City Project: design and methods, *Am. J. Epidemiol.*, 122: 323–334.

Filozof, C. and Gonzalez, C. (2000) Perdictors of weight gain: the biological behavioural debate, *Obes. Rev.*, 1: 21–26.

Flegal, K.M., Carroll, M.D., Ogden, C.L. and Johnson, C.L. (2002) Prevalence and trends in obesity among US adults 1999–2000, *JAMA*, 288: 1723–1727.

Ford, E.S., Giles, W.H. and Dietz, W.H. (2002) Prevalence of the metabolic syndrome among US adults: findings from the third National Health and Nutrition Examination Survey, *JAMA*, 287: 356–359.

Ford, E.S., Williamson, D.F. and Liu, S. (1997) Weight change and diabetes incidence: findings from a national cohort of US adults, *Am. J. Epidemiol.*, 146: 214–222.

Franz, I.W., van-der-Meyden, J., Tönnesmann, U., Müller, J.F.M., Röcker, L. and Hopfenmüller, W. (2002) Blood coagulation in normotensives and hypertensives in relation to their body mass index, Dtsch Med Wochenschr, 127: 2374–2378 (in German).

Frohlich, E.D. (2002) Clinical management of the obese hypertensive patient, *Cardiol. Rev.*, 10: 127–138.

Goodpaster, B.H., Krishnaswami, S., Resnick, H., Kelley, D.E., Haggerty, C., Harris, T.B., Schwartz, A.V., Kritchevsky, S. and Newman, A.B. (2003) Association between regional adipose tissue distribution and both type 2 diabetes and impaired glucose tolerance in elderly men and women, *Diabetes Care*, 26: 372–379.

Gotto, A.M. (2002) High-density lipoprotein cholesterol and triglycerides as therapeutic targets for preventing and treating coronary artery disease, *Am. Heart J.*, 144 (Suppl. 6): S33–S42.

Guy–Grand, B., Crepaldi, G., Lefebvre, P., Apfelbaum, M., Gries, A. and Turner, P. (1989) International trial of long-term dexfenfluramine in obesity, *Lancet*, II: 1142–1144.

Gwinup, G. (1975) Effect of exercise alone on the weight of obese women, *Arch. Intern. Med.*, 135: 676–680.

Halbert, J.A., Silagy, C.A., Finucane, P., Withers, R.T. and Hamdorf, P.A. (1999) Exercise training and blood lipids in hyperlipidemic and normolipidemic adults: a meta-analysis of randomized, controlled trials, *Eur. J. Clin. Nutr.*, 53: 514–522.

Hall, J.E., Crook, E.D., Jones, D.W., Wofford, M.R. and Dubbert, P.M. (2002) Mechanisms of obesity-associated cardiovascular and renal disease, *Am. J. Med. Sci.*, 324: 127–137.

Hauner, H. (2002) Insulin resistance and the metabolic syndrome-a challenge of the new millennium, *Eur. J. Clin. Nutr.*, 56 (Suppl. 1): S25–S29.

Heyden, S. (1978) The workinghman's diet. II. Effect of weight reduction in obese patients with hypertension, diabetes, hyperuricemia and hyperlipidemia, *Nutr. Metab.*, 22: 141–158.

Hoffmann, I.S., Jimenez, E. and Cubeddu, L.X. (2001) Urinary albumin excretion in lean, overweight and obese glucose tolerant individuals: its relationship with dyslipidaemia, hyperinsulinaemia and blood pressure, *J. Hum. Hypertens.*, 15: 407–412.

Hokanson, J.E. (2002) Hypertriglyceridemia and risk of coronary heart disease, *Curr. Cardiol. Rep.*, 4: 488–493.

Holden, J.H., Darga, L.L., Olson, S.M., Stettner, D.C., Ardito, E.A. and Lucas, C.P. (1992) Long-term follow up of patients attending a combination very-low calorie diet and behaviour therapy weight loss programme, *Int. J. Obesity*, 16: 605–613.

Hubert, H.B., Feinleib, M., McNamara, P.M. and Castelli, W.P. (1983) Obesity as an independent risk factor for cardiovascular disease: a 26-year follow-up of participants in the Framingham Heart Study, *Circulation*, 67: 968–977.

Jeffery, R.W. (1993) Minnesota studies on cummunity-based approaches to weight loss and control, *Ann. Intern. Med.*, 119 (7 pt 2): 719–721.

Jeffery, R.W., Forster, J.L., French, S.A., Kelder, S.H., Lando, H.A., McGovern, P.G., Jacobs, D.R. and Baxter, J.E. (1993) The Healthy Worker Project: a work-site intervention for weight control and smoking cessation, *Am. J. Public Health*, 83: 395–401.

Jeppesen, J., Hein, H.O., Suadicani, P. and Gyntelberg, F. (1997) Relation of high TG-low HDL cholesterol and LDL cholesterol to the incidence of ischemic heart disease. An 8-year follow-up in the Copenhagen Male Study, *Arterioscler. Thromb. Vasc. Biol.*, 17: 1114–1120.

Jeppesen, J., Hein, H.O., Suadicani, P. and Gyntelberg, F. (2003) High triglycerides/low high-density lipoprotein cholesterol, ischemic electrocardiogram changes, and risk of ischemic heart disease, *Am. Heart J.*, 145: 103–108.

Jeukendrup, A.E. (2002) Regulation of fat metabolism in skeletal muscle, *Ann. N.Y. Acad. Sci.*, 967: 217–235.

Jones, P.H. (2000) Diet and pharmacologic therapy of obesity to modify atherosclerosis, *Curr. Atheroscler. Rep.*, 2: 314–320.

Kim, Y.I., Kim, C.H., Choi, C.S., Chung, Y.E., Lee, M.S., Lee, S.I., Park, J.Y., Hong, S.K. and Lee, K.U. (2001) Microalbuminuria is associated with the insulin resistance syndrome independent of hypertension and type 2 diabetes in the Korean population, *Diabetes Res. Clin. Pract.*, 52: 145–152.

Klesges, R. and Klesges, L. (1988) Smoking and fear of weight gain, *Int. J. Eating Disord.*, 7: 413–419.

Knowler, W.C., Barrett-Connor, E., Fowler, S.E., Hamman, R.F., Lachin, J.M., Walker, E.A. and Nathan, D.M. (2002) Reduction in the incidence of type 2 diabetes with life style intervention of metformin, *N. Engl. J. Med.*, 346: 393–403.

Kohler, H.P. (2002) Insulin resistance syndrome: ineraction with coagulation and fibrinolysis, *Swiss Med. Wkly.*, 132: 241–252.

Kuczmarski, R.J., Flegal, K.M., Campbell, S.M. and Johnson, C.L. (1994) Increasing prevalence of overweight among US adults. The National Health and Nutrition Examination Surveys, 1960–1991, *JAMA*, 272: 205–211.

Lahmann, P.H., Lissner, L., Gullberg, B. and Berglund, G. (2000) Sociodemographic factors associated with long-term weight gain, current body fatness and central adiposity in Swedish women, *Int. J. Obes. Relat. Metab. Disord.*, 24: 685–694.

Lakka, H.M., Salonen, J.T., Tuomilehto, J., Kaplan, G.A. and Lakka, T.A. (2002) Obesity and weight gain are associated with increased incidence of hyperinsulinemia in non-diabetic men, *Horm. Metab. Res.*, 34: 492–498.

Lamarche, N., Lemieux, I. and Despres, J.P. (1999) The small, dense LDL phenotype and the risk of coronary heart disease: epidemiology, patho-physiology and therapeutic aspects, *Diabetes Metab.*, 25: 199–211.

Lee, I.M., Blair, S.N., Allison, D.B., Folsom, A.R., Harris, T.B., Manson, J.A. and Wing, R.R. (2001) Epidemiologic data on the relationship of caloric intake, energy balance, and weight gain over the life span with longevity and morbidity, *J. Gerontol.* (Series A), 56A (special issue 1): 7–19.

Leinonen, E., Hurt–Camejo, E., Wiklund, O., Hulten, L.M., Hiukka, A. and Taskinen, M.R. (2003) Insulin resistance and adiposity correlate with acute-phase reaction and soluble cell adhesion molecules in type 2 diabetes, *Atherosclerosis*, 166: 387–394.

Levine, J.A., Eberhardt, N.L. and Jensen, M.D. (1999) Role of nonexercise activity thermogenesis in resistance to fat gain in humans, *Science*, 283: 212–214.

Liese, A.D., Hense, H.W., Doring, A., Stieber, J. and Keil, U. (2001) Microalbuminuria, central adiposity and hypertension in the non-diabetic urban population of the MONICA Augsburg survey 1994/95, *J. Hum. Hypertens.*, 15: 799–804.

Long, S.D., O'Brien, K., MacDonald, K.G., Leggett–Frazier, N., Swanson, M.S., Pories, W.J. and Caro, J.F. (1994) Weight loss in severely obese subjects prevents progression of impaired glucose tolerance to type II diabetes: a longitudinal interventional study, *Diabetes Care*, 17: 372–375.

Looker, H.C., Knowler, W.C. and Hanson, R.L. (2001) Changes in BMI and weight before and after the development of type 2 diabetes, *Diabetes Care*, 24: 1917–1922.

MacMahon, S., Cutler, J., Brittain, E. and Higgins, M. (1987) Obesity and hypertension: epidemiological and clinical issues, *Eur. Heart J.*, 8 (Suppl. B): 57–70.

McGandy, R.B., Barrows, C.H., Spanias, A., Meredith, A., Stone, J.L. and Norris, A.H. (1966) Nutrient intakes and energy expenditure in men of different ages, *J. Gerontol.*, 4: 581–587.

McLaughlin, T., Abbasi, F., Lamendola, C., Liang, L., Reaven, G., Schaaf, P. and Reaven, P. (2000) Differentiation between obesity and insulin resistance in the association with C-reactive protein, *Circulation*, 106: 2908–2912.

McLellan, F. (2002) Obesity rising to alarming levels around the world, *Lancet*, 359: 1412.

Melinek, J., Livingston, E., Cortina, G. and Fishbein, M.C. (2002) Autopsy findings following gastric bypass surgery for morbid obesity, *Arch. Pathol. Lab. Med.*, 126: 1091–1095.

Mertens, I. and Van-Gaal, L.F. (2002) Obesity, haemostasis and the fibrinolytic system, *Obes. Rev.*, 3: 85–101.

Mokdad, A.H., Ford, E.S., Bowman, B.A., Dietz, W.H., Vinicor, F., Bales, V.S. and Marks, J.S. (2003) Prevalence of obesity, diabetes, and obesity-related health risk factors, 2001, *JAMA*, 289: 76–79.

Mokdad, A.H., Serdula, M.K., Dietz, W.H., Bowman, B.A., Marks, J.S.l. and Koplan, J.P. (1999) The spread of the obesity epidemic in the United States, 1991–1998, *JAMA*, 282: 1519–1522.

Moore, L.L., Visioni, A.J., D'Agostino, R.B., Finkle, E.D. and Ellison, R.C. (2000) Can sustained weight loss in overweight individuals reduce the risk of diabetes mellitus, *Epidemiology*, 11: 269–273.

Mulrow, C.D., Chiquette, E., Angel, L., Cornell, J., Summerbell, C., Anagnostelis, B., Grimm, R. and Brand, M.B. (2000) Dieting to reduce body weight for controlling hypertension in adults, *Cochrane Database Syst. Rev.*, 2: CD000484.

Mulyadi, L., Stevens, C., Munro, S., Lingard, J. and Bermingham, M. (2001) Body fat distribution and total body fat as risk factors for microalbuminuria in the obese, *Ann. Nutr. Metab.*, 45: 67–71.

Naidoo, D.P. (2002) The link between microalbuminuria, endothelial dysfunction and cardiovascular disease in diabetes, *Cardiovasc. J. S. Afr.*, 13: 194–199.

Nakanishi, N., Yoshida, H., Nakamura, K., Suzuki, K. and Tatara, K. (2001) Predictors for the development of hyperuricemia: an 8-year longitudinal study in middle-aged Japanese men, *Metabolism*, 50: 621–626.

Newburgh, L. (1942) Control of hyperglycaemia of obese "diabetics" by weight reduction, *Ann. Intern. Med.*, 17: 935–942.

Nguyen–Duy, T.B., Nichaman, M.Z., Church, T.S., Blair, S.N. and Ross, R. (2003) Visceral fat and liver fat are independent predictors of metabolic risk factors in men, *Am. J. Physiol. Endocrinol. Metab.* (in press).

Noakes, M. and Clifton, P.M. (2000) Weight loss and plasma lipids, *Curr. Opinion Lipidol.*, 11: 65–70.

Ohashi, H., Oda, H., Ohno, M. and Watanabe, S. (2001) Weight reduction improves high blood pressure and microalbuminuria in hypertensive patients with obesity, *Nippon Jinzo Gakkai Shi*, 43: 333–339 (English abstract).

Olson, M.B., Kelsey, S.F., Bittner, V., Reis, S.E., Reichek, N., Handberg, E.M. and Merz, C.N. (2000) Weight cycling and high-density lipoprotein cholesterol in women: evidence of an adverse effect: a report from the NHLBI-sponsored WISE study. Women's Ischemia Syndrome Evaluation Study Group, *J. Am. Coll. Cardiol.*, 36: 1565–1571.

Ornish, D., Brown, S.E., Scherwitz, L.W., Billings, J.H., Armstrong, W.T., Ports, T.A., McLanahan, S.M., Kirkeeide, R.L., Brand, R.J. and Gould, K.L. (1990) Can lifestyle changes reverse coronary artery disease?, *Lancet*, 336: 129–133.

Parati, G. (2002) Obesity, hypertension and the sympathetic nervous system, *J. Hypertens.*, 20: 835–837.

Parks, E.J. (2001) Recent findings in the study of postprandial lipemia, *Curr. Atheroscler. Rep.*, 3: 462–470.

Pasanisi, F., Contaldo, F., di-Simone, G. and Mancini, M. (2001) Benefits of sustained moderate weight loss in obesity, *Nutr. Metab. Cardiovasc. Dis.*, 11: 401–406.

Pedersen, B.K. and Bruunsgaard, H. (2003) Possible beneficial role of exercise in modulating low-grade inflammation in the elderly, *Scand. J. Med. Sci. Sports*, 13: 56–62.

Peeters, A., Barendregt, J.J., Willekens, F., Mackenbach, J.P., Al-Mamun, A. and Bonneux, L. (2003) Obesity in adulthood and its consequences for life expectancy: a life-table analysis, *Ann. Intern. Med.*, 138: 24–32.

Pischon, T. and Sharma, A.M. (2002) Optimizing blood pressure control in the obese patient, *Curr. Hypertens. Rep.*, 4: 358–362.

Poirier, P. and Eckel, R.H. (2002) Obesity and cardiovascular disease, *Curr. Atherosclerosis Rep.*, 4: 448–453.

Ravnikar, V.A. (1993) Diet, exercise, and lifestyle in preparation for menopause, *Obstet. Gynaecol. Clin. North Am.*, 2: 365–378.

Reid, M., Bennett, F., Wilks, R. and Forrester, T. (1998) Microalbuminuria, renal function and waist:hip ratio in black hypertensive Jamaicans, *J. Hum. Hypertens.*, 12: 221–227.

Resnick, H.E., Valsania, P., Halter, J.B. and Lin, X. (2000) Relation of weightr gain and weight loss on subsequent diabetes risk in overweight adults, *J. Epidemiol. Community Health*, 54: 596–602.

Reusch, J.E. (2002) Current concepts in insulin resistance, type 2 diabetes mellitus, and the metabolic syndrome, *Am. J. Cardiol.*, 90 (5A): 19G–26G.

Rhoads, G.G. and Kagan, A. (1983) The relation of coronary artery disease, stroke and mortality to weight in young and middle-age, *Lancet*, 1: 492–495.

Ridker, P.M., Buring, J.E., Cook, N.R. and Rifai, N. (2003) C-reactive protein, the metabolic syndrome, and risk of incident cardiovascular events: an 8-year follow-up of 14,719 initially healthy American women, *Circulation*, 107: 391–397.

Rissanen, A.M., Heliövaara, M., Knekt, P., Reunanen, A. and Aromaa, A. (1991) Determinants of weight gain and overweight in adult Finns, *Eur. J. Clin. Nutr.*, 45: 419–430.

Rissanen, P., Vahtera, E., Krusius, T., Uusitupa, M. and Rissanen, A. (2001) Weight change and blood coagulability and fibrinolysis in healthy obese women, *Int. J. Obes. Relat. Metab. Disord.*, 25: 212–218.

Roessner, S. (1989) Weight cycling — a "new" risk factor? *J. Int. Med.*, 226: 209–211.

Sea, M.M., Fong, W.P., Huang, Y. and Chen, Z.Y. (2000) Weight cycling-induced alteration in fatty acid metabolism, *Am. J. Physiol. Regul. Integr. Comp. Physiol.*, 279: R1145–1155.

Sharma, A.M., Pischon, T., Engeli, S. and Scholze, J. (2001) Choice of drug treatment for obesity-related hypertension: where is the evidence? *J. Hypertens.*, 19: 667–674.

Shepard, T.Y., Jensen, D.R., Blotner, S., Zhi, J., Guerciolini, R., Pace, D. and Eckel, R.H. (2000) Orlistat fails to alter postprandial lipid excursions or plasma lipases in normal weight volunteers, *Int. J. Obesity*, 24: 187–194.

Shimokata, N., Muller, D.C. and Andres, R. (1989) Studies on the distribution of body fat. III. Effect of cigarette smoking, *JAMA*, 261: 1169–1173.

Sjöström, L., Rissanen, A., Andersen, T., Boldrin, M., Golay, A., Koppeschaar, H.P.F. and Krempf, M. (1998) Randomised placebo-controlled trial of orlistat for weight loss and prevention of weight gain in obese patients, *Lancet*, 352: 167–172.

Skyler, J.S. and Oddo, C. (2002) Diabetes trends in the USA, *Diabetes Metab. Res. Rev.*, 18: S21–S26.

Smith, S.R. and Zachwieja, J.J. (1999) Visceral adipose tissue: A critical review of intervention strategies, *Int. J. Obesity*, 23: 329–335.

Somes, G.W., Kritchevsky, S.B., Shorr, R.I., Pahor, M. and Applegate, W.B. (2002) Body mass index, weight change, and death in older adults. The Systolic Hypertension in the Elderly Program, *Am. J. Epidemiol.*, 156: 132–138.

Sorof, J. and Daniels, S. (2002) Obesity Hypertension in Children. A problem of epidemic proportions, *Hypertension*, 40: 441–447.

Stevens, V.J., Corrigan, S.A., Obarzanek, E., Bernauer, E., Cook, N.R., Herbert, P., Mattfeldt–Berman, M., Oberman, A., Sugars, C., Dalcin, A.T. and Whelton, P.K. (1993) Weight loss intervention in phase 1 of the trials of hypertension prevention, *Arch. Intern. Med.*, 153: 849–858.

Sudi, K., Gallistl, S., Payerl, D., Aigner, R., Moller, R., Tafeit, E. and Borkenstein, M.H. (2001) Interrelationship between estimates of adiposity and body fat distribution with metabolic and hemostatic parameters in obese children, *Metabolism*, 50: 681–617.

Suter, P.M., Gerritsen Zehnder, M., Häsler, E., Gürtler, M., Vetter, W. and Hänseler, E. (2001) Effect of alcohol on postprandial lipemia with and without preprandial exercise, *J. Am. Coll. Nutr.*, 20: 58–64.

Suter, P.M., Locher, R., Häsler, E. and Vetter, W. (1997a) Is there a role of the ob-gene product leptin in essential hypertension? Abstract 746, 8th European Meeting on Hypertension (June 1997).

Suter, P.M., Maire, R. and Vetter, W. (1995) Is an increased waist:hip ratio the cause of alcohol-induced hypertension. The AIR94 study, *J. Hypertens.*, 13: 1857–1862.

Suter, P.M., Maire, R. and Vetter, W. (1997b) Alcohol consumption: a risk factor for abdominal fat accumulation in men, *Add. Biol.*, 2: 101–103.

Suter, P.M. and Vetter, W. (1995) Metabolic effects of antihypertensive drugs, *J. Hypertens.*, 13 (Suppl.4): S11–S17.

Swinburn, B.A., Noyomba, B.L., Saad, M.F., Zurlo, F., Raz, I., Knowler, W.C., Lillioja, S., Bogardus, C. and Ravussin, E. (1991) Insulin resistance associated with lower rates of weight gain in Pima Indians, *J. Clin. Invest.*, 88: 168–173.

Taylor, C.B., Fortmann, S.P., Flora, J., Kayman, S., Barrett, D.C., Jatulis, D. and Farquhar, J.W. (1991) Effect of long-term community health education on body mass index, *Am. J. Epidemiol.*, 134: 235–249.

Ter-Maaten, J.C., Voorburg, A., Heine, R.J., Ter-Wee, P.M., Donker, A.J. and Gans, R.O. (1997) Renal handling of urate and sodium during acute physiological hyperinsulinemia in healthy subjects, *Clin. Sci.*, 92: 51–58.

Thakur, V., Richards, R. and Reisin, E. (2001) Obesity, hypertension, and the heart, *Am. J. Med. Sci.*, 321: 242–248.

Tsunoda, S., Kamide, K., Minami, J. and Kawano, Y. (2002) Decreases in serum uric acid by amelioration of insulin resistance in overweight hypertensivde patients: effect of a low-energy diet and an insulin-sensitizing agent, *Am. J. Hypertens.*, 15: 697–701.

Tuomilehto, J., Lindstrom, J., Eriksson, J.G., Valle, T.T., Hamalainen, H., Ilanne–Parikka, P., Keinanen–Kiukaanniemi, S., Laakso, M., Louheranta, A., Rastas, M., Salminen, V., Uusitupa, M. et al., Finnish Diabetes Prevention Study Group (2001) Prevention of type 2 diabetes mellitus by changes in lifestyle among subjects with impaired glucose tolerance, *N. Engl. J. Med.*, 344: 1343–1350.

Ukkola, O. and Bouchard, C. (2001) Clustering of metabolic abnormalities in obese individuals: the role of genetic factors, *Ann. Med.*, 33: 79–90.

UKPDS Group (1990) U.K. Prospective Diabetes Study 7: response of fasting plasma glucose to diet therapy in newly presenting type II diabetic patients, *Metabolism*, 39: 905–912.

Valensi, P., Assayag, M., Busby, M., Paries, J., Lormeau, B. and Attali, J.R. (1996) Microalbuminuria in obese patients with or without hypertension, *Int. J. Obes. Relat. Metab. Disord.*, 20: 574–579.

Vambergue, A., Rugeri, L., Gaveriaux, V., Devos, P., Martin, A., Fermon, C., Fontaine, P. and Jude, B. (2001) Factor VII, tissue factor pathway inhibitor, and monocyte tissue factor in diabetes mellitus: influence of type of diabetes, obesity index, and age, *Thromb. Res.*, 101: 367–375.

van Italie, T.B. (1985) Health implications of overweight and obesity in the United States, *Ann. Intern. Med.*, 103: 983–989.

Van-Liew, J.B., Davis, F.B., Davis, P.J., Noble, B. and Bernardis, L.L. (1992) Calorie restriction decreases microalbuminuria associated with aging in barrier-raised Fischer 344 rats, *Am. J. Physiol.*, 263: F554–F556.

Vidal, J. (2002) Uptated review of the benefits of weight loss, *Int. J. Obes.*, 26 (Suppl. 4): S25–S28.

Vorster, H.H. (2002) The emergence of cardiovascular disease during urbanisation of Africans, *Public Health Nutr.*, 5(1A): 239–243.

Wajchenberg, B.L. (2000) Subcutaneous and visceral adipose tissue: their relation to the metabolic syndrome, *Endocr. Rev.*, 21: 697–738.

Walker, A.R., Adam, F. and Walker, B.F. (2001) World pandemic of obesity: the situation in Southern African populations, *Public Health*, 115: 368–372.

Wannamethee, S.G., Shaper, G. and Walker, M. (2002) Weight change, weight fluctuation, and mortality, *Arch. Intern. Med.*, 162: 2575–2580.

Weinsier, R.L., Hunter, G.R., Desmond, R.A., Byrne, N.M., Zuckerman, P.A. and Darnell, B.E. (2002) Free-living activity energy expenditure in women successful and unsuccessful at maintaining a normal body weight, *Am. J. Clin. Nutr.*, 75: 499–504.

Weintraub, M. (1992) Long-term weight control: the National Heart, Lung and Blood Institute Funded Multimodal Intervention Study, *Clin. Pharmacol. Ther.*, 51: (Supplement) 581–646.

Wierzbicki, A.S., Reynolds, T.M. and Crook, M.A. (2002) Usefulness of Orlistat in the treatment of severe hypertriglyceridemia, *Am. J. Cardiol.*, 89: 229–231.

Will, J.C., Williamson, D.F., Ford, E.S., Calle, E.E. and Thun, M.J. (2002) Intentional weight loss and 13-year diabetes incidence in overweight adults, *Am. J. Public Health*, 92: 1245–1248.

Williamson, D.F., Madans, J., Anda, R.F., Kleinman, J.C., Giovino, G.A. and Byers, T. (1991) Smoking cessation and severity of weight gain in a national cohort, *N. Engl. J. Med.*, 324: 739–745.

Wilson, P.W., Anderson, K.M., Harris, T., Kannel, W.B. and Castelli, W.P. (1994) Determinants of change in total cholesterol and HDL-C with age: the Framingham Study, *J. Gerontol.*, 49: M252–M257.

Wing, R.R. (1995) Changing diet and exercise behaviors in individuals at risk for weight gain, *Obes. Res.*, 3: (Suppl. 2) 277S–282S.

Wolf, A.M. (1998) What is the economic case for treating obesity?, *Obes. Res.*, 6 (Suppl I): 2S–7S.

Yaari, S. and Goldbourt, U. (1998) Voluntary and involuntary weight loss: associations with long term mortality in 9228 middle-aged and elderly men, *Am. J. Epidemiol.*, 148: 546–555.

Ziccardi, P., Nappo, F., Giugliano, G., Esposito, K., Marfella, R., Cioffi, M., D'Andrea, F., Molinari, A.M. and Giugliano, D. (2002) Reduction of inflammatory cytokine concentrations and improvement of endothelial functions in obese women after weight loss over one year, *Circulation*, 105: 804–809.

Zilversmit, D.B. (1979) Atherosclerosis: a postprandial phenomenon, *Circulation*, 60: 473–485.

10

Weight Loss and Metabolic Diseases

F. Xavier Pi–Sunyer

CONTENTS

10.1   Introduction

Obesity is increasing rapidly throughout the world (Flegal et al. 2002; World Health Organization 1998). As it does so, it leads to an increased disease burden (Must et al. 1999; Pi–Sunyer 1993a), leading to an increased mortality (Allison et al. 1999) and shortened life span (Fontaine et al. 2003). It brings with it an increased incidence of type 2 diabetes,

TABLE 10.1

ATP III: The Metabolic Syndome[a]

Risk Factor	Defining Level
Abdominal obesity (waist circumference)	
Men	>102 cm (>40 in.)
Women	>88 cm (>35 in.)
TG	≥150 mg/dl
HDL-C	
Men	<40 mg/dl
Women	<50 mg/dl
Blood pressure	≥130/≥85 mmHg
Fasting glucose	≥110 mg/dl

[a] Diagnosis is established when ≥3 of these risk factors are present.

Source: From Adult Treatment Panel III 2003, *JAMA*, 285:2486–2497, 2001.

TABLE 10.2

1998 World Health Organization Definition of the Metabolic Syndrome[a]

Antihypertensive treatment and/or elevated blood pressure (>160 mmHg systolic or >90 mmHg diastolic)

Elevated plasma triglycerides (>1.7 mmol/l) and/or low HDL cholesterol (<0.9 mmol/l in men; <1.0 mmol/l in women)

Elevated BMI (>30 kg/m²) and/or WHR (>0.90 in men; >0.85 in women)

Microalbuminuria (urinary albumin excretion rate [AER]) > 20 mg/min

[a] Defined as insulin resistance (IR) plus any two of the following IR defined as having type 2 diabetes, impaired fasting glucose, impaired glucose tolerance or (for those with normal fasting glucose values < 110 mg/dl) or being in the highest quartile of the homeostasis model (HO-MA–IR) index.

Source: From Alberti, K.G. and Zimmet, P.Z., *Diabetic Med.*, 15:539–553, 1998.

dyslipidemia, hypertension, and cardiovascular disease. Some of the conditions named have recently been clustered together and named the "metabolic syndrome" by U.S. (Adult Treatment Panel III 2003) and international (Alberti and Zimmet 1998) expert groups. The National Cholesterol Education Program (NCEP) and World Health Organization (WHO) definitions of the metabolic syndrome are shown in Table 10.1 and Table 10.2. The aim of this chapter is to relate weight loss to changes in these conditions. Type 2 diabetes mellitus will be discussed initially and then dyslipidemia. (Hypertension, although very important, will not be discussed here because it is covered in another chapter.) Cardiovascular disease will be cited next and then other disease risks will be mentioned.

10.2 Abnormal Glucose Metabolism and Type 2 Diabetes

A frequent manifestation of the metabolic syndrome is abnormal glucose metabolism, expressed as an elevated fasting glucose (Adult Treatment Panel III 2003) or impaired glucose tolerance (Alberti and Zimmet 1998). The ability to measure glucose disposal, first by the euglycemic hyperinsulinemic clamp (DeFronzo et al. 1979) and then by the minimal model of Bergman et al. (1979), allowed for a quantitation of total body glucose disposal.

Once the ability to define those who are insulin sensitive and those who are insulin resistant became available, an effort to elucidate the pathophysiology began.

Obesity has a major effect on the prevalence and severity of type 2 diabetes. The prevalence of reported diabetes is 2.9 times higher in overweight than nonoverweight persons in the NHANES (National Health Examination Survey) data (Harris et al. 1998). A strong cross-sectional correlation exists between relative weight and prevalence of diabetes in population groups. Obesity is associated with type 2 diabetes mellitus in women (Colditz et al. 1990) and men (Chan et al. 1994). Increasing weight has been associated with increasing insulin resistance (Bogardus et al. 1984a, b) and central or upper body fat deposition has been found to be independently associated with insulin resistance (Bonora 2000).

As obesity prevalence increases, the incidence of diabetes rises (Mokdad et al. 2001). Prospective studies have described this in Israel (Medalie et al. 1974), Norway (Westlund and Nicolaysen 1972), and Sweden (Larsson et al. 1984). In fact, over 85% of type 2 diabetic patients are overweight or obese (Maggio and Pi–Sunyer 1997). Risk of developing diabetes increases with increasing weight gain and is enhanced the higher the baseline BMI is in an individual adult (Chan et al. 1994; Colditz et al. 1990). In cross-sectional (Després et al. 1989; Haffner et al. 1991; Sparrow et al. 1986) and longitudinal (Lundgren et al. 1989; Ohlson et al. 1985; Olefsky 1981) studies, fat distribution has been found also to be important in diabetes risk. The greater the amount of central, upper body, or abdominal obesity, the greater the risk is for diabetes and cardiovascular disease (Lapidus et al. 1984; Larsson et al. 1984). Overall, by enhancing insulin resistance and its sequelae, glucose intolerance, hypertension, dyslipidemia, coagulation abnormalities, inflammation, and endothelial dysfunction, obesity leads to type 2 diabetes and cardiovascular disease.

The reason for this increasing insulin resistance has been a subject of much controversy. A "portal hypothesis" postulates that free fatty acids are actively released, primarily from the visceral fat depot, because the insulin does not shut off lipolysis appropriately (Bjorntorp 1990). These fatty acids enter the portal vein, go to the liver, and there initiate a number of events. Production of VLDL increases, which leads to greater amounts of circulating triglycerides; a drop in HDL cholesterol; and an increase in small, dense LDL particles. The increased FFA flux leads to an inhibition of glucose utilization by skeletal muscle (Boden 1997). This seems to be primarily due to a decrease of glucose transporters (Shulman 2000) and a decrease in glycogen synthase activity (Roden et al. 1996). Evidence from epidemiological studies indicates that intra-abdominal fat is a strong, positive, significant predictor of type 2 diabetes (Boyko et al. 1996).

Insulin resistance occurs in adipose tissue, liver, and muscle (DeFronzo 1988); glucose transport (Hissin et al. 1982) and glucose oxidation (Bogardus et al. 1984a; Segal et al. 1991) are affected. Activation of tyrosine kinase is impaired after insulin locks to its receptor in insulin-sensitive cells (Caro et al. 1989). The net effect is a requirement for an increased insulin secretion by the β-cells of the pancreas and higher prevailing insulin levels (Kreisberg et al. 1967; Polonsky et al. 1988). In obese persons with the appropriate genetic make-up, β-cell secretion eventually begins to exhaust and carbohydrate tolerance begins to become impaired. Eventually, frank diabetes supervenes.

The relationship of appropriate glucose disposal in obese individuals may also be related to a widespread problem of ectopic fat in tissues important in insulin action. This ectopic fat is due to the increased FFA flux in these individuals. There is now good evidence that fat in skeletal muscle can have a negative impact on glucose uptake (Kelley et al. 1999), as well as growing evidence that fat in the liver can lead to increased insulin resistance and type 2 diabetes (Yki–Jarvinen 2002). Finally, evidence also indicates increased fat deposits in the β-cell that may cause interference with insulin production and may lead to β-cell apoptosis (Unger and Zhou 2001).

10.3 Weight Loss Effects in Persons with Abnormal Glucose Metabolism and Type 2 Diabetes

The effect of weight loss on insulin resistance is clear. An improvement in insulin sensitivity occurs that translates into lower risk factors for diabetes and cardiovascular disease (Goldstein 1992; Pi–Sunyer 1993b, 1996). Some of the randomized trials carried out in this regard are summarized next.

10.3.1 Diabetes Prevention Trials in Persons with Impaired Glucose Tolerance

Three longitudinal diabetes prevention trials were long enough, large enough, and well enough conducted to be reviewed here as evidence for the proposition that weight loss helps to prevent the onset of type 2 diabetes.

- The Da Qing Trial (Pan et al. 1997) was conducted in 33 centers in China. It was unusual in that the cohort of 577 persons was randomized by center; some centers assigned their patients to dietary change, some to exercise change, some to both, and one (the control) to none. The results of the study are presented in Table 10.3 (Pan et al. 1997). It can be seen that diet, exercise, and the combination of diet and exercise all prevented the development of diabetes to a much greater extent than at the control site.
- The Finnish Diabetes Prevention Study (Tuomilehto et al. 2001) of 523 people was carried out in five centers in Finland. Subjects were randomized into two arms: usual care and life-style intervention. The goals of the life-style intervention are listed in Table 10.4. After 5 years, the development of diabetes was 58% less in the intervention group compared to the usual care group, as shown in Figure 10.1.

TABLE 10.3

Da Qing IGT and Diabetes Study[a]

Intervention	6-Year Incidence of NIDDM (%)	Reduction from Control (%)
Control	67.7	—
Diet	43.8	31 ($p < .03$)
Exercise	41.1	46 ($p < .0005$)
Diet + exercise	46.0	42 ($p < .005$)

[a] Adjusted for BMI and fasting glucose.

Source: From Pan, X.R. et al., *Diabetes Care*, 20, 537–544, 1997.

TABLE 10.4

Goals for Intervention

Weight reduction >5%
Fat intake <30% energy intake
Saturated fat intake <10% energy intake
Fiber intake >15 g/1000 kcal
Exercise >4 h/week

Source: From Tuomilehto, J. et al., *N. Engl. J. Med.*, 344, 1343–1350, 2001.

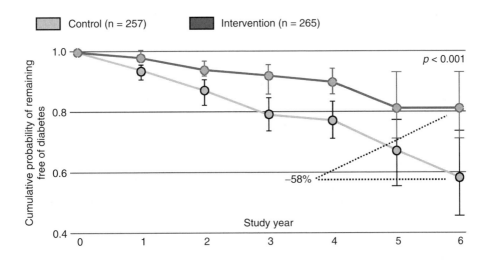

FIGURE 10.1
Finnish diabetes prevention (IGT) study. (From Tuomilehto, J. et al., *N. Engl. J. Med.*, 344, 1343–1350.)

- The Diabetes Prevention Program (Diabetes Prevention Program Research Group 2002) was a randomized trial that engaged 26 centers in the U.S. and included 4000 individuals (The Diabetes Prevention Program 1999). Individuals were randomized to a life-style arm; a metformin arm; a troglitazone arm; and a placebo usual-care arm. The troglitazone arm was stopped after about a year because of hepatic toxicity. The life-style intervention goals were very similar to the goals of the Finnish study, although the weight loss goal was a little greater — 7% from baseline. The weight results are shown in Figure 10.2 and the physical activity results in Figure 10.3. It can be seen that the goal of 7% weight loss from baseline was reached at 6 months, with a gradual return thereafter toward baseline weight. With this amount of weight loss in the life-style arm, development of diabetes in the life-style intervention group was reduced 58% compared to the usual-care

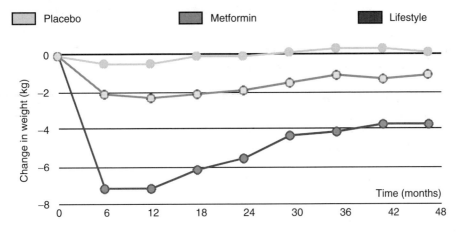

FIGURE 10.2
DPP — effect of interventions on weight. (From Knowler, W.C., *N. Engl. J. Med.*, 2002, 346:393–403.)

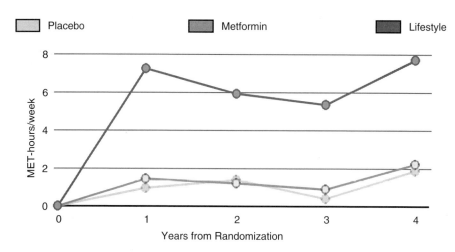

FIGURE 10.3

DPP — mean change in leisure physical activity. (From Knowler, W.C., *N. Engl. J. Med.*, 2002, 346:393–403.)

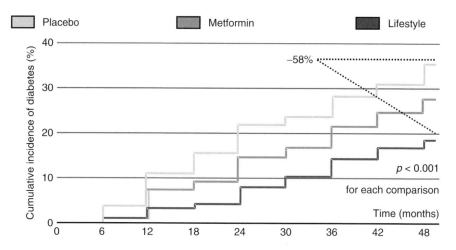

FIGURE 10.4

DPP — cumulative incidence of diabetes according to study group. (From Knowler, W.C., *N. Engl. J. Med.*, 2002, 346:393–403.)

group. The metformin group had a reduction of diabetes of 31%. The progression to diabetes in the three arms is shown in Figure 10.4.

These three studies show that it is possible to have a significant impact on the development of diabetes in overweight and obese persons with a program of a hypocaloric diet and exercise that will drop weight about 7% and is at least partially sustained for the following 4 years. This has caused the American Diabetes Association and the National Institute of Diabetes and Digestive and Kidney Disease to suggest life-style intervention as the first line of treatment in attempting to prevent diabetes (American Diabetes Association 2003).

10.3.2 Weight Loss Studies for Prevention of Diabetes in Persons without IGT

More recently, a study was done in Europe to evaluate weight loss effects on the progression to diabetes in a group of obese patients, with and without IGT. The weight loss was induced with Xenical in combination with life-style change in comparison with life-style change alone over a period of 4 years. Xenical is a lipase inhibitor, a new class of antiobesity agent. It causes a dose-dependent reduction in dietary fat absorption in the gut, with a maximum 30% inhibition of fat absorption utilizing a dosage of 120 mg tid (Hauptman et al. 1992; Zhi et al. 1994). This action tends to counteract the excess fat intake characteristic of many obese individuals (Jebb 1997). The drug has been shown to be effective in large, long-term (1 and 2 year) randomized clinical trials in inducing and maintaining weight loss in obese patients without (Davidson et al. 1999; Sjöström et al. 2000) and with (Hollander et al. 1998) diabetes.

Xenical significantly reduced the incidence of type 2 diabetes. The hazard ratio showed a 37.5% decrease with Xenical compared to placebo over 4 years. Approximately 50% more Xenical than placebo patients achieved weight loss of 5 and 10% from baseline. Waist circumference, LDL cholesterol, and blood pressure decreased significantly more in the drug group. The adverse event profile in this study was not serious and was equivalent to that previously reported in other long-term trials (Davidson et al. 1999; Hollander et al. 1998; Sjöström et al. 2000).

Will et al. (2002) examined retrospectively the 13-year incidence of diabetes in a large cohort of subjects from the first Cancer Prevention Study. The authors found that intentional weight loss was associated with a significant reduction in the rate of developing diabetes. Also, Colditz et al. (1995) found in the Nurses Health Study that women who lost more than 5 kg reduced their risk for diabetes by more than 50%.

10.3.3 Weight Loss for the Improvement of Type 2 Diabetes Mellitus

As mentioned earlier, weight loss leads to an improvement in insulin resistance. As a result, it is not surprising that weight loss improves type 2 diabetes because this disease is characterized by a combination of insulin resistance and β-cell dysfunction. Numerous studies have reported the improvement of insulin sensitivity with weight loss, including better peripheral glucose disposal; decreased hepatic glucose output; and improved β-cell insulin secretory response (DeFronzo 1988). Low-calorie diets quickly cause elevated blood glucose levels to drop whether with moderate caloric restriction (Anderson et al. 1992; Doar et al. 1975; Hadden et al. 1975; Liu et al. 1985; Bogardus et al. 1984c) or with more severe caloric deficits (Amatruda et al. 1998; Genuth et al. 1974; Henry et al. 1986; Kirschner et al. 1988; Wing et al. 1991). Not only do blood glucose levels improve, but also antidiabetic medications may be decreased or eliminated altogether in many instances (Anderson et al. 1992; Bistrian et al. 1976; Kirschner et al. 1988; Liu et al. 1985; Wing et al. 1991).

Because the onset and progression of diabetic complications are strongly associated with poor glycemic control (The Diabetes Control and Complications Trial Research Group 1993), better glycemic control has now become the standard of care for diabetic patients (American Diabetes Association 2003). Kirschner et al. (1988) reported that a 23-kg weight loss (22% of baseline weight) allowed all patients taking oral agents and 82% of patients taking insulin to discontinue medication. Fitz et al. (1983) obtained similar results with an average weight loss of 9.3 kg.

10.4 Dyslipidemia

The association of dyslipidemia with obesity has been described in a number of epidemiological studies. Although most have related overall obesity to dyslipidemia, some have reported that the dyslipidemia is primarily related to central fat distribution (Després et al. 1990; Walton et al. 1995). About one third of obese patients have abnormal lipids. The triad includes high levels of triglycerides; low HDL cholesterol; and small, dense LDL particles (Krauss 1998a; Krauss 1998b). The first two have been listed as part of the metabolic syndrome (see Table 10.1).

The most common pattern includes elevations of VLDL levels; increased small, dense LDL particles; and low HDL cholesterol (Austin et al. 1988; Grundy 1995, 1997). This pattern is considered atherogenic because it is common in patients with premature coronary heart disease (Austin et al. 1988, 1990). It is particularly common in patients who are obese and have type 2 diabetes (Betteridge 1999; Verges 1999). Because these patients have elevated triglyceride-rich lipoproteins, they generally have elevated serum triglycerides (Krauss 1998). These lipoproteins are primarily made up of VLDL remnants, which have been reported to be particularly atherogenic (Gianturco and Bradley 1999; Ooi and Ooi 1998; Packard 1999; Phillips et al. 1993; Steiner 1998). A number of studies have also shown an association between small, dense LDL particles and CHD (Austin et al. 1988, 1990; Krauss 1998a; Lamarche et al. 1998). The risk from these small particles is greater than one might expect from the level of LDL cholesterol (Griffin 1999; Lamarche et al. 1997). HDL cholesterol levels are low because HDL particles are depleted of cholesterol and the number of particles is reduced. Because HDL is protective against CHD (Adult Treatment Panel III 2003), these low levels enhance risk.

Obese persons tend to have a fatty liver. With fatty liver comes an overproduction of VLDL particles and of apoB100, the major apolipoprotein of VLDL particles (Moberly et al. 1990; Sparks et al. 1997; White et al. 1992; Wu et al. 1994). The high apo-B is due to the elevated VLDL and the small, dense LDL because each of these particles contains a single molecule of apo B. Apolipoprotein C is also overproduced, which retards the uptake of VLDL particles by the liver (Aalto–Setala et al. 1992; Clavey et al. 1995) and impairs the action of lipoprotein lipase (Ginsberg et al. 1986). Overactivity and overproduction of hepatic lipase (Cohen et al. 1999; Nie et al. 1998; Vega and Grundy 1996) also occur, as well as increased synthesis of LDL receptors (Egusa et al. 1985; Howard et al. 1986).

10.5 Weight Loss in Dyslipidemia

Weight loss improves the lipid triad, lowering triglycerides, increasing LDL-cholesterol particle size, and raising HDL cholesterol (Pi–Sunyer 1993b). Short-term studies have reported considerable improvement in these risk factors (Carmena et al. 1984; Fachnie and Foreback 1987; Follick et al. 1984; Rossner and Bjorvell 1987; Schieffer et al. 1991; Zimmerman et al. 1984).

Long-term studies have been fewer (Pi–Sunyer 1996), but some are available. Hall et al. (1972) reported that in a trial in which patients lost an average of 10 lbs and changed to a cholesterol-lowering diet, serum cholesterol dropped by 12.1% and triglycerides by 17.3% in one year. Mancini et al. (1981) studied obese patients who lost an average of 12.4 lbs after 30 months and 10.2 lbs after 54 months and found a significant drop in triglycerides but not cholesterol. A study by Wood et al. (1988) comparing diet, exercise, and controls, showed a significant drop in triglycerides and an increase in HDL cholesterol at 1 year in the diet group, which lost 5.9 kg. In a long-term study conducted by Weintraub et al. (1992), patients at 54 weeks had lost 15% of their baseline body weight. This was associated with an improvement in serum triglycerides, LDL, and HDL.

Patients who have undergone bariatric surgery and lost considerable amounts of weight have also shown an improvement of lipid levels. Brolin et al. (1990) reported on 38 obese persons with dyslipidemia who underwent gastric by-pass surgery. Lipid profiles became normal in 32 of 38 patients. Improvements in lipid profile were sustained at 12 months in all patients who lost more than 50% of their excess weight. A more complete study is the Swedish Obesity Surgery Study (Sjöström et al. 1999). Patients underwent vertical-banded gastroplasty and were followed over time. The control group was matched for weight, age, and sex and followed medically. The surgical group had lost an average of 23.2 kg in men and 20.3 kg in women at 2 years. Total cholesterol, HDL cholesterol, and triglycerides significantly improved in the surgical group, whereas no change took place in the group treated medically.

10.6 Hypertension

Hypertension has been known to be associated with obesity for many years (Ferrannini et al. 1990, 1997). The mechanism for this is not clear, but may include increased sodium reasbsorption; increased sympathetic nervous system activation; H^+/K^+ and Ca^{++} cation exchange; and angiotensin II production by enlarged adipose cells. Whatever the mechanisms, the relationship between increasing weight and increasing blood pressure has been well established in a number of population groups (Stamler et al. 1978). The effect of weight loss on blood pressure is discussed in another chapter.

10.7 Cardiovascular Disease

Cardiovascular disease (CVD) is increased in obese subjects. The manifestations include coronary artery disease, sudden death, congestive heart failure, and arrhythmias. Because many obese persons also manifest hypertension and dyslipidemia, it has sometimes been difficult to assign causality for the cardiovascular disease to obesity independent of these other conditions. Because obesity is associated with a number of cardiovascular risk factors, it is not surprising that it has been related directly to greater cardiovascular risk (Calle et al. 1999; Rexrode et al. 1998). In the Framingham study, obesity was found to be an independent risk factor for cardiovascular disease (Hubert et al. 1983). In the Nurses Health Study, overweight and obesity increased the risk of coronary heart disease (Manson et al. 1990). In a more recent report, Wilson et al. (2002) have shown increased relative and population-attributable risk for hypertension and cardiovascular sequelae in Framingham Heart Study participants (Wilson et al. 2002).

10.8 Weight Loss in Cardiovascular Disease

Few studies of the effect of weight loss on cardiovascular disease have been conducted. Williamson et al. (1995, 1999) carried out retrospective analyses in women and men on the effect of intentional weight loss on mortality. They examined the life expectancy of more than 43,000 white U.S. women in the American Cancer Society Study. Overweight women with obesity-related health conditions had significantly higher mortality rates compared with women with no pre-existing illness. Women with obesity-related conditions who intentionally lost weight showed a significant reduction in all-cause mortality compared with women whose weight remained stable. The risk of cardiovascular mortality was reduced by 14 to 24% in obese women who intentionally lost weight. Williamson et al. (1999) then carried out a similar study in men, using the same American Cancer Society database. Again, they found that men with obesity-related conditions who lost weight had a reduced all-cause and cardiovascular mortality.

A 4-year prospective study of over 7500 middle-aged men found an independent decrease in cardiovascular mortality of almost 50% in those whose weight loss brought them below a BMI of 28 and a reduction of 77% in those who had associated hypertension (Wannamethee and Shaper 1990). Keys et al. (1972) suggested that coronary heart disease mortality could be reduced by 15% if everyone had a BMI between 21 and 25.

10.9 Congestive Heart Failure

Congestive heart failure occurs with greater frequency in obese patients. Left ventricular hypertrophy is common and is often related to the hypertension that occurs in many of these patients. However, even in the absence of hypertension, left ventricular mass can be increased and dysfunction occurs (Alpert and Hashimi 1993; Duflou et al. 1995; Messerli 1982). Dilated cardiomyopathy can also occur, leading to concomitant cardiac arrhythmias (Duflou et al. 1995). Prolonged QT intervals in many of these patients may add to the risk of arrhythmia and sudden death (Frank et al. 1986). Right heart failure also occurs, particularly in those persons with obstructive sleep apnea (Burwell et al. 1956; Menashe et al. 1965). In fact, heart failure is often biventricular (Alpert and Hashimi 1993).

10.10 Weight Loss in Congestive Heart Failure

Small reductions in weight, along with sodium restriction, can greatly improve cardiac function (Estes et al. 1957). Also, the QT interval can be shortened, thus decreasing the risk of arrhythmias (Carella et al. 1996). MacMahon et al. (1986) reported a decrease in left ventricular mass in obese patients who lost an average of 8.3 kg. Greater weight loss, as occurs in gastrointestinal surgery, can decrease not only type 2 diabetes, but also cardiovascular mortality (MacDonald et al. 1997; Matts et al. 1995).

10.11 Obstructive Sleep Apnea

The risk of obstructive sleep apnea is greatly increased in obese individuals, particularly those who are morbidly obese. An increase of one standard deviation in BMI is accompanied by a fourfold increase in apnea and hypoventilation (Young et al. 1993). In a group of 250 obese persons with an average BMI of 45.3, 40% of the men and 3% of the women had sleep apena, while none was found in a control group of lean people (Vgontzas et al. 1994). Deposition of fat centrally, and particularly intra-abdominally, seems to enhance the risk for sleep apnea (Shinohara et al. 1997; Vgontzas et al. 2000). Although women at a similar weight have a much lower risk than men for developing sleep apnea, those with polycystic ovary syndrome have a greatly increased risk (Vgontzas et al. 2001).

10.12 Weight Loss in Obstructive Sleep Apnea

Weight loss has been found to reduce sleep apnea greatly. For example, in the SOS study previously mentioned, the loss of weight through surgical intervention caused significant improvement in those who had the condition (Karason et al. 2000). Sugerman et al. (1992) found the same thing. Life-style-induced weight loss also reduces sleep apnea, although the results are less dramatic. Reports by Smith et al. (1985), Suratt et al. (1987, 1992), and Kansanen et al. (1998) showed that weight loss improved sleep apnea symptoms. Unfortunately, the relief of symptoms is not always sustained, even if the weight loss is maintained (Sampol et al. 1998). This may be true also of surgically induced weight loss (Charuzi et al. 1992). Nevertheless, the bulk of patients is greatly helped, with major improvement of symptoms.

10.13 Inflammation

Evidence that inflammation plays a key role in obesity and the progression of coronary heart disease is growing. Prospective studies have shown an association between elevated markers of inflammation and risk of coronary heart disease. For example, a study of 159 men aged 22 to 63 years showed that C-reactive protein (CRP) levels correlated with central adiposity and that significant increases in visceral adipose tissue and waist circumference occurred with increasing quintiles of CRP (Lemieux et al. 2001). Other studies have also shown an association between inflammatory markers and obesity (Blake and Ridker 2001; Das 2002; Resnick and Howard 2002). Hotamisligil et al. (1993, 1995) reported an increased expression of tumor necrosis factor in adipose tissue of obese persons. If TNF-α is neutralized in obese animals with diabetes, insulin-stimulated peripheral glucose uptake is enhanced (Hotamisligil et al. 1993).

10.14 Weight Loss in Relation to Inflammatory Markers

A number of investigators studying the effect of weight loss on inflammation and inflammatory markers have reported that C-reactive protein levels drop with weight loss (Heilbronn et al. 2001; Laimer et al. 2002; Tchernof et al. 2002). A drop in IL-6 (Bastard et al. 2000a; Gallistl et al. 2001; Ziccardi et al. 2002) and in TNF-α (Bastard et al. 2000a;

Mingrone et al. 2002) has also been described with weight loss. Also, Ziccardi et al. (2002) have shown that intercellular adhesion molecule-1 (ICAM-1); vascular adhesion molecule-1 (VCAM-1); and P-selectin improved in 56 obese women after an average weight loss of 9.8 kg. Thus, it is clear that weight loss improves the activated inflammatory state present with obesity and, one would assume, slows down the progression of coronary artery disease.

10.15   Coagulation Defects

The relationship of insulin resistance to coagulation abnormalities has been uncovered in the last few years. The best data are available for prothrombin activator inhibitor 1 (PAI-1), which, by inhibiting the activation of prothrombin, tends to delay clotting. PAI-1 is elevated with insulin resistance (Juhan–Vague et al. 1991); it has also been reported to be elevated in obesity (Hamsten et al. 1987). In a study of overweight and obese diabetic and nondiabetic women, Mertens et al. (2001) reported that PAI-1 activity was significantly higher in diabetic women than in nondiabetic ones. They also reported that visceral fat was the most important variable determining PAI-1 activity. On the other hand, Bastard et al. (2000b) reported that a decrease in abdominal subcutaneous adipose tissue was associated with a decrease in plasma PAI-1 levels. Landin et al. (1990) and Lee et al. (1990) also reported that abdominal obesity is associated with impaired fibrinolytic activity and elevated PAI-1. Also, fibrinogen is elevated and fibrinolytic activity is decreased (Meade et al. 1993; Vague et al. 1986).

10.16   Weight Loss in Relation to Coagulation Defects

With weight loss, PAI-1, fibrinogen, and factor VII decrease (Folsom et al. 1993). More recently, Svendsen et al. (1996) and Calles–Escandon et al. (1996) have reported lower PAI-1 and lower fibrinogen in patients losing weight. Bastard et al. (2000b) have shown that PAI-1 levels in plasma and PAI-1 mRNA and protein in subcutaneous abdominal adipose tissue drop after weight loss.

10.17   Weight Loss and Mortality

An early study by Lean et al. (1990) found that type 2 diabetic patients who lost weight had an increased life expectancy. Also, Singh et al. (1992) put patients who had had a myocardial infarction on a cardioprotective diet for a year. Those who lost more than 0.5 kg had the largest reduction in total and cardiovascular mortality. Williamson et al. (1995, 1999) also have reported the improvement of mortality in obese persons with health risks who intentionally lost weight.

10.18 Conclusion

Obesity is associated with a number of health risks, including insulin resistance; diabetes mellitus; hypertension; dyslipidemia; coagulation abnormalities; inflammatory markers; coronary heart disease; sleep apnea; congestive heart failure; and arthritis. These all improve with weight loss. A decrease of 10% or more from baseline weight can have a significant positive effect on these associated conditions (National Heart Lung and Blood Institute 1998; World Health Organization 1998).

References

Aalto–Setala, K., Fisher, E.A., Chen, X., Chajek-Shaul, T., Hayek, T., Zechner, R., Walsh, A., Ramakrishnan, R., Ginsberg, H.N., and Breslow, J.L. 1992, Mechanism of hypertriglyceridemia in human apolipoprotein (apo) CIII transgenic mice. Diminished very low density lipoprotein fractional catabolic rate associated with increased apo CIII and reduced apo E on the particles, *J. Clin. Invest.*, 90(5), 1889–1900.

Adult Treatment Panel III 2003, Executive summary of the third report of the National Cholesterol Education Program (NCEP) Expert Panel on Detection, Evaluation, and Treatment of High Blood Cholesterol in Adults, *JAMA*, 285, 2486–2497.

Alberti, K.G. and Zimmet, P.Z. 1998, Definition, diagnosis and classification of diabetes mellitus and its complications. Part 1: diagnosis and classification of diabetes mellitus provisional report of a WHO consultation, *Diabet. Med.*, 15(7), 539–553.

Allison, D.B., Fontaine, K.R., Manson, J.E., Stevens, J., and VanItallie, T.B. 1999, Annual deaths attributable to obesity in the United States, *JAMA*, 282, 1530–1538.

Alpert, M. and Hashimi, M. 1993, Obesity and the heart, *Am. J. Med. Sci.*, 306, 117–123.

Amatruda, J.M., Richeson, J.F., Welle, S.L., Brodows, R., and Lockwood, D.H. 1998, The safety and efficacy of a controlled low-energy (very-low-calorie) diet in the treatment of non-insulin dependent diabetes and obesity, *Arch. Intern. Med.*, 148, 873–877.

American Diabetes Association 2003, Standards of medical care for patients with diabetes, *Diabetes Care*, 26, S62–S69.

Anderson, J., Hamilton, C., and Brinkman–Kaplan, V. 1992, Benefits and risks of an intensive very-low-calorie-diet program for severe obesity, *Am. J. Gastroenterol.*, 87, 6–15.

Austin, M.A., Breslow, J.L., Hennekens, C.H., Buring, J.E., Willett, W.C., Krasnow, N., and Krauss, R.M. 1988, Low density lipoprotein subclass patterns and risk of myocardial infarction, *J. Am. Med. Assoc.*, 260, 1917–1921.

Austin, M.A., King, M.C., Vranizan, K.M., and Krauss, R.M. 1990, Atherogenic lipoprotein phenotype: a proposed genetic marker for coronary heart disease, *Circulation*, 82, 495–506.

Bastard, J.P., Jardel, C., Bruckert, E., Blondy, P., Capeau, J., Laville, M., Vidal, H., and Hainque, B. 2000a, Elevated levels of interleukin 6 are reduced in serum and subcutaneous adipose tissue of obese women after weight loss, *J. Clin. Endocrinol. Metab.*, 85(9), 3338–3342.

Bastard, J.P., Vidal, H., Jardel, C., Bruckert, E., Robin, D., Vallier, P., Blondy, P., Turpin, G., Forest, C., and Hainque, B. 2000b, Subcutaneous adipose tissue expression of plasminogen activator inhibitor-1 gene during very low calorie diet in obese subjects, *Int. J. Obes. Relat. Metab. Disord.*, 24(1) 70–74.

Bergman, R.N., Ider, Y.Z., Bowden, C.R., and Cobelli, C. 1979, Quantitative estimation of insulin sensitivity, *Am. J. Physiol.*, 236(6) E667–E677.

Betteridge, D.J. 1999, Diabetic dyslipidaemia, *Eur. J. Clin. Invest.*, 29 (Suppl 2) 12–16.

Bistrian, B.R., Blackburn, G.L., Flatt, J.P., Sizer, J., Scrimshaw, N.S., and Sherman, M. 1976, Nitrogen metabolism and insulin requirements in obese diabetic adults on a protein-sparing modified fast, *Diabetes*, 25(6), 494–504.

Bjorntorp, P. 1990, Portal adipose tissue as a generator of risk factors for cardiovascular disease and diabetes, *Arteriosclerosis*, 10, 493–496.

Blake, G.J. and Ridker, P.M. 2001, Novel clinical markers of vascular wall inflammation, *Circ. Res.*, 89(9), 763–771.

Boden, G. 1997, Role of fatty acids in the pathogenesis of insulin resistance and NIDDM, *Diabetes*, 46(1), 3–10.

Bogardus, C., Lillioja, S., Stone, K., and Mott, D. 1984a, Correlation between muscle glycogen synthase activity and *in vivo* insulin action in man, *J. Clin. Invest.*, 73(4), 1185–1190.

Bogardus, C., Lillioja, S., Mott, D., Reaven, G.R., Kashiwagi, A., and Foley, J.E. 1984b, Relationship between obesity and maximal insulin-stimulated glucose uptake *in vivo* and *in vitro* in Pima Indians, *J. Clin. Invest.*, 73(3), 800–805.

Bogardus, C., Ravussin, E., Robbins, D.C., Wolfe, R.R., Horton, E.S., and Sims, E.A. 1984c, Effects of physical training and diet therapy on carbohydrate metabolism in patients with glucose intolerance and non-insulin-dependent diabetes mellitus, *Diabetes*, 33(4), 311–318.

Bonora, E. 2000, Relationship between regional fat distribution and insulin resistance, *Int. J. Obes. Relat. Metab. Disord.*, 24 (Suppl 2), S32–S35.

Boyko, E.J., Leonetti, D.L., Bergstrom, R.W., Newell–Morris, L., and Fujimoto, W.Y. 1996, Visceral adiposity, fasting plasma insulin, and lipid and lipoprotein levels in Japanese Americans, *Int. J. Obes. Relat. Metab. Disord.*, 20(9), 801–808.

Brolin, R.E., Kenler, H.A., Wilson, A.C., Kup, P.T., and Cody, R.P. 1990, Serum lipids after gastric bypass surgery for morbid obesity, *Int. J. Obes.*, 14, 939–950.

Burwell, C.S., Robin, E.D., Whaley, R.D., and Bickleman, A.G. 1956, Extreme obesity associated with alveolar hypoventilation: a Pickwickian syndrome, *Am. J. Med.*, 21, 811–818.

Calle, E.E., Thun, M.J., Petrelli, J.M., Rodriguez, C., and Heath, C.W., Jr. 1999, Body-mass index and mortality in a prospective cohort of U.S. adults, *N. Engl. J. Med.*, 341(15), 1097–1105.

Calles–Escandon, J., Ballor, D., Harvey–Berino, J., Ades, P., Tracy, R., and Sobel, B. 1996, Amelioration of the inhibition of fibrinolysis in elderly, obese subjects by moderate energy intake restriction, *Am. J. Clin. Nutr.*, 64(1), 7–11.

Carella, M.J., Mantz, S.L., Rovner, D.R., Willis, P.W., III, Gossain, V.V., Bouknight, R.R., and Ferenchick, G.S. 1996, Obesity, adiposity, and lengthening of the QT interval: improvement after weight loss, *Int. J. Obes. Relat. Metab. Disord.*, 20(10), 938–942.

Carmena, R., Ascaso, J., Tebar, J., and Soriano, J. 1984, Changes in plasma high-density lipoproteins after body weight reduction in obese women, *Int. J. Obes.*, 8, 135–140.

Caro, J.F., Dohm, L.G., Pories, W.J., and Sinha, M.K. 1989, Cellular alterations in liver, skeletal muscle, and adipose tissue responsible for insulin resistance in obesity and type II diabetes, *Diabetes/Metab. Rev.*, 5, 665–689.

Chan, J.M., Rimm, E.B., Colditz, G.A., Stampfer, M.J., and Willett, W.C. 1994, Obesity, fat distribution, and weight gain as risk factors for clinical diabetes in men, *Diabetes Care*, 17, 961–969.

Charuzi, I., Lavie, P., Peiser, J., and Peled, R. 1992, Bariatric surgery in morbidly obese sleep-apnea patients: short- and long-term follow-up, *Am. J. Clin. Nutr.*, 55(2 Suppl), 594S–596S.

Clavey, V., Lestavel–Delattre, S., Copin, C., Bard, J.M., and Fruchart, J.C. 1995, Modulation of lipoprotein B binding to the LDL receptor by exogenous lipids and apolipoproteins CI, CII, CIII, and E, *Arterioscler. Thromb. Vasc. Biol.*, 15(7), 963–971.

Cohen, J.C., Vega, G.L., and Grundy, S.M. 1999, Hepatic lipase: new insights from genetic and metabolic studies, *Curr. Opin. Lipidol.*, 10(3), 259–267.

Colditz, G.A., Willett, W.C., Rotnitzky, A., and Manson, J.E. 1995, Weight gain as a risk factor for clinical diabetes mellitus in women, *Ann. Intern. Med.*, 122(7), 481–486.

Colditz, G.A., Willett, W.C., Stampfer, M.J., Manson, J.E., Hennekens, C.H., Arky, R.A., and Speizer, F.E. 1990, Weight as a risk factor for clinical diabetes in women, *Am. J. Epidemiol.*, 132(3), 501–513.

Das, U.N. 2002, Obesity, metabolic syndrome X, and inflammation, *Nutrition*, 18(5), 430–432.

Davidson, M.H., Hauptman, J., DiGirolamo, M., Foreyt, J.P., Halsted, C.H., Heber, D., Heimburger, D.C., Lucas, C.P., Robbins, D.C., Chung, J., and Heymsfield, S.B. 1999, Weight control and risk factor reduction in obese subjects treated for 2 years with orlistat: a randomized controlled trial, *JAMA*, 281(3), 235–242.

DeFronzo, R.A. 1988, The triumvirate; β cell, muscle, liver: a collusion responsible for NIDDM, *Diabetes*, 37, 644–667.

DeFronzo, R.A., Tobin, J.D., and Andres, R. 1979, Glucose clamp technique: a method for quantifying insulin secretion and resistance, *Am. J. Physiol.*, 237(3), E214–E223.

Després, J.P., Moorjani, S., Lupien, P.J., Tremblay, A., Nadeau, A., and Bouchard, C. 1990, Regional distribution of body fat, plasma lipoproteins, and cardiovascular disease, *Arteriosclerosis*, 10(4), 497–511.

Després, J.P., Nadeau, A., Tremblay, A., Ferland, M., Moorjani, S., Lupien, P.J., Theriault, G., Pinault, S., and Bouchard, C. 1989, Role of deep abdominal fat in the association between regional adipose tissue distribution and glucose tolerance in obese women, *Diabetes*, 38(3), 304–309.

Diabetes Control and Complications Trial Research Group 1993, The effect of intensive treatment of diabetes on the development and progression of long-term complications in insulin-dependent diabetes mellitus, *N. Engl. J. Med.*, 329(14), 977–986.

Diabetes Prevention Program 1999, The diabetes prevention program. Design and methods for a clinical trial in the prevention of type 2 diabetes, *Diabetes Care*, 22(4), 623–634.

Diabetes Prevention Program Research Group 2002, Reduction in the incidence of type 2 diabetes with lifestyle intervention or metformin, *N. Engl. J. Med.*, 346, 393–403.

Doar, J.W., Wilde, C.E., Thompson, M.E., and Sewell, P.F. 1975, Influence of treatment with diet alone on oral glucose-tolerance test and plasma sugar and insulin levels in patients with maturity-onset diabetes mellitus, *Lancet*, 1(7919), 1263–1266.

Duflou, J., Virmani, R., Rabin, I., Burke, A., Farb, A., and Smialek, J. 1995, Sudden death as a result of heart disease in morbid obesity, *Am. Heart J.*, 130(2), 306–313.

Egusa, G., Beltz, W.F., Grundy, S.M., and Howard, B.V. 1985, Influence of obesity on the metabolism of apolipoprotein B in humans, *J. Clin. Invest.*, 76(2), 596–603.

Estes, E.H., Jr., Seider, H.O., and McIntosh, H.D. 1957, Reversible cardiopulmonary syndrome with extreme obesity, *Circulation*, 16, 179–187.

Fachnie, J.D. and Foreback, C.C. 1987, Effects of weight reduction, exercise, and diet modification on lipids and apolipoproteins A-1 and B in severely obese persons, *Henry Ford Hosp. Med. J.*, 35(4), 216–220.

Ferrannini, E., Haffner, S.M., and Stern, M.P. 1990, Essential hypertension: an insulin-resistant state, *J. Cardiovasc. Pharmacol.*, 15 (Suppl 5), S18–S25.

Ferrannini, E., Natali, A., Capaldo, B., Lehtovirta, M., Jacob, S., and Yki-Jarvinen, H. 1997, Insulin resistance, hyperinsulinemia, and blood pressure: role of age and obesity. European Group for the Study of Insulin Resistance (EGIR), *Hypertension*, 30(5), 1144–1149.

Fitz, J.D., Sperling, E.M., and Fein, H.G. 1983, A hypocaloric high-protein diet as primary therapy for adults with obesity-related diabetes: effective long-term use in a community hospital, *Diabetes Care*, 6(4), 328–333.

Flegal, K.M., Carroll, M.D., Ogden, C.L., and Johnson, C.L. 2002, Prevalence and trends in obesity among US adults, 1999–2000, *JAMA*, 288(14), 1723–1727.

Follick, M., Abrams, D., Smith, T., Henderson, L.O., and Herbert, P.N. 1984, Contrasting short- and long-term effects of weight loss on lipoprotein levels, *Arch. Intern. Med.*, 144, 1571–1574.

Folsom, A.R., Qamhieh, H.T., Wing, R.R., Jeffery, R.W., Stinson, V.L., Kuller, L.H., and Wu, K.K. 1993, Impact of weight loss on plasminogen activator inhibitor (PAI-1), factor VII, and other hemostatic factors in moderately overweight adults, *Arterioscler. Thromb.*, 13(2), 162–169.

Fontaine, K.R., Redden, D.T., Wang, C., Westfall, A.O., and Allison, D.B. 2003, Years of life lost due to obesity, *JAMA*, 289(2), 187–193.

Frank, S., Colliver, J.A., and Frank, A. 1986, The electrocardiogram in obesity: statistical analysis of 1,029 patients, *J. Am. Coll. Cardiol.*, 7(2), 295–299.

Gallistl, S., Sudi, K.M., Aigner, R., and Borkenstein, M. 2001, Changes in serum interleukin-6 concentrations in obese children and adolescents during a weight reduction program, *Int. J. Obes. Relat. Metab. Disord.*, 25(11), 1640–1643.

Genuth, S.M., Castro, J.H., and Vertes, V. 1974, Weight reduction in obesity by outpatient semistarvation, *JAMA*, 230, 987–991.

Gianturco, S.H. and Bradley, W.A. 1999, Pathophysiology of triglyceride-rich lipoproteins in atherothrombosis: cellular aspects, *Clin. Cardiol.*, 22(6 Suppl), II7–14.

Ginsberg, H.N., Le, N.A., Goldberg, I.J., Gibson, J.C., Rubinstein, A., Wang–Iverson, P., Norum, R., and Brown, W.V. 1986, Apolipoprotein B metabolism in subjects with deficiency of apolipo-proteins CIII and AI. Evidence that apolipoprotein CIII inhibits catabolism of triglyceride-rich lipoproteins by lipoprotein lipase *in vivo, J. Clin. Invest.*, 78(5), 1287–1295.

Goldstein, D.J. 1992, Beneficial health effects of modest weight loss, *Int. J. Obes.*, 16, 397–415.

Griffin, B.A. 1999, Lipoprotein atherogenicity: an overview of current mechanisms, *Proc. Nutr. Soc.*, 58(1), 163–169.

Grundy, S.M. 1995, Atherogenic dyslipidemia: lipoprotein abnormalities and implications for ther-apy, *Am. J. Cardiol.*, 75(6), 45B–52B.

Grundy, S.M. 1997, Small LDL, atherogenic dyslipidemia, and the metabolic syndrome, *Circulation*, 95(1), 1–4.

Hadden, D.R., Montgomery, D.A., Skelly, R.J., Trimble, E.R., Weaver, J.A., Wilson, E.A., and Bucha-nan, K.D. 1975, Maturity onset diabetes mellitus: response to intensive dietary management, *Br. Med. J.*, 3(5978), 276–278.

Haffner, S.M., Mitchell, B.D., Hazuda, H.P., and Stern, M.P. 1991, Greater influence of central distri-bution of adipose tissue on incidence of non–insulin-dependent diabetes in women than men, *Am. J. Clin. Nutr.*, 53(5), 1312–1317.

Hall, Y., Stamler, J., Cohen, D.B., Mojonnier, L., Epstein, M.B., Berkson, D.M., Whipple, I.T., and Catchings, S. 1972, Effectiveness of a low saturated fat, low cholesterol, weight-reducing diet for the control of hypertriglyceridemia, *Atherosclerosis*, 16, 389–403.

Hamsten, A., de Faire, U., Walldius, G., Dahlen, G., Szamosi, A., Landou, C., Blomback, M., and Wiman, B. 1987, Plasminogen activator inhibitor in plasma: risk factor for recurrent myocardial infarction, *Lancet*, 2(8549), 3–9.

Harris, M., Flegal, K., Cowie, C., Eberhardt, M., Golstein, D., Little, R., Wiedmeyer, H., and By-rd–Holt, D. 1998, Prevalence of diabetes: impaired fasting glucose and impaired glucose tolerance in U.S. adults, *Diabetes Care*, 21, 518–524.

Hauptman, J.B., Jeunet, F.S., and Hartmann, D. 1992, Initial studies in humans with the novel gastrointestinal lipase inhibitor Ro 18-0647 (tetrahydrolipstatin), *Am. J. Clin. Nutr.*, 55(1 Suppl), 309S–313S.

Heilbronn, L.K., Noakes, M., and Clifton, P.M. 2001, Energy restriction and weight loss on very-low-fat diets reduce C-reactive protein concentrations in obese, healthy women, *Arterioscler. Thromb. Vasc. Biol.*, 21(6), 968–970.

Henry, R.R., Wiest–Kent, T.A., Scheaffer, L., Kolterman, O.G., and Olefsky, J.M. 1986, Metabolic consequences of very-low-calorie diet therapy in obese non-insulin-dependent diabetic and non-diabetic subjects, *Diabetes*, 35, 155–164.

Hissin, P.J., Foley, J.E., Wardzala, L.J., Karnieli, E., Simpson, I.A., Salans, L.B., and Cushman, S.W. 1982, Mechanism of insulin-resistant glucose transport activity in the enlarged adipose cell of the aged, obese rat, *J. Clin. Invest.*, 70, 780–790.

Hollander, P.A., Elbein, S.C., Hirsch, I.B., Kelley, D., McGill, J., Taylor, T., Weiss, S.R., Crockett, S.E., Kaplan, R.A., Comstock, J., Lucas, C.P., Lodewick, P.A., Canovatchel, W., Chung, J., and Hauptman, J. 1998, Role of orlistat in the treatment of obese patients with type 2 diabetes, *Diabetes Care*, 21(8), 1288–1294.

Hotamisligil, G.S., Arner, P., Caro, J.F., Atkinson, R.L., and Spiegelman, B.M. 1995, Increased adipose tissue expression of tumor necrosis factor-alpha in human obesity and insulin resistance, *J. Clin. Invest.*, 95(5), 2409–2415.

Hotamisligil, G.S., Shargill, N.S., and Spiegelman, B.M. 1993, Adipose expression of tumor necrosis factor-alpha: direct role in obesity-linked insulin resistance, *Science*, 259(5091), 87–91.

Howard, B.V., Egusa, G., Beltz, W.F., Kesaniemi, Y.A., and Grundy, S.M. 1986, Compensatory mech-anisms governing the concentration of plasma low density lipoprotein, *J. Lipid Res.*, 27(1), 11–20.

Hubert, H.B., Feinlieb, M., McNamara, P.M., and Castelli, W.P. 1983, Obesity as an independent risk factor for cardiovascular disease: a 26-year follow-up of participants in the Framingham Heart Study, *Circulation*, 67, 968–977.

Jebb, S.A. 1997, Aetiology of obesity, *Br. Med. Bull.*, 53(2), 264–285.

Juhan–Vague, I., Alessi, M.C., and Vague, P. 1991, Increased plasma plasminogen activator inhibitor 1 levels. A possible link between insulin resistance and atherothrombosis, *Diabetologia*, 34(7), 457–462.

Kansanen, M., Vanninen, E., Tuunainen, A., Pesonen, P., Tuononen, V., Hartikainen, J., Mussalo, H., and Uusitupa, M. 1998, The effect of a very low-calorie diet-induced weight loss on the severity of obstructive sleep apnoea and autonomic nervous function in obese patients with obstructive sleep apnoea syndrome, *Clin. Physiol.*, 18(4), 377–385.

Karason, K., Lindroos, A.K., Stenlof, K., and Sjöström, L. 2000, Relief of cardiorespiratory symptoms and increased physical activity after surgically induced weight loss: results from the Swedish obese subjects study, *Arch. Intern. Med.*, 160(12), 1797–1802.

Kelley, D.E., Goodpaster, B., Wing, R.R., and Simoneau, J.A. 1999, Skeletal muscle fatty acid metabolism in association with insulin resistance, obesity, and weight loss, *Am. J. Physiol.*, 277(6) Pt 1, E1130–E1141.

Keys, A., Aravanis, C., Blackburn, H., Van Buchem, F.S., Buzina, Djordjevic, B.S., Fidanza, F., Karvonen, M.J., Menotti, A., Puddu, V., and Taylor, H.L. 1972, Coronary heart disease: overweight and obesity as risk factors, *Ann. Inter. Med.*, 77(1), 15–27.

Kirschner, M.A., Schneider, G., Ertel, N.H., and Gorman, J. 1988, An eight-year experience with a very-low-calorie formula diet for control of major obesity, *Int. J. Obes.*, 12(1), 69–80.

Knowler, W.C., Barrett-Connor, E., Fowler, S.E., Hamman, R.F., Lachin, J.M., Walker, E.A., Nathan, D.M. 2002, Reduction in the incidence of type 2 diabetes with lifestyle intervention metformin, *N. Engl. J. Med.*, 346(6), 393–403.

Krauss, R.M. 1998a, Triglycerides and atherogenic lipoproteins: rationale for lipid management, *Am. J. Med.*, 105, 58S–62S.

Krauss, R.M. 1998b, Atherogenicity of triglyceride-rich lipoproteins, *Am. J. Cardiol.*, 81(4A), 13B–17B.

Kreisberg, R.A., Boshell, B.R., DiPlacido, J., and Roddam, R.F. 1967, Insulin secretion in obesity, *N. Engl. J. Med.*, 276(6), 314–319.

Laimer, M., Ebenbichler, C.F., Kaser, S., Sandhofer, A., Weiss, H., Nehoda, H., Aigner, F., and Patsch, J.R. 2002, Markers of chronic inflammation and obesity: a prospective study on the reversibility of this association in middle-aged women undergoing weight loss by surgical intervention, *Int. J. Obes. Relat. Metab. Disord.*, 26(5), 659–662.

Lamarche, B., Tchernof, A., Mauriege, P., Cantin, B., Dagenais, G.R., Lupien, P.J., and Després, J.P. 1998, Fasting insulin and apolipoprotein B levels and low-density lipoprotein particle size as risk factors for ischemic heart disease, *JAMA*, 279(24), 1955–1961.

Lamarche, B., Tchernof, A., Moorjani, S., Cantin, B., Dagenais, G.R., Lupien, P.J., and Després, J.P. 1997, Small, dense low-density lipoprotein particles as a predictor of the risk of ischemic heart disease in men. Prospective results from the Quebec Cardiovascular Study, *Circulation*, 95(1), 69–75.

Landin, K., Stigendal, L., Eriksson, E., Krotkiewski, M., Risberg, B., Tengborn, L., and Smith, U. 1990, Abdominal obesity is associated with an impaired fibrinolytic activity and elevated plasminogen activator inhibitor-1, *Metab.: Clin. Exp.*, 39(10), 1044–1048.

Lapidus, L., Bengtsson, C., Larsson, B., Pennert, K., Rybo, E., and Sjöström, L. 1984, Distribution of adipose tissue and risk of cardiovascular disease and death: a 12 year follow up of participants in the population study of women in Gothenburg, Sweden, *Br. Med. J.*, 289, 1257–1261.

Larsson, B., Svärdsudd, K., Welin, L., Wilhelmsen, L., Björntorp, P., and Tibblin, G. 1984, Abdominal adipose tissue distribution, obesity, and risk of cardiovascular disease and death: 13 year follow up of participants in the study of men born in 1913, *Br. Med. J.*, 288, 1401–1404.

Lean, M., Powrie, J., Anderson, A., and Garthwaite, P. 1990, Obesity, weight loss and prognosis in type 2 diabetes, *Diabetic Med.*, 7, 228–233.

Lee, A.J., Smith, W.C., Lowe, G.D., and Tunstall–Pedoe, H. 1990, Plasma fibrinogen and coronary risk factors: the Scottish Heart Health Study, *J. Clin. Epidemiol.*, 43(9), 913–919.

Lemieux, I., Pascot, A., Prud'homme, D., Almeras, N., Bogaty, P., Nadeau, A., Bergeron, J., and Després, J.P. 2001, Elevated C-reactive protein: another component of the atherothrombotic profile of abdominal obesity, *Arterioscler. Thromb. Vasc. Biol.*, 21(6), 961–967.

Liu, G.C., Coulston, A.M., Lardinois, C.K., Hollenbeck, C.B., Moore, J.G., and Reaven, G.M. 1985, Moderate weight loss and sulfonylurea treatment of non-insulin-dependent diabetes mellitus. Combined effects, *Arch. Intern. Med.*, 145(4), 665–669.

Lundgren, H., Bengtsson, C., Blohme, G., Lapidus, L., and Sjöström, L. 1989, Adiposity and adipose tissue distribution in relation to incidence of diabetes in women: results from a prospective population study in Gothenburg, Sweden, *Int. J. Obes.*, 13(4), 413–423.

MacDonald, K.G., Jr., Long, S.D., Swanson, M.S., Brown, B.M., Morris, P., Dohm, G.L., and Pories, W.J. 1997, The gastric bypass operation reduces the progression and mortality of non-insulin-dependent diabetes mellitus, *J. Gastrointest. Surg.*, 1(3), 213–220.

MacMahon, S.W., Wilcken, D.E., and Macdonald, G.J. 1986, The effect of weight reduction on left ventricular mass. A randomized controlled trial in young, overweight hypertensive patients, *N. Engl. J. Med.*, 314(6), 334–339.

Maggio, C. and Pi–Sunyer, F.X. 1997, The prevention and treatment of obesity, *Diabetes Care*, 20(11), 1744–1766.

Mancini, M., Di Biase, G., Contaldo, F., Fischetti, A., Grasso, L., and Mattioli, P.L. 1981, Medical complication of severe obesity: importance of treatment by very-low-calorie diets: intermediate and long-term effects, *Int. J. Obesity*, 5, 341–352.

Manson, J.E., Colditz, G.A., Stampfer, M.J., Willett, W.C., Rosner, B., Monson, R.R., Speizer, F.E., and Hennekens, C.H. 1990, A prospective study of obesity and risk of coronary heart disease in women, *N. Engl. J. Med.*, 322(13), 882–889.

Matts, J.P., Buchwald, H., Fitch, L.L., Campos, C.T., Varco, R.L., Campbell, G.S., Pearce, M.B., Yellin, A.E., Smink, R.D., Jr., Sawin, H.S., Jr. 1995, Subgroup analyses of the major clinical endpoints in the program on the surgical control of the hyperlipidemias (POSCH): overall mortality, atherosclerotic coronary heart disease (ACHD) mortality, and ACHD mortality or myocardial infarction, *J. Clin. Epidemiol.*, 48(3), 389–405.

Meade, T.W., Ruddock, V., Stirling, Y., Chakrabarti, R., and Miller, G.J. 1993, Fibrinolytic activity, clotting factors, and long-term incidence of ischaemic heart disease in the Northwick Park Heart Study, *Lancet*, 342(8879), 1076–1079.

Medalie, J.H., Papier, C., Herman, J.B., Goldbourt, U., Tamir, S., Neufeld, H.N., and Riss, E. 1974, Diabetes mellitus among 10,000 adult men. I. Five-year incidence and associated variables, *Isr. J. Med. Sci.*, 10(7), 681–697.

Menashe, V.D., Farrehi, C., and Miller, M. 1965, Hypoventilation and cor pulmonale due to chronic upper airway obstruction, *J. Pediatr.*, 67, 198–203.

Mertens, I., Van der Planken, M., Corthouts, B., Wauters, M., Peiffer, F., DeLeeuw, I., and Van Gaal, L. 2001, Visceral fat is a determinant of PAI-1 activity in diabetic and non-diabetic overweight and obese women, *Horm. Metab. Res.*, 33(10), 602–607.

Messerli, F.H. 1982, Cardiovascular effects of obesity and hypertension, *Lancet*, 1(8282), 1165–1168.

Mingrone, G., Rosa, G., Di Rocco, P., Manco, M., Capristo, E., Castagneto, M., Vettor, R., Gasbarrini, G., and Greco, A.V. 2002, Skeletal muscle triglycerides lowering is associated with net improvement of insulin sensitivity, TNF-alpha reduction and GLUT4 expression enhancement, *Int. J. Obes. Relat. Metab. Disord.*, 26(9), 1165–1172.

Moberly, J.B., Cole, T.G., Alpers, D.H., and Schonfeld, G. 1990, Oleic acid stimulation of apolipoprotein B secretion from HepG2 and Caco-2 cells occurs post-transcriptionally, *Biochim. Biophys. Acta*, 1042(1), 70–80.

Mokdad, A.H., Bowman, B.A., Ford, E.S., Vinicor, F., Marks, J.S., and Koplan, J.P. 2001, The continuing epidemics of obesity and diabetes in the United States, *JAMA*, 286(10), 1195–1200.

Must, A., Spadano, J., Coakley, E.H., Field, A.E., Colditz, G., and Dietz, W.H. 1999, The disease burden associated with overweight and obesity, *JAMA*, 282(16), 1523–1529.

National Heart Lung and Blood Institute 1998, Clinical guidelines on the identification, evaluation, and treatment of overweight and obesity in adults — the evidence report, *Obesity Res.*, 6 (suppl 2), 51S–210S.

Nie, L., Wang, J., Clark, L.T., Tang, A., Vega, G.L., Grundy, S.M., and Cohen, J.C. 1998, Body mass index and hepatic lipase gene (LIPC) polymorphism jointly influence postheparin plasma hepatic lipase activity, *J. Lipid Res.*, 39(5), 1127–1130.

Ohlson, L.O., Larsson, B., Svardsudd, K., Welin, L., Eriksson, H., Wilhelmsen, L., Björntorp, P., and Tibblin, G. 1985, The influence of body fat distribution on the incidence of diabetes mellitus. 13.5 years of follow-up of the participants in the study of men born in 1913, *Diabetes*, 34(10), 1055–1058.

Olefsky, J.M. 1981, Insulin resistance and insulin action: an *in vivo* and *in vitro* perspective, *Diabetes*, 38, 148–162.

Ooi, T.C. and Ooi, D.S. 1998, The atherogenic significance of an elevated plasma triglyceride level, *Crit. Rev. Clin. Lab. Sci.*, 35(6), 489–516.

Packard, C.J. 1999, Understanding coronary heart disease as a consequence of defective regulation of apolipoprotein B metabolism, *Curr. Opin. Lipidol.*, 10(3), 237–244.

Pan, X.R., Li, G.W., Hu, Y.H., Wang, J.X., Yang, W.Y., An, Z.X., Hu, Z.X., Lin, J., Xiao, J.Z., Cao, H.B., Liu, P.A., Jiang, X.G., Jiang, Y.Y., Wang, J.P., Zheng, H., Zhang, H., Bennett, P.H., and Howard, B.V. 1997, Effects of diet and exercise in preventing NIDDM in people with impaired glucose tolerance. The Da Qing IGT and Diabetes Study, *Diabetes Care*, 20, 537–544.

Phillips, N.R., Waters, D., and Havel, R.J. 1993, Plasma lipoproteins and progression of coronary artery disease evaluated by angiography and clinical events, *Circulation*, 88(6), 2762–2770.

Pi–Sunyer, F.X. 1993a, Medical hazards of obesity, *Ann. Intern. Med.*, 119, 655–660.

Pi–Sunyer, F.X. 1993b, Short-term medical benefits and adverse effects of weight loss, *Ann. Intern. Med.*, 119, 722–726.

Pi–Sunyer, F.X. 1996, A review of long-term studies evaluating the efficacy of weight loss in ameliorating disorders associated with obesity, *Clin. Therap.*, 18(6), 1006–1035.

Polonsky, K.S., Given, B.D., Hirsch, L.J., Tillil, H., Shapiro, E.T., Beebe, C., Frank, B.H., Galloway, J.A., and Van Cauter, E. 1988, Abnormal patterns of insulin secretion in non-insulin-dependent diabetes mellitus, *N. Engl. J. Med.*, 318(19), 1231–1239.

Resnick, H.E. and Howard, B.V. 2002, Diabetes and cardiovascular disease, *Annu. Rev. Med.*, 53:245–67, 245–267.

Rexrode, K.M., Carey, V.J., Hennekens, C.H., Walters, E.E., Colditz, G.A., Stampfer, M.J., Willett, W.C., and Manson, J.E. 1998, Abdominal adiposity and coronary heart disease in women, *JAMA*, 280(21), 1843–1848.

Roden, M., Price, T.B., Perseghin, G., Petersen, K.F., Rothman, D.L., Cline, G.W., and Shulman, G.I. 1996, Mechanism of free fatty acid-induced insulin resistance in humans, *J. Clin. Invest.*, 97(12), 2859–2865.

Rossner, S. and Bjorvell, H. 1987, Early and late effects of weight loss on lipoprotein metabolism in severe obesity, *Atherosclerosis*, 64(2–3), 125–130.

Sampol, G., Munoz, X., Sagales, M.T., Marti, S., Roca, A., Dolors, D.l.C., Lloberes, P., and Morell, F. 1998, Long-term efficacy of dietary weight loss in sleep apnoea/hypopnoea syndrome, *Eur. Respir. J.*, 12(5), 1156–1159.

Schieffer, B., Moore, D., Funke, E., Hogan, S., Alphin, F., Hamilton, M., and Heyden, S. 1991, Reduction of atherogenic risk factors by short-term weight reduction. Evidence of the efficacy of National Cholesterol Education Program guidelines for the obese, *Klin Wochenschr*, 69, 163–167.

Segal, K.R., Edano, A., Abalos, A., Albu, B., Tomas, M., and Pi-Sunyer, F. 1991, Effect of exercise training on insulin sensitivity and glucose metabolism in lean, obese, and diabetic men, *J. Appl. Physiol.*, 71, 2402–2411.

Shinohara, E., Kihara, S., Yamashita, S., Yamane, M., Nishida, M., Arai, T., Kotani, K., Nakamura, T., Takemura, K., and Matsuzawa, Y. 1997, Visceral fat accumulation as an important risk factor for obstructive sleep apnoea syndrome in obese subjects, *J. Intern. Med.*, 241(1), 11–18.

Shulman, G.I. 2000, Cellular mechanisms of insulin resistance, *J. Clin. Invest.*, 106(2), 171–176.

Singh, R.B., Rastogi, S.S., Verma, R., Laxmi, B., Singh, R., Ghosh, S., and Niaz, M.A. 1992, Randomized controlled trial of cardioprotective diet in patients with recent acute myocardial infarction: results of one year follow up, *Br. Med. J.*, 304(6833), 1015–1019.

Sjöström, L., Rissanen, A., Andersen, T., Boldrin, M., Golay, A., Koppeschaar, H., and Krempf, M. 2000, Randomized placebo-controlled trial of orlistat for weight loss and prevention of weight regain in obese patients, *Ter. Arkh.*, 72(8), 50–54.

Sjöström, C.D., Lissner, L., Wedel, H., and Sjöström, L. 1999, Reduction in incidence of diabetes, hypertension and lipid disturbances after intentional weight loss induced by bariatric surgery: the SOS Intervention Study, *Obesity Res.*, 7, 477–484.

Smith, P.L., Gold, A.R., Meyers, D.A., Haponik, E.F., and Bleecker, E.R. 1985, Weight loss in mildly to moderately obese patients with obstructive sleep apnea, *Ann. Intern. Med.*, 103(6) Pt 1, 850–855.

Sparks, J.D., Collins, H.L., Sabio, I., Sowden, M.P., Smith, H.C., Cianci, J., and Sparks, C.E. 1997, Effects of fatty acids on apolipoprotein B secretion by McArdle RH-7777 rat hepatoma cells, *Biochim. Biophys. Acta*, 1347(1), 51–61.

Sparrow, D., Borkan, G.A., Gerzof, S.G., Wisniewski, C., and Silbert, C.K. 1986, Relationship of fat distribution to glucose tolerance. Results of computed tomography in male participants of the normative aging study, *Diabetes*, 35(4), 411–415.

Stamler, R., Stamler, J., Riedlinger, W.F., Algera, G., and Roberts, R.H. 1978, Weight and blood pressure. Findings in hypertension screening of 1 million Americans, *JAMA*, 240, 1607–1610.

Steiner, G. 1998, Intermediate-density lipoproteins, diabetes and coronary artery disease, *Diabetes Res. Clin. Pract.*, 40, S29–S33.

Sugerman, H.J., Fairman, R.P., Sood, R.K., Engle, K., Wolfe, L., and Kellum, J.M. 1992, Long-term effects of gastric surgery for treating respiratory insufficiency of obesity, *Am. J. Clin. Nutr.*, 55(2), 597S–601S.

Suratt, P.M., McTier, R.F., Findley, L.J., Pohl, S.L., and Wilhoit, S.C. 1987, Changes in breathing and the pharynx after weight loss in obstructive sleep apnea, *Chest*, 92(4), 631–637.

Suratt, P.M., McTier, R.F., Findley, L.J., Pohl, S.L., and Wilhoit, S.C. 1992, Effect of very-low-calorie diets with weight loss on obstructive sleep apnea, *Am. J. Clin. Nutr.*, 56(1 Suppl), 182S–184S.

Svendsen, O.L., Hassager, C., Christiansen, C., Nielsen, J.D., and Winther, K. 1996, Plasminogen activator inhibitor-1, tissue-type plasminogen activator, and fibrinogen: effect of dieting with or without exercise in overweight postmenopausal women, *Arterioscler. Thromb. Vasc. Biol.*, 16(3), 381–385.

Tchernof, A., Nolan, A., Sites, C.K., Ades, P.A., and Poehlman, E.T. 2002, Weight loss reduces C-reactive protein levels in obese postmenopausal women, *Circulation*, 105(5), 564–569.

Tuomilehto, J., Lindstrom, J., Eriksson, J.G., Valle, T.T., Hamalainen, H., Ilanne–Parikka, P., Keinanen–Kiukaanniemi, S., Laakso, M., Louheranta, A., Rastas, M., Salminen, V., Uusitupa, M., and Finnish Diabetes Prevention Study Group 2001, Prevention of type 2 diabetes mellitus by changes in lifestyle among subjects with impaired glucose tolerance, *N. Engl. J. Med.*, 344, 1343–1350.

Unger, R.H. and Zhou, Y.T. 2001, Lipotoxicity of beta-cells in obesity and in other causes of fatty acid spillover, *Diabetes*, 50 (Suppl 1) S118–S121.

Vague, P., Juhan–Vague, I., Aillaud, M.F., Badier, C., Viard, R., Alessi, M.C., and Collen, D. 1986, Correlation between blood fibrinolytic activity, plasminogen activator inhibitor level, plasma insulin level, and relative body weight in normal and obese subjects, *Metab.: Clin. Exp.*, 35(3), 250–253.

Vega, G.L. and Grundy, S.M. 1996, Hypoalphalipoproteinemia (low high density lipoprotein) as a risk factor for coronary heart disease, *Curr. Opin. Lipidol.*, 7(4), 209–216.

Verges, B.L. 1999, Dyslipidaemia in diabetes mellitus. Review of the main lipoprotein abnormalities and their consequences on the development of atherogenesis, *Diabetes Metab.*, 25 (Suppl 3), 32–40.

Vgontzas, A.N., Legro, R.S., Bixler, E.O., Grayev, A., Kales, A., and Chrousos, G.P. 2001, Polycystic ovary syndrome is associated with obstructive sleep apnea and daytime sleepiness: role of insulin resistance, *J. Clin. Endocrinol. Metab.*, 86(2), 517–520.

Vgontzas, A.N., Papanicolaou, D.A., Bixler, E.O., Hopper, K., Lotsikas, A., Lin, H.M., Kales, A., and Chrousos, G.P. 2000, Sleep apnea and daytime sleepiness and fatigue: relation to visceral obesity, insulin resistance, and hypercytokinemia, *J. Clin. Endocrinol. Metab.*, 85(3), 1151–1158.

Vgontzas, A.N., Tan, T.L., Bixler, E.O., Martin, L.F., Shubert, D., and Kales, A. 1994, Sleep apnea and sleep disruption in obese patients, *Arch. Intern. Med.*, 154(15), 1705–1711.

Walton, C., Lees, B., Crook, D., Worthington, M., Godsland, I.F., and Stevenson, J.C. 1995, Body fat distribution, rather than overall adiposity, influences serum lipids and lipoproteins in healthy men independently of age, *Am. J. Med.*, 99(5), 459–464.

Wannamethee, G. and Shaper, A.G. 1990, Weight change in middle-aged British men: implications for health, *Eur. J. Clin. Nutr.*, 44(2), 133–142.

Weintraub, M., Sundaresan, P., and Schuster, B. 1992, Long-term weight control study VII (weeks 0–210), *Clin. Pharmacol. Ther.*, 51, 634–641.

Westlund, K. and Nicolaysen, R. 1972, Ten-year mortality and morbidity related to serum cholesterol. A follow-up of 3751 men aged 40–49, *Scand. J. Clin. Lab. Invest.*, 30(Suppl 127), 1–24.

White, A.L., Graham, D.L., LeGros, J., Pease, R.J., and Scott, J. 1992, Oleate-mediated stimulation of apolipoprotein B secretion from rat hepatoma cells. A function of the ability of apolipoprotein B to direct lipoprotein assembly and escape presecretory degradation, *J. Biol. Chem.*, 267(22), 15657–15664.

Will, J.C., Williamson, D.F., Ford, E.S., Calle, E.E., and Thun, M.J. 2002, Intentional weight loss and 13-year diabetes incidence in overweight adults, *Am. J. Public Health*, 92(8), 1245–1248.

Williamson, D.F., Pamuk, E., Thun, M., Flanders, D., Byers, T., and Heath, C. 1995, Prospective study of intentional weight loss and mortality in never-smoking overweight US white women aged 40–64 years, *Am. J. Epidemiol.*, 141(12), 1128–1141.

Williamson, D.F., Pamuk, E., Thun, M., Flanders, D., Byers, T., and Heath, C. 1999, Prospective study of intentional weight loss and mortality in overweight white men aged 40–64 years, *Am. J. Epidemiol.*, 149(6), 491–503.

Wilson, P.W., D'Agostino, R.B., Sullivan, L., Parise, H., and Kannel, W.B. 2002, Overweight and obesity as determinants of cardiovascular risk: the Framingham experience, *Arch. Intern. Med.*, 162(16), 1867–1872.

Wing, R.R., Marcus, M.D., Salata, R., Epstein, L.H., Miaskiewicz, S., and Blair, E.H. 1991, Effects of a very-low-calorie diet on long-term glycemic control in obese type 2 diabetic subjects, *Arch. Intern. Med.*, 151(7), 1334–1340.

Wood, P.D., Stefanick, M.L., Dreon, D.M., Frey–Hewitt, B., Garay, S.C., Williams, P.T., Superko, H.R., Fortmann, S.P., Albers, J.J., and Vranizan, K.M., 1988, Changes in plasma lipids and lipoproteins in overweight men during weight loss through dieting as compared with exercise, *N. Engl. J. Med.*, 319(18), 1173–1179.

World Health Organization 1997, Obesity: preventing and managing the global epidemic. Report of a WHO consultation on obesity; Geneva, 3–5 June 1997.

Wu, X., Sakata, N., Dixon, J., and Ginsberg, H.N. 1994, Exogenous VLDL stimulates apolipoprotein B secretion from HepG2 cells by both pre- and post-translational mechanisms, *J. Lipid Res.*, 35(7), 1200–1210.

Yki–Jarvinen, H. 2002, Ectopic fat accumulation: an important cause of insulin resistance in humans, *J. R. Soc. Med.*, 95 (Suppl 42), 39–45.

Young, T., Palta, M., Dempsey, J., Skatrud, J., Weber, S., and Badr, S. 1993, The occurrence of sleep-disordered breathing among middle-aged adults, *N. Engl. J. Med.*, 328(17), 1230–1235.

Zhi, J., Melia, A.T., Guerciolini, R., Chung, J., Kinberg, J., Hauptman, J.B., and Patel, I.H. 1994, Retrospective population-based analysis of the dose-response (fecal fat excretion) relationship of orlistat in normal and obese volunteers, *Clin. Pharmacol. Ther.*, 56(1), 82–85.

Ziccardi, P., Nappo, F., Giugliano, G., Esposito, K., Marfella, R., Cioffi, M., D'Andrea, F., Molinari, A.M., and Giugliano, D. 2002, Reduction of inflammatory cytokine concentrations and improvement of endothelial functions in obese women after weight loss over one year, *Circulation*, 105(7), 804–809.

Zimmerman, J., Kaufmann, N.A., Fainaru, M., Eisenberg, S., Oschry, Y., Friedlander, Y., and Stein, Y. 1984, Effect of weight loss in moderate obesity on plasma lipoprotein and apolipoprotein levels and on high density lipoprotein composition, *Arteriosclerosis*, 4(2), 115–123.

Part IV

Drugs on the Market

11

Orlistat

Hans Hauner

CONTENTS

SUMMARY   Orlistat is a hydrogenated derivative of a bacterial lipase inhibitor that also blocks gastric and pancreatic lipases in humans. At a dose of 120 mg three times daily,

0-415-30321-4/04/$0.00+$1.50
© 2004 by CRC Press LLC

orlistat was found to reduce the hydrolysis and absorption of orally ingested dietary triglycerides by approximately 30%. Several clinical trials over up to 2 years demonstrated that orlistat in combination with a hypocaloric diet produces a weight loss of 6 to 10% after 1 year compared to 4 to 6% under placebo treatment in obese subjects with and without type 2 diabetes. When the drug is administered for weight maintenance, weight regain is significantly smaller under orlistat than under placebo treatment. However, the response to orlistat varies considerably, and it is the responsibility of the treating team to decide whether the effect is clinically significant. Due to its mechanism of action, the main adverse effects of orlistat are oily spotting, fecal urgency, and increased defecation, but due to mitigation of these side effects over time, the drug is generally well tolerated by most patients. Long-term studies are lacking, so it is unknown whether orlistat is able to reduce cardiovascular morbidity and mortality.

11.1 Introduction

There is general agreement among experts and growing recognition among physicians that obesity is a severe chronic disease that carries along the burden of multiple long-term complications such as type 2 diabetes mellitus, hypertension, and osteoarthritis. The recent acceleration in the epidemic of obesity is particularly alarming, because it has occurred despite growing public awareness and strengthened efforts to promote a healthy life-style and prevent weight gain of the general population in many countries (WHO 2000).

In view of this threatening development, pharmacological options that support the conventional strategies for decreasing excess body weight by reducing energy intake, increasing energy expenditure, or both are undoubtedly desirable (National Task Force 1996). Most drugs developed so far for the treatment of obesity have a central mechanism of action by directly addressing the hypothalamic center of appetite and satiety regulation (Bray and Greenway 1999). However, the clinical application of such centrally acting drugs may include unpredictable risks. In the past, clinical use of some of these drugs was associated with severe adverse effects, which led ultimately to withdrawal from the market. In light of this catastrophic history, the issue of adjunct use of drugs for long-term management of obesity remains an open and much debated question.

To date, only one drug is available that aims at reducing food intake by a peripheral mechanism of action. Orlistat, available under the trade name Xenical®, is a modified bacterial product that inhibits gastrointestinal lipases and thereby reduces fat absorption. High fat intake is considered a major cause of obesity because this nutrient has the highest energy density and is abundantly consumed in many populations (Bray and Popkin 1998). Orlistat is currently the only drug with a peripheral mechanism of action that has been approved for the adjunct treatment of obesity in many countries.

11.2 Pharmacology

Orlistat, or tetrahydrolipstatin (N-formyl-L-leucine(S)-1-[[(2S,3S)-3-hexyl-4-oxooxetan-2-yl]methyl]dodecylester), is the hydrogenated derivative of lipstatin, a naturally occurring lipase inhibitor produced by the bacterium *Streptomyces toxytricini*. The chemical structure

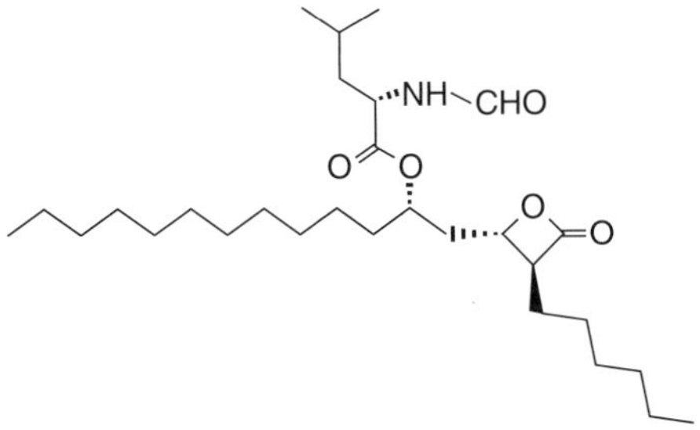

FIGURE 11.1
Chemical structure of orlistat. (From Guerciolini, R., *Int. J. Obes. Relat. Metab. Disord.* 21 (Suppl.), S12–S23, 1997.)

contains an aliphatic hydrocarbon backbone bearing a β-lactone ring and an *N*-formyl-L-leucyl ester side chain (Figure 11.1). The molecular formula is $C_{29}H_{53}NO_5$, and the molecular weight is 495.74.

The compound is highly lipophilic, and its solubility in water at 23°C is extremely low: <1 mg/100 ml (Guerciolini 1997). Orlistat is a selective and potent inhibitor of gastric and pancreatic lipases (Hadvary et al. 1988, 1991; Guerciolini 1997). To understand the action of orlistat it is necessary to introduce briefly the physiology of fat digestion and absorption with particular reference to the role of gastrointestinal lipases. Lipases constitute a subgroup of a large category of enzymes that catalyze hydrolytic reactions (hydrolases) and are formally referred to as triacylglycerol ester hydrolases. They differ from classical esterases in that their substrates are insoluble in water, and their activity is dependent on enzyme adsorption to an oil–water interface (Guerciolini 1997). Classical lipases display activity only when their substrates are aggregated in an emulsified or micellar state.

Lipases play a central role in the digestion of long-chain triacylglycerides, which account for more than 95% of dietary lipids that are consumed in amounts between 50 and 150 g daily, depending on the type of diet. In habitual Western diets, the lipid content is usually high, ranging from 80 to 150 g. Triacylglycerides are considered to represent the nutrient component that contributes mostly to high energy intake and subsequent passive over-consumption of calories (Bray and Popkin 1998). Apart from triacylglycerides, other dietary lipids in the Western diet consist of phospholipids (2 to 4 g are consumed daily) and cholesterol (normal intake of 200 to 600 mg daily), but are not important for the energy balance.

In humans, four lipases are known to take part in the digestion of dietary lipids: gastric lipase; pancreatic lipase; carboxylester lipase; and phospholipase A_2. The digestion of lipids starts in the stomach under the control of gastric lipase. This enzyme is remarkably stable and active under acid conditions; by its action, 10 to 20% of dietary lipids are hydrolyzed in the stomach. However, the major part of fat digestion occurs in the duodenum, in which the dominant lipolytic enzyme is pancreatic lipase. The enzyme is secreted in great excess relative to the amount needed for complete hydrolysis of triacylglycerides in the upper small intestine. Although under normal physiological conditions carboxylester lipase and phospholipase A_2 play only a minor role in triacylglyceride hydrolysis, these enzymes are able largely to compensate for pancreatic lipase if this enzyme is absent or deficient.

Pancreatic lipase is a 449-amino acid enzyme that shares a folded structure with other lipases. In the folded structure, the enzyme is inactive. In this state, the N-terminal domain contains the catalytic site that includes serine, histidine, and aspartate residues. Evidence for the importance of these amino acids for catalytic activity comes from site-directed mutagenesis studies (Lowe 1992). Binding of the enzyme to triacylglycerides is facilitated by colipase in the presence of bile salts. This interaction serves to expose the active site by opening the lid.

It is important to note that the intestinal digestion and absorption of triglycerides is a highly complex process that is not yet fully understood. The sequential steps include emulsification; hydrolysis of fatty acid ester bonds by lipases; aqueous dispersion of lipolytic products; and, finally, their absorption in the upper small intestine. The hydrolysis of the various lipid components involves different enzymes and results in different products. Before absorption becomes possible, each triacylglyceride molecule must be hydrolyzed into two fatty acid molecules and one monoacylglycerol molecule.

After a lipid meal, an oil emulsion phase develops in the duodenum in dynamic equilibrium with lipids in the aqueous phase. In the aqueous phase, mixed micelles containing the products of lipolysis coexist with liposomes. Fatty acids, monoacylglycerides, cholesterol, and other lipids are taken up by the brush border of the upper intestinal tract — mainly from mixed micelles but also from liposomes. As absorption progresses, the mixed micelles become depleted but are continuously replenished by products of the ongoing lipolysis. This process depends on the presence of colipase, which binds the enzyme and induces the conformational change required for its anchoring to the substrate interface and subsequent activation (Guerciolini 1997).

11.3   Action of Orlistat

In view of the physiology of the digestion of dietary lipids, inhibition of this process represents a logical target for pharmacological intervention. Orlistat is a compound that exerts a potent inhibitory activity against all lipases in the human gastrointestinal tract. Lipases recognize the inhibitor as a normal substrate and catalyze the opening of the β-lactone ring. The lipases are progressively inactivated through the formation of a long-lived covalent acyl-type intermediate, probably with a 1:1 stoichiometry. This inhibition is based on an almost irreversible reaction between the β-lactone secondary ester, which is the reactive part of orlistat, and the serine residue 152 at the catalytic site of the enzyme that is exposed at the oil–water interface (Hadvary et al. 1988, 1991). During interaction with the normal substrate, the covalent acyl-type intermediate is rapidly cleaved, and the enzymatic reaction can continue with new substrate molecules. In the case of orlistat, the covalent lipase-inhibitor complex is relatively stable and only slowly degraded.

In contrast to its inhibition of lipases, orlistat does not inhibit other intestinal hydrolases such as trypsin; chymotrypsin; pancreatic α-amylase; pancreatic phospholipase A_2; phosphoinositol-specific phospholipase C; acetylcholinesterase; or nonspecific liver carboxyesterase, even at concentrations that are 100-fold higher than those suppressing lipase activity (Guerciolini 1997). This finding may lead to the assumption that no major interference exists between orlistat and hydrolysis and absorption of carbohydrates, proteins, and phospholipids (Meyer et al. 1986).

The inhibition of intestinal lipases by orlistat leads to a fecal loss of dietary fat. Thus, the amount of excreted fecal fat is considered representative of the extent of gastrointestinal lipase inhibition and can be used as a noninvasive method to quantify the pharmacological effect of orlistat. Such studies have demonstrated that applying orlistat to humans results in partial inhibition of triacylglyceride hydrolysis and reduction of the subsequent absorption of fatty acids and monoacylglycerides (Zhi et al. 1994). In a small randomized, crossover study involving six healthy volunteers, administration of 120 mg orlistat with a liquid

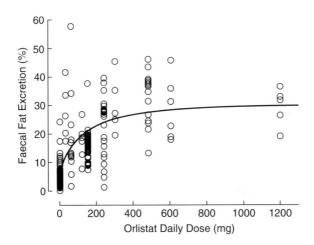

FIGURE 11.2
Dose–response relationship for the effect of orlistat on fecal fat excretion (percent of fat intake) in healthy volunteers. (From Zhi, J. et al., *Clin. Pharmacol. Ther.* 56, 82–85, 1994.)

fat meal significantly reduced postprandial pancreatic lipase activity in the small intestine by approximately 75% (Borovicka et al. 2000). During short-term treatment with orlistat, the fecal fat loss rises rapidly during the active treatment period. Fat excretion reaches maximum levels within 2 days from the start of orlistat administration (Guerciolini 1997). This effect is maintained throughout the active treatment period, whereas discontinuation of the drug is followed by a rapid normalization of fat absorption (Hussain et al. 1994; Guerciolini 1997).

When orlistat is taken in conjunction with a mildly hypocaloric diet with 30% of the total energy coming from dietary fat (the usual recommendation), a variable part of the ingested fat is excreted (Figure 11.2). It can be calculated that an additional caloric deficit of about 200 to 300 kcal per day will result from administration of 120 mg orlistat three times daily, depending on the amount of dietary fat intake. Fecal fat excretion is already seen at a dose of 60 mg three times daily. At increasing doses, fecal fat loss increases rapidly and reaches a plateau at a daily dose between 400 and 600 mg. At this dose, approximately 32% of dietary fat is lost in the stools under conditions in which patients ingested between 50 and 80 g of fat per day. Larger doses will not result in substantial increases of the pharmacological effect (Zhi et al. 1994) (Figure 11.2). This dose–response relationship as assessed by fecal fat excretion can be described by a simple E_{max} model (Guerciolini 1997).

It is noteworthy that the response to orlistat as assessed by determination of fecal fat excretion in healthy volunteers (Figure 11.2) varies considerably. This observation is important because the clinical trials have also demonstrated a high variability in weight loss in response to orlistat treatment. As addressed later in detail, careful monitoring of the effect of orlistat is essential to avoid ineffective treatment of obese patients.

11.3.1 Systemic Absorption of Orlistat

After oral application, nearly all of the administered drug is excreted in the feces, mostly as intact orlistat. Because orlistat is a potent inhibitor of a large number of mammalian lipases, the clinically relevant question may arise as to whether the drug reaches the systemic circulation and whether it has systemic effects. Uptake of the compound into the blood could imply that, in addition to its effect on lipid absorption, orlistat also interferes with other pathways of lipid metabolism. In particular, the question is whether absorbed orlistat or its metabolites inhibit lipoprotein or hepatic lipases or other lipases located in the endothelium or adipose tissue. However, recent studies indicate that the low systemic absorption has no significant effect on circulating lipase activity. In a randomized, placebo-controlled study involving 24 healthy men who received 120 mg orlistat three times daily, no inhibition of plasma lipases was detectable (Shephard et al. 2000).

Investigations of the systemic absorption of orlistat revealed a rather low uptake. In an early pharmacokinetic study in eight healthy lean volunteers, orlistat was not measurable in the circulation (Zhi et al. 1995). In overweight or obese volunteers between 23 and 68 years of age receiving a dose of 360 mg ^{14}C-labeled orlistat, serial blood samples were collected over 10 h after administration of orlistat for determination of total radioactivity in plasma. In addition, urine samples were collected over 24 h. Maximum observed concentration (Cmax) and time to Cmax values of plasma total radioactivity were 150 ± 51 ng.eq/ml and 6.8 ± 1.5 h, respectively. Urinary and fecal recovery of the administered dose of total radioactivity was 1.13 ± 0.50% and 96.4 ± 18.1%, respectively. These parameters obtained in overweight/obese subjects were similar to those reported previously in lean, healthy subjects (Zhi et al. 1996).

Subsequent pharmacokinetic screening of obese patients from five double-blind, placebo-controlled, long-term studies suggested that systemic exposure to orlistat is not required for its efficacy. This systematic analysis also demonstrated that administration of orlistat at doses ranging from 90 to 720 mg daily results only in a sporadic detection of intact orlistat. The measurable plasma concentrations in the orlistat recipients were low (<10 ng/ml or 0.02 μmol/l) without evidence of accumulation, consistent with only minimal absorption (Zhi et al. 1999). Other multiple-dose studies demonstrated an extent of systemic absorption similar to that of single-dose studies with the exception of one investigation in which a concentration of <40 ng/ml was measured at a maximum dose of 400 mg orlistat three times daily.

Thus, single- and multiple-dose studies indicated an extremely low degree of systemic absorption of orlistat as well as a lack of accumulation (Guerciolini 1997). Data from additional studies in rats and dogs suggested a moderate volume of distribution and hepatic extraction and a high degree of gastrointestinal wall metabolism and biliary excretion of absorbed orlistat. Thus, the most likely explanation for the low plasma concentrations is a limited absorption of orlistat (Guerciolini 1997); the elimination half-life of orlistat was reported to be about 1 to 2 h (Roche 1999). It is, however, important to note that these studies were performed in healthy subjects. Nothing is known about the absorption and circulating levels of orlistat in patients with gastrointestinal diseases, or renal or hepatic impairment. The same is true for elderly and pediatric patients.

After absorption, orlistat is degraded into two major metabolites. The metabolite M1 is formed by hydrolysis of the β-lactone ring of orlistat, whereas M3 is the result of cleavage of the *N*-formyl leucine side chain on M1. It has been demonstrated that M1 and M3 have only a very weak lipase inhibitory activity and are therefore considered to be pharmacologically inactive (Zhi et al. 1996, 1999). In addition, three other metabolites of orlistat were found in the urine: M9, M13, and M13 glucuronic acid conjugate (Zhi et al. 1996).

11.3.2 Interaction with Other Drugs

Different types of drug–drug interaction studies have been performed with orlistat. Most studies were conducted in an open-label, placebo-controlled, randomized, two-way crossover study in healthy volunteers. Serial blood samples were collected before and at appropriate intervals after each dose of the interacting drug. These studies in healthy volunteers have demonstrated that orlistat does not alter the pharmacokinetic properties of single oral doses of digoxin and phenytoin (Melia et al. 1995) and warfarin (Zhi et al. 1995) with regard to maximum concentration and areas under the curve. These drugs have a narrow therapeutic window and alteration of their pharmacokinetic properties is of critical importance.

Another series of pharmacokinetic studies in healthy volunteers has been performed to investigate the interaction between orlistat and frequent concomitant medications. Such studies have indicated that the absorption of glyburide is not significantly altered by treatment with orlistat with regard to various metabolic parameters. In addition, there was no apparent difference in the postprandial glucose profile (Zhi et al. 1995). In a study of four antihypertensive drugs, orlistat did not affect the pharmacokinetic properties of furosemide; captopril; nifedipine; or atenolol (Weber et al. 1996). In a study on the interaction between orlistat and pravastatin, orlistat had no significant effect on all characteristics of pravastatin uptake and clearance, including maximum concentration, time to maximum concentration, and area under the curve (Guerciolini 1997). In a recent pharmacokinetic evaluation, orlistat did not affect the pharmacokinetics of atorvastatin; amitriptyline; losartan; metformin; phentermine; and sibutramine (Zhi et al. 2002). Another study showed that orlistat did not influence the systemic availability of combination oral contraceptives (Güzelhan et al. 1994). Finally, orlistat administration was found to have no significant influence on alcohol pharmacokinetics. Concomitant ingestion of social amounts of ethanol did not alter the inhibitory effect of orlistat on dietary fat absorption during short-term (6 days) treatment with 120 mg orlistat three times daily (Melia et al. 1998).

Recent case reports indicated that administration of orlistat together with cyclosporine A is associated with reduced plasma concentrations of the immunosuppressant drug. In two renal transplant patients, treatment with orlistat resulted in a considerable reduction of circulating cyclosporine A levels by 40 to 50%. After stopping orlistat treatment, the cyclosporine A levels rose in both patients without modification of the dose (Errasti et al. 2002). In a heart transplant patient, coadministration of orlistat and cyclosporine was reported to be associated with a similar decrease in the circulating level of cyclosporine (Le Beller et al. 2000).

In another study, evidence was provided that orlistat-induced reduction of cyclosporine levels was responsible for the development of acute organ rejection (Schnetzler et al. 2000). In a pharmacokinetic study, a reduction of serum concentrations of cyclosporine by 70 to 80% was demonstrated when orlistat was simultaneously administered with the immunosuppressant (Nägeli et al. 2001). Another pharmacokinetic evaluation confirmed this observation but indicated a smaller reduction of the absorption of cyclosporine by approximately one third (Zhi et al. 2002). The explanation for this phenomenon may be that orlistat interferes with cyclosporine A absorption in the small intestine leading to increased excretion via fatty stools. The logical conclusion is that orlistat should not be used in renal transplant patients or other patients taking cyclosporine A to avoid under-immunosuppression.

11.3.3 Effect on Other Organ Functions

Other studies dealt with the effect of orlistat on selected physiological parameters, mainly in conjunction with digestion. It turned out that orlistat does not cause significant disturbances of gastric emptying and acidity; gallbladder motility; bile lithogenicity; pancreatic secretion; and gastrointestinal transit time (Guerciolini 1997).

11.3.4 Absorption of Fat-Soluble Vitamins and Electrolytes

Due to its mechanism of action, there was some concern that the use of orlistat could be associated with a reduced absorption of fat-soluble vitamins. Now the bulk of data from numerous clinical studies indicates that administration of orlistat results in a modestly reduced uptake of the vitamins D, E, and β-carotene (Zhi et al. 1996; Melia et al. 1995, 1996). For example, in healthy volunteers, the absorption of tocopherol (vitamin E) and β-carotene was compromised by the administration of orlistat 120 mg three times daily, but the absorption of vitamin A was not altered (Zhi et al. 1996; Melia et al. 1996).

Similar observations were made in prospective clinical trials including large groups of overweight and obese patients. Between 2 and 10% of the patients treated with orlistat had two consecutive low levels of β-carotene and vitamins D and E, although circulating levels of vitamin A were usually not reduced (Sjöström et al. 1998; Davidson et al. 1999; Hauptman et al. 2000). However, when vitamin E levels were corrected for LDL cholesterol, the vitamin levels remained unchanged in the orlistat-treated patients (Sjöström et al. 1998; Davidson et al. 1999). In one of these studies, vitamin supplementation was required in 14% of the subjects treated with orlistat for 2 years vs. 6.5% of the placebo recipients (Davidson et al. 1999). In the other two studies, the percentage of patients receiving vitamin supplementation was slightly lower (Sjöström et al. 1998; Hauptman et al. 2000).

The clinical significance of reduced absorption of fat-soluble vitamins is currently unclear. These vitamins exert a variety of specific functions, e.g., by increasing the antioxidative capacity in the case of vitamin E or by supporting calcium homeostasis in the case of vitamin D. Therefore, an incalculable risk is that a reduced supply with fat-soluble vitamins under orlistat treatment could have long-term adverse health consequences. Obesity is considered to be a state of increased oxidative stress that may even require an increased supply of antioxidative vitamins. Although a significant decrease in circulating levels of fat-soluble vitamins was only seen in a small percentage of patients taking orlistat, it is, unfortunately, not possible to identify patients at risk of decreased vitamin concentrations in advance.

This dilemma makes it rather difficult to solve this problem properly. One possibility would be to supplement fat-soluble vitamins to all patients who receive orlistat. However, this would mean that the majority of patients are overtreated. Another possibility would be to measure fat-soluble vitamins in plasma before and at least once during treatment, e.g., after 4 weeks to identify those who would require supplementation of fat-soluble vitamins. However, this alternative is expensive and depends on specific laboratory facilities. A compromise could be to advocate dietary recommendations that lead to a preferential high intake of fat-soluble vitamins. However, it is currently unknown whether this strategy is effective.

In a recent 21-day randomized controlled trial of obese men, the effect of 120 mg orlistat three times daily on mineral balance was examined. Subjects consumed a hypocaloric diet with a constant daily mineral content. At the end of the study, differences in mineral absorption, urinary mineral loss, or mineral balance (calcium, phosphorus, magnesium, iron, copper, zinc) were not significant between both groups. In addition, markers of bone turnover and serum and urine electrolytes did not differ (Pace et al. 2001).

11.4 Clinical Trials

11.4.1 Dose-Ranging Studies

In a 12-week randomized, placebo-controlled, double-blind study in five European out-patient clinics, 188 obese subjects were randomized to treatment with orlistat 10, 60, 120 mg, or placebo three times daily in combination with a mildly hypocaloric diet. Researchers observed a mean additional weight loss of 0.6 ± 0.5 kg with orlistat 30 mg per day; 0.7 ± 0.6 kg with orlistat 180 mg per day; and 1.8 ± 0.5 kg with orlistat 360 mg per day compared to placebo. Mild gastrointestinal side effects were more frequently seen in the orlistat groups, but caused premature withdrawal from the study in only four patients (Drent et al. 1995).

In another multicenter, dose-ranging study, 676 obese males and females were randomized to receive orlistat 30, 60, 120, 240 mg or matching placebo three times a day for 24 weeks. The resulting weight loss was 6.5% in the placebo group; 8.5% in the orlistat 30-mg group; and 8.8, 9.8, and 9.3%, respectively, in the 60-, 120-, and 240-mg groups. A central conclusion from this large study was that orlistat 120 mg three times daily represents the optimal dosage regimen (van Gaal et al. 1998).

11.4.2 Randomized Controlled Trials of Orlistat for Weight Loss and Maintenance in Obese Patients

11.4.2.1 Trials with Duration up to 1 Year

The first clinical trial on orlistat was a 12-week randomized, double-blind, parallel group comparison between 50 mg orlistat three times daily and placebo in addition to an energy-reduced diet in 52 healthy obese subjects. Total weight loss in the orlistat group was 4.3 ± 3.4 kg vs. 2.1 ± 2.8 kg in the placebo group ($p < .05$), thereby proving the principle of weight loss by inhibition of gastrointestinal lipases (Drent and van der Veen 1993).

In a small randomized, double-blind, placebo-controlled single-center study, 46 obese patients with a BMI between 30 and 43 kg/m^2 were allocated to treatment with orlistat 120 mg three times daily or placebo in combination with a mildly hypocaloric diet with an energy deficit of approximately 600 kcal/day. Body weight was reduced by 5.5 ± 4.5 kg in the placebo group and 8.6 ± 5.4 kg in the orlistat-treated group by 6 months. Thereafter, the placebo group tended to relapse, whereas the orlistat group maintained their weight loss (2.6 vs. 8.4% reduction from baseline at 52 weeks) (James et al. 1997).

In another randomized, placebo-controlled multicenter study, 228 patients with a BMI between 30 and 43 kg/m^2 received orlistat 120 mg three times daily or placebo for 52 weeks after a 4-week placebo run-in period. All patients were placed on an individually calculated diet containing approximately 30% of calories as fat and causing an energy deficit of approximately 600 kcal/day. After the first 24 weeks, the prescribed daily energy intake was further reduced by 300 kcal per day. The difference between the two groups for mean percentage weight loss was statistically significant (8.5 vs. 5.4% in the orlistat and the placebo group, respectively, $p < .016$) (Finer et al. 2000).

11.4.2.2 2-Year Trials

Most clinical studies on the effect of orlistat were performed over a period of 2 years. The five clinical trials published so far were characterized by a 1-year weight loss program followed by a 1-year weight maintenance period (Sjöström et al. 1998; Davidson et al. 1999; Hauptman et al. 2000 Rössner et al. 2000; Karhunen et al. 2000).

In a large European multicenter trial, 688 patients with a BMI between 28 and 47 kg/m^2 were assigned double-blind treatment with orlistat 120 mg three times a day or placebo for 1 year in conjunction with a moderately hypocaloric diet. In the second 52-week double-blind period, patients were reassigned orlistat or placebo with a weight-maintaining diet. In the first year of treatment, the orlistat group lost significantly more body weight than the placebo group (10.2 vs. 6.1%, $p < .001$). During the second year, patients who

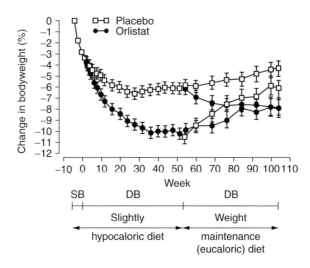

FIGURE 11.3
Change in body weight during a 2-year randomized placebo-controlled trial on the effect of orlistat vs. placebo. After year 1, patients were reassigned orlistat or placebo with a eucaloric diet. SB = single blind; DB = double blind. (From Sjöström, L. et al., *Lancet* 352, 167–172, 1998.)

continued with orlistat regained half as much weight as those patients switched to placebo (difference in weight loss orlistat vs. placebo 2.4 kg, $p < 0.001$). Patients who switched from placebo to orlistat lost body weight in the second year while patients who continued on placebo gained weight. At the end of year 2, the difference in weight loss between the two groups was 3.6 kg ($p < .001$; Figure 11.3) (Sjöström et al. 1998).

A similar 2-year randomized, placebo-controlled, clinical study was conducted in the U.S. A 1-year treatment with orlistat 120 mg three times a day or a placebo was randomly assigned to 892 subjects with a BMI ranging from 30 to 43 kg/m². In the second year, participants followed a weight-maintaining diet and received orlistat 60 mg three times a day, 120 mg three times daily, or placebo. During the first year, orlistat-treated patients lost significantly more weight than placebo-treated subjects (8.8 ± 0.4 kg vs. 5.8 ± 0.7 kg, $p < 0.001$). Subjects treated with orlistat 120 mg three times daily in the second year regained less weight (3.2 ± 0.5 kg) than those who received orlistat 60 mg three times daily (4.3 ± 0.6 kg) or those who received placebo (5.6 ± 0.4 kg) (Davidson et al. 1999).

Another 2-year clinical trial was carried out to evaluate the long-term efficacy and tolerability of orlistat within primary care settings. In this randomized, placebo-controlled study, 796 obese patients with a BMI between 30 and 44 kg/m² were cared for in 17 primary care centers. Patients received orlistat 60 mg, orlistat 120 mg, or placebo, each three times daily, in conjunction with an energy-reduced diet for the first year and a weight-mainte-nance diet during the second year. Patients treated with orlistat lost significantly more weight (7.1 ± 0.5 kg and 7.9 ± 0.6 kg for the 60- and 120-mg orlistat group, respectively) than those treated with placebo (4.1 ± 0.6 kg, each $p < .001$) in year 1 and sustained more of this weight loss during year 2. This study further indicated that orlistat is an effective adjunct to dietary intervention in the treatment of obesity (Hauptman et al., 2000).

In the fourth randomized, placebo-controlled study performed in Europe, 729 obese subjects with a BMI between 28 and 43 kg/m² were allocated to placebo or orlistat 60 or 120 mg three times daily, combined with a hypocaloric diet during the first year and a weight maintenance diet in the second year of treatment to prevent weight regain. Orlistat-treated patients lost significantly more weight than placebo-treated patients after year 1 (6.6, 8.6, and 9.7% for the placebo group, orlistat 60 mg, and the orlistat 120 mg groups, respectively). During the second year, orlistat therapy produced significantly less weight regain than placebo (p = .005 for orlistat 60 mg; p < .001 for orlistat 120 mg) (Rössner et al. 2000).

In a randomized, controlled study from Finland, 96 obese men and women were treated with orlistat 120 mg three times daily or placebo three times daily in conjunction with a mildly hypoenergetic balanced diet for 1 year. This was followed by a 1-year double-blind period with reassignment of the participating subjects to receive orlistat or placebo in conjunction with a weight maintenance diet. During the first year, the orlistat-treated group had a greater reduction of body weight (13.1 vs. 8.6 kg at 12 months, p < .001) and fat mass but not of fat-free mass or resting energy expenditure (REE) compared to placebo. During the second year, orlistat treatment was associated with a smaller regain of body weight and fat mass with no significant differences in the changes of fat-free mass or REE compared to placebo (Karhunen et al. 2000).

11.4.2.3   Orlistat for Weight Maintenance

To further evaluate the potential of orlistat for long-term maintenance of weight loss, a study was designed to test the hypothesis that orlistat is more effective than placebo in preventing weight regain. Originally, 1313 subjects with a BMI between 28 and 43 kg/m² were recruited. During a 6-month lead-in phase, a hypoenergetic diet (4180 kJ/day deficit) was prescribed. Those participants who lost >8% of their initial body weight on this conventional diet (n = 729) were randomly assigned to receive placebo or 30, 60, or 120 mg orlistat three times daily for 1 year in combination with a maintenance diet to prevent weight regain. After 1 year, subjects treated with 120 mg orlistat three times daily regained significantly less weight than the placebo-treated subjects ($32.8 \pm 4.5\%$ compared with $58.7 \pm 5.8\%$ regain of lost weight, p < .001). This effect could be attributed to the partial inhibition of fat absorption. Fecal fat content in the orlistat 120 mg group was 20.6 g per day compared to 0.5 g per day in the placebo group (Hill et al.1999).

11.5   Effect of Orlistat on Cardiovascular Risk Factors

In all of the preceding studies, changes in cardiovascular risk factors such as blood lipids, serum glucose, and blood pressure were regularly documented. As expected, the additional weight loss induced by administration of orlistat was associated with a greater improvement in cardiovascular risk factors (Sjöström et al. 1998; Davidson et al. 1999; Hill et al. 1999; Hauptman et al. 2000; Rössner et al. 2000; Finer et al. 2000). Apart from these trials, further studies were conducted that followed particular changes in cardiovascular risk factors in patients treated with orlistat. These studies differed from the former ones because obese subjects with defined risk factors or comorbid conditions were selected and assigned to treatment with orlistat or placebo. Some of these studies will be described in more detail.

In the Swedish Multimorbidity Study, 376 obese Swedish adults with concomitant type 2 diabetes, hypercholesterolemia, and/or hypertension were recruited to receive 120 mg orlistat three times daily or placebo, in addition to a mildly hypocaloric diet. After 1 year, a moderately greater weight loss took place with orlistat compared with placebo (5.9 vs. 4.6%, p < .05). Orlistat treatment was also associated with significantly greater improvements than placebo administration in total serum cholesterol (−3.3% vs. −0.5%, p < .05); LDL cholesterol (−7.0 vs. −1.1%, p < .05); fasting glucose (−5.1 vs. −0.1%, p < .01); and

HbA1c (–2.7 vs. –0.5%, $p < .05$), whereas systolic and diastolic blood pressure were reduced to a similar degree in both treatment groups (Lindgärde 2000).

In a study from China, obese patients with or without type 2 diabetes were given 120 mg orlistat three times daily without a concomitant hypocaloric diet for 6 months. Despite less weight reduction in the diabetic subjects, there was a significantly greater reduction in HbA1c levels; fasting plasma glucose; and systolic blood pressure compared to nondiabetic subjects. Obese subjects without diabetes had greater improvements in triglyceride levels; albuminuria; and insulin sensitivity as assessed by the homeostasis model (Tong et al. 2002).

A retrospective analysis included five double-blind, randomized, placebo-controlled trials that examined the effect of orlistat on cardiovascular risk. A total of 3132 obese patients (BMI 28 to 43 kg/m²) were evaluated. Patients followed a mildly hypocaloric diet and were randomized to double-blind treatment with orlistat 120 mg three times a day or placebo for 1 year. Orlistat produced greater weight loss than placebo (9.2 vs. 5.8%, $p < .001$) and orlistat-treated patients had significantly greater improvements than placebo-treated patients in several lipid parameters, including total cholesterol; LDL cholesterol; triglycerides; and apolipoprotein B. In addition, orlistat had a beneficial effect on oral glucose tolerance, waist circumference, and systolic and diastolic pressure (Zavoral 1998).

An abdominal pattern of body fat distribution usually assessed by waist circumference or waist/hip ratio is a good marker for cardiovascular risk (Despres et al. 2001). In some of the clinical studies, these indices were used to follow changes in the pattern of fat distribution under treatment with orlistat. The results show no or only small reductions of abdominal fat by adjunct treatment with orlistat (Hollander et al. 1998; Davidson et al. 1999). In addition, visceral fat area was studied by computer tomography scanning at the level of L4. In this particular study, the greater weight loss by orlistat treatment was associated with a significantly greater reduction in the visceral fat area (Keating and Jarvis 2001).

11.6 Orlistat in Diabetes

11.6.1 Weight Loss Using Orlistat in Obese Subjects with Type 2 Diabetes

Type 2 diabetes mellitus is one of the most frequent comorbidities and certainly the most expensive adverse consequence of obesity (Wolf and Colditz 1998). Therefore, measures to prevent diabetes or improve glucose homeostasis are central to reduce morbidity and mortality in obese subjects. Evidence of the potential of orlistat concerning this challenge is growing. Numerous randomized, placebo-controlled studies have been performed on the effect of orlistat in overweight and obese patients with impaired glucose tolerance or type 2 diabetes (see reviews in Keating and Jarvis, 2001, and Scheen and Ernest, 2002).

The results of these studies show that orlistat effectively supports weight loss in this patient group and significantly improves glycemic control compared to placebo treatment. The mean weight loss in these studies was 2.6 to 6.2 kg under orlistat vs. 1.3 to 4.3 kg in the placebo groups. In addition, in randomized controlled studies of a duration of up to 52 weeks, obese patients with type 2 diabetes receiving orlistat experienced significantly greater reductions from baseline in glycated hemoglobin levels compared to placebo treatment. The change in HbA1c in the orlistat-treated patients was –0.28 to –0.93% vs. +0.27 to –0.64% in the placebo-treated patients (Keating and Jarvis 2001). The three fully published large multicenter studies in obese patients with type 2 diabetes under different types of hypoglycemic agents and treated with orlistat or placebo are presented in more detail next (Hollander et al. 1998; Kelley et al. 2002; Miles et al. 2002).

In the first study, conducted by Hollander et al. (1998), 391 obese men and women with type 2 diabetes (BMI range from 28 to 40 kg/m²) received orlistat 120 mg or placebo three times a day in addition to a mildly hypocaloric diet. Another inclusion criterion was that the patients were under stable metabolic control on oral sulfonylureas. After 1 year of treatment, weight loss compared to baseline was 6.2% in the orlistat-treated patients and 4.3% in the placebo-treated patients ($p < .001$). In the orlistat-treated group, 43% decreased the amount of oral sulfonylureas and 12% discontinued antidiabetic medication. In the placebo-treated patients, the respective figures were 29 and 2.5%. Despite this difference, decrease in HbA1c levels was greater in the orlistat-treated patients compared to the controls (−0.28 vs. +0.18%, $p < .001$). Interestingly, orlistat therapy resulted in greater improvements than placebo in total cholesterol, LDL cholesterol, triglycerides, and LDL-to-HDL cholesterol ratio (Hollander et al. 1998).

In a similar randomized, placebo-controlled design, 503 overweight and obese patients with type 2 diabetes treated with metformin were assigned to orlistat 120 mg or placebo three times daily combined with a mildly hypocaloric diet. After 1 year of treatment, weight loss was greater in the orlistat than in the placebo group (4.6 vs. 1.7%, $p < .001$). Orlistat treatment caused a greater improvement in glycemic control than placebo, as demonstrated by change in HbA1c (−0.90 vs. −0.61%, $p = .014$) and a greater reduction in fasting serum glucose (−2.0 vs. −0.7 mM, $p = .001$).

Due to the well-known gastrointestinal side effects of metformin and orlistat, some concern was that this combination could lead to a greater frequency and severity of adverse effects as well as to a higher rate of premature study withdrawal. However, the overall rate of study withdrawal was in fact higher in the placebo than in the orlistat group (43 vs. 35%, $p < .05$). The overall difference in the incidence of gastrointestinal side effects between the orlistat and placebo groups in this study was similar to that previously observed between orlistat and placebo treatment in type 2 diabetic patients receiving sulfonylurea monotherapy (Hollander et al. 1998). Therefore, the decision to use orlistat in management of overweight and obese subjects with type 2 diabetes should not be based on the type of diabetes medication (Miles et al. 2002).

In another 1-year multicenter, randomized, placebo-controlled trial, orlistat 120 mg three times a day or placebo combined with a reduced-calorie diet was given to overweight or obese patients with type 2 diabetes treated with insulin alone or a combination of insulin with oral antidiabetic agents. At the end of the study, the orlistat group had lost significantly more weight than the placebo group (−3.9 vs. −1.3 kg, $p < .001$). Orlistat treatment also produced greater decreases in HbA1c (−0.62 vs. −0.27%, $p = 0.002$) (Figure 11.4); fasting serum glucose (−1.63 vs. −1.08 mM, $p = .02$) and the doses of insulin and other diabetic medications. In addition, orlistat produced greater improvements than placebo in total and LDL cholesterol (Kelley et al. 2002). Thus, randomized controlled trials offer good evidence that orlistat demonstrates beneficial effects in the management of patients with orally or insulin-treated type 2 diabetes.

11.6.2 Orlistat and Prevention of Type 2 Diabetes

Another important question in the context of glucose metabolism is whether orlistat has a potential to reduce the risk of developing impaired glucose tolerance and type 2 diabetes in obese subjects. To answer this question, data from 675 obese adults (BMI 30 to 43 kg/m²) at U.S. and European research centers in three randomized, placebo-controlled, clinical trials were pooled. A standard 3-h oral glucose tolerance test was performed on day 1

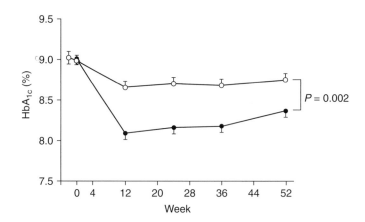

FIGURE 11.4
Effect of orlistat 120 mg three times daily (●) compared to placebo treatment (○) on HbA1c in obese adults with type 2 diabetes treated with insulin over 52 weeks. (From Kelley, D.E. et al., *Diabetes Care* 25, 1033–1041, 2002.)

and at the end of treatment. After a mean follow-up of 582 days, subjects treated with orlistat had lost more weight than subjects who had received placebo (6.7 kg vs. 3.8 kg, $p < .001$). A smaller percentage of subjects with impaired glucose tolerance at baseline progressed to type 2 diabetes in the orlistat vs. the placebo groups (3.0 vs. 7.6%, $p < .05$). In addition, among subjects with impaired glucose tolerance at baseline, glucose levels normalized in more subjects after orlistat treatment than after placebo treatment (71.6 vs. 49.1%, $p = .04$). At the end of treatment, fewer patients with normal glucose tolerance at baseline developed impaired glucose tolerance or type 2 diabetes under orlistat treatment than under placebo (6.6 vs. 12.0%, $p = .04$).

Thus, the addition of orlistat to a conventional weight loss regimen in the first year of treatment and a eucaloric weight-maintaining diet in the second year significantly improves glucose tolerance and diminishes the rate of progression to overt type 2 diabetes (Heymsfield et al. 2000). Although this study has some limitations, e.g., retrospective data analysis, it is important to note that an improvement in glucose tolerance depends on relatively small changes in body weight. Despite the small difference in weight loss between the orlistat and the placebo groups, the diabetes risk was substantially reduced.

In a recent study from Sweden, 3304 obese patients with a BMI ≥ 30 kg/m² were enrolled in a prospective study to investigate the potential of orlistat to prevent the development of impaired glucose tolerance and progression from impaired glucose tolerance to overt type 2 diabetes. Weight loss over a period of 4 years was significantly greater in the orlistat group compared to the placebo group (6.9 vs. 4.1 kg, $p < .001$). This difference in weight reduction resulted in a significant difference in the cumulative incidence of type 2 diabetes (6.2 vs. 9.0%, $p = .003$) corresponding to a relative risk reduction of 37.3%. In the subgroup of patients with impaired glucose tolerance, the conversion to type 2 diabetes was reduced from 28.8% in the placebo group to 18.8% in the orlistat group. In addition, greater reductions in cardiovascular risk factors were observed in the orlistat group compared to the placebo group (according to Scheen and Ernest, 2002).

These results are in agreement with recent data from two large prospective studies from Finland and the U.S. in which intensive life-style intervention programs were found to reduce the risk for the development of diabetes markedly in overweight and obese subjects with impaired glucose tolerance (Tuomilehto et al. 2001; Knowler et al. 2002). In these studies, the prevention of diabetes was dependent on the extent of weight reduction. Thus, antiobesity pharmacotherapy may offer an additional effective option for the prevention of diabetes in obese subjects at increased risk.

11.6.3 Effect of Orlistat on Insulin Resistance

Another interesting finding in these and other studies was that treatment with orlistat was associated with a greater decrease in fasting serum insulin levels and the insulin area under the curve than placebo treatment. Because fasting insulin levels are considered to be an indirect correlate of insulin sensitivity, decreasing plasma concentrations may indicate a reduction of insulin resistance (Heymsfield et al. 2000). Some additional studies are in favor of a beneficial effect of orlistat on insulin resistance in obese patients independent of weight loss. In a small euglycemic hyperinsulinemic glucose clamp study published in abstract form (Bachmann et al. 2000), a 3-month treatment of six obese men with orlistat 120 mg three times daily resulted in a significant improvement of insulin sensitivity compared to baseline. After discontinuation of orlistat administration, insulin resistance returned to baseline levels within 3 months.

In another study of 150 obese women, a 6-month treatment with orlistat 120 mg three times daily diminished insulin resistance by 33% compared to placebo treatment, as assessed by homeostasis model assessment (HOMA) (Gokcel et al. 2001). Additional studies reported similar improvements in insulin sensitivity dependent on or independent of the extent of weight loss produced by orlistat (Keating and Jarvis 2001). It is currently difficult to understand how orlistat is exerting this favorable effect on insulin resistance. One possibility is that this is simply a consequence of weight loss because any measure to reduce body weight may improve insulin sensitivity. Another possibility is that the reduced uptake of dietary fat may be responsible for this improvement because a high-fat diet can directly deteriorate insulin sensitivity and increase the risk of developing diabetes (Hu et al. 2001). In addition, lipids may also be detrimental to β-cells, a phenomenon called lipotoxicity (Unger 1995).

11.7 Orlistat and Lipid Disorders

The effect of dietary fat on blood lipids is well documented (Grundy and Denke 1990). Restriction and favorable modification of dietary fat intake is associated with lowering of serum cholesterol and triglyceride concentrations and may even induce regression of atherosclerosis (Ornish et al. 1990). Therefore, it would not be surprising that a drug that limits the intestinal absorption of dietary fat could have a beneficial effect on serum lipids and may support normalization of at least mild lipid disorders. Many data are now available that demonstrate the potential of orlistat to influence lipid metabolism in lean and obese humans.

In an early study, the effect of orlistat on serum lipids and lipoproteins was studied in patients with primary hyperlipidemia defined by baseline serum cholesterol ≥ 6.2 mmol/l and triglycerides ≤ 5.0 mmol/l, not responsive to dietary changes alone. In this randomized, placebo-controlled study, 103 men and 70 women received 30, 90, 180, or 360 mg orlistat or placebo three times daily for 8 weeks. Total and LDL cholesterol levels were reduced respectively by 4 and 5% with 30 mg orlistat; 7 and 8% with 90 mg orlistat; 7 and 7% with 180 mg orlistat; and 11 and 10% with 360 mg orlistat compared to placebo. HDL cholesterol levels significantly decreased by 11% in the 360-mg orlistat group. Triglyceride levels significantly increased in the placebo group but not in the drug group. Minor decreases were also found for apolipoprotein A1 and B concentrations. These changes were due not only to a reduced fat absorption but also to a decrease of body weight by 1.2 kg in the 360-mg orlistat group, despite a weight maintenance diet (Tonstad et al. 1994).

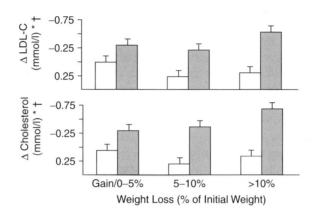

FIGURE 11.5

Effect of orlistat, 120 mg three times daily (hatched bars), vs. placebo treatment (open bars) on total (lower panel) and LDL cholesterol (upper panel) in obese subjects with type 2 diabetes after a 1-year treatment period, according to the extent of weight loss. (From Hollander, P. et al., *Diabetes Care* 21, 1288–1294, 1998.)

Consistent beneficial changes in lipid variables were found in various clinical studies on the effect of orlistat on body weight in obese subjects. For example, in the European multicenter trial, serum total and LDL cholesterol decreased by 0.4 and 0.35 mmol/l, respectively, in the orlistat group at the end of year 1 and remained stable during year 2. No significant change was seen for HDL cholesterol, while minor but significant improvements were seen for the LDL/HDL ratio (Sjöström et al. 1998). Similar changes in the lipid variables were also reported in many other studies, including those performed in patients with type 2 diabetes (Hollander et al. 1998; Davidson et al. 1999; Hauptman et al. 2000; Rössner et al. 2000; Kelley et al. 2002).

Because weight loss is a strong determinant of changes in serum lipids, it is important to examine whether the improvement in serum lipids is simply due to the greater weight loss produced by orlistat or due to the specific pharmacological action of the drug. In the study of Hollander et al. (1998) in overweight patients with type 2 diabetes, the patients of both treatment groups (120 mg orlistat vs. placebo three times daily) were categorized according to whether they lost >10% of their initial weight; 5 to 10% of their initial weight; <5% of their initial weight; or even gained weight. This analysis revealed that orlistat treatment reduced total and LDL cholesterol to a significantly greater extent than placebo within all three categories of weight loss (Figure 11.5) (Hollander et al. 1998).

In a recent randomized, placebo-controlled study from Belgium, 294 patients with a BMI between 27 and 40 kg/m^2 and hypercholesterolemia (LDL cholesterol between 4.1 and 6.7 mM) were submitted to a hypocaloric diet and randomly assigned to orlistat 120 mg or placebo three times daily. After the 24-week period, weight loss was greater in the orlistat-treated patients compared to the placebo recipients (6.8 vs. 3.8%, $p < 0.001$). Treatment with orlistat was also associated with significantly greater changes in total cholesterol (–11.9 vs. –4.0%, $p < 0.001$) and LDL cholesterol (–17.6 vs. –7.6%, $p < 0.001$). For any category of weight loss, the change in LDL cholesterol was more pronounced in orlistat-treated patients than in placebo recipients, indicating that orlistat has a direct cholesterol-lowering effect independent of weight reduction (Muls et al. 2001). It is tempting to speculate that this independent lipid-lowering effect of orlistat is related to reduced absorption of dietary fat.

Because orlistat reduces dietary fat absorption, it was postulated that orlistat treatment may also cause beneficial changes in postprandial lipid metabolism. This topic was recently addressed in a study of overweight patients with type 2 diabetes who received a standard mixed meal containing 70 g of fat. Orlistat treatment was followed by significantly lower triglyceride concentrations after 2 h, as well as significantly lower concentrations of plasma remnant-like particle cholesterol and free fatty acids after 2 and 4 h, respectively. The incremental areas under the curves were more reduced after orlistat than placebo, indicating that this drug induces favorable changes in lipid variables during the early postprandial period (Tan et al. 2002).

11.8 Orlistat and Changes in Eating Pattern

A topic of high practical relevance is whether orlistat changes eating habits and diet composition in obese patients. In a subgroup analysis of a multicenter trial, Franson and Rössner (2000) analyzed changes in these variables over a 2-year treatment period. Irrespective of the general underestimation of energy intake, total fat intake (g) and fat energy percentage were not different between the orlistat and the placebo groups, indicating that the lipase inhibitor does not change the amount and sources of fat intake (Franson and Rössner 2000). However, clinical experience with orlistat suggests that an increased fat intake may be followed by more severe adverse effects, thereby causing better compliance to the recommendations of a low-fat diet in many patients. In the long run, this educatory effect of orlistat may lead to a stricter control of fat consumption and thus greater weight loss. On the other hand, in women with a low fat intake, the effect of orlistat on energy intake may be smaller and associated with only a modest loss or no weight loss at all.

11.9 Adverse Effects

11.9.1 Frequent Adverse Effects

Due to its mechanism of action and absence of significant systemic absorption, the adverse effects of orlistat are largely restricted to the gastrointestinal tract. In the European multicenter trial, the overall frequency of adverse events in the orlistat group was only slightly higher than in the placebo group during year 1 (94 vs. 82%) and similar in the four treatment groups (two were on orlistat, two on placebo) during year 2. The frequencies of the most relevant adverse effects under orlistat compared to placebo treatment in year 1 were:

- Fatty/oily stools (31 vs. 5%)
- Increased defecation (20 vs. 7%)
- Oily spotting (18 vs. 1%)
- Soft stool (15 vs. 9%)
- Liquid stools (13 vs. 10%)
- Abdominal pain (7 vs. 9%)
- Fecal urgency (10 vs. 3%)
- Flatulence (7 vs. 3%)
- Flatus with discharge (7 vs. 0%)

- Fecal incontinence (7 vs. 0%)
- Oily evacuation (6 vs. 1%)

Most of the gastrointestinal side effects happened early during orlistat treatment and were of short duration. It is also noteworthy that patients treated with orlistat experienced fewer gastrointestinal adverse events during year 2 than year 1. The good tolerance of orlistat is also indicated by the drop-out rates. The total number of premature withdrawals was lower in the orlistat group than in the placebo group during year 1 (61 vs. 83 subjects) and virtually the same in both groups during year 2 (46 vs. 45). In this study, 12 subjects dropped out in the first year due to gastrointestinal adverse effects in the orlistat group compared to 2 in the placebo group. In the second year, the respective numbers of subjects dropping out due to gastrointestinal adverse events were 7 and 2, respectively (Sjöström et al. 1998). Similar rates of adverse events and similar or slightly higher rates of premature study withdrawal were reported in the other 1- and 2-year trials with orlistat (Davidson et al. 1999; Hauptman et al. 2000; Rössner et al. 2000).

11.9.2 Rare Adverse Effects and Adverse Effects under Debate

Few cases of hypersensitivity (rash, urticaria, angiooedema) have been reported with orlistat treatment (Ballinger and Peikin 2002). In a case report, an increase in blood pressure was found under administration of orlistat, which was reversible after discontinuation (Persson et al. 2000). The reason for this finding is presently unknown and there is no additional evidence for an increase in blood pressure by orlistat. With these exceptions, adverse effects of orlistat do not appear to be related to systemic exposure to the compound or its metabolites.

Treatment with orlistat was recently observed to be associated with a decreased postprandial release of cholecystokinin. Because cholecystokinin is an important mediator of gallbladder emptying, an increased risk of gallstone formation could be a possible consequence. At present, no evidence suggests enhanced induction of this complication by orlistat (Trouillot et al. 2001). However, a recent study suggested that reduced cholecystokinin levels are associated with an increase in hunger and a decrease in fullness, which could at least partially counteract the weight loss induced by lipase inhibition (Feinle et al. 2001).

In some early trials with orlistat, more breast malignancies were observed in women treated with orlistat than those treated with placebo. A total of 11 women on orlistat (120 mg three times daily); 1 woman on orlistat (60 mg three times daily); and 2 women on placebo were reported to have breast cancer (FDA 1998). For example, in a large 2-year U.S. trial, three breast malignancies were identified in women taking orlistat compared to one woman in the placebo group. These reports, together with all available data, were thoroughly reviewed by an independent expert committee. Eight of the 11 patients on orlistat 120 mg were classified as having had a pre-existing lesion based on histopathology; six patients had a mammogram prior to the start of the study and four of these confirmed the pre-existing nature of the tumor.

The complete analysis of these reviews provided no evidence that orlistat or its metabolites, directly or indirectly, initiate or promote the growth of breast tumors (FDA 1998). In addition, animal studies did not indicate any carcinogenic potential of orlistat. In a carcinogenicity study, rats and mice were treated with orlistat at doses up to 1000 mg/kg/day and 1500 mg/kg/day, respectively, which is equivalent to 100 to 200 times higher doses than those used in humans. The results showed no carcinogenic potential of orlistat. Other animal experiments using similarly high doses of orlistat did not demonstrate embryotoxicity or teratogenicity. Also interesting in this context is that a thorough review of toxicological data concluded that orlistat exerts no estrogen-stimulating effect in women (FDA 1998).

11.9.3 Misuse of Orlistat

Misuse of orlistat has also been reported in a few clinical situations. Patients with bulimia nervosa are usually characterized by frequent binging episodes, feelings of guilt, and compensatory purging behaviors to avoid weight gain; they are therefore eager for drugs that support weight loss or prevent weight gain. Some reports now indicate that such patients may also misuse orlistat for this purpose, usually without severe adverse effects (Fernandez–Aranda et al. 2001). Because up to 30% of women who attend weight loss programs have some form of eating disorder (mostly binge eating), it is necessary to pay attention to this possibility.

11.10 Current Indications for Treatment with Orlistat

Based on the results of many clinical trials, orlistat was approved for treatment of obese patients with an initial body mass index of $\geq 30 \ kg/m^2$ or patients with a BMI $\geq 28 \ kg/m^2$ in the presence of risk factors such as hypertension, type 2 diabetes, dyslipidemia, and obstructive sleep apnea. In addition to these criteria, the National Institute for Clinical Excellence (NICE) in the U.K. recently published guidelines that contain additional recommendations for the use of orlistat (NICE 2001). These recommendations include:

- Orlistat should only be prescribed for obese patients as defined previously who have lost at least 2.5 kg in weight by dietary control and increased physical activity alone in the month prior to treatment.
- When drug treatment is offered, arrangements should be made for appropriate health professionals to offer specific concomitant advice, support, and counseling on diet, physical activity, and behavioral strategies.
- Continuation of orlistat therapy beyond 3 months should be supported by evidence of a loss of at least a further 5% of body weight from the start of treatment.
- Continuation of treatment beyond 6 months should be supported by evidence of a cumulative weight loss of at least 10% of body weight from the start of drug treatment.
- Treatment should usually not be continued beyond 12 months and never beyond 24 months.

These extended guidelines are more restrictive than those for use of orlistat approved by the U.S. Food and Drug Administration, in which prior weight loss using a hypocaloric diet and exercise alone is not required. In addition, continuation of drug treatment beyond 3 and 6 months does not require the achievement of defined weight loss categories.

The predictive value of such guidelines has been recently examined in a retrospective analysis of pooled data from two randomized controlled trials. Considering the NICE recommendations, Rissanen et al. (2003) studied the prediction of weight loss after 2 years in patients completing 2-year orlistat trials after a weight loss ≥ 2.5 kg during a 4-week dietary lead-in period; a weight loss ≥ 5% after 3 months; and weight loss ≥ 10% after 6 months of combined dietary and orlistat treatment, respectively. It turned out that only weight loss ≥ 5% after 3 months of diet and orlistat was a good indicator of 2-year weight loss, whereas weight loss ≥ 2.5 kg during the 4-week run-in period and weight loss ≥ 10% after 6 months did not add significantly to the predictive value. Thus, the conclusion from this study was that among the criteria currently suggested for assessing the response to orlistat treatment, only weight loss ≥ 5% at 3 months predicts sustained improvement in weight and major risk factors at 2 years; the other suggested criteria proved less useful (Rissanen et al. 2003).

11.11   Recommendations for Orlistat Use in Clinical Practice

The recommended dose for orlistat in adults is 120 mg with each main meal; the drug is available as a 120-mg capsule. One capsule is taken immediately before, during, or even up to 1 h after a meal. The obese patient should keep a mildly hypocaloric well-balanced diet that contains not more than 30% of total calories from fat sources. When a meal with a higher fat content is consumed, the occurrence of gastrointestinal adverse effects may increase. On the other hand, in patients with a rather low fat consumption, the effect of orlistat may be diminished or even missing. Usually, the effect of orlistat is seen within 2 to 3 days of treatment; after discontinuation, fat excretion returns to baseline levels within the same period.

The simplest way to prevent decreased intake of fat-soluble vitamins is to recommend that the patient take a multivitamin supplement. The supplement should be taken once a day at least 2 h before or after administration of orlistat; another prudent piece of advice is to take the supplement at bedtime. The opinion also exists that a well-balanced diet containing adequate amounts of fat-soluble vitamins in its natural foods would also be sufficient to compensate for the loss of fat-soluble vitamins and cover the essential requirements.

11.12   Experience with Orlistat Use in Clinical Practice

The clinical trials required for drug approval by medical and government authorities do not reflect real-life conditions. Usually, study participants undergo a high selection bias and close monitoring, sometimes associated with specific incentives for compliance that may affect behavior. On the other hand, patients recruited in specialized obesity clinics are frequently characterized by failure of previous therapeutic approaches and may be more resistant to new options than treatment-naïve subjects would be. In the case of orlistat, this phenomenon could lead to an underestimation of the clinical effect of the drug. To be able to assess the actual benefit from treatment by a specific drug, additional clinical studies are required that better resemble the real-life situation than approval studies do.

To date, little information is available on the prescription pattern and clinical use of orlistat in primary care. However, in a recent study from Sweden, the prescription pattern, as well as the use of orlistat in general medicine, were studied by using an anonymous postal questionnaire survey of prescribers. Useful information was obtained for 789 patients. It was found that orlistat was prescribed for 4% of the patients despite a BMI of less than 28 kg/m². Only 24% of the patients had a diet period with a weight loss of 2.5 kg or greater before the start of treatment; only half with a weight loss of less than 5% after 3 months continued the therapy. Ten percent gained weight or had no weight loss at all, while 43% lost less than 5%. At least one quarter of the patients stopped treatment within the 3-month observation period. These findings brought the authors to the conclusion that orlistat was not prescribed according to the approved indication in the majority of cases. Thus, the gain from drug treatment was considered to be minor for most patients (Beermann et al. 2001).

In most countries, the use of orlistat is not reimbursed by health insurance funds, which has led to a situation in which most patients take orlistat only for a few weeks. For this reason, it would be necessary to perform additional research to determine how these circumstances may affect the clinical effectiveness of orlistat prescription and how obese subjects outside of obesity clinics respond to the drug. Another problem that needs to be addressed in the future is the longer-term effectiveness and safety of orlistat. The maximum duration of administration of orlistat in published clinical trials is 2 years, which is a rather short period in view of the chronic and deteriorating nature of obesity. Therefore, data on long-term intake of orlistat are urgently needed. Such studies should also consider the effect of orlistat on complications of obesity, including cardiovascular disease. Unfortunately, such outcome studies are unavailable now or in the near future.

11.13 Cost Effectiveness of Treatment with Orlistat

As adjunct treatment of obese subjects with orlistat produces additional costs, it is essential to assess the cost effectiveness of this treatment option. Any health economic evaluation is strongly influenced by the presence of comorbid conditions. In a recent analysis in obese type 2 diabetic patients, a Markow model was developed to predict over a 10-year period the complication rates and mortality with and without a 2-year orlistat treatment assuming a 5-year catch-up period after treatment. Four subgroups were studied based on the presence of risk factors. The cost effectiveness varied between 3462 euros per life-year gained (LYG) for obese diabetic patients with hypertension and hypercholesterolemia and 19,986 euros per LYG for obese diabetic patients without other risk factors. These results suggest that orlistat is cost effective in the management of obese type 2 diabetic patients, particularly in those with hypertension and hypercholesterolemia (Lamotte et al. 2002). However, different results may be obtained in obese subjects without comorbid conditions or with another weight course, e.g., more rapid weight regain. Thus, additional studies are required to better define the conditions under which orlistat treatment is cost effective.

11.14 Conclusions

Administration of the gastrointestinal lipase inhibitor orlistat at a dosage of 120 mg three times daily produces an additional 2- to 4-kg weight loss on average in large clinical trials with duration of up to 2 years. The response to the drug is highly variable for only partially understood reasons and, therefore, it remains the responsibility of the physician to decide whether an effect is clinically significant and whether the use of orlistat should be continued. In obese patients with comorbid conditions, orlistat treatment was found to be accompanied by small, but significant, reductions in total and LDL cholesterol; LDL/HDL ratio; systolic and diastolic blood pressure; and, in patients with type 2 diabetes, glycated hemoglobin and fasting plasma glucose and insulin levels. However, these effects were not consistent across the clinical trials and the clinical significance of the reported results is to some extent questionable. In this context, the possibility of adverse effects of orlistat administration must be taken into account. Nevertheless, current data suggest that the drug is well tolerated, and most adverse effects are mild and transient. Unfortunately, long-term outcome studies on the effect of orlistat on cardiovascular events are not available.

References

Bachmann, O.P., Dahl, D.B., Brechtel, K. et al. Orlistat (Xenical®) improves insulin sensitivity in obese intentionally weight maintaining subjects. *Diabetes Res. Clin. Pract.* 50 Suppl. 1, 2000, 70.

Ballinger, A. and Peikin, S.R. Orlistat: its current status as an anti-obesity drug. *Eur. J. Pharmacol.* 440, 2002, 109–117.

Beermann, B., Melander, H., Säwe, J., Ulleryd, C., and Dahlqvist, R. Incorrect use and limited weight reduction of orlistat (Xenical) in clinical practice. *Eur. J. Clin. Pharmacol.* 57, 2001, 309–311.

Borovicka, J., Schwizer, W., Guttmann, G. et al. Role of lipase in the regulation of postprandial gastric acid secretion and emptying of fat in humans: a study with orlistat, a highly specific lipase inhibitor. *Gut* 46, 2000, 774–781.

Bray, G.A. and Popkin, B.M. Dietary fat intake does affect obesity! *Am. J. Clin. Nutr.* 68, 1998, 1157–1163.

Bray, G.A. and Greenway, F.L. Current and potential drugs for treatment of obesity. *Endocr. Rev.* 20, 1999, 805–875.

Davidson, M.H., Hauptman, J., DiGirolamo, M., Foreyt, J.P., Halsted, C.H., Heber, D., Heimburger, D.C., Lucas, C.P., Robbins, D.C., Chung, J., and Heymsfield, S.B. Long-term weight control and risk factor reduction in obese subjects treated with orlistat, a lipase inhibitor. *JAMA* 281, 1999, 235–242.

Despres, J-P., Lemieux, I. and Prud'homme D. Treatment of obesity: need to focus on high risk abdominally obese patients. *Br. Med. J.* 326, 2001, 716–720.

Drent M.L. and van der Veen, E.A. Lipase inhibition: a novel concept in the treatment of obesity. *Int. J. Obes. Relat. Metab. Disord.* 17, 1993, 241–244.

Drent, M.L., Larsson, I., William–Olsson, T., Quadde, F., Czubayko, F., von Bergmann, K., Strobel, W., Sjöström, L. and van der Veen, E.A. Orlistat (Ro18-0647), a lipase inhibitor, in the treatment of human obesity: a multiple dose study. *Int. J. Obes. Relat. Metab. Disord.* 19, 1995, 221–226.

Errasti, P., Garcia, I., Lavilla, J., Ballester, B., Manrique, J., and Purroy, A. Reduction in blood cyclosporine cencentration by orlistat in two renal transplant patients. *Transplant Proc.* 34, 2002, 139–149.

Feinle, C., Rades, T., Otto, B., and Fried, M. Fat digestion modulates gastrointestinal sensations induced by gastric distension and duodenal lipid in humans. *Gastroenterology* 120, 2001, 1100–1107.

Fernandez–Aranda, F., Amor, A., Jimenez–Murcia, S., Gimenez–Martinez, L., Turon–Gil, V., and Vallejo–Ruiloba, J. Bulimia nervosa and misuse of orlistat: two case reports. *Int. J. Eat. Disord.* 30, 2001, 458–461.

Finer, N., James, W.P.T., Kopelman, P.G., Lean, M.E.J., and Williams, G. One-year treatment of obesity: a randomized, double-blind placebo-controlled, multi-center study of orlistat (Xenical®), a gastrointestinal lipase inhibitor. *Int. J. Obes. Relat. Metab. Disord.* 23, 2000, 1–8.

FDA (Food and Drug Administration), Center for Drug Evaluation. NDA 20-766, Xenical (orlistat). Presented at the Endocrinological and Metabolic Drugs Advisory Committee Meeting 69, March 1998, Gaithersburg, MD.

Franson, K. and Rössner, S. Fat intake and food choices during weight reduction with diet, behavioural modification and a lipase inhibitor. *J. Intern. Med.* 247, 2000, 607–614.

Gokcel, A., Gumurdulu, Y., Karakose, H., Melek Ertorer, E., Tanaci, N., Bascil Tutuncu, N., and Guvener, N. Evaluation of the safety and efficacy of sibutramine, orlistat and metformin in the treatment of obesity. *Diabetes Obes. Metab.* 4, 2002, 49–55.

Grundy, S.M. and Denke, M.A. Dietary influences on serum lipids and lipoproteins. *J. Lipid Res.* 31, 1990, 1149–1172.

Guerciolini, R. Mode of action of orlistat. *Int. J. Obes. Relat. Metab. Disord.* 21 (Suppl.), 1997, S12–S23.

Güzelhan, C., Odink, J., Niestijl Jansen–Zuidema, J.J., and Hartmann, D. Influence of dietary composition on the inhibition of fat absorption by orlistat. *J. Int. Med. Res.* 22, 1994, 255–265.

Hadvary, P., Lengsfeld, H., and Wolfer, H. Inhibition of pancreatic lipase *in vitro* by the covalent inhibitor tetrahydrolipstatin. *Biochem. J.* 256, 1988, 357–361.

Hadvary, P., Sidler, W., Meister, W., Vetter, W., and Wolfer, H. The lipase inhibitor tetrahydrolipstatin binds covalently to the putative active site serine of pancreatic lipase. *J. Biol. Chem.* 266, 1991, 2021–2027.

Hauptman, J., Lucas, C., Boldrin, M.N., and Collins, H., for the Orlistat Primary Care Study Group. Orlistat in the long-term treatment of obesity in primary care. *Arch. Fam. Med.* 9, 2000, 160–167.

Hill, J.O., Hauptman, J., Anderson, J.W., Fujioka, K., O'Neil, P.M., Smith, D.K., Zavoral, J.H., and Aronne, L.J. Orlistat, a lipase inhibitor, for weight loss after conventional dieting: a 1-y study. *Am. J. Clin. Nutr.* 69, 1999, 1108–1116.

Heymsfield, S.B., Segal, K.R., Hauptman, J., Lucas, C.P., Boldrin, M.N., Rissanen, A., Wilding, J.P.H., and Sjöström, L. Effects of weight loss with orlistat on glucosetolerance and progression to type 2 diabetes in obese adults. *Arch. Intern. Med.* 160, 2000, 1321–1326.

Hollander, P., Elbein, S.C., Hirsch, I.B., Kelley, D., McGill, J., Taylor, T., Weiss, S.R., Crockett, S.E., Kaplan, R.A., Comstock, J., Lucas, C.P., Lodewick, P.A., Canovatchel, W., Chung, J., and Hauptman, J. Role of orlistat in the treatment of obese patients with type 2 diabetes. *Diabetes Care* 21, 1998, 1288–1294.

Hu, F.B., van Dam, R.M., and Liu, S. Diet and risk of type 2 diabetes: the role of types of fat and carbohydrate. *Diabetologia* 2001, 44: 805–817.

Hussain, Y., Güzelhan, C., Odink, J., van der Beek, E.J., and Hartmann, D. Comparison of the inhibition of dietary fat absorption by full vs. divided doses of orlistat. *J. Clin. Pharmacol.* 34, 1994, 1121–1125.

James W.P.T., Avenell, A., Broom, J., and Whitehead, J. A one-year trial to assess the value or orlistat in the management of obesity. *Int. J. Obes. Relat. Metab. Disord.* 21 (Suppl.), 1997, S24–S30.

Karhunen, L., Franssila–Kallunki, A., Rissanen, P., Valve, R., Kolehmainen, M., Rissanen, A., and Uusitupa, M. Effect of orlistat treatment on body composition and resting energy expenditure during a two-year weight reduction program in obese Finns. *Int. J. Obes. Relat. Metab. Disord.* 24, 2000, 1567–1572.

Keating, G.M. and Jarvis, B. Orlistat in the prevention and treatment of type 2 diabetes mellitus. *Drugs* 61, 2001, 2107–2119.

Kelley, D.E., Hill, J., Bray, G.A., Miles, J., Pi–Sunyer, F.X., Klein, S., and Hollander, P. Clinical efficacy of orlistat therapy in overweight and obese patients with insulin-treated type 2 diabetes. *Diabetes Care* 25, 2002, 1033–1041.

Knowler, W.C., Barrett–Conner, E., Fowler, S.E., Hamman, R.F., Lachin, J.M., Walker, E.A., and Nathan, D.M. Reduction in the incidence of type 2 diabetes with lifestyle intervention or metformin. *N. Engl. J. Med.* 346, 2002, 393–403.

Lamotte, M., Annemans, L., Lefever, A., Nechelput, M., and Masure, J. A health economic model to assess the long-term effects and cost-effectiveness of orlistat in obese type 2 diabetic patients. *Diabetes Care* 25, 2002, 303–308.

Le Beller, C., Bezie, Y., Chabatte, C., Guillemain, R., Amrein, C., and Billaud, E.M. Co-administration of orlistat and cyclosporine in a heart transplant recipient. *Transplantation* 70, 2000, 1541–1542.

Lindgärde, F., on behalf of the Orlistat Swedish Multimorbidity Study Group. The effect of orlistat on body weight and coronary heart disease risk factor profile in obese patients: the Swedish Multimorbidity Study. *J. Intern. Med.* 248, 2000, 245–254.

Lockene, A., Skottova, N., and Olivecrona, G. Interactions of lipoprotein lipase with the active site inhibitor tetrahydrolipstatin (orlistat). *Eur. J. Biochem.* 222, 1994, 395–403.

Lowe, M.E. The catalytic site residues and interfacial binding of human pancreatic lipase. *J. Biol. Chem.* 267, 1992, 17069–17073.

Melia, A.T., Zhi, J., Koss–Twardy, S.G., Min, B., Guerciolini, R., Freundlich, N.L., Arora, S., and Passe, S.M. The influence of reduced dietary fat absorption induced by orlistat on the pharmacokinetics of digoxin in healthy volunteers. *J. Clin. Pharmacol.* 35, 1995, 840–843.

Melia, A.T., Koss–Twardy, S.G., and Zhi, J. The effect of orlistat, an inhibitor of dietary fat absorption, on the absorption of vitamins A and E in healthy volunteers. *J. Clin. Pharmacol.* 36, 1996, 647–653.

Melia, A.T., Zhi, J., Zelasko, R., Hartmann, D., Güzelhan, C., Guerciolini, R., and Odink, J. The interaction of the lipase inhibitor orlistat with ethanol in healthy volunteers. *Eur. J. Clin. Pharmacol.* 54, 1998, 773–777.

Meyer, J.H., Mayer, E.A., Jehn, D., Gu, Y., Fink, A.S., and Fried, M. Gastric processing and emptying of fat. *Gastroenterology* 90, 1986, 1176–1187.

Miles, J.M., Leiter, L., Hollander, P., Wadden, T., Anderson, J.W., Doyle, M., Foreyt, J., Aronne, L., and Klein, S. Effect of orlistat in overweight and obese patients with type 2 diabetes treated with metformin. *Diabetes Care* 2002, 25: 1123–1128.

Muls, E., Kolanowski, J., Scheen, A., and van Gaal, L. The effects of orlistat on weight and on serum lipids in obese patients with hypercholesterolemia: a randomized, double-blind, placebo-controlled, multicentre trial. *Int. J. Obes. Relat. Metab. Disord.* 2001, 25: 1713–1721.

Nägeli, H., Peterson, B., Bonacker, U., and Rodiger, W. Effect of orlistat on blood cyclosporine concentration in an obese heart transplant patient. *Eur. J. Clin. Pharmacol.* 55, 1999, 667–669.

National Institute for Clinical Excellence. (2001) Orlistat for treatment of obesity in adults. 2001, http://www.nice.org.uk.

National Task Force on the Prevention and Treatment of Obesity. Long-term pharmacotherapy in the management of obesity. *JAMA* 276, 1996, 1907–1915.

O'Meara, S., Riemsa, R., Shirran, L., Mather, L., and ter Riet, G. A rapid and systematic review of the clinical effectiveness and cost-effectiveness of orlistat in the management of obesity. *Health Technol. Assessment* 5(18), 2001.

Ornish, D., Brown, S.E., Scherwitz, L.W., Billings, J.H., Armstrong, W.T., Ports, T.A., McLanahan, S.M., Kirkeeide, R.L., Brand, R.J., and Gould, K.L. Can lifestyle changes reverse coronary heart disease? *Lancet* 336, 1990, 129–133.

Pace, D., Blotner, S., and Guerciolini, R. Short-term orlistat treatment does not affect mineral balance and bone turnover in obese men. *J. Nutr.* 131, 2001, 1694–1699.

Persson, M., Vitols, S., and Yue, Q.Y. Orlistat associated with hypertension. *Br. Med. J.* 321, 2000, 87.

Rissanen, A., Lean, M., Rössner, S., Segal, K.R., and Sjöström, L. Predictive value of early weight loss in obesity management with orlistat: an evidence-based assessment of prescribing guidelines. *Int. J. Obes. Relat. Metab. Disord.* 27, 2003, 103–109.

Roche. Xenical (Orlistat). Complete product information. 1999.

Rössner, S., Sjöström, L., Noack, R., Meinders, A.E., and Noseda, G. Weight loss, weight maintenance, and improved cardiovascular risk factors after 2 years of treatment with orlistat for obesity. *Obes. Res.* 2000, 8: 49–61.

Scheen, A.J. and Ernest, P. New antiobesity agents in type 2 diabetes: overview of clinical trials with sibutramine and orlistat. *Diabetes Metab.* 2002, 28: 437–445.

Schnetzler, B., Kondo–Oestreicher, M., Vala, D., Khatchatourian, G., and Faidutti, B. Orlistat decreases the plasma levels of cyclosporine and may be responsible for the development of acute rejection episodes. *Transplantation* 70, 2000, 1540–1541.

Shephard, T.Y., Jensen, D.R., Blotner, S., Zhi, J., Guerciolini, R., Pace, D., and Eckel, R.H. Orlistat fails to alter postprandial plasma lipid excursions or plasma lipases in normal-weight male volunteers. *Int. J. Obes. Relat. Metab. Disord.* 24, 2000, 187–194.

Sjöström, L., Rissanen, A., Andersen, T., Boldrin, M., Golay, A., Koppeschaar, H.P., and Krempf, M. Randomized placebo-controlled trial of orlistat for weight loss and prevention of weight regain in obese patients. European Multicentre Orlistat Study Group. *Lancet* 352, 1998, 167–172.

Tan, K.C.B., Tso, A.W.K., Tam, S.C.F., Pang, R.W.C., and Lam, K.S.L. Acute effect of orlistat on postprandial lipemia and free fatty acids in overweight patients with type 2 diabetes mellitus. *Diabet. Med* 19, 2002, 944–948.

Tong, P.C.Y., Lee, Z.S.K., Sea, M-M., Chow, C-C., Ko, G.T.C., Chan, W-B., So, W-Y., Ma, R.C.W., Ozaki, R., Woo, J., Cockram, C.S., and Chan, J.C.N. The effect of orlistat-induced weight loss, without concomitant hypocaloric diet, on cardiovascular risk factors and insulin sensitivity in young obese Chinese subjects with or without type 2 diabetes. *Arch. Intern. Med.* 162, 2002, 2428–3245.

Tonstad, S., Pometta, D., Erkelens, D.W., Ose, L., Moccetti, T., Schouten, J.A., Golay, A., Reitsma, J., Del Bufalo, A., Pasotti, E., and van der Wal, P. The effect of the gastrointestinal lipase inhibitor, orlistat, on serum lipids and lipoproteins in patients with primary hyperlipidaemia. *Eur. J. Clin. Pharmacol.* 46, 1994, 405–410.

Trouillot, T.E., Pace, D.G., McKinley, C., Cockey, L., Zhi, J., Häussler, J., Guerciolini, R., Showalter, R., and Everson, G.T. Orlistat maintains biliary lipid composition and hepatobiliary function in obese subjects undergoing moderate weight loss. *Am. J. Gastroenterol.* 96, 2001, 1888–1894.

Tuomilehto, J., Lindström, J., Eriksson, J.G., Valle, T.T., Hamalainen, H., Ilanne–Parikka, P., Keinanen–Kiukaanniemi, S., Laakso, M., Louheranta, A., Rastas, M., Salminen, V., and Uusitupa, M. Prevention of type 2 diabetes mellitus by changes in lifestyle among subjects with impaired glucose tolerance. *N. Engl. J. Med.* 344, 2001, 1343–1350.

Unger, R.H. Lipotoxicity in the pathogenesis of obesity-dependent NIDDM. Genetic and clinical implications. *Diabetes* 1995, 44: 863–870.

van Gaal, L.F., Broom, J.I., Enzi, G., and Toplak, H. Efficacy and tolerability of orlistat in the treatment of obesity — a 6-month dose-ranging study. *Eur. J. Clin. Pharmacol.* 54, 1998, 125–132.

Weber, C., Tam, Y.K., Schmidtke–Schrezenmeier, D., Jonkmann, J.H., and van Brummelen, P. Effect of the lipase inhibitor orlistat on the pharmacokinetics of four different antihypertensive drugs in healthy volunteers. *Eur. J. Clin. Pharmacol.* 51, 1996, 87–90.

Wolf, A.M. and Colditz, G.A. Current estimates of the economic costs of obesity in the United States. *Obes. Res.* 1998, 6: 97–106.

WHO (World Health Organization). Obesity: preventing and managing the global epidemic. Report of a WHO Consultation. WHO Technical Report Series 894, 2000.

Zavoral, J.H. Treatment with orlistat reduces cardiovascular risk in obese patients. *J. Hypertension* 16, 1998, 2013–2017.

Zhi, J., Melia, A.T., Guerciolini, R., Chung, J., Kinberg, J., Hauptman, J.B., and Patel, I.H. Retrospective population-based analysis of the dose–response (fecal fat excretion) relationship of orlistat in normal and obese volunteers. *Clin. Pharmacol. Ther.* 56, 1994, 82–85.

Zhi, J., Melia, A.T., Koss–Twardy, S.G., Min, B., Guerciolini, R., Freundlich, N.L., Milla, G., and Patel, I.H. The influence of orlistat on the pharmacokinetics and pharmacodynamics of glyburide in healthy volunteers. *J. Clin. Pharmacol.* 35, 1995, 521–525.

Zhi, J., Melia, A.T., Funk, C., Viger–Chougnet, A., Hopfgartner, C., Lausecker, B., Wang, K., Fulton, J.S., Gabriel, L., and Mulligan, T.E. Metabolic profiles of minimally absorbed orlistat in obese/overweight volunteers. *J. Clin. Pharmacol.* 36, 1996, 1006–1011.

Zhi, J., Mulligan, T.E., and Hauptman, J.B. Long-term systemic exposure of orlistat, a lipase inhibitor, and its metabolites in obese patients. *J. Clin. Pharmacol.* 39, 1999, 41–46.

Zhi, J., Moore, R., Kanitra, L., and Mulligan, T.E. Pharmacokinetic evaluation of the possible interaction between selected concomitant medications and orlistat at steady state in healthy subjects. *J. Clin. Pharmacol.* 42, 2002, 1011–1019.

12

Sibutramine

Donna H. Ryan

CONTENTS

ABSTRACT Sibutramine is a centrally acting reuptake inhibitor of monoamines that has approval from the U.S. Food and Drug Administration and the European Committee for Proprietary Medicinal Products for use in long-term obesity treatment. The amount of weight lost with sibutramine corresponds to the drug dose as well as the intensity of the behavioral approach to dieting used concomitantly with pharmacotherapy. Sibutramine has demonstrated efficacy in weight loss maintenance, with studies documenting significant advantages compared to placebo at 18 months follow-up. The medication has been used successfully in obese diabetic patients and obese patients with well-controlled hypertension. The tolerability profile of sibutramine is acceptable, with common side effects (insomnia, constipation, asthenia, and dry mouth) usually being self-limited.

The drug should not be used by patients with a history of seizures, and it should not be prescribed for patients taking monoamine oxidase inhibitors or serotonergic or noradrenergic medications. Its use in patients with pre-existing cardiovascular disease has not been established. Sibutramine use is not associated with primary pulmonary hypertension or with valvular heart disease. Weight loss with sibutramine has been shown to be associated with improvement in waist circumference; blood lipids; indices of glycemic control; symptoms of sleep apnea; and measures of quality of life.

The chief barrier to the use of sibutramine is the reported elevation in heart rate and blood pressure that can be associated with its use. In clinical trials, <2% of patients have had to be discontinued from the drug because of clinically significant blood pressure increase; however, not all patients experience blood pressure increase. Still, the concern is that even the small increase in mean resting blood pressure observed in clinical trials could result in adverse effects if the drug were prescribed widely. The clinical significance of the small increase in mean resting blood pressure values has recently been called into question by the observation of paradoxical attenuation of blood pressure in response to pressors when sibutramine is compared to placebo. Because the risk factor response associated with sibutramine-induced weight loss may be mixed, plans are underway to evaluate more advanced endpoints in clinical trials as a measure of sibutramine efficacy. Sibutramine can be a useful adjunct to diet and physical activity to produce weight loss and concomitant health benefits.

12.1 Pharmacology and Mechanism of Action

Sibutramine (marketed as Meridia in the U.S. and Reductil in Europe) is a selective reuptake inhibitor for norepinephrine, serotonin, and dopamine. The drug is rapidly metabolized to two active metabolites, whose half-life is 14 to 16 h, with the peak concentration at 3 to 4 h and a plateau from 3 to 7 h (Luque and Rey 1999). The chemical structures of sibutramine and those of its two active metabolites are illustrated in Figure 12.1. The pharmacological profile allows for dosing once a day, an advantage when appetite regulation is the aim. The drug was first evaluated as a potential antidepressant in three phase II clinical trials, with disappointing results in depression (Kelly et al. 1995). However, striking weight loss was observed in the enrolled depressed patients (Kelly et al. 1995), and the drug has been developed and marketed for weight loss.

The mechanisms by which sibutramine produces its pharmacological effects are thought to be through the actions of serotonin and norepinephrine in combination, acting within the central nervous system (Heal et al. 1998). Sibutramine's dopaminergic action is minimal (Heal et al. 1998). When administered to experimental animals, sibutramine has dual mechanisms to induce weight reduction: decrease in food intake and increase in energy expenditure (Stock 1997). The increase in energy expenditure is prominent in rodents, with sustained (>6 h) increase in metabolic rate up to 30%, and is based upon sympathetic activation of thermogenesis in brown adipose tissue (Stock 1997; Connoley et al. 1995).

In clinical trials with humans, sibutramine decreases food intake in nondieting men (Chapelot et al. 2000) and women (Rolls et al. 1998) by increasing meal-induced satiety (Chapelot et al. 2000; Rolls et al. 1998; Hansen et al. 1998). Sibutramine also affects energy

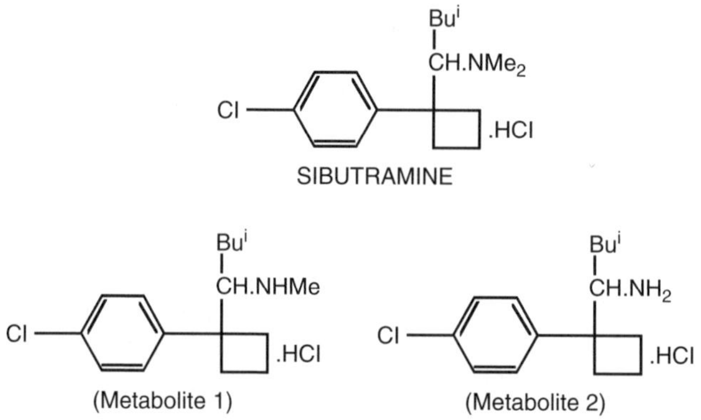

FIGURE 12.1
Structure formulas for sibutramine and the two active metabolites.

expenditure in humans, but the effect on thermogenesis is not as great as that seen in rodents. Considering all investigations of sibutramine's thermogenic effect in humans, it can be estimated on the order of 2 to 4% increase in metabolic rate beginning 3 h from ingestion and lasting less than 24 h. A well-designed study is required to demonstrate the increase in energy expenditure with the drug because the pharmacologic profile must be taken into account and because of the inherent variability of human metabolic rate measurements.

Two such well-designed studies document sibutramine's enhancement of metabolic rate. In a study of the acute effects of sibutramine on energy expenditure, Hansen et al. (1998) measured energy expenditure for 5.5 h after dosing with 30 mg sibutramine compared to placebo in fed and fasted men. Sibutramine induced an increase in energy expenditure by about 3 to 5%. In a study of the thermogenic effects of sibutramine when taken over a longer course, Walsh et al. (1999) studied obese females receiving 12 weeks of a calorie-reduced diet, and 15 mg/day sibutramine or a placebo. The expected decline in resting energy expenditure usually observed with weight loss and documented in the placebo-treated participants was blunted in the sibutramine-treated patients. The authors suggest that the sibutramine effect is equivalent to 100 kcal/day and might be enough to promote weight loss maintenance over the long term.

12.2 Clinical Efficacy

When pharmacological approaches are included in a weight control plan, they should be part of a comprehensive treatment plan that includes diet and physical activity measures in a long-term approach of life-style modification (National Institutes of Health, National Heart, Lung and Blood Institute, 1998). Medications are no longer recommended for use for just a few weeks — when the FDA reviews weight loss medications, clinical data describing their use for 2 years are required. This chapter will therefore focus primarily on sibutramine clinical efficacy reports that document the drug's use for 24 weeks or longer.

The first reported clinical trial with sibutramine (Weintraub et al. 1991) enrolled 21 men and women who were 130 to 180% of the ideal body weight. After a 3-week run-in period in which a calorie-reduced diet was employed, participants were randomized to 20 mg/day sibutramine, 5 mg/day sibutramine, or a placebo. At 8 weeks, statistically significant differences ($p < .05$) were found for all comparisons of weight loss, with −5.0 kg (20 mg sibutramine dose), −2.9 kg (5 mg dose), and −1.4 kg (placebo). Additional studies with an 8-week or a 12-week endpoint have been reviewed elsewhere (O'Meara et al. 2002).

Since the early short-term trials, sibutramine has been extensively evaluated in otherwise healthy men and women of all ethnic groups with ages ranging from 18 to 65 years and with a body mass index (BMI) between 27 and 40 kg/m^2 in single-center and multicenter trials lasting 6 to 24 months; these are summarized in Table 12.1 (Bray et al. 1996, 1999; Fanghanel et al. 2000; Cuellar et al. 2000; Smith and Goulder 2001; Dujovne et al. 2001; Halpern et al. 2002; Apfelbaum et al. 1999; James et al. 2000; Wirth and Krause 2001). These are randomized, placebo-controlled, double-blind clinical trials enrolling primarily obese but otherwise healthy adults. The experience with sibutramine in patients with hypertension and diabetes will be discussed later.

From the clinical experiences outlined in Table 12.1, several observations regarding sibutramine's efficacy can be made:

TABLE 12.1

Clinical Trials[a] Using Sibutramine for ≥24 Weeks in Otherwise Healthy Obese Subjects

| No. Subjects | | Dose | Duration of | Initial Wt. (kg) | | Wt. Loss (kg) | | Wt. Loss (%) | | Comments | Ref. |
Started	Completed	(mg/d)	Study (wks)	Placebo	Drug	Placebo	Drug	Placebo	Drug		
24	23	0	24	92.0		-0.75		-0.77		Part of multicenter study (Bray et al., 1999); data described are for completing men and women	Bray et al., 1996
24	21	1			95.8		-2.96		-3.20		
25	24	5			90.9		-2.87		-3.07		
25	22	10			87.2		-6.19		-6.91		
25	20	15			89.7		-6.89		-7.77		
24	22	20			90.9		-7.30		-8.06		
26	23	30			91.4		-8.24		-9.17		
148	87	0	24	95.0		-1.3		-1.2		Multicenter phase III trial	Bray et al., 1999
149	95	1			94.0		-2.4		-2.7		
151	107	5			94.0		-3.7		-3.9		
150	99	10			91.0		-5.7		-6.1		
152	98	15			93.0		-7.0		-7.4		
146	96	20			93.0		-8.2		-8.8		
151	101	30			95.0		-9.0		-9.4		
55	44	0	26	86.4		-4.6		-4.8		BMI > 30 kg/m². Diet 30 kcal/kg of ideal body weight	Fanghanel et al., 2000
54	40	10			87.5		-8.8		-9.9		
34	9	0	24	90.1		-1.3		-1.4			Cuellar et al., 2000
35	22	15			86.0		-10.4		-10.4		
163	80	0	52	87.0		-1.6		-1.8			Smith and Goulder, 2001
161	94	10			87.0		-4.4		-5.0		
161	82	20			87.0		-6.4		-7.3		
160	54	0	24	102.0		-0.6		-0.6		Obese subjects with dyslipidemia	Dujovne et al., 2001
162	48	20			99.7		-4.9		-4.9		
31	23	0	6 months	88.9		-2.6		-2.8		60 females and 1 male; echocardiograms performed	Halpern et al., 2002
30	23	10			91.1		-7.3		-8.0		

Sibutramine Clinical Trials of Weight Loss Maintenance

N		Dose (mg)	Wk							Comments	Reference
181	48	0	52	97.7	+0.2	95.7	-6.1	+0.2	-6.4	Multicenter; those with wt. loss ≥ 6 kg after 4 wk VLCD were randomized; 75% of sibutramine treated vs. 42% on placebo maintained all wt. lost on VLCD	Apfelbaum et al., 1999
82	60	10									
115	57	0	78	102.1	-4.7	102.3	-10.2	-4.4	-10.0	Multicenter trial in subjects who lost ≥ 5% on 10 mg sibutramine in 6 months	James et al., 2000
352	204	10–20									
201	146	0	48	98.2	-3.8	98.6	-7.8	-3.9	-8.2	After > 2% loss at 4 weeks, subjects randomized to placebo vs. 15 mg sibutramine daily vs. 15 mg intermittent (weeks 1–12; 19–30; 37–48); no changes in blood pressure observed for any groups	Wirth and Krause, 2001
405	325	15				98.2			-8.1		
	315	15[b]									

[a] Randomized, placebo-controlled, double-blind studies.
[b] Intermittent (weeks 1 to 12; 19 to 30; 37 to 48).

- A dose–response relationship is present, with higher sibutramine doses producing greater weight loss.
- The "dose" of the diet and exercise approach, used adjunctively with the drug, also influences degree of weight loss.
- Although active weight loss occurs in the first 6 months of use, the drug is efficacious in maintaining weight loss.

The dose–response relationship between sibutramine 1, 5, 10, 15, 20, and 30 mg and weight loss is illustrated by Figure 12.2 and Figure 12.3, which show the results of a double-blind, placebo-controlled study conducted in seven centers and enrolling 1047 subjects (Bray et al. 1999). Figure 12.2 shows mean weight loss over time displayed graphically for all treatment groups in this trial and demonstrates a clear dose–response relationship. The recommended dose levels for use in clinical practice are 5 to 15 mg/day and these doses produced –3.9, –6.1, and –7.4% loss from baseline at week 24.

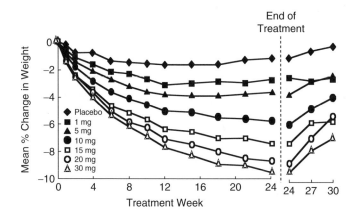

FIGURE 12.2
Weight loss in patients completing 24 weeks of treatment. $P < .05$ vs. placebo for all time points for sibutramine doses 5 to 30 mg, nonparametric Williams' test. $N = 87$ to 107 per group. Posttreatment follow-up data are also shown for those patients in whom it was available ($N = 50$ to 61 per group). (From Bray, G.A. et al., *Obes Res*, 7:189–198, 1999.)

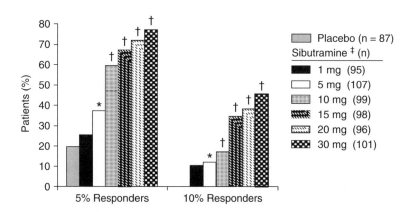

FIGURE 12.3
Percentage of patients losing at least 5 or 10% of baseline weight after 24 weeks treatment. †$P < 0.001$ vs. placebo. ‡Recommended dose of sibutramine 10 or 15 mg once daily.

As can be observed in Figure 12.2 and Figure 12.3, the behavioral approach used with pharmacotherapy in this study was relatively weak because the mean weight loss associated with placebo was only 1.2% from baseline at 24 weeks and <20% of patients on placebo achieved ≥5% weight loss from baseline. Weight losses of 5 and 10% from baseline are useful benchmarks because these are associated with significant health benefits. Figure 12.3 illustrates that 37.4, 59.5, and 63.7% of persons taking 5, 10, and 15 mg sibutramine doses achieved 5% weight loss from baseline compared to only 19.5% of those taking placebo. Other placebo-controlled studies of ≥24-week duration using sibutramine in healthy obese individuals are presented in Table 12.1; these studies add additional evidence for the sibutramine dose–weight loss response relationship.

Another sibutramine study is of interest by virtue of the magnitude of weight lost. In that study (Apfelbaum et al. 1999), 159 obese subjects who initially lost 7.2% from baseline weight with a very low calorie liquid diet for 1 month were then randomized to receive a behavioral modification program with placebo or 10 mg/day sibutramine. The usual pattern with cessation of very low calorie diet programs is rapid weight regain, unless a strong behavioral program is in place. The total magnitude of weight loss that resulted by combining the very low calorie diet followed by sibutramine (–16% from baseline at 1 year) is among the largest demonstrated in clinical trial. This trial and the one discussed next attest to the role of the intensity of the behavioral component in maximizing weight loss.

The intensity of the behavioral component of the weight loss program influences the amount of weight loss with sibutramine. Because sibutramine enhances satiety, a dietary program that takes advantage of this mechanism is likely to produce greater weight loss. Wadden et al. (2001) illustrated the advantage of a highly structured dietary intervention in combination with sibutramine. In that study, 53 women were randomized to receive 10 to 15 mg sibutramine daily vs. the same dosing scheme, with a group life-style modification program, vs. the same dosing scheme with a highly structured portion-controlled diet included in the first 4 months of the life-style modification program. (This study is not listed in Table 12.1 because it does not contain a placebo arm.)

As can be observed in Figure 12.4, the group that received an initial 4 months of a highly structured diet (four servings of nutritional supplements and an evening meal of a frozen

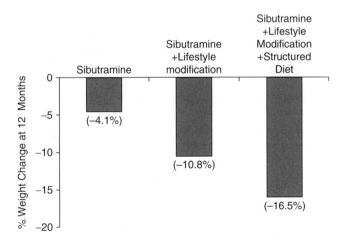

FIGURE 12.4
Percentage reduction in initial body weight for women treated with sibutramine alone; sibutramine plus group life-style modification; or sibutramine and a highly structured diet for 4 months plus group life-style modification. All three groups differed significantly ($p < .05$) at 6 months and at 12 months; the 19 women in the drug alone group lost significantly ($p < .05$) less than the other two groups, which did not differ significantly from each other.

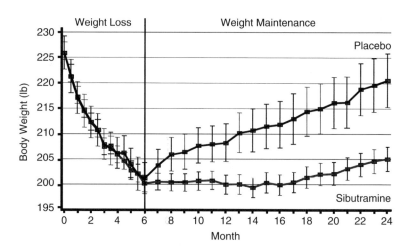

FIGURE 12.5
Mean (SE) sequential body weight change during weight loss and weight maintenance phases of the STORM trial for sibutramine and placebo groups. At month 24, mean (SE) kilogram weight loss was –8.9 (8.1) for sibutramine and –4.0 (5.9) for placebo (p < .001). *Same diet, exercise for sibutramine, placebo; P ≤ 0.001, sibutramine vs. placebo for weight maintenance. (From James, W.P.T. et al., *Lancet*, 356:2119–2125, 2000.)

entrée, fruit, and salad) lost the greatest amount at 6 months (17.7% from baseline) compared to the other two groups who lost 5.5% (drug alone) and 11.0% (drug + life-style).

Another advantage of sibutramine is its efficacy in weight loss maintenance. The three trials that have been designed to address this issue are listed in Table 12.1. After inducing weight loss with very low calorie liquid diet (Apfelbaum et al. 1999) or with sibutramine (James et al. 2000; Wirth and Krause 2001), patients were randomized to placebo or sibutramine for maintenance of weight loss for up to 18 months. The STORM trial (James et al. 2000; see Figure 12.5) illustrates that sibutramine is quite effective for inducing and maintaining weight loss for up to 2 years. In this multicenter European study, patients received 10 mg sibutramine and a calorie deficit diet for 6 months. Of the 605 obese patients who entered the trial, 467 (77%) achieved weight loss of at least 5% from baseline. Those patients were then randomized to receive sibutramine (doses could be titrated from 10 to 20 mg daily) or placebo. Following 24 months of observation, weight loss of the sibutramine-treated group averaged 10.2 kg baseline compared to 4.7 kg for placebo.

A number of observations from the STORM trial are worthy of note. Practitioners might infer from this study that about three fourths of obese patients prescribed 10 mg/day sibutramine with a diet program will achieve clinically meaningful weight loss (i.e., ≥5% from baseline). If medication is continued, almost half of those will maintain 80% of the weight loss at 18 months' follow-up. The fate of subjects randomized to placebo during the 18-month double-blind portion of the trial offers a lesson: the placebo-treated patients steadily regained weight, maintaining only 20% of their weight loss at the end of the trial.

Weight loss maintenance is a major challenge in obesity treatment. Figure 12.6 shows the results of an interesting study by Wirth and Krause (2001) evaluating an intermittent therapy approach to weight loss maintenance. In that study, patients who had lost 2% or 2 kg after 4 weeks of treatment with 15 mg/day sibutramine were randomized to placebo vs. continuous sibutramine vs. sibutramine prescribed intermittently (weeks 1 to 12, 19 to 30, and 37 to 48). Both sibutramine treatment regimens gave equivalent results and were significantly better than placebo. The effect of stopping sibutramine is illustrated in Figure 12.6 by a small increase in weight, which is then reversed when the medication is restarted.

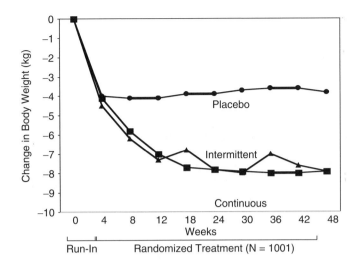

FIGURE 12.6
Mean change in body weight during the study period. Patients (n = 1102) received 15 mg sibutramine/day. Those who lost 2% or 2 kg in 4 weeks were randomized to placebo (n = 395) vs. continued sibutramine (n = 405) vs. intermittent sibutramine (weeks 1 to 12, 19 to 30, and 37 to 48) (n = 395). (From Wirth, A. and Krause, J., *JAMA*, 286(11):1331–1339, 2001.)

In clinical practice, it is difficult to obtain long-term medication compliance for weight loss agents. Patients will report that "the medication is not working, since I am no longer losing weight." Patients will discontinue weight loss medications with subsequent weight regain. This study emphasizes the value of restarting medications before weight regain is advanced and the necessity of continued therapy for weight loss maintenance.

12.3 Efficacy in Special Populations (Diabetes and Hypertension)

Obesity is associated with increased risk for type 2 diabetes and for hypertension; in clinical practice, these co-morbidities are frequently encountered. The experience with sibutramine in obese patients with diabetes is presented in Table 12.2 and with hypertension in Table 12.3.

In the case of diabetes, weight loss is expected to improve indices of glycemic control; the expected changes are a reduction in fasting insulin, glucose, and HbA1c. Four studies using sibutramine in obese patients with type 2 diabetes have been published (see Table 12.2). With the exception of the study by Gokcel et al. (2002), the weight loss observed is somewhat disappointing. In most of the studies, <50% of patients achieved a reduction of 5% body weight, reflecting the difficulty in managing complicated obesity. Still, in all of the studies, the percentage of patients on sibutramine who achieved meaningful weight loss was significantly greater than that of those on placebo; analysis of glycemic control showed benefit corresponding to the degree of weight loss.

In the study by Gokcel et al. (2002), 60 female patients with diabetes who had poorly controlled glucose levels (HbA1c > 8%) on maximal doses of sulfonylureas and metformin were randomly assigned to 10 mg sibutramine twice daily or placebo. The weight loss at 24 weeks was striking: –9.6 kg in sibutramine-treated patients compared to –0.9 kg with placebo. The improvements in glycemic control were equally striking. In the sibutramine-

TABLE 12.2

Sibutramine: Trials in Patients with Diabetes

Population/Run-In	Duration	Dose (mg/day)	Sibutramine N Completers/ N Starting	Sibutramine >5% Weight Loss	Sibutramine Efficacy	Placebo N Completers/ N Starting	Placebo >5% Weight Loss	Placebo Efficacy	Notes	Author
Obese patients with poorly controlled diabetes; 5-week placebo run-in period	24 weeks	20	60/89 (67%)	33%	5% responders had HbA1c −0.53%; HbA1c for all patients was +0.17%	61/86 (71%)	0%	Hb Ab1c for all patients was +0.27%	Mean weight change −4.5% for sibutramine vs. −0.1% for placebo	Fujioka et al., 2000
Obese with diabetes	12 weeks	15	43/47 (91%)	19%	Mean HbA1c −0.3%; 33% of patients achieved decreased HbA1c	40/44 (91%)	0%	Mean HbA1c unchanged; 5% achieved decrease in HbA1c	Mean weight change −2.4 kg for sibutramine vs. −0.1 kg for placebo	Finer et al., 2000
Obese females with poorly controlled diabetes	6 months	20	29/30 (97%)	NR*	Mean HbA1c −2.73%; fasting glucose −124.9 mg/dl	25/30 (83%)	NR	Mean HbA1c unchanged; fasting glucose −15.8 mg/dl	Mean weight change −9.6 kg for sibutramine vs. −0.9 kg for placebo	Gokcel et al., 2001
Obese with diabetes; stable on sulphonyl-urea therapy	6 months	15	53/69 (77%)	49%	Mean HbA1c −0.78%;	57/65 (88%)	29%	Mean HbA1c −0.68%	Mean weight change −4.5 kg for sibutramine vs. −1.7 kg for placebo	Serrano–Rios et al., 2002

Note: NR = not reported.

TABLE 12.3

Sibutramine: Trials in Patients with Hypertension

Duration	Population	Dose (mg/day)	Sibutramine			Placebo			Notes	Author
			N Completed/ N Enrolled	DBP[1]	SBP[2]	N Completed/ N Enrolled	DBP[a]	SBP[b]		
52 weeks	Calcium channel blocker ± diuretic ± β blocker medications	20	NR/150	+2.0	+2.7	NR/74	−1.3	+1.5	Weight loss favoring sibutramine: −4.7 vs. −0.7% for placebo; 40% achieved >5% weight loss with sibutramine vs. 8.7% with placebo	McMahon et al., 2000
12 weeks	All hypertension medications permitted	10	50/62 (81%)	−3.7	−4.1	56/65 (86%)	−5.2	−4.2	Weight loss favoring sibutramine: −4.7 vs. −2.3% at 12 weeks	Hazenberg, 2000
12 weeks	β-blocker medications	20	27/29 (93%)	+1.8	+1.5	28/32 (88%)	−0.8	+0.3	Weight loss favoring sibutramine: −4.5 vs. +0.4%	Sramek et al., 2002
52 weeks	ACE-inhibitor ± diuretic medications	20	84/146 (58%)	+3.0	+3.8	36/74 (49%)	−0.1	+1.1	Weight loss favoring sibutramine: −4.8 vs. −0.3%; 42.8 vs. 8.3% achieved 5% response	McMahon et al., 2002

[a] Diastolic blood pressure change from baseline (mmHg).

[b] Systolic blood pressure change from baseline (mmHg).

Note: NR = not reported.

treated patients, HbA1c fell –2.73%, compared to –0.53% with placebo. Insulin levels fell 5.66 U/ml compared to 0.68 for placebo; fasting glucose fell –124.88 mg/dl compared to –15.76 for placebo. Although weight loss in most of the studies of patients with diabetes does not appear as great as in nondiabetic patients, in all of the studies the percentage of patients who achieved weight loss ≥ 5% from baseline was statistically significantly greater than placebo. In all studies, the degree of weight loss corresponds to the degree of improvement in glycemic control.

Two trials using sibutramine for ≥1 year have been reported in obese hypertensive patients (McMahon et al. 2000, 2002) (Table 12.3), and two additional studies provide data on 12 weeks of treatment (Hazenberg 2000; Sramek et al. 2002). In all instances, the weight loss pattern favors sibutramine. However, except for one study (Sramek et al. 2002), mean weight loss, although favorable, was associated with small increases in mean blood pressure. In one 3-month trial, all patients were receiving β-blockers with or without thiazides for their hypertension (Hazenberg 2000). The sibutramine-treated patients lost –4.2 kg (4.5%) compared to a loss of –0.3 kg (0.3%) in the placebo-treated group. Mean supine and standing diastolic and systolic blood pressure were not statistically significantly different between drug-treated and placebo-treated patients. Heart rate, however, increased +5.6 ± 8.25 (M ± SD) bpm in the sibutramine-treated patients compared to an increase in heart rate of +2.2 ± 6.43 (M ± SD) bpm in the placebo group.

McMahon et al. (2000) reported a 52-week trial in hypertensive patients whose blood pressure was controlled with calcium channel blockers with or without β-blockers or thiazides (Table 12.3). Sibutramine doses were increased from 5 to 20 mg/d during the first 6 weeks. Weight loss was significantly greater in the sibutramine-treated patients, averaging –4.4 kg (4.7%) compared to –0.5 kg (0.7%) in the placebo-treated group. Diastolic blood pressure (DPP) decreased –1.3 mmHg in the placebo-treated group and increased by 2.0 mmHg in the sibutramine-treated group. The systolic blood pressure (SBP) increased +1.5 mmHg in the placebo-treated group and by +2.7 in the sibutramine-treated group. Heart rate was unchanged in the placebo-treated patients, but increased + 4.9 bpm in the sibutramine-treated patients (McMahon et al. 2000). One small study in eight obese men demonstrated that an aerobic exercise program mitigated silbutramine's adverse effects on resting blood pressure (Berube–Parent et al. 2001).

12.4 Effect on Obesity-Related Risk Factors

With the exception of resting blood pressure and pulse, the weight loss induced with sibutramine is associated with improvement in all other obesity-related risk factors, including lipids, uric acid, indices of glycemic control, and waist circumference. These positive changes are related to weight loss; the drug does not have an independent effect on these factors. Figure 12.7 demonstrates a meta-analysis of four long-term obesity studies (Van Gaal et al. 1998) and shows statistically and clinically significant improvement in waist circumference with sibutramine use.

The lipid profile improvement with sibutramine is related to the amount of weight lost. Table 12.4 shows a combined analysis of 11 placebo-controlled trials with sibutramine. The degree of improvement in lipids is proportional to the amount of weight lost (Aronne 2001). Sibutramine has been used in obese patients with hyperlipidemia. In a study by Dujovne et al. (2001), 322 obese men and women with triglycerides ≥250 and ≤1000 mg/dl and serum HDL cholesterol <40 mg/dl (men) or ≤45 mg/dl (women) were put on a

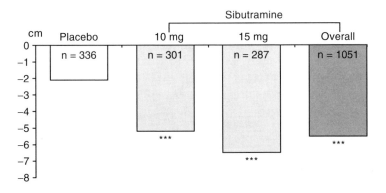

FIGURE 12.7
Mean change in waist circumference from baseline to endpoint in a meta-analysis of four long-term obesity studies involving sibutramine. ***$P < .001$ vs. placebo; n = number of patients. (From Van Gaal, L.F. et al., *Int. J. Obes. Relat. Metab. Disord.*, 22(Suppl 1):S38–40, 1998.)

Step 1 American Heart Association diet and randomized to 20 mg sibutramine ($n = 162$) or placebo ($n = 160$). The mean weight loss at 24 weeks favored sibutramine (–4.9 vs. 0.6 kg) and 42% of sibutramine-treated patients achieved ≥5% reduction in weight, compared to only 8% of those on placebo. For those patients on sibutramine who achieved ≥5% loss from baseline weight, serum triglycerides decreased 33.4 mg/dl and HDL cholesterol increased 4.9 mg/dl.

Sibutramine's weight loss efficacy in patients with diabetes has been previously discussed. A meta-analysis (Krejs 2002) of sibutramine-induced weight loss in patients with type 2 diabetes showed an overall 0.4% reduction in HbA1c with sibutramine use. In patients who lost 10% of baseline body weight, the HbA1c reduction was 0.7% ($p < .003$).

One study (Zannad et al. 2002) has evaluated ventricular dimensions and heart valves in obese patients during weight reduction with sibutramine. In this fairly large study, 184 patients were randomized to 10 or 20 mg sibutramine or a placebo in a double-blind fashion. After 6 months, the reductions in ventricular mass in the sibutramine groups were statistically significant compared to baseline ($p < .01$) but results of pair-wise comparisons to placebo were not statistically significant.

TABLE 12.4

Changes in Serum Lipids: Combined Analysis of 11 Placebo-Controlled Sibutramine Studies

		Sibutramine		
	Placebo (mg/dL)	All Patients (mg/dL)	<5% Weight Loss (mg/dL)	≥5% Weight Loss (mg/dL)
Triglycerides	+0.53	–8.75[a]	–0.54	–16.59[a]
Total cholesterol	–1.53	–2.21	–0.17	–4.87[a]
LDL cholesterol	–0.09	–1.85	–0.37	–4.56[b]
HDL cholesterol	–0.56	+4.13[a]	+3.19[a]	+4.68[a]

[a] $p \leq .001$ vs. placebo.
[b] $p \leq .05$, $p \leq .01$ vs. placebo.

Note: LDL = low density lipoprotein; HDL = high-density lipoprotein. Pooled trial data.

Source: Adapted from Aronne, L.J., *Prog. Cardiovasc. Nurs.*, 16(3):98, 2001.

In addition to improvement in obesity-related risk factors, weight loss with sibutramine can produce improvements in health-related quality of life (HRQOL). Samsa et al. (2001) combined data from four double-blind, randomized, controlled trials of 20 mg/dl sibutramine vs. placebo. Moderate weight loss (5.01 to 10%) was associated with a statistically significant improvement in HRQOL.

12.5 Safety and Tolerability

Sibutramine is available in 5-, 10-, and 15-mg pills; 10 mg/d as a single daily dose is the recommended starting level with titration up or down based on response. Doses above 15 mg/d are not recommended by the FDA. Sibutramine is not recommended for use in patients with a history of coronary artery disease, congestive heart failure, cardiac arrhythmias, or stroke. There should be a 2-week interval between termination of monoamine oxidase inhibitors (MAOIs) and beginning sibutramine. Sibutramine should not be used with selective serotonin reuptake inhibitors (SSRIs). Because sibutramine is metabolized by the cytochrome P_{450} enzyme system (isozyme CYP3A4), when drugs like erythromycin and ketoconazole are taken, competition for this enzymatic pathway and prolonged metabolism can result.

The side effects of sibutramine (insomnia, asthenia, dry mouth, and constipation) are generally mild and transient. Sibutramine is not associated with valvulopathy (Bach et al. 1999; Halpern et al. 2002; Zannad et al. 2002). Although the drug is scheduled as a Class IV substance, a study of 31 male recreational stimulant users provided no evidence for abuse potential (Cole et al. 1998). In that study, the volunteers were questioned about "street value"; 20 and 30 mg dextroamphetamine had higher street values ($2.80 and $3.30, respectively) than 20 and 30 mg sibutramine ($0.50 and $0.70, respectively) or placebo ($0.20). The p value was significant ($p < .001$) for dextroamphetamine doses compared to placebo or sibutramine doses, but no significant difference between placebo and both sibutramine doses was found. No evidence has been found for a clinically relevant interaction of sibutramine with alcohol in impairment of cognitive function (Wesnes et al. 2000).

If sibutramine acts via central nervous system stimulation of norepinephrine and serotonin and through the sympathetic nervous system to increase thermogenesis, then cardiostimulatory effects are to be expected. The principal concerns with sibutramine safety have been the observed increase in mean resting blood pressure and pulse rate that averages 1 to 3 mm Hg for BP and a four- to six-beat/minute increase in pulse (Bray et al. 1996, 1999; Lean 1997). The mean increases do not tell the whole story. Some patients are sensitive to sibutramine and will experience resting blood pressure and pulse increases to unacceptable levels. In the clinical trials reviewed in this chapter, that usually represents <2% of patients exposed to sibutramine.

One published (Sharma 2001) composite of data from clinical trials describes withdrawals for cardiovascular events (shown in Table 12.5). For long-term studies, withdrawals for hypertension between placebo and sibutramine do not differ, according to Sharma's analysis; however, this overall integrated database shows a significant difference in withdrawals for tachycardia and for palpitations. Still, total withdrawals for hypertension, palpitations, tachycardia, and vasodilation in this database are ≤2%. It is recommended in the prescribing information that patients be monitored for blood pressure and pulse changes at 2 to 4 weeks after initiating the medication. If blood pressure is in the hyper-

TABLE 12.5

Incidence of Patient Withdrawals from Sibutramine Clinical Studies

COSTART Preferred Term	Overall Integrated Database			Long-Term Studies		
	Placebo (n = 2335)	Sibutramine (n = 4748)	P<	Placebo (n = 770)	Sibutramine (n = 1741	P<
Hypertension	0.6%	1.1%	0.21	0.6%	1.1%	0.21
Palpitations	0.04%	0.3%	0.02	0.0%	0.2%	0.22
Tachycardia	0.04%	0.5%	0.02	0.0%	0.6%	0.048
Vasodilation	0.0%	0.04%	0.32	0.0%	0.1%	0.48
Total	6.4%	8.9%		8.7%	9.0%	

Source: Adapted from Sharma, A.M., *Int. J. Obes. Relat. Metab. Disord.*, 25(Suppl 4):S20–23, 2001.

tensive range or pulse >100 beats per minute, the drug should be stopped. Less severe increases in blood pressure and heart rate should prompt consideration of dose reduction.

It has been suggested that the blood pressure effects of sibutramine are mitigated by greater weight loss (Sharma 2001). That is, with increasing amounts of weight loss, the blood pressure change may actually be a net decrease, albeit less than that observed with similar nonpharmacological weight loss. Thus, for an individual patient who has successfully achieved weight loss with sibutramine, the blood pressure may be reduced from baseline, although the reduction may not be as great as that associated with the same degree of weight lost without medications.

Another strategy to deal with the cardiostimulatory effects of sibutramine has been described by Berube–Parent (2001). In this intervention, an aerobic exercise program was added to a weight loss program that combined diet and 10 mg sibutramine. This small (*n* = 8 men) observational study should not be extrapolated to a larger, more diverse population. However, the study did show promise in terms of enhanced weight loss (10.7 kg in 12 weeks) and a benefit in mitigating the blood pressure and pulse side effects of sibutramine with the aerobic exercise component.

The mean increase in blood pressure and pulse is problematic on another level in addition to the tendency to cause clinically significant changes in some patients and represents a therapeutic dilemma when viewed from a population perspective. Weight loss is usually associated with beneficial effects on risk factors such as lipids, indices of glycemic control, waist circumference, and blood pressure. If sibutramine has mixed effects on risk factors — increasing resting blood pressure while producing decreases in cholesterol and improvement in other risk factors associated with weight reduction — how can the net result be judged? Indeed, a recent study has called into question the adversity of sibutramine's blood pressure effects.

Birkenfeld et al. (2002) conducted a double-blind crossover study in 11 healthy men and women comparing placebo to sibutramine effects on cardiovascular response to autonomic reflex tests. In these subjects, supine and upright blood pressure and pulse did indeed increase with sibutramine. These effects were abolished with metoprolol. However, the increase in blood pressure observed with the cold pressor test and in response to handgrip testing was attenuated with sibutramine, compared to placebo. These changes are illustrated graphically in Figure 12.8. Sibutramine was also associated with decreased levels of norepinephrine in the plasma while supine. The authors propose that sibutramine may have an inhibitory clonidine-like effect centrally and a peripheral stimulatory effect. These findings must be investigated further in obese hypertensive and obese nonhypertensive patients before definitive conclusions can be drawn regarding sibutramine's safety profile. Furthermore, ambulatory blood pressure monitoring of these types of individuals may provide additional helpful information regarding this important issue.

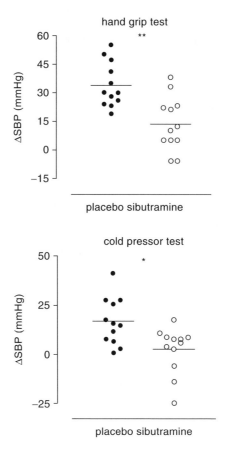

FIGURE 12.8
Individual changes in systolic blood pressure (SBP) after 3 min handgrip testing (top) and 1 min of cold pressor testing on placebo and on sibutramine. Sibutramine blunted response to handgrip and to cold pressor testing. $*p < .05$. $**P < .01$. (From Birkenfeld, A.L. et al., *Circulation*, 106:2459-2465, 2002.)

12.6 Predicting Response

Not all patients will experience weight loss with sibutramine. Therefore, it is important to recognize nonresponders and responders early, before prolonged exposure to an ineffective drug. A useful benchmark is "4 lb lost in 4 weeks" as a criterion for predicting ultimate successful weight loss. Figure 12.9 shows the chances of achieving ≥5% greater weight loss with sibutramine compared to placebo. Early weight loss (4 lb in the first 4 weeks) was predictive of success at 6 months for all doses (including placebo!). Another benchmark sometimes used is ≥5% weight loss in 3 months.

12.7 Role in Clinical Practice

The burden of managing obesity (30.5% of Americans in 1999 to 2000) (Flegal et al. 2002) and metabolic syndrome (24% of Americans in an analysis of the 1996 NHANES survey)

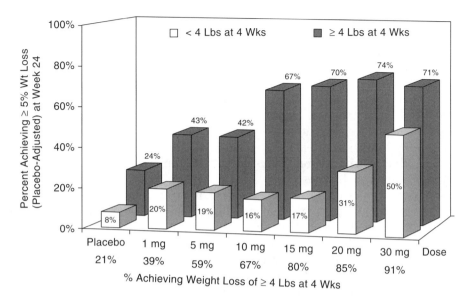

FIGURE 12.9
Weight loss at 24 weeks in patients losing more or less than 4 lb in the first 4 weeks of treatment. Because mean weight loss in the placebo group was 1.2%, 5% placebo-adjusted weight loss = 6.2% total weight loss. (From Bray, G.A. et al., *Obes Res*, 7:189–198, 1999.)

(Ford et al. 2002) can be daunting to physicians who are not adequately compensated for the time they take counseling for life-style change. Physicians can help patients lose weight and improve their health risk profile by judicious use of medications for obesity.

Medications can help by reinforcing the patient's intent to follow a behavioral (diet) approach. If sibutramine is prescribed with a reduced calorie diet plan, satiety will be aided, and the patient is more likely to comply with the plan. The studies discussed in this chapter demonstrate that when sibutramine is used with a more structured, portion-controlled diet plan, greater weight loss is more likely than when the drug is used with a less structured diet. If the patient is motivated and ready to embark on a program of life-style change, the physicians can "coach" him or her to the more successful diet plan. The physician should also coach the patient to set an achievable goal (5 to 10% weight loss in 6 months).

If the patient meets prescribing guidelines (BMI ≥30 or ≥27 with a comorbidity) and is motivated and ready to make reasonable lifestyle modifications, and if there are no con-traindications, sibutramine can be prescribed, starting at a dose of 10 mg daily. Then the patient should be seen at 4 weeks to check for safety, tolerability, and efficacy. At the 4-week visit, the physician will want to see 4 lb lost as a reasonable criterion to predict ultimate efficacy. The safety profile should also be acceptable. Two authors (Sharma 2001; Narkiewicz 2002) recommend following the summary of product characteristics for clinical management of blood pressure and pulse responses to sibutramine. That recommendation is to withdraw sibutramine treatment if, on two consecutive visits, systolic or diastolic blood pressure increases by >10 mmHg or >145/90, heart rate increases by >10 bpm, or progressive dyspnea, chest pain, or ankle edema is present. If any of these criteria is exceeded, sibutramine should be reduced or discontinued.

Of course, inadequate weight loss is also an indication to discontinue the drug. Patients should be followed monthly for the first 6 months and then at least every 6 months as long as the medication is continued. If tolerability issues arise, the dose can be reduced to 5 mg; if weight is regained, the dose can be increased to 15 mg. As long as weight maintenance continues and as long as blood pressure and pulse meet the preceding guidelines, sibutramine may be continued. If lack of efficacy appears with pronounced weight gain, if blood pressure or pulse exceeds the previous guidelines, or if other tolerability issues become problematic, then sibutramine should be discontinued.

Even though some studies have demonstrated long-term weight maintenance with medication (Weintrabu et al., 1992a–e), patients will often discontinue weight loss medications on their own, without seeking physician advice. Physicians should caution patients regarding the weight regain that occurs when sibutramine is discontinued. Because the nature of obesity is such that relapse is frequent, physicians need to counsel patients to seek medical advice early in a relapse cycle, rather than later, so that appropriate interventions can be discussed.

Obesity is a chronic, incurable condition. The primary care physician can help patients manage their conditions by acting as a coach in the patient's obesity management attempts. Physicians should take their prescribing responsibility seriously and address the patient's need for assistance in aiding behavioral weight loss approaches. Sibutramine plays a role in promoting satiety and in blunting the reduction of metabolic rate that occurs with weight loss. It can help selected patients achieve and maintain meaningful weight loss with the attendant improvement in certain obesity-related health risk factors. If a conservative approach is used, blood pressure elevation need not be a barrier to successful weight management with this drug.

12.8 Future Directions

A number of clinical trials are underway that will add to the knowledge base of sibutramine's clinical use. The AWESOME trial evaluates sibutramine's use in obese adolescents. It will include data on ambulatory blood pressure monitoring; left ventricular wall thickness by echocardiography; pharmacokinetics; body composition by dual emission x-ray absorptiometry; and quality of life measures. A 1-year study of sibutramine's use with a commercial meal replacement is underway.

There is also a 5-year randomized, double-blind, placebo-controlled study of 15 mg sibutramine used for up to 5 years. In this study, patients who have achieved 10% weight loss without pharmacotherapy assistance and maintained it for 6 months are randomized to placebo or 15 mg sibutramine and observed for 5 years. The Sibutramine Cardiovascular Outcomes Study (SCOUT) plans to enroll over 9000 obese or overweight patients with diabetes or existing cardiovascular risk factors. This double-blind, randomized, placebo-controlled multicenter study will have as its endpoint the time to first occurrence of a nonfatal myocardial infarction, nonfatal stroke, resuscitated cardiac arrest, or cardiovascular death. This study's "hard endpoint" is designed to address the issue of mixed risk factor response to sibutramine.

12.9 Conclusion

Sibutramine is a reuptake inhibitor of norepinephrine and serotonin that produces weight loss by a dual mechanism of action. It promotes satiety and reduces food intake while increasing thermogenesis and blunting the reduction in metabolic rate associated with weight loss. It has a favorable pharmacologic profile requiring dosing once daily, has no abuse potential, and is not associated with valvulopathy or primary pulmonary hypertension. The weight loss with sibutramine is dose related and at the recommended doses of 5 to 15 mg will produce 2 to 6% weight loss from baseline above that seen with placebo. By using stronger behavioral approaches with sibutramine, initial weight loss can approach 16% from baseline. Weight loss with sibutramine is associated with improvement in measures of metabolic control, lipids, uric acid, and quality of life.

The chief barrier to sibutramine's use is the elevation in mean resting blood pressure and heart rate that is observed in clinical trials. Although <5% of patients who take sibutramine require discontinuation for clinically significant blood pressure increases, concern over small mean blood pressure increases persists and is stimulating further study. Sibutramine is contraindicated with monoamine oxidase inhibitors, serotonergic agents, and noradrenergic agents. It should not be used in those with congestive heart failure, cardiac arrhythmias, and seizures and should be used with caution in those with other cardiovascular diseases. Clinical trials are underway to expand the clinical profile of this drug. To date, sibutramine has been demonstrated to be a useful tool in the clinical toolbox for obesity management.

References

Apfelbaum, M., Vague, P., Ziegler, O., Hanotin, C., Thomas, F. and Leutenegger, E. (1999) Long-term maintenance of weight loss after a very-low-calorie diet: a randomized blinded trial of the efficacy and tolerability of sibutramine, *Am. J. Med.*, 106:179–184.

Aronne, L.J. (2001) Treating obesity: a new target of prevention of coronary heart disease, *Prog. Cardiovasc. Nurs.*, 16(3):98–106, 115.

Bach, D.S., Rissanen, A.M., Mendel, C.M., Shepherd, G., Weinstein, S. and Kelly, F. (1999) Absence of cardiac valve dysfunction in obese patients treated with sibutramine, *Obes. Res.*, 7(4):363–369.

Birkenfeld, A.L., Schroeder, C., Boschmann, M., Tank, J., Franke, G., Luft, F.C., Biaggioni, I., Sharma, A.M. and Jordan, J. (2002) Paradoxical effect of sibutramine on autonomic cardiovascular regulation, *Circulation*, 106:2459–2465.

Berube–Parent, S., Prud'homme, D., St-Pierre, S., Doucet, E. and Tremblay, A. (2001) Obesity treatment with a progressive clinical tri-therapy combining sibutramine and a supervised diet — exercise intervention, *Int. J. Obes. Relat. Metab. Disord.*, 25(8):1144–1153.

Bray, G.A. (1991) Barriers to the treatment of obesity (editorial), *Ann. Int. Med.*, 115:152–153.

Bray, G.A. (1999) Uses and misuses of the new pharmacotherapy of obesity (editorial), *Ann. Med.*, 31:1–3.

Bray, G.A., Blackburn, G.L., Ferguson, J.M., Greenway, F.L., Jain, A.K., Mendel, C.M., Mendels, J., Ryan, D.H., Schwartz, S.L., Scheinbaum, M.L. and Seaton, T.B. (1999) Sibutramine produces dose-related weight loss, *Obes. Res.*, 7:189–198.

Bray, G.A., Ryan, D.H., Gordon, D., Heidingsfelder, S., Cerise, F. and Wilson, K. (1996) A double-blind randomized placebo-controlled trial of sibutramine, *Obes. Res.*, 4:263–270.

Calle, E., Thun, M.J., Petrelli, J.M., Rodriguez, C. and Heath, C.S. (1999) Body mass index and mortality in a prospective cohort of U.S. adults, *N. Engl. J. Med.*, 344:1097–1105.

Chapelot, D., Marmonier, C., Thomas, F. and Hanotin, C. (2000) Modalities of the food intake-reducing effect of sibutramine in humans, *Physiol. Behav.*, 68:299–308.

Cole, J.O., Levin, A., Beake, B., Kaiser, P.E. and Scheinbaum, M.L. (1998) Sibutramine: a new weight loss agent without evidence of the abuse potential associated with amphetamines, *J. Clin. Psychopharmacol.*, 18(3):231–236.

Connoley, I.P., Heal, D.J. and Stock, M.J. (1995) A study in rats of the effects of sibutramine on food intake and thermogenesis, *Br. J. Pharmacol.*, 114:388P.

Connolly, H.M., Crary, J.L., McGoon, M.D., Hensrud, D.D., Edwards, B.S., Edwards, W.D. and Schaff, H.V. (1997) Valvular heart disease associated with fenfluramine-phentermine, *N. Engl. J. Med.*, 337:581–588.

Cuellar, G.E.M., Ruiz, A.M., Monsalve, M.C.R. and Berber, A. (2000) Six-month treatment of obesity with sibutramine 15 mg/a double-blind, placebo-controlled monocenter clinical trial in a Hispanic population, *Obes. Res.*, 8(1):71–82.

Dujovne, C.A., Zavoral, J.H., Rowe, E. and Mendel, C.M. (2001) Effects of sibutramine on body weight and serum lipids: a double blind, randomized, placebo-controlled study in 322 over-weight and obese patients with dyslipidemia, *Am. Heart J.*, 142(3):489–497.

Fanghanel, G., Cortinas, L., Sanchez–Reyes, L. and Berber, A. (2001) Second phase of a double blind study clinical trial on sibutramine for the treatment of patients suffering essential obesity: 6 months after treatment cross-over, *Int. J. Obes. Relat. Metab. Disord.*, 25(5):741–747.

Finer, N., Bloom, S.R., Frost, G.S., Banks, L.M. and Griffiths, J. (2000) Sibutramine is effective for weight loss and diabetic control in obesity with type 2 diabetes: a randomised, double blind, placebo-controlled study, *Diabetes, Obesity Metab.*, 2:105–112.

Flegal, K.M., Carroll, M.D., Ogden, C. L. and Johnson C.L. (1998) Prevalence and trends in obesity among US adults, 1999–2000, *JAMA*, 288:1723–1727.

Ford, E.S., Giles, W.H. and Dietz, W.H. (2002) Prevalence of the metabolic syndrome among U.S. adults: findings from the third National Health and Nutrition Examination Survey, *JAMA*, 287:356–359.

Fujioka, K., Seaton, T.B., Rowe, E., Jelinek, C.A., Raskin, P., Lebovitz, H.E. and Weinstein, S.P. (2000) Weight loss with sibutramine improves glycaemic control and other metabolic parameters in obese patients with type 2 diabetes mellitus, *Diabetes Obes. Metab.*, 2:175–187.

Gokcel, A., Bumurdulu, Y., Karakose, H., Melek Ertorer, E., Tanaci, N., Bascil Tutuncu, N. and Guvener, N. (2002) Evaluation of the safety and efficacy of sibutramine, orlistat and metformin in the treatment of obesity, *Diabetes Obes. Metab.*, 4(1):49–55.

Gokcel, A., Karakose, H., Ertorer, E.M., Tanaci, N., Tutuncu, N.B. and Guvener, N. (2001) Effects of sibutramine in obese female subjects with type 2 diabetes and poor blood glucose control, *Diabetes Care*, 24(11):1957–1960.

Halpern A., Leite, C.C., Herszkowicz, N., Barbato, A., and Costa. A.P. (2002) Evaluation of efficacy, reliability, and tolerability of sibutramine in obese patients, with an echocardiographic study, *Rev. Hosp. Clin.*, 57(3):98–102.

Hansen, D.L., Toubro, S., Stock, M.J., Macdonald, I.A. and Astrup, A. (1998) Thermogenic effects of sibutramine in humans, *Am. J. Clin. Nutr.*, 6:1180–1186.

Hazenberg, B.P. (2000) Randomized, double-blind, placebo-controlled, multicenter study of sibutra-mine in obese hypertensive patients, *Cardiology*, 94:152–158.

Heal, D.J., Aspley, S., Prow, M.R., Jackson, H.C., Martin, K.F. and Cheetham, S.C. (1998) Sibutramine: a novel anti-obesity drug. A review of the pharmacological evidence to differentiate it from d-amphetamine and d-fenfluramine, *Int. J. Obes. Relat. Metab. Disord.*, 22(Suppl 1):S19–S28.

Hensrud, D.D., Connolly, H.M., Grogan, M., Miller, F.A., Bailey, K.R. and Jensen, M.D. (1999) Echocardiographic improvement over time after cessation of use of fenfluramine and phen-termine, *Mayo Clin. Proc.*, 74:1191–1197.

James, W.P.T., Astrup, A., Finer, N., Hilsted, J., Kopelman, P., Rossner, S., Saris, W.H. and Van Gaal, L.F. for the STORM Study Group. (2000) Effect of sibutramine on weight maintenance after weight loss: a randomised trial, *Lancet*, 356:2119–2125.

Jick, H. (2000) Heart valve disorders and appetite-suppressant drugs, *JAMA*, 283:1738–1740.

Kelly, F., Jones, S.P. and Lee, J.K. (1995) Sibutramine weight loss in depressed patients, *Int. J. Obes.*, 19(Suppl2):P397.

Krejs, G.J. (2002) Metabolic benefits associated with sibutramine therapy, *Int. J. Obes.*, 26(Suppl 4):S34-37.

Lean, M.E. (1997) Sibutramine — a review of clinical efficacy, *Int. J. Obes.*, 21:S30–36.

Luque, C.A. and Rey, J.A. (1999) Sibutramine: A serotonin-norepinephrine reuptake-inhibitor for the treatment of obesity, *Ann. Pharmacother.*, 33:968–978.

McMahon, F.G., Fujioka, K., Singh, B.N., Mendel, C.M., Rowe, E., Rolston, K., Johnson, F. and Mooradian, A.D. (2000) Efficacy and safety of sibutramine in obese white and African American patients with hypertension, *Arch. Intern. Med.*, 160:2185–2191.

McMahon, F.G., Weinstein, S.P., Rowe, E., Ernst, K.R., Johnson, F. and Fujioka, K. (2002) Sibutramine is safe and effective for weight loss in obese patients whose hypertension is well controlled with angiotensin-converting enzyme inhibitors, *J. Hum. Hypertens.*, 16(1):5–11.

Narkiewicz, K. (2002) Sibutramine and its cardiovascular profile, *Int. J. Obes.*, 26(4)S38–41.

National Center for Health Statistics (2000) www.cdc.gov/nchs/products/pubs/pubd/hestats/obese/obse99.htm.

National Institutes of Health. (2001) Third Report of the National Cholesterol Education Program Expert Panel on Detection, Evaluation, and Treatment of High Blood Cholesterol in Adults (Adult Treatment Panel III). Bethesda, Maryland: National Institutes of Health. NIH Publication 01-3670.

National Institutes of Health, National Heart, Lung, and Blood Institute. (1998) Clinical guidelines on the identification, evaluation, and treatment of overweight and obesity in adults — the evidence report, *Obes. Res.*, 6(Supplement 2):51S–210S.

National Institutes of Health, National Heart, Lung, and Blood Institute, North American Association for the Study of Obesity. (2000) *The Practical Guide: Identification, Evaluation, and Treatment of Overweight and Obesity in Adults.* NIH Publication Number 00-4084.

O'Meara, S., Riemsma, R., Shirran, L., Mather, L. and ter Reit, G. (2002) The clinical effectiveness of sibutramine in the management of obesity: a technology assessment, *Health Technol. Assess.*, 6:1–97.

Rolls, B.J., Shide, D.J., Thorwart, M.L. and Ulbrecht, J.S. (1998) Sibutramine reduces food intake in non-dieting women with obesity, *Obes. Res.*, 6:1–11.

Ryan D.H., Kaiser, P., and Bray, G.A. (1995) Sibutramine: A novel new agent for obesity treatment, *Obes. Res.*, 3(Suppl 4):553S-559S.

Samsa, G.P., Kolotkin, R.L., Williams, G.R., Nguyen, M.H. and Mendel, C.M. (2001) Effect of moderate weight loss on health-related quality of life: an analysis of combined data from 4 randomized trials of sibutramine vs. placebo, *Am. J. Manag. Care*, 7(9):875–883.

Serrano–Rios, M., Melchionda, N., Moreno–Carretero, E. (2002) Role of sibutramine in the treatment of obese Type 2 diabetic patients receiving sulphonylurea therapy, *Diabet. Med.*, 19(2):119–124.

Sharma, A.M. (2001) Sibutramine in overweight/obese hypertensive patients, *Int. J. Obes. Relat. Metab. Disord.*, 25(Suppl 4):S20–23.

Smith, I.G. and Goulder, M.A. (2001) Randomized placebo-controlled trial of long-term treatment with sibutramine in mild to moderate obesity, *J. Fam. Pract.*, 50(6):505–512.

Sramek, J.J., Leibowitz, M.T., Weinstein, S.P., Rowe, E.D., Mendel, C.M., Levy, B., McMahon, F.G., Mullican, W.S., Toth, P.D. and Cutler, N.R. (2002) Efficacy and safety of sibutramine for weight loss in obese patients with hypertension well controlled by beta-adrenergic blocking agents: a placebo-controlled, double-blind, randomised trial, *J. Hum. Hypertens.*, 16(1):13–19.

Stock, M.J. (1997) Sibutramine: a review of the pharmacology of a novel antiobesity agent, *Int. J. Obes.*, 21:S25–29.

Van Gaal, L.F., Wauters, M.A., Peiffer, F.W. and De Leeuw, I.H. (1998) Sibutramine and fat distribution: is there a role for pharmacotherapy in abdominal/visceral fat reduction? *Int. J. Obes. Relat. Metab. Disord.*, 22(Suppl 1):S38–40.

Wadden, T.A., Berkowitz, R.I., Sarwer, D.B., Prus–Wisniewski, R. and Steinberg, C. (2001) Benefits of lifestyle modification in the pharmacologic treatment of obesity, *Arch. Intern. Med.*, 161:218–227.

Walsh, K.M., Leen, E. and Lean, M.E.J. (1999) The effect of sibutramine on resting energy expenditure and adrenaline-induced thermogenesis in obese females, *Int. J. Obes. Rel. Met. Dis.*, 23(10):1009–1015.

Weintraub, M., Rubio, A., Golik, A., Bryne, L., Scheinbaum, L.L. (1991) Sibutramine in weight control: a dose-ranging, efficacy study, *Obes. Res.*, 3: 553–559.

Weintraub, M., Sundaresan, P.R., Madan, M., Schuster, B., Balder, A., Lasagna, L. and Cox, C. (1992a) Long-term weight control study. I (weeks 0 to 34). The enhancement of behavior modification, caloric restriction, and exercise by fenfluramine plus phentermine versus placebo, *Clin. Pharmacol. Ther.*, 51:586–594.

Weintraub, M., Sundaresan, P.R., Schuster, B., Ginsberg, G., Madan, M., Balder, A., Stein, E.C. and Byrne L. (1992b) Long-term weight control study. II (weeks 34 to 104). An open-label study of continuous fenfluramine plus phentermine versus targeted intermittent medication as adjuncts to behavior modification, caloric restriction, and exercise, *Clin. Pharmacol. Ther.,* 51:595–601.

Weintraub, M., Sundaresan, P.R., Schuster, B., Moscucci, M. and Stein, E.C. (1992c) Long-term weight control study. III (weeks 104 to 156). An open-label study of dose adjustment of fenfluramine and phentermine, *Clin. Pharmacol. Ther.,* 51:602–607.

Weintraub, M., Sundaresan, P.R., Schuster, B., Averbuch, M., Stein, E.C., Cox, C. and Byrne, L. (1992d) Long-term weight control study. IV (weeks 156 to 190). The second double-blind phase, *Clin. Pharmacol. Ther.,* 51:608–614.

Weintraub, M., Sundaresan, P.R., Schuster, B., Averbuch, M., Stein, E.C. and Byrne, L. (1992e) Long-term weight control study. V (weeks 190 to 120). Follow-up of participants after cessation of medication, *Clin. Pharmacol. Ther.,* 51:615–618.

Wesnes, K.A., Garratt, C., Wickens, M., Gudgeon, A. and Oliver, S. (2000) Effects of sibutramine alone and with alcohol on cognitive function in healthy volunteers, *Br. J. Clin. Pharmacol.,* 49(2):110–17.

Wirth, A. and Krause, J. (2001) Long-term weight loss with sibutramine, *JAMA,* 286(11):1331–1339.

Yanovski, S.Z. and Yanovski, J.A. (2002) Obesity, *N. Engl. J. Med.,* 346(8):591–602.

Zannad, F., Gille, B., Grentzinger, G., Bruntz, J-F., Hammadi, M., Boivin, J-M., Hanotin, C., Igau, B., and Drouin, B. (2002) Effects of sibutramine on ventricular dimensions and heart valves in obese patients during weight reduction, *Am. Heart J.,* 144:508–515.

13

Noradrenergic, Serotonergic, Antiepileptic, and Herbal Drugs

George A. Bray

CONTENTS

ABSTRACT   Drugs on the market to treat overweight individuals are limited. Sibutramine (Meridia or Reductil) and orlistat (Xenical) are the only drugs approved by the regulatory agencies in the U.S. and Europe. However, a number of other noradrenergic drugs (phentermine, diethylpropion, benzphetamine, and phendimetrazine) are approved only for short-term use in some countries. In the U.S., purchases of phentermine make it the most widely used of the drugs for treating obesity. Two other groups of drugs are also used. The first is the thermogenic combination of ephedrine and caffeine; the other is the over-the-counter drugs sold directly to the consumer. In terms of total sales, these eclipse all of the prescription items.

13.1   Introduction

Obesity is an important and growing problem. The prevalence of obesity has increased from 27.5 to 30.5% of the adult American population over a period of a few years. Because it is a stigmatized problem that causes great distress, a large market exists for agents that can help combat the problem. These range from diet foods and diet beverages to medical and surgical techniques. This chapter deals with some of the older drugs that have been used to treat obesity. The currently approved drugs for long-term use, orlistat and sibutramine, will be discussed in other chapters.

To put the problem in perspective, Table 13.1 lists expenditures for many antiobesity drugs currently on the market in the U.S. In the year 2000, sales of three of these older medications exceeded those of sibutramine and were only a little less than those of orlistat. Because these older medications are not protected by patents, their costs are low; thus, in terms of total usage, the numbers of these agents prescribed significantly exceeds those of orlistat and sibutramine combined. This chapter discusses these agents and tries to put the field of drug treatment into perspective.

TABLE 13.1

Expenditures for Weight Loss Drugs

| Antiobesity | Sales ($ Million) | | |
Medication	1999	2000	2001
Xenical	153	295	243
Meridia	127	116	166
Phentermine	52	69	120
Dexedrine	67	77	78
Didrex	8.3	8.8	8.4
Total	467.6	662.9	705.8

Source: Adapted from LaRosa, J., *Bariatrician* 2002, 17: 25–52.

Drug treatment for obesity has been tarnished by a number of unfortunate problems.[1] Since the introduction of thyroid hormone to treat obesity in 1893, almost every drug tried in obese patients has led to undesirable outcomes resulting in termination. Thus, caution must be used in accepting any new drug for treatment of obesity unless the safety profile would make it acceptable for almost everyone.

An additional serious negative aspect to the use of drug treatment for obesity is the negative halo spread by the addictive properties of amphetamine.[2] Amphetamine stands for alpha-methyl-phenethylamine. It is an addictive β-phenethylamine that reduces food intake. The addictiveness of amphetamine is probably related to its effects on dopaminergic neurotransmission. On the other hand, its anorectic effects appear to result from modulation of noradrenergic neurotransmission. Because amphetamine is addictive, other β-phenethylamine compounds were presumed to be addictive — whether addictive or not, they were guilty by association. This has led to restrictions on the use of this entire class of drugs by the U.S. Drug Enforcement Agency (DEA).

Drugs such as phentermine; diethylpropion; fenfluramine; sibutramine; and the antidepressant venlafaxine are β-phenethylamines. Phentermine and diethylpropion are sympathomimetic amines, like amphetamine, but differ from amphetamine in having little or no effect on dopamine release or reuptake at the synapse. Abuse of phentermine or diethylpropion is rare.[1] Fenfluramine, on the other hand, has no effect on reuptake or release of either norepinephrine or dopamine in the brain. Rather, it increases serotonin release and partially inhibits serotonin reuptake. Sibutramine, likewise, has no evident abuse potential. Thus, derivatives of β-phenethylamine have a wide range of pharmacological effects and highly variable potential for abuse. However, if examined uncritically, they all should be lumped with amphetamine and carry its negative halo. It is thus misleading to use "amphetamine-like" in reference to appetite suppressant β-phenethylamine drugs, except amphetamine and methamphetamine, because of negative linguistic images and inaccurate linguistic content.

A third issue surrounding drug treatment of obesity is the perception that the drugs are ineffective because patients regain weight when they are stopped.[3] Quite the contrary is true. Overweight is a chronic disease that has many causes and is rarely cured; treatment is thus aimed at palliation. Clinicians do not expect to cure such diseases as hypertension or hypercholesterolemia with medications, but rather to palliate them. When the medications for any of these diseases are discontinued, clinicians expect the disease to recur — medications only work when used. The same arguments apply to medications used to treat overweight — a chronic, incurable disease for which drugs work only when used.

Reports of valvular heart disease associated with the use of fenfluramine, dexfenfluramine, and phentermine have provided the most recent problem for drug treatment of obesity.[4] This is an example of the "law of unintended consequences." The report of valvulopathy in up to 35% of patients treated with a combination of fenfluramine and phentermine was totally unexpected. The finding, however, will add caution to any future drugs marketed to treat obesity and will provide support for those who believe drug treatment of obesity is inappropriate and risky.

The final issue is the plateau of weight that occurs with all treatments for obesity.[5–11] Figure 13.1 shows the weight loss that can be achieved by various treatments in relation to patients' expectations when they enter treatment. At the beginning of treatment, a weight loss of less than 15% is considered unsatisfactory by most patients.[12] Yet the reality is that none of the treatments, except gastric bypass,[11] reaches this level of effectiveness. When weight loss reaches a plateau, as it invariably does with all treatments, patients usually blame the treatment. The perceived loss of effectiveness often leads patients to terminate treatment with the inevitable slow regain of weight. Currently available medications are reviewed with these limitations in mind.

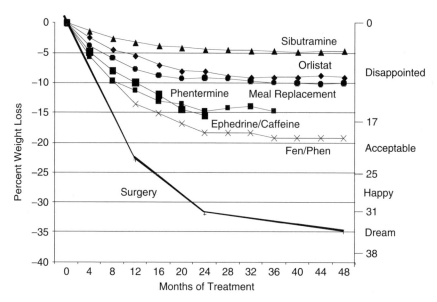

FIGURE 13.1
Relation of plateaued weight during treatment for obesity and participant expectations in a weight loss program. The left hand ordinate shows the percent weight loss for each treatment; the right hand ordinate shows the cut points for weight loss expectations for each category. Only surgical treatment[11] produced a "dream" level of weight loss. The combination of fenfluramine and phentermine[9] produced acceptable weight loss, but the other treatments, including ephedrine combined with caffeine,[10] phentermine,[8] meal replacement,[7] orlistat,[6] and sibutramine[5] left patients disappointed. (From Bray, G.A., 2001.)

13.2 Mechanisms for Drug Treatment of Obesity

Obesity results from an imbalance between energy intake and energy expenditure (EE). Drugs can shift this balance in a favorable way by reducing food intake, altering metabolism, and/or increasing EE. These three mechanisms will be used to classify the drugs used for treating obesity.[1,13]

13.2.1 Reducing Food Intake

13.2.1.1 Noradrenergic Receptors

A number of monoamines and neuropeptides are known to modulate food intake. Noradrenergic receptors and serotonergic receptors have served as sites for clinically useful drugs to decrease food intake[1,13] (Table 13.2). Activation of the α_1- and β_2-adrenoceptors decreases food intake.[14] On the other hand, stimulation of the α_2-adrenoceptor in experimental animals increases food intake. Direct agonists and drugs that release norepinephrine (NE) or block NE reuptake at the neuronal junction can activate one or more of these receptors, depending on where the NE is released.

Phenylpropanolamine is an α_1-agonist that decreases food intake by acting on α_1-adrenergic receptors in the paraventricular nucleus. The weight gain seen in patients treated with α_1-adrenergic antagonists for hypertension or prostatic hypertrophy indicates that the α_1-adrenoceptor is clinically important in regulation of body weight. Stimulation of the β_2-adrenoceptor by NE or agonists like terbutaline, clenbuterol, or salbutamol reduces

TABLE 13.2

Monoamine Mechanisms That Reduce Food Intake

Neurotransmitter System	Action Mechanism	Examples
Noradrenergic	α_1-Agonist	Phenylpropanolamine
	β_2-Agonist	Clenbuterol
	Stimulate NE release	Phentermine
	Block NE reuptake	Mazindol
Serotonergic	5-HT$_{1B}$ or 5-HT$_{2C}$ Agonist	Quipazine
	Stimulate 5-HT release	Fenfluramine
	Block 5-HT reuptake	Fluoxetine
Dopaminergic	D$_1$-Agonist	Apomorphine
Histaminergic	HT$_2$-Antagonist	Chlorpheniramine

food intake. The weight gain in patients treated with some β_2-adrenergic antagonists also indicates that this is a clinically important receptor for regulation of body weight.

13.2.1.2 Serotonergic Receptors

The serotonin receptor system consists of seven families of receptors. Stimulation of receptors in the hydroxytryptamine 5-HT$_1$ and 5-HT$_2$ families produces the major effects on feeding. Activation of the 5-HT$_{1A}$ receptor increases food intake; however, this acute effect is rapidly down-regulated and is not clinically significant in control of body weight. Activation of the 5-HT$_{2C}$, and possibly 5-HT$_{1B}$, receptors decreases food intake. Direct agonists such as quipazine or drugs that block serotonin reuptake, such as fluoxetine, sertraline, or fenfluramine, will reduce food intake by acting on these receptors or by providing the serotonin that modulates them.

13.2.2 Altering Metabolism

Excess fat is the visible sign of obesity. Metabolic strategies have been directed at preabsorptive and postabsorptive mechanisms for modifying fat, carbohydrate absorption, or metabolism. Preabsorptive mechanisms that influence digestion and absorption of macronutrients are the basis for orlistat, a drug that inhibits intestinal digestion of fat and lowers body weight. The second strategy is to affect intermediary metabolism. Enhancing lipolysis, inhibiting lipogenesis, and affecting fat distribution between subcutaneous and visceral sites are strategies that can be developed.[1,15]

13.2.3 Increasing Energy Expenditure

Increasing energy expenditure through exercise would be an ideal approach to treating obesity. Drugs that have the same physiological thermogenic consequences as exercise could provide a useful pharmaceutical alternative for treating this intractable problem.[1,15]

13.3 Drugs on the Market that Reduce Food Intake

Table 13.3 summarizes the effects of a number of drugs currently available in the U.S. for treating obesity.[1,16] They are discussed in more detail next.

TABLE 13.3

Prescription Drugs Currently Marketed for Treatment of Obesity

Drug Name	Trade Name(s)	Dosage	DEA Schedule	Cost/d	Side Effects and Comments
Pancreatic Lipase Inhibitor					
Orlistat	Xenical	120 mg tid before meals	None	$3.56/d	Daily vitamin pill in the evening; may interact with cyclosporine
Norepinephrine–Serotonin Reuptake Inhibitor					
Sibutramine	Meriedia; Reductil	5–15 mg/d	IV	$2.98 to $3.56/d	Raises blood pressure slightly; do not use with monoamine oxidase inhibitors; SSRIs (sumatriptan, dihydroergotamine, meperidine); methadon; pentazocine; fentanyl; lithium; tryptophan
Sympathomimetic Drugs					
Diethylpropion	Tenuate; Tepanil; Tenuate dospan	25 mg tid 25 mg tid 75 mg in AM	IV	$1.27 to $1.52/d	All sympathomimetic drugs are similar; do not use with monoamine oxidase inhibitors; guanethidine; alcohol; sibutramine; tricyclic antidepressants
Phentermine	Standard release: Adipex-P; Fastin; Obenix; Oby-Cap; Oby-Trim; Zantryl Slow release: Ionamin	18.75–37.5 mg/d tid (standard); 15–30 mg/d in A.M. (slow)	IV	$0.67 to $1.60/d (standard); $0.75 to $2.01/d (slow)	All sympathomimetic drugs are similar; do not use with monoamine oxidase inhibitors; guanethidine; alcohol; sibutramine; tricyclic antidepressants
Benzphetamine	Didrex	25–50 mg 1–3 times/d	III	$1.19 to $2.38/d	All sympathomimetic drugs are similar; do not use with monoamine oxidase inhibitors; guanethidine; alcohol; sibutramine; tricyclic antidepressants
Phendimetrazine	Standard release: Bontril PDM; Plegine; X-Trozine; Slow release: Bontril; Prelu-2; X-Trozine	35 mg tid before meals (standard); 105 mg/d in A.M. (slow)	III	$1.20 to $5.25/d	All sympathomimetic drugs are similar; do not use with monoamine oxidase inhibitors; guanethidine; alcohol; sibutramine; tricyclic antidepressants

13.3.1 Sympathomimetic Drugs Approved by the Food and Drug Administration to Treat Obesity

13.3.1.1 Pharmacology

The sympathomimetic drugs are grouped together because they can increase blood pressure and, in part, act like NE. Drugs in this group work by a variety of mechanisms, including the release of NE from synaptic granules (benzphetamine, phendimetrazine, phentermine, and diethylpropion); blockade of NE reuptake (mazindol); blockade of reuptake of NE and 5-HT (sibutramine); or direct action on α_1 adrenoceptors (phenylpropanolamine).

All of these drugs are absorbed orally and reach peak blood concentrations within a short time. The half-life in blood is also short for all except the metabolites of sibutramine, which have a long half-life.[1] The two metabolites of sibutramine are active, but this is not true for the metabolites of other drugs in this group. Liver metabolism inactivates a large fraction of these drugs before excretion. Side effects include dry mouth, constipation, and insomnia. Food intake is suppressed by delaying the onset of a meal or by producing early satiety. Sibutramine and mazindol (which has been removed from the market) increase thermogenesis.

13.3.1.2 Efficacy

The efficacy of an appetite-suppressing drug can be established through randomized double-blind clinical trials that show a significant weight loss of at least 5% in addition to that observed in the placebo group.[1] This is the basic criterion for approval by the U.S. Food and Drug Administration (FDA). A decrease in weight 10% below baseline and significantly greater than placebo is the major criterion for the European Committee on Proprietary Medicinal Products (CPMP). Clinical trials of sympathomimetic drugs carried out before 1975 were generally short term because it was widely believed that short-term treatment would "cure obesity."[1,17] This was unfounded optimism, but because the trials were of short duration and often crossover in design, they provided little long-term data. This review will focus on longer-term trials lasting 24 weeks or more and only those trials in which the control group is adequate.

Phentermine, Diethylpropion, Benzphetamine, and Phendimetrazine. Most of the data on these drugs comes from short-term trials that were often crossover in design. Table 13.4 provides a summary of the long-term clinical trials on the first generation of sympathomimetic drugs.[1,13,18–23] The best and one of the longest of these clinical trials lasted 36 weeks and compared placebo treatment against continuous phentermine or intermittent phentermine (Figure 13.2).[8] Continuous and intermittent phentermine therapy produced more weight loss than did placebo. In the drug-free periods, the patients treated intermittently slowed their weight loss only to lose more rapidly when the drug was reinstituted. Phentermine and diethylpropion are classified by the U.S. DEA as schedule IV drugs, and benzphetamine and phendimetrazine as schedule III drugs. This regulatory classification indicates the government's belief that they have the potential for abuse, although this potential appears to be very low. Phentermine and diethylpropion are only approved for a "few weeks," which is usually interpreted as up to 12 weeks. Weight loss with phentermine and diethylpropion persists for the duration of treatment, suggesting that tolerance does not develop to these drugs. If tolerance were to develop, the drugs would be expected to lose their effectiveness or require increased amounts of drug for patients to maintain weight loss. This does not occur.

Sibutramine. In contrast to the other sympathomimetic drugs, sibutramine has been extensively evaluated in several multicenter trials lasting 6 to 18 months. These are presented in detail in an earlier chapter.[5,24–38]

13.3.1.3 Safety

The side effect profile of the marketed sympathomimetic drugs is similar.[1] They produce insomnia, dry mouth, asthenia, and constipation. The safety of the older sympathomimetic appetite-suppressant drugs has been the subject of considerable controversy because dextroamphetamine is addictive. The sympathomimetic drugs phentermine, diethylpropion, benzphetamine, and phendimetrazine have very little abuse potential as assessed by the low rate of reinforcement when the drugs are self-injected intravenously to test animals.[1]

TABLE 13.4

Marketed Appetite Suppressants Other Than Sibutramine

Start Placebo	Start Drug	Complete Placebo	Complete Drug	mg/d	No. Weeks	Baseline Weight (kg) Placebo	Baseline Weight (kg) Drug	Weight Loss (kg) Placebo	Weight Loss (kg) Drug	Weight Loss (%) Placebo	Weight Loss (%) Drug	Comments	Ref
Diethylpropion													
16	16	6	5	75	52	78.8	80.7	−10.5	−8.9	−13.3	−11.0	Medication given on alternate months	Silverstone and Solomon, 1965
10	10	6	10	75	24	84.5	92.3	−2.5	−11.7	−2.8	−12.3		McKay, 1973
Phentermine													
36	36	25	17	30	36	92.3	94.1	−4.8	−12.2	−5.9	−15.0	Continuous Rx group (top) lost as much as intermittent therapy (bottom)	Munro et al., 1968
	36		22				97.3		−13.0		−16.0		
35	35	29	30	30	14	87.0	85.1	−1.8	−7.3	−2.1	−8.5	1000 kcal/d diet	Langlois et al., 1974
10	10	11	10	30	16	84.1	85.0	−2.9	−7.8	−3.4	−9.2	Obese diabetics	Gershberg et al., 1977
35	36	32	34	30	24	N/A	N/A	−1.5	−5.3	N/A	N/A	Obese diabetics; diet, biguanide, or insulin	Campbell et al., 1977
15	15	11	11	30	24	73.6	73.6	−4.5	−6.3	−9.2	−12.6	Elderly with osteoarthritis	Williams and Foulsham, 1981
20	20	10	14	30 (resin)	20	No baseline weights given	No baseline weights given	−4.4	−10.0			4-Arm trial: placebo; fenfluramine (F); phentermine (P); and F + P	Weintraub, 1992

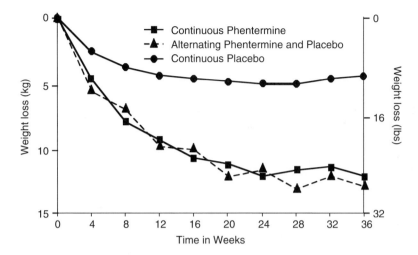

FIGURE 13.2

Comparison of weight loss with continuous and intermittent therapy using phentermine.[8] Overweight patients were randomized to receive placebo or one of two dosing regimens with phentermine. One regimen provided 15 mg/d each morning for 9 months and the other provided 15 mg/d for 1 month and then a month of no treatment.

In this same paradigm, neither phenylpropanolamine nor fenfluramine showed any reinforcing effects and no clinical data show any abuse potential for either of these drugs. Sibutramine, likewise, has no abuse potential, but it is nonetheless a schedule IV drug.

Sympathomimetic drugs can increase blood pressure. Phenylpropanolamine is an α_1-agonist and, at doses of 75 mg or more, it can increase blood pressure. Phenylpropanolamine has been associated with hemorrhagic stroke in women,[39] and the FDA has removed it from the market for weight loss and decongestant treatments. Phenylpropanolamine has also been reported in association with cardiomyopathy. Sibutramine increases blood pressure in normotensive patients[28] or prevents the fall that might have occurred with weight loss. These effects and related precautions are discussed in more detail in the chapter on sibutramine.

13.3.2 Sympathomimetic Drugs Not Approved by the FDA to Treat Obesity

Several other sympathomimetic agents carry warning labels (amphetamine and methamphetamine) or have never been approved by the FDA for treatment of obesity (fenproporex, chlobenzorex). In December, 2000, the FDA requested manufacturers of products such as cold remedies and weight loss drugs that contain phenylpropanolamine (PPA) to remove the PPA from these products because of its alleged relation to development of hemorrhagic strokes.[39]

13.3.3 Serotonergic Drugs (None Approved by the FDA to Treat Obesity)

No drugs working by this mechanism are currently approved by the FDA to treat obesity. Serotonergic drugs that act on specific serotonin receptors (5-HT$_{1B}$ or 5-HT$_{2C}$) reduce food intake and specifically reduce fat intake. Several drugs that influence serotonin release (fenfluramine and dexfenfluramine) or serotonin reuptake (fluoxetine and sertraline) have been used in obese patients. The clinical trial data are reviewed in detail elsewhere.[1] At

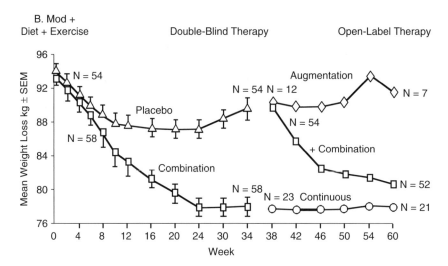

FIGURE 13.3
Effect of fenfluramine and phentermine on weight loss. This figure is the first year of the 4-year clinical trial of Weintraub. During the first 6 weeks, all patients received a single-blind treatment and a program of behavior modification, diet, and exercise (B Mod + Diet + Exercise). The left-hand part, from weeks 0 to 34, is the initial double-blind, placebo-controlled period. Following the initial 6 weeks, the patients were randomized to placebo or the combination therapy. Weight loss was significantly greater in those treated with the combination therapy and had reached a plateau by 24 weeks. After week 34, therapy was continued for those who responded (continuous group). Individuals treated with placebo were switched to the combination therapy and lost weight. Individuals who had not lost weight initially on the combination therapy received increased doses (augmentation), which failed to produce weight loss. (From Weintraub, M., *Clin. Pharmacol. Ther.* 1992, 51:581–585.)

present, no drug that acts on the serotonin receptor system directly or indirectly is approved for the treatment of obesity in the U.S.

13.3.4 Combining Serotonergic and Noradrenergic Drugs

13.3.4.1 *Efficacy*

Drugs that act on the noradrenergic or the serotonergic feeding system can reduce body weight. The possibility that combining a drug that acts on the serotonergic system with a drug that acts on the noradrenergic system was evaluated by Weintraub.[40] Such a combination might produce more weight loss and/or have fewer side effects if submaximal doses of one drug from each group were combined than if full doses of a single agent were used.[37] During the baseline run-in, patients received a program of behavior therapy, diet, and exercise that was demonstrably effective because they lost weight. When the patients were randomized, the drug-treated group lost 15.9% from baseline compared to the placebo-treated group that lost only 4.9% from baseline during the first 34 weeks. When the placebo-treated patients began active drug therapy in the open label period, they, too, lost weight, indicating that the drug was active. Some patients received long-term benefit by maintaining their weight at lower levels for up to 3.5 years during the time that the drug treatment was continued (Figure 13.3).

13.3.4.2 *Safety*

Following the report by Weintraub,[40] the combination of phentermine and fenfluramine to treat obesity spread rapidly. More than 18 million prescriptions were written in 1996 and an estimated 3 to 4 million people were treated with this drug combination. In July,

1997, 24 patients with a regurgitant type of valvular heart disease were reported to the medical profession.[41] In the three patients in whom histopathology of the heart valves was available, the valvular changes were similar to the changes seen in the carcinoid syndrome. Because early reports indicated that this valvulopathy might be present in more than 30% of treated patients, fenfluramine and dexfenfluramine were withdrawn from the market on September 15, 1997. A series of 233 patients, including 91 with echocardiograms done before treatment, have been followed in the author's institution[4] and many reports have been published from other institutions.[41] Of the patients in this series, 8% had preexisting lesions and 16.5% developed new lesions. With continued follow-up, some of the lesions have improved and a few have completely regressed.[4,42]

The current recommendations are that all symptomatic patients treated with fenfluramine or dexfenfluramine, alone or in combination with phentermine, have an echocardiogram. Because careful clinical examination fails to detect a murmur in more than half of the patients with documented regurgitant lesions, it would be prudent to do an echocardiogram on any patient who might need prophylactic antibiotics as recommended by the American Heart Association.

13.3.5 Drugs Marketed for Other Purposes That Produce Weight Loss in Controlled Trials

13.3.5.1 *Bupropion*

Bupropion is a drug approved by the FDA for treatment of depression. In a short-term clinical trial, it was found to reduce body weight, prompting a 6-month multicenter trial. In this trial, a dose-related decrease in body weight occurred.[43]

13.3.5.2 *Topiramate*

Topiramate is an anticonvulsant drug, approved for monotherapy and for combination with other antiepileptic drugs. It is a carbonic anhydrase inhibitor that also has effects on the $GABA_A$ receptor. In a placebo-controlled, double-blind, randomized dose-ranging clinical trial, it showed a mean percent weight loss from baseline to week 24 of –2.6% in placebo-treated patients vs. –5.0, –4.8, –6.3, and –6.3% in the 64-, 96-, 192-, and 384-mg/d topiramate groups, respectively. Greater percentages of topiramate-treated patients lost at least 5 or 10% of body weight compared with placebo. The most frequent adverse events were related to the central or peripheral nervous system, including paresthesia, somnolence, and difficulty with memory, concentration, and attention. Most events were dose related, occurred early in treatment, and usually resolved spontaneously; only 21% receiving topiramate withdrew due to adverse events compared with 11% on placebo. Thus, topiramate produced significantly greater weight loss than placebo at all doses.[44]

13.3.5.3 *Zonisamide*

Zonisamide is an antiepileptic drug that blocks sodium and calcium channels as well as affecting the activity of the dopaminergic and serotonergic neurotransmitter systems. It is approved by the FDA as an antieplipetic. In a 16-week randomized, double-blind, placebo-controlled trial, 51 of 60 patients completed the 16-week acute phase. The zonisamide-treated group lost more body weight than the placebo group — 5.9 ± 0.8 kg (6.0% loss) vs. 0.9 ± 0.4 kg (1.0% loss). Zonisamide was tolerated well, with few adverse effects. Thus, in one short-term, preliminary trial, zonisamide and a hypocaloric diet resulted in more weight loss than placebo and hypocaloric diet in the treatment of obesity.[45]

13.4   Drugs That Alter Metabolism

13.4.1   Drugs Approved by the U.S. FDA

13.4.1.1   Orlistat (Xenical®)

Orlistat is a potent selective inhibitor of pancreatic lipase that reduces intestinal digestion of fat. The drug has a dose-dependent effect on fecal fat loss, increasing it to about 30% of a diet that has 30% of energy as fat.[46] Orlistat has little effect in subjects eating a low-fat diet as might be anticipated from the mechanism by which this drug works.[46] A number of long-term clinical trials with orlistat lasting 6 months to 2 years have been published. They are described in detail in another chapter.

13.4.2   Drugs Approved by the U.S. FDA for Indications Other Than Obesity

13.4.2.1   Androgens and Androgen Antagonists

Dehydroepiandrosterone (DHEA) is a weak androgen that induces weight loss in several animal species. Clinical trials in humans have shown no effect.[1] In men, *testosterone* and the anabolic steroid oxandrolone have been reported to reduce visceral fat. A trial of an antiandrogen and nandrolone in women did not show any effects on visceral fat.[1]

13.5   Comparison of Available Drugs

Of the drugs discussed in this review, three, phentermine, orlistat, and sibutramine, are the most widely used in the U.S. and in other countries. The other drugs in the sympathomimetic category, benzphetamine, phendimetrazine, and diethylpropion, are less widely used and have less long-term information. Two other drugs in this category, mazindol and phenylpropanolamine, are no longer manufactured or are under a request from the FDA to be removed from diet-drug and cold preparations.

To provide a comparison of the three drugs that are available to the clinician, weight loss of the placebo and drug-treated groups has been plotted in Figure 13.4. All of the trials included in this figure lasted 6 months or more. The weight loss of the placebo group is at the beginning of the arrow on the right, and the weight loss of the drug-treated group at the tip of the arrowhead to the left. The length of the arrow is the magnitude of the difference between drug and placebo. In all of the studies plotted, the difference between the two groups was greater than 4 kg, except for one study with phentermine and one study with orlistat. Three trials with phentermine had weight losses exceeding 5 kg whereas most of the others were around 5 kg.

The effect size, expressed as the difference between the drug-treated and placebo-treated group in each study, is plotted in Figure 13.5. The weight loss of the phentermine and orlistat groups was greater than the sibutramine group, but so was the weight loss of the placebo-treated group. When the difference is plotted on the right side of each of the three groups, sibutramine and phentermine produced a similar amount of weight loss that was slightly greater than with orlistat.

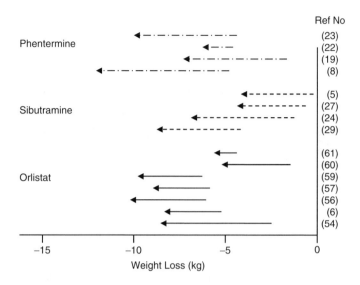

FIGURE 13.4
Effect sizes for three weight loss drugs. Each line is a separate study with phentermine, sibutramine, or orlistat. Reference to each study is in parentheses. The right-hand end of the arrow is the weight loss of the placebo-treated group and the tip of the arrow is the weight loss of the drug-treated group. (From Bray, G.A., 2001.)

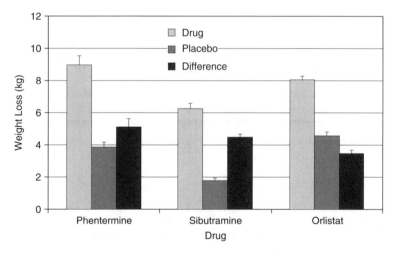

FIGURE 13.5
Effect size of weight loss. The drug effect, placebo effect, and the difference are plotted for the studies shown in Figure 13.4. (From Bray, G.A., 2001.)

13.6 Drugs That Increase Energy Expenditure

13.6.1 Drugs Approved by the U.S. FDA for Indications Other Than Obesity

13.6.1.1 *Ephedrine and Caffeine*

- *Pharmacology.* Ephedrine is a derivative of phenylpropanolamine and is used to relax bronchial smooth muscles in patients with asthma. It also stimulates ther-

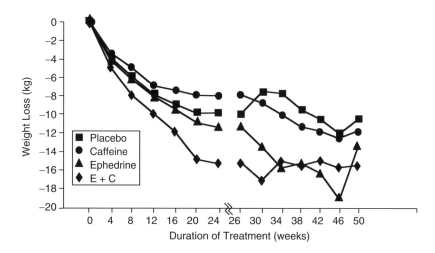

FIGURE 13.6
Effect of ephedrine and caffeine alone and in combination on weight loss. This figure combined the initial randomized, double-blind comparison of 20 mg ephedrine three times a day; 200 mg caffeine given 3 times a day; placebo; and a combination of ephedrine and caffeine. The combination produced significantly more weight loss than caffeine or ephedrine alone. When the patients who chose to continue were given the combination therapy during the second 6 months, they all reached the same weight. The symbols in the second half were continued from the first half to show the continuation of individual groups.

mogenesis in human subjects.[47] Caffeine is a xanthine that blocks adenosine receptors and inhibits phosphodiesterase. In experimental animals, the combination of ephedrine and caffeine reduces body weight, probably through stimulation of thermogenesis and reduction in food intake.

- *Efficacy.* One long-term placebo-controlled clinical trial treated 180 patients with ephedrine, caffeine, or the combination of ephedrine and caffeine.[10] Patients treated with the combination of ephedrine and caffeine lost more weight than did patients treated with ephedrine alone (Figure 13.6). In a 6-month open-label extension, subjects who completed the initial trial were offered additional treatment with ephedrine and caffeine. Nearly two thirds of the group opted for this treatment and were able to maintain their initial weight loss for the next 6 months. No other long-term data using ephedrine and caffeine are available. During controlled metabolic studies, patients treated with ephedrine and caffeine lost less lean tissue than did those in the placebo-treated group. Using the changes in body composition from these studies, Astrup and his colleagues have estimated the contribution of thermogenesis and food intake to the weight loss.[48] They concluded that 60 to 75% of the weight loss was due to a decrease in food intake and 25 to 40% was due to the thermogenic effects of ephedrine and caffeine.

- *Safety.* Although caffeine and ephedrine have a long record of clinical use separately, neither drug alone nor the combination is approved for treatment of obesity.

13.7 Herbal Preparations for Treatment of Obesity

Several different herbal preparations have been recommended for use in treating obesity. These include chromium picolinate; garcinia cambogia as a source of hydroxycitrate;

chitosan as a fiber source claiming to reduce fat absorption; and ma huang as a source of ephedra alkaloids with or without guarana as a source of caffeine. Clinically controlled trials with these agents are few; they do not carry FDA approval because the law allows them to be sold directly to the public over the counter.

- *Chromium picolinate.* There are no clinical trials in human subjects with chromium picolinate as a single agent that would allow evaluation of its effectiveness as a treatment for obesity.[1]
- *Garcinia cambogia.* A single randomized 3-month clinical trial with Garcinia cambogia as a source of hydroxycitrate has been published.[49] The herbal-treated group and the placebo group showed no difference in weight loss.
- *Chitosan.* A recent study has evaluated the effect of this material on fecal fat loss. Using human subjects in whom fecal fat samples were collected, Guerciolini et al.[50] showed that chitosan did not increase fecal fat loss. In a 4-week dietary study, chitosan or placebo was given to subjects randomly with no dietary advice. At the end of this time, no difference was found in weight loss between the two groups, suggesting that chitosan has no effect independent of a lower calorie diet.[51]
- *Ma huang and guarana.* This combination is among the most widely used over-the-counter preparations for weight loss. Two randomized, placebo-controlled clinical trials have been done with these herbal preparations, but the data have so far only appeared in abstract form. In an 8-week study with Metabolife 356,[52] the patients treated with the herbal preparation lost more weight and body fat, but the authors commented on the number of side effects and urged caution until longer studies were available. A second trial was presented in November 2000.[53] This was a 6-month trial comparing 90 mg of ephedra alkaloids from ma huang in three divided doses with 200 mg of guarana as a source of caffeine. The patients treated with the herbal medications again lost significantly more weight than the placebo-treated group. In this trial, Holter monitors were used to evaluate changes in cardiac rhythmicity at 1 week and 4 weeks of treatment. Compared to baseline, no significant changes took place in any of the cardiac parameters measured. Pulse rate increased 4 bpm from baseline in the groups treated with ephedra and guarana, but blood pressure did not change significantly.

A recent meta-analysis of safety data for ephedra and ephedrine concluded that "ephedrine and ephedra promote modest short-term weight loss in clinical trials. Use of ephedra or ephedrine and caffeine is associated with increased risk of psychiatric, autonomic, or gastrointestinal symptoms, and heart palpitations."[54]

13.8 Summary

At present only two drugs are approved for long-term treatment of obesity. Sibutramine inhibits the reuptake of serotonin and norepinephrine. In clinical trials, it produces a dose-dependent 5 to 10% decrease in body weight. Its side effects include dry mouth, insomnia, asthenia, and constipation. In addition, sibutramine produces a small increase in blood pressure and pulse contraindicative to its use in some individuals with heart disease.

Orlistat is the other drug approved for long-term use in the treatment of obesity. It works by blocking lipase and thus increasing the fecal loss of triglyceride. One valuable consequence of this mechanism of action is reduction of serum cholesterol averaging about 5% more than can be accounted for by weight loss alone. In clinical trials, it produces a 5 to 10% weight loss. Its side effects are entirely due to undigested fat in the intestine that can lead to increased frequency and change in the character of stools. It can also lower fat-soluble vitamins. The ingestion of a vitamin supplement before bedtime is a reasonable treatment strategy.

The effect on weight loss during long-term trials with these two drugs is shown in Figure 13.4 and Figure 13.5. Also in this figure are data on phentermine used in trials of 6 months or more. Although differences in mean weight losses with these drugs were found, when the placebo effect was taken into account they had a surprisingly similar magnitude of weight loss.

References

1. Bray, G.A. and Greenway, F.L. Current and potential drugs for treatment of obesity (review). *Endocr. Rev.* 1999; 20:805–875.
2. Weintraub, M. and Bray, G.A. Drug treatment of obesity (review). *Med. Clin. North. Am.* 1989; 73:237–249.
3. Bray, G.A. Obesity — a time-bomb to be defused. *Lancet* 1998; 352:160–161.
4. Ryan, D.H., Bray, G.A., Helmcke, F. et al. Serial echocardiographic and clinical evaluation of valvular regurgitation before, during, and after treatment with fenfluramine or dexfenfluramine and mazindol or phentermine. *Obes. Res.* 1999; 7:313–322.
5. McMahon, F.G., Fujioka, K., Singh, B.N., Mendel, C.M., Rowe, E., Rolston, K., Johnson, F. and Mooradian, A.D. Efficacy and safety of sibutramine in obese white and African–American patients with hypertension. *Arch. Int. Med.* 2000; 160:2185–2191.
6. Finer, N., James, W.P., Kopelman, P.G., Lean, M.E. and Williams, G. One-year treatment of obesity: a randomized, double-blind, placebo-controlled, multicentre study of orlistat, a gastrointestinal lipase inhibitor. *Int. J. Obes. Relat. Metab. Disord.* 2000; 24:306–313.
7. Flechtner–Mors, M., Ditschuneit, H.H., Johnson, T.D., Suchard, M.A. and Adler, G. Metabolic and weight loss effects of long-term dietary intervention in obese patients: four-year results. *Obes. Res.* 2000; 8:399–402.
8. Munro, J.F., MacCuish, A.C., Wilson, E.M. et al. Comparison of continuous and intermittent anorectic therapy in obesity. *Br. Med. J.* 1968; 1:352–354.
9. Greenway, F.L., Ryan, D.H., Bray, G.A., Rood, J.C., Tucker, E.W. and Smith, S.R. Pharmaceutical cost savings of treating obesity with weight loss medications. *Obes. Res.* 1999; 7:523–531.
10. Astrup, A., Breum, L., Tourbro, S. et al. The effect and satiety of an ephedrine/caffeine compound compared to ephedrine, caffeine and placeo in obese subjects on an energy restricted diet. A double blind trial. *Int. J. Obes.* 1992; 16:260–277.
11. Sjostrom, C.D., Lissner, L., Wedel, H. and Sjostrom, L. Reduction in incidence of diabetes, hypertension and lipid disturbances after intentional weight loss induced by bariatric surgery: the SOS Intervention Study. *Obes. Res.* 1999; 7:477–484.
12. Foster, G.D., Wadden, T.A., Vogt, R.A. et al. What is a reasonable weight loss? Patients' expectations and evaluations of obesity treatment outcomes. *J. Consult. Clin. Psychol.* 1997; 65:79–85.
13. Bray, G.A. Evaluation of drugs for treating obesity (review). *Obes. Res.* 1995; 3 Suppl 4:425S–434S.
14. Tsujii, S. and Bray, G.A. Food intake of lean and obese Zucker rats following ventricular infusions of adrenergic agonists. *Brain Res.* 1992; 587:226–232.
15. Bray, G.A. and Tartaglia, L.A. Medicinal strategies in the treatment of obesity (review). *Nature* 2000; 404(6778):672–677.
16. National Task Force Prevention and Treatment of Obesity. Long-term pharmacotherapy in the management of obesity (review). *JAMA* 1996; 276:1907–1915.

17. Scoville, B. Review of amphetamine-like drugs by the Food and Drug Administration: clinical data and value judgments. In: *Obesity in Perspective.* Washington: Department of Health, Education, and Welfare, Publication no. 75–708, 1975; 441–443.

18. Silverstone, J.J. and Solomon T. The long-term management of obesity in general practice. *Br. J. Clin. Pract.* 1965; 19:395–398.

19. McKay, R.H.G. Long-term use of diethylpropion in obesity. *Curr. Med. Res. Opin.* 1973; 1:489–493.

20. Langlois, K.J., Forbes, J.A., Bell, G.W. and Grant, G.F., Jr. A double-blind clinical evaluation of the safety and efficacy of phentermine hydrochloride (Fastin) in the treatment of exogenous obesity. *Curr. Ther. Res.* 1974; 16:289–296.

21. Gershberg, H., Kane, R., Hulse, M. and Pensgen, E. Effects of diet and an anorectic drug (phentermine resin) in obese diabetics. *Curr. Ther. Res.* 1977; 22:814–820.

22. Campbell, C.J., Bhalla, I.P., Steel, J.M. and Duncan, L.J.P. A controlled trial of phentermine in obese diabetic patients. *Practitioner* 1977; 218:851–855.

23. Williams, R.A. and Foulsham, B.M. Weight reduction in osteoarthritis using phentermine. *Practitioner* 1981; 225:231–232.

24. Weintraub, M., Rubio, A., Golik, A., Byrne, L. and Scheinbaum, M.L. Sibutramine in weight control: a dose-ranging, efficacy study. *Clin. Pharmacol. Ther.* 1991; 50:330–337.

25. Jones, S.P., Smith, I.G., Kelly, F. and Gray, J.A. Long-term weight loss with sibutramine. *Int. J. Obes.* 1995; 19(Suppl 2):40.

26. Bray, G.A., Ryan, D.H., Gordon, D., Heidingsfelder, S., Cerise, F. and Wilson, K. 1996 A double-blind randomized placebo-controlled trial of sibutramine. *Obes. Res.* 1996; 4:263–270.

27. Hanotin, C., Thomas, F., Jones, S.P., Leutenegger, E. and Drouin, P. Efficacy and tolerability of sibutramine in obese patients: a dose-ranging study. *Int. J. Obes. Relat. Metab. Disord.* 1998; 22:32–58.

28. Bray, G.A., Blackburn, G.L., Ferguson, J.M., Greenway, F.L., Jain, A.K., Mendel, C.M., Mendels, C.M., Mendels, J., Ryan, D., Schwartz, S.L., Scheinbaum, M.L. and Seaton, T.B. Sibutramine produces dose-related weight loss. *Obes. Res.* 1999; 7:189–198.

29. Apfelbaum, M., Vague, P., Ziegler, O., Hanotin, C., Thomas, F. and Leutenegger, E. Long-term maintenance of weight loss after a very-low-calorie diet: a randomized blinded trial of the efficacy and tolerability of sibutramine. *Am. J. Med.* 1999; 106:179–184.

30. Fanghanel, G., Cortinas, L., Sanchez–Reyes, L. and Berber, A. A clinical trial of the use of sibutramine for the treatment of patients suffering essential obesity. *Int. J. Obes.* 2000; 24:144–150.

31. James, W.P.T., Astrup, A., Finer, N., Hilsted, J., Kopelman, P., Rossner, S., Saris, W.H.M. and van Gaal, L., for the STORM study group. Effect of sibutramine on weight maintenance after weight loss: a randomized trial. *Lancet* 2000; 356:2119–2125.

32. McMahon, F.G., Weinstein, S.P., Rowe, E., Ernst, K.R., Johnson, F. and Fujioka, K. Sibutramine is safe and effective for weight loss in obese patients whose hypertension is well controlled with angiotensin-converting enzyme inhibitors. *J. Hum. Hypertens.* 2002; 16:5–11.

33. Sramek, J.J., Seiowitz, M.T., Weinstein, S.P., Rowe, E.D., Mendel, C.M., Levy, B., McMahon, F.G., Mullican, W.S., Toth, P.D. and Cutler, N.R. Efficacy and safety of sibutramine for weight loss in obese patients with hypertension well controlled by β-adrenergic blocking agents: a placebo-controlled, double-blind, randomized trial. *Am. J. Hypertension* 2002; 16:13–19.

34. Finer, N., Bloom, S.R., Frost, G.S., Banks, L.M. and Griffiths, J. Sibutramine is effective for weight loss and diabetic control in obesity with type 2 diabetes: a randomised, double-blind placebo-controlled study. *Diab. Obes. Metab.* 2000; 2:105–112.

35. Fujioka, K., Seaton, T.B., Rowe, E., Jelinek, C.A., Raskin, P., Lebovitz, H.E., Weinstein, S.P. and the Sibutramine/Diabetes clinical study group. Weight loss with sibutramine improves glycemic control and other metabolic parameters in obese type 2 diabetes mellitus. *Diab. Obes. Metab.* 2000; 2:1–13.

36. Gockel, A., Karakose, H., Ertorer, E.M., Tanaci, N., Tutuncu, N.B. and Guvener, N. Effects of sibutramine in obese female subjects with type 2 diabetes and poor blood glucose control. *Diabetes Care* 2001; 24:1957–1960.

37. Wadden, R.A., Berkowitz, R.I., Sarwer, D.B., Prus–Wisniewski, R. and Steinberg, C.M. Benefits of lifestyle modification in the pharmacologic treatment of obesity: a randomized trial. *Arch. Intern. Med.* 2001; 161:218–227.
38. Wirth, A. and Krause, J. Long-term weight loss with sibutramine: a randomized controlled trial. *JAMA* 2001; 286:1331–1339.
39. Kernan, W.N., Viscoli, C.M., Brass, L.M., Broderick, J.P., Brott, T., Feldmann, E., Morgenstern, L.B., Wilterdink, J.L. and Horwitz, R.I. Phenylpropanolamine and the risk of hemorrhagic stroke. *N. Engl. J. Med.* 2000; 343(25):1826–1832.
40. Weintraub, M. Long term weight control: the National Heart, Lung, and Blood Institute funded multimodal intervention study. *Clin. Pharmacol. Ther.* 1992; 51:581–585.
41. Connolly, H.M., Crary, J.L., McGoon, M.D. et al. Valvular heart disease associated with fen-fluramine–phentermine. *N. Engl. J. Med.* 1997; 337:581–588.
42. Mast, S.T., Jollis, J.G., Ryan, T., Anstrom, K.J. and Crary, J.L. The progression of fenflu-ramine–associated valvular heart disease assessed by echocardiography. *Ann. Intern. Med.* 2001; 134:261–266.
43. Anderson, J.W., Greenway, F.L. Fujioka, K., Gadde, K.M., McKenney, J. and O'Neil, P.M. Bupropion SR significantly enhances weight loss: a 24-week double-blind, placebo-controlled trial with placebo group randomzed to bupropion SR during 24-week extension. *Obes. Res.* 2002; 10:633–641.
44. Bray, G.A., Hollander, P., Klein, S., Kushner, R., Levy, B., Fitchet, M. and Perry, B.H. A 6-month randomized, placebo-controlled, dose-ranging trial of topiramate for weight loss in obesity. *Obes. Res.* 2003 Jun; 11(6):722–733.
45. Gadde, K.M., Franciscy, D.M., Wagner, H.R., II and Krishnan, K.R. Zonisamide for weight loss in obese adults: a randomized controlled trial. *JAMA* 2003 Apr 9; 289(14):1820–1825.
46. Hauptmann, J.B., Jeunet, F.S. and Hartmann, D. Initial studies in humans with the novel gastrointestinal lipase inhibitor Ro18-0647 (tetrahydrolipstatin). *Am. J. Clin. Nutr.* 1992; 5:309S–313S.
47. Astrup, A., Bulow, J., Madsen, J. and Christensen, N.J. Contribution of BAT and skeletal muscle to thermogenesis induced by ephedrine in man. *Am. J. Physiol.* 1985; 248(5 Pt 1):E507–E515.
48. Astrup, A., Breum, L. and Toubro, S. Pharmacological and clinical studies of ephedrine and other thermogenic agonists (review). *Obes. Res.* 1995; 3 Suppl 4:537S–540S.
49. Heymsfield, S.B., Allison, D.B., Vasselli, J.R., Pietrobelli, A., Greenfield, D. and Nunez, C. Garcinia cambogia (hydroxycitric acid) as a potential antiobesity agent: a randomized con-trolled trial. *JAMA* 1998; 280:1596–1600.
50. Guerciolini, R., Radu–Radulescu, L., Boldrin, M. and Moore, R. Fecal fat excretion induced by treatment with orlistat or chitosan: A 3-week randomized crossover design study. *Obes. Res.* 2000; 8(Suppl 1):43S.
51. Pittler, M.H., Abbot, N.C., Harkness, E.F. and Ernst, E. Randomized, double-blind trial of chitosan for body weight reduction. *Eur. J. Clin. Nutr.* 1999; 53(5):379–381.
52. Boozer, C.N., Nasser, J.A., Heymsfield, S.B., Wang, V., Chen, G. and Solomon, J.L. An herbal supplement containing Ma Huang–Guarana for weight loss: a randomized, double-blind trial. *Int. J. Obes. Relat. Metab. Disord.* 2001; 25:316–324.
53. Boozer, C.N., Daly, P.A., Blanchard, D., Nasser, J.A., Solomon, J.L. and Homel, P. Herbal ephedra/caffeine for weight loss: a 6-month safety and efficacy trial. *Int. J. Obes. Metab. Disorders* 2002; 26:593–604.
54. Shekelle, P.G., Hardy, M.L., Morton, S.C., Maglione, M., Mojica, W.A., Suttorp, M.J., Rhodes, S.L., Jungvig, L. and Gagne, J. Efficacy and safety of ephedra and ephedrine for weight loss and athletic performance: a meta-analysis. *JAMA* 2003 Mar 26; 289(12):1537–1545.
55. LaRosa, J. 2002 outlook for the U.S. weight loss market, *Bariatrician* 2002; 17:25–52.

14

Adverse Effects and Drug–Drug Interactions

Stephan Krähenbühl

CONTENTS

ABSTRACT Drugs currently used most frequently for weight reduction include noradrenaline liberators and/or reuptake inhibitors and lipase inhibitors. The serotonin reuptake inhibitors fenfluramine and dexfenfluramine, which had been used widely, have been withdrawn from the market in many countries due to pulmonary hypertension and valvular heart disease. The use of amphetamine and derivatives as anorectic drugs is decreasing due to their dose-dependent, cardiovascular and cerebral toxicity, and their abuse potential. Sibutramine is a prodrug that acts as a powerful noradrenaline reuptake inhibitor after N-demethylation by cytochrome P450 3A4 (CYP3A4). Dose-dependent adverse effects of this drug include increased heart rate and increased blood pressure. So far, valvular heart disease has not been described in patients using this drug. Possible interacting drugs include inhibitors of CYP3A4 (inhibition of sibutramine activation); serotonin reuptake inhibitors (possible serotonin syndrome); and monoamine oxidase inhibitors and yohimbine, which may increase systemic blood pressure. Orlistat is a specific, irreversible lipase inhibitor of which only 1% reaches systemic circulation. Gastrointestinal adverse effects are frequent, but can be minimized by ingesting a fat-reduced diet. Other adverse effects include a decrease in the serum concentration of some fat-soluble vitamins and hepatotoxicity, for which some case reports have been published. Orlistat can decrease the blood concentration of cyclosporine due to interference with the intestinal absorption of this drug and should therefore not be administered to patients

TABLE 14.1

Drugs Used for Weight Reduction

Noradrenaline Releasing Agents and/or Reuptake Inhibitors

Amphetamine derivatives
    Dexamphetamine (not approved by FDA)
    Diethylpropion (approved by FDA)
Mazindol (approved by FDA)
Phentermine (approved by FDA)
Phenylpropanolamine (d,l-Norephedrine) (not approved by FDA)
d-Norpseudoephedrine (cathine) (not approved by FDA)
Sibutramine (approved by FDA, also inhibits reuptake of serotonin and dopamine)

Serotonin Reuptake Inhibitors

Fenfluramine (not approved by FDA)
Dexfenfluramine (not approved by FDA)

Lipase Inhibitors

Orlistat (approved by FDA)

---

treated with cyclosporine. Further research is necessary for the development of efficient and safe anorectic drugs.

14.1 Introduction

Considering the increase in the proportion of obese persons in Western countries, safe drugs leading to a significant decrease in body weight would be highly beneficial and welcome (Korner and Aronne, 2003). So far, this goal has not been achieved. Drugs currently used for this purpose are listed in Table 14.1. This chapter will discuss their safety profiles, including adverse reactions, drug–drug interactions, and potential for abuse.

14.2 Drugs Associated with Noradrenaline Release and/or Inhibition of Noradrenaline Reuptake

14.2.1 Amphetamine Derivatives

Dexamphetamine (dextroamphetamine) and diethylpropion have marked stimulant effects on the central nervous system (CNS). Dexamphetamine is therefore used primarily to treat patients with narcolepsy or the attention-deficit/hyperactivity disorder. More recently, dexamphetamine has also been studied in patients with stroke (Martinsson and Wahlgren, 2003) and in patients with chronic fatigue syndrome (Olson et al., 2003).

Amphetamine derivatives suppress appetite (Rogers and Blundell, 1979) and can therefore be used for weight loss in obese patients. The site of action is probably the feeding center in the hypothalamus. Because of rapid development of tolerance for the appetite suppressing action of amphetamine, the beneficial effect of amphetamine derivatives in weight reduction is doubtful. Dexamphetamine is partially metabolized in the liver (oxidative deamination and ring hydroxylation). In the urine, 50% of the drug is excreted nonmetabolized; excretion is enhanced when the urine is acidic.

Acute toxicity from dexamphetamine is most often due to overdosage, resulting in central and cardiovascular toxicity and mental alterations. Central effects include restlessness; tremor; hyperactive reflexes; insomnia; fever; and euphoria. Cardiovascular toxicity includes palpitations; cardiac arrhythmias; hypertension; angina pectoris symptoms; and finally collapse. Common mental alterations are increased aggressiveness; anxiety; delirium; and hallucinations. Gastrointestinal symptoms are also predominant, including dry mouth; metallic taste; abdominal cramps; and diarrhea. Overdosage can result in convulsions and coma, often due to cerebral hemorrhage (Delaney and Estes, 1980; Salanova and Taubner, 1984).

Besides these predictable (type A) reactions, idiosyncratic (type B) adverse reactions have also been described. Very rarely, patients ingesting high doses of dexamphetamine can develop rhabdomyolysis with renal failure (Scandling and Spital, 1982). Interstitial nephritis with renal failure has also been described in the absence of rhabdomyolysis (Foley et al., 1984). There are reports of cardiomyopathy in the literature, but pulmonary hypertension has not been reported (Smith et al., 1976; Call et al., 1982).

Amphetamines are abused due to their euphoriant effects. Although tolerance can develop to central effects, amphetamines are not associated with significant physical dependence. Regarding dexamphetamine, the literature contains some reports of pharmacodynamic, but not pharmacokinetic, drug–drug interactions. Hydroxylation of dexamphetamine is probably performed by CYP2D6 in humans (Bach et al., 1999b), but the literature offers no reports of increased action or toxicity of dexamphetamine in the presence of CYP2D6 inhibitors (e.g., quinidine) or in slow metabolizers of CYP2D6. In patients with refractory depression, the combination of dexamphetamine and monoamine oxidase inhibitors has been used and described to be safe (Fawcett et al., 1991). Nevertheless, due to the possibility of developing a hypertensive crisis, such combinations should be avoided. Because amphetamine derivatives can induce symptoms of mania in humans, the effect of lithium or neuroleptics has been investigated in such situations. In normal volunteers treated with amphetamine derivatives, neither lithium (Silverstone et al., 1998) nor pimozide (Brauer and De Wit, 1997) was able to alter manic symptoms, suggesting that the biochemical mechanisms for mania are different between dexamphetamine and patients with bipolar disorders.

14.2.2 Mazindol

Besides its use as an anorectic drug, mazindol has been investigated in patients with narcolepsy (Shindler et al., 1985; Alvarez et al., 1991) and, due to its inhibitory effect on dopamine reuptake, in patients with Parkinson's disease (Delwaide et al., 1983). Dose-dependent adverse effects of mazindol are mainly cardiovascular, similar to those of dexamphetamine. One case reported testicular pain after ingestion of mazindol in several individuals, representing a possible idiosyncratic reaction to this drug (McEwen and Meyboom, 1983).

Considering drug–drug interactions, there was one report of a probable pharmacokinetic interaction in a woman treated with lithium. She developed lithium toxicity shortly after starting the ingestion of mazindol (Hendy et al., 1980). The mechanism of this interaction is not clear. Interestingly, mazindol has been proposed as a treatment for suppressing craving in cocaine abusers (Berger et al., 1989). Based on studies in rodents that showed a pharmacodynamic interaction between mazindol and cocaine leading to convulsions and death (Jaffe et al., 1989), this combination should be avoided in humans.

14.2.3   d-Norpseudoephedrine (Cathine)

d-Norpseudoephedrine is the main alkaloid in the leaves of *catha edulis* and is therefore also called cathine. Most of the drug is eliminated nonmetabolized in the urine. Although the drug is generally considered to be safe and is used widely in European countries a considerable number of cases report severe adverse effects. Such adverse effects include

- Severe headache; hypertensive crises associated with intracranial hemorrhage; seizures; and death (Arauz et al., 2003; Morgenstern et al., 2003; La Grenade et al., 2001; Hamilton and Sharieff; 2000; Kernan et al., 2000)
- Cardiac arrhythmias; myocardial infarction; and cardiopulmonary arrest (Ooster-baan and Burns, 2000)
- Psychotic episodes (Marshall and Douglas, 1994; Goodhue et al., 2000; Dewsnap and Libby, 1992)
- Rhabdomyolysis and acute tubular necrosis (Kasamatsu et al., 1998)
- Fulminant liver failure (Favreau et al., 2002)

In addition, a chronic dyskinetic syndrome (spasmodic torticollis and cranial dystonia) has been described in two patients ingesting the drug (Thiel and Dressler, 1994). These symptoms persisted even after cessation of the intake of d-norpseudoephedrine.

Because the drug is not metabolized, no pharmacokinetic interactions take place. Pharmacodynamic interactions are identical with those described for dexamphetamine. Tolerance has been reported in patients ingesting d-norpseudoephedrine, but physical dependence does not seem to occur (Woolverton, 1986).

14.2.4   Phentermine

Dose-dependent adverse effects are similar to those of dexamphetamine. In an open study assessing the effect of phentermine on weight reduction in 50 obese women over 20 weeks, 34 patients finished the study, achieving a mean weight reduction of 6.7 kg (Douglas et al., 1983). Seven patients had to be withdrawn from the study due to adverse effects. Of these, three had disabling, intractable headache, representing a severe adverse effect of this drug. Occasionally, patients may develop urticaria. Interactions and abuse potential are similar to those described for dexamphetamine.

14.2.5   Phenylpropanolamine (d,l-Norephedrine)

Phenylpropanolamine is an indirect sympathomimetic agent that exerts only a minor stimulatory effect on the CNS and is used primarily for symptomatic treatment of nasal congestion. Less frequently, it is used for short-term reduction of body weight, but it is not approved for this indication by the FDA. The majority of the drug is excreted unchanged by the kidneys.

D,l-norephedrine shows a similar spectrum of adverse effects as d-norpseudoephedrine, but they may be less frequent (Lake et al., 1990). Due to the risk of hemorrhagic stroke in young individuals, the FDA has issued a public warning about the risk of this drug and has asked manufacturers of over-the-counter preparations containing d,l-norephedrine to stop marketing them (SoRelle, 2000). Subsequently, the drug was also withdrawn from the market in other countries (Figueras and Laporte, 2002). Other toxicities are rare, but cutaneous reactions have been described (Heikkila et al., 2000).

Because the drug is not metabolized, no pharmacokinetic interactions take place. Pharmacodynamic interactions are identical with those described for dexamphetamine. In contrast to the other amphetamine derivatives, if used at therapeutic dosages, phenylpropanolamine has not been associated with the development of addiction (Griffiths et al., 1978; Williams, 1990).

14.2.6 Sibutramine

Sibutramine is a monoamine reuptake inhibitor showing powerful activity *in vivo*, but only a weak activity *in vitro*. The drug is a tertiary amine metabolized primarily through N-demethylation by cytochrome P450 (CYP) 3A4. The secondary and primary amine metabolites of sibutramine are potent noradrenaline reuptake inhibitors (approximately 10 times more potent for noradrenaline than for dopamine or serotonin), thus explaining the weak activity of sibutramine *in vitro* (Nisoli and Carruba, 2000). Because the demethylated metabolites of sibutramine are primarily reuptake inhibitors of noradrenaline (to a lesser extent also for serotonin and dopamine), the pharmacological action and the spectrum of adverse effects are different from the serotonin reuptake inhibitors fenfluramine and dexfenfluramine.

Sibutramine is associated with a decrease in body weight by inducing satiety (Rolls et al., 1998) and by stimulating thermogenesis (Connoley et al., 1999). The recommended dose is 10 to 15 mg per day in a single dose in the morning. The effect of sibutramine on body weight has been shown in several double-blind, randomized studies (Rolls et al., 1998; Wirth and Krause, 2001; Dujovne et al., 2001) and is of a similar magnitude to the one observed with dexfenfluramine (Nisoli and Carruba, 2000).

The adverse effects reported most often are headache, constipation, and nausea, followed by dizziness, xerostomia, and insomnia (>5% of patients treated) (Bray et al., 1999; Nisoli and Carruba, 2000) (see Table 14.2). Single doses up to 75 mg appear to be well tolerated, as well as 20 mg/day for up to 6 weeks. Dose-dependent effects observed include tachycardia (increase of 6 to 13 beats per minute) and palpitations (Sramek et al., 2002; Nisoli

TABLE 14.2

Adverse Effects and Drug Interactions of Sibutramine

Adverse Effects

General: headache (30%)
Heart and circulation: tachycardia; flush; hypertension; palpitations (5%)
Gastrointestinal: anorexia (13%); obstipation (12%); emesis (6%); increased appetite (9%)
Central nervous system: xerostomia (17%); insomnia (11%); dizziness (7%); nervosity (5%)
Skin: rash (5%)
Case reports: interstitial nephritis; glomerulonephritis; thrombocytopenia; seizures

Possible Drug Interactions

CYP3A4 inhibitors: decreased N-demethylation of sibutramine and norsibutramine (clinical significance uncertain)
CYP3A4 inducers: increased production of active metabolites (clinical effect possibly increased)
Monoamine oxidase inhibitors: increased noradrenergic and/or serotoninergic activity (risk for hypertensive crisis and/or serotonin syndrome)
Selective serotonin reuptake inhibitors (SSRI): risk for serotonin syndrome

Source: From Sramek et al., 2002; Nisoli and Carruba, 2000; Benazzi, 2002.

and Carruba, 2000). These events led to drug withdrawal in 0.3 to 0.4% of patients treated in controlled studies. In addition, doses of 10 mg/day or more are associated with an increase in systolic and/or diastolic blood pressure of about 2 mmHg (Sramek et al., 2002; Nisoli and Carruba, 2000). In obese patients treated with sibutramine, this adverse effect may be offset by the positive effect of weight reduction on blood pressure (Narkiewicz, 2002). Nevertheless, pulse rate and blood pressure should be monitored in patients treated with this drug. Sibutramine should not be used in patients with uncontrolled arterial hypertension or coronary heart disease. Controlled studies show, however, that sibutramine can be used safely in obese patients when blood pressure is controlled by β-blockers (Sramek et al., 2002) or ACE-inhibitors (McMahon et al., 2002).

Because fenfluramine and dexfenfluramine have been withdrawn from the market due to associations with valvulopathies, heart anatomy and function have been studied in detail in patients treated with sibutramine. In a placebo-controlled study, patients treated with sibutramine (n = 133) or with placebo (n = 77) were investigated by transthoracic echocardiographic imaging for the presence of valvular heart disease. After treatment for 7.7 months, valvular defects were found in 2.3% in the sibutramine group and 2.6% in the placebo group (Bach et al., 1999a), suggesting that sibutramine does not affect cardiac valves. This may be explained by the fact that sibutramine and its metabolites have no high affinity for cardiac $5-HT_{2B}$ receptors, which appear to be activated by norfenfluramine (Fitzgerald et al., 2000). Further studies are necessary, however, to be sure that sibutramine has no effect on cardiac structure and function.

Because sibutramine is a prodrug activated by N-demethylation via CYP3A4, it is evident that CYP3A4 inhibitors (e.g., ketoconazole, itraconazole, and fluconazole; macrolide antibiotics [except azithromycin]; verapamil; and diltiazem) should be avoided in patients treated with this drug because they could decrease the pharmacological effects of sibutramine. However, so far no reports of such interactions are found in the literature.

Although inhibition of serotonin reuptake is not the primary mechanism of action of sibutramine, the combination with serotoninergic drugs such as selective serotonin reuptake inhibitors (SSRI) should be avoided, due to possible development of a serotonin syndrome. A patient with a possible serotonin syndrome who ingested sibutramine and citalopram has recently been described (Benazzi, 2002). Similarly, the combination of sibutramine with monoamine oxidase inhibitors may lead to an increase of noradrenaline in the synaptic cleft, possibly resulting in hypertensive crises (Nisoli and Carruba, 2000). Sibutramine should also not be combined with other drugs increasing the noradrenaline concentration in the synaptic cleft, e.g., amphetamine and derivatives; ephedrine and derivatives; mazindol; phentermine; and phenylpropanolamine.

An interesting possibility for an interaction has been proposed recently with yohimbine, a drug that may also be used for weight control (Jordan and Sharma, 2003). Sibutramine increases the noradrenaline concentration in the brain, decreasing satiety but also stimulating cerebral α_2-receptors and thereby attenuating the cerebral output of the sympathetic nervous system (clonidine-like effect). Yohimbine is an inhibitor of cerebral α_2-receptors, possibly leading to a strong increase in peripheral sympathetic activity in patients treated with sibutramine and potentially leading to cardiac arrhythmias and/or hypertensive crises. This combination should therefore be avoided.

According to studies in rats (Heal et al., 1992) and in humans (Cole et al., 1998), sibutramine has no abuse potential. The abuse potential of sibutramine was investigated in recreational users of stimulant drugs using the validated addiction research center inventory (ARCI) scale (Cole et al., 1998). In this double-blind study, 20 mg sibutramine was indistinguishable from placebo, whereas the abuse potential of amphetamine (positive control) could be demonstrated.

14.3 Serotonin Reuptake Inhibitors

14.3.1 Fenfluramine and Dexfenfluramine

Fenfluramine and dexfenfluramine (d-fenfluramine) have been withdrawn from the market due to the development of pulmonary hypertension and valvular heart defects. These drugs are indirect serotoninergic agents, stimulating the release of serotonin and inhibiting its reuptake, thus resulting in increased serotonin concentrations in the CNS. In contrast to amphetamine, they suppressed activity of the CNS.

The association between intake of these drugs and development of pulmonary hypertension has been described in detail. Pulmonary hypertension could be reversible or irreversible, in this case eventually with fatal outcome (Abenhaim et al., 1996; McMurray et al., 1986). Because case reports and case series suggested that the risk of developing pulmonary hypertension was increased with the length of treatment and repetitive treatment, most countries allowed no longer than 3 months of treatment.

Shortly after the risk for pulmonary hypertension had been recognized, a series of 24 cases was published suggesting a risk for the development of valvular heart disease in patients treated with the combination fenfluramine–phentermine (Connolly et al., 1997). Subsequently, more cases with valvular heart disease using these drugs were published (Khan et al., 1998; Jick et al., 1998; Weissman et al., 1998); all were treated with the combination but not with phentermine alone. These publications eventually led to the worldwide withdrawal of fenfluramine and dexfenfluramine.

14.4 Lipase Inhibitors

14.4.1 Orlistat

Orlistat is a naturally occurring lipase inhibitor produced by *Streptomyces toxytricini* (Guerciolini, 1997). This drug forms a covalent bond with the serine residue at the active site of gastric and pancreatic lipases, leading to a reduction in fat absorption of about 30%. Other intestinal enzymes, e.g., amylase, pepsin, trypsin, chymotrypsin, and phospholipases, are not inhibited. Approximately 1% of orlistat reaches systemic circulation, thus rendering dose-dependent systemic adverse reactions and systemic lipase inhibition very unlikely.

The effect of orlistat on body weight has been demonstrated in several placebo-controlled clinical trials (Ballinger and Peikin, 2002). The usual dose of orlistat is 120 mg before or during each meal. Obese patients treated for 12 months with orlistat and a fat-reduced (hypocaloric) diet lose 2 to 5 kg more weight than obese patients treated with placebo and hypocaloric diet. After discontinuation of the hypocaloric diet, orlistat reduces weight regain of body weight (Ballinger and Peikin, 2002; Davidson et al., 1999; Sjostrom et al., 1998).

The safety of orlistat has not been established for treatments lasting longer than 2 years. As expected from the mode of action, patients ingesting orlistat have dose- and diet-dependent gastrointestinal adverse effects (see Table 14.3). In clinical trials, most patients had one to two gastrointestinal events such as increased defecation; soft stools; abdominal pain; fatty evacuation; and flatulence (Ballinger and Peikin, 2002; Sjostrom et al., 1998; McNeely and Benfield, 1998). These symptoms are usually mildly to moderately intense and tend to resolve spontaneously. In clinical trials, orlistat had to be withdrawn due to

TABLE 14.3

Adverse Effects and Drug Interactions of Orlistat

Adverse Effects

Gastrointestinal: discharge of oily liquid (27%); flatulence with fecal incontinence (24%); abdominal pain (20%);
  oily and fatty feces (20%); increased frequency of defecation (11%); fecal incontinence (8%). These adverse
  effects are dependent on the intake of fat, which should not be more than 30% of the calories ingested.
Case reports: hepatocellular and/or cholestatic liver injury; hepatic failure; effects on the skin (vasculitis, rash,
  urticaria, and angioedema)

Drug Interactions

Decreased intestinal absorption of vitamin A (β-carotene), vitamin D; and vitamin K
Decreased absorption of cyclosporine

Source: From McNeely and Benfield, 1998; Ballinger and Peitkin, 2002; Persson et al., 2000.

adverse effects in 1.1 to 6% of the patients. This figure is in the same range as for patients treated with placebo, where the drop-out rate was 0.6 to 1.3% (Ballinger and Peikin, 2002).

Weight loss is usually associated with a decrease in blood pressure, which is also true for orlistat. In some case reports, however, individual patients treated with orlistat experienced an increase in blood pressure (Persson et al., 2000). The mechanism for this adverse effect is not clear.

Cholecystokinin is an important gastrointestinal hormone for gallbladder emptying. Because the release of cholecystokinin from the small intestine is dependent on the presence of intestinal long-chain fatty acids, orlistat might decrease gallbladder emptying and thereby increase the risk for gallstone formation. In a double-blind, placebo-controlled trial, obese patients ingesting a hypocaloric diet were treated with orlistat (3 × 120 mg/day) or with placebo for 4 weeks (Trouillot et al., 2001). At the end of the treatment period, the biliary phospholipid and bile salt concentrations were decreased in the placebo group; no differences were detectable between the two groups regarding biliary cholesterol concentration, presence of sludge in the bile, or gallbladder motility. However, the safety of orlistat regarding longer treatment periods has so far not been investigated.

Because orlistat affects intestinal absorption of fatty acids, lipid-soluble vitamins (A, D, E, K, and β-carotene) may also be affected (Ballinger and Peikin, 2002). In a study by Sjöström et al. (1998), 11.9% of the patients in the orlistat group and 5.3% of the patients in the placebo group had low serum vitamin levels at two or more occasions during the first year of the study. Davidson et al. (1999) found that lipid-soluble vitamins had to be replaced in 14.1% of patients treated with orlistat, compared to 6.5% of patients treated with placebo, over a treatment period of 2 years. In a recent study, in patients with daily ingestion of multivitamin preparation, serum levels of lipid soluble vitamins were determined after 3 to 6 months of treatment with orlistat (McDuffie et al., 2002). Although the serum levels of vitamins A and E remained unchanged, the levels for vitamin K and D dropped significantly, suggesting that monitoring vitamin D levels might be necessary in patients receiving a long-term treatment with this drug. Vitamin supplementation should be performed 2 h after orlistat administration, ideally in the evening before sleep.

Dose-independent systemic toxicity of orlistat is rare, with some reports of hypersensitivity (vasculitis, rash, urticaria, and angioedema) (Ballinger and Peikin, 2002; Gonzalez–Gay et al., 2002). Orlistat may affect liver function, as evidenced by patients developing cholestatic (Kim et al., 2002) or hepatocellular (Lau and Chan, 2002; Montero et al., 2001) liver injury. One patient developed subacute hepatic failure while being treated with orlistat as the only drug and had to receive a transplant (Montero et al., 2001). It is important to realize, however, that obesity is a risk factor for hepatic steatosis and steatohepatitis, which are associated with increased serum transaminase activity (Meier et al., 2002). Therefore, increased transaminases in patients treated with orlistat do not necessarily reflect drug toxicity.

Regarding drug–drug interactions, orlistat may interfere with the absorption of lipophilic drugs, as described earlier for lipophilic vitamins. A large pharmacokinetic study has shown that, with the exception of cyclosporine, orlistat does not interfere with drugs commonly used in this population (amitriptyline, atorvastatin, losartan, metformin, phentermine, sibutramine) (Zhi et al., 2002). As revealed by two case reports, orlistat can decrease markedly the intestinal absorption of cyclosporine, leading to very low cyclosporine blood concentrations with the potential for organ rejection in patients who have received transplants (Nagele et al., 1999; Evans et al., 2003). Orlistat should therefore be avoided in patients treated with cyclosporine.

Because orlistat can interfere with intestinal absorption of vitamin K, the coagulation parameters should be monitored closely in patients treated with oral anticoagulants (MacWalter et al., 2003). Similarly, as discussed before, vitamin D serum levels should be checked in patients receiving long-term treatment with orlistat (McDuffie et al., 2002).

14.5 Conclusions

The two drugs currently used most often for weight reduction are sibutramine and orlistat. Regarding their limited long-term effectiveness and adverse effects, neither represents the ideal drug for weight reduction. Further research is therefore necessary to find new pharmacological treatments of obesity.

References

Abenhaim, L., Moride, Y., Brenot, F., Rich, S., Benichou, J., Kurz, X., Higenbottam, T., Oakley, C., Wouters, E., Aubier, M., Simonneau, G. and Begaud, B. (1996) Appetite-suppressant drugs and the risk of primary pulmonary hypertension. International Primary Pulmonary Hypertension Study Group. *N. Engl. J. Med.*, 335, 609–616.

Alvarez, B., Dahlitz, M., Grimshaw, J. and Parkes, J.D. (1991) Mazindol in long-term treatment of narcolepsy. *Lancet*, 337, 1293–1294.

Arauz, A., Velasquez, L., Cantu, C., Nader, J., Lopez, M., Murillo, L. and Aburto, Y. (2003) Phenylpropanolamine and intracranial hemorrhage risk in a Mexican population. *Cerebrovasc. Dis.*, 15, 210–214.

Bach, D.S., Rissanen, A.M., Mendel, C.M., Shepherd, G., Weinstein, S.P., Kelly, F., Seaton, T.B., Patel, B., Pekkarinen, T.A. and Armstrong, W.F. (1999a) Absence of cardiac valve dysfunction in obese patients treated with sibutramine. *Obes. Res.*, 7, 363–369.

Bach, M.V., Coutts, R.T. and Baker, G.B. (1999b) Involvement of CYP2D6 in the in vitro metabolism of amphetamine, two N-alkylamphetamines and their 4-methoxylated derivatives. *Xenobiotica*, 29, 719–732.

Ballinger, A. and Peikin, S.R. (2002) Orlistat: its current status as an anti-obesity drug. *Eur. J. Pharmacol.*, 440, 109–107.

Benazzi, F. (2002) Organic hypomania secondary to sibutramine-citalopram interaction. *J. Clin. Psychiatry.*, 63, 165.

Berger, P., Gawin, F. and Kosten, T.R. (1989) Treatment of cocaine abuse with mazindol. *Lancet*, 1, 283.

Brauer, L.H. and De Wit, H. (1997) High dose pimozide does not block amphetamine-induced euphoria in normal volunteers. *Pharmacol. Biochem. Behav.*, 56, 265–272.

Bray, G.A., Blackburn, G.L., Ferguson, J.M., Greenway, F.L., Jain, A.K., Mendel, C.M., Mendels, J., Ryan, D.H., Schwartz, S.L., Scheinbaum, M.L. and Seaton, T.B. (1999) Sibutramine produces dose-related weight loss. *Obes. Res.*, 7, 189–198.

Call, T.D., Hartneck, J., Dickinson, W.A., Hartman, C.W. and Bartel, A.G. (1982) Acute cardiomyopathy secondary to intravenous amphetamine abuse. *Ann. Intern. Med.*, 97, 559–560.

Cole, J.O., Levin, A., Beake, B., Kaiser, P.E. and Scheinbaum, M.L. (1998) Sibutramine: a new weight loss agent without evidence of the abuse potential associated with amphetamines. *J. Clin. Psychopharmacol.*, 18, 231–236.

Connoley, I.P., Liu, Y.L., Frost, I., Reckless, I.P., Heal, D.J. and Stock, M.J. (1999) Thermogenic effects of sibutramine and its metabolites. *Br. J. Pharmacol.*, 126, 1487–1495.

Connolly, H.M., Crary, J.L., McGoon, M.D., Hensrud, D.D., Edwards, B.S., Edwards, W.D. and Schaff, H.V. (1997) Valvular heart disease associated with fenfluramine-phentermine. *N. Engl. J. Med.*, 337, 581–588.

Davidson, M.H., Hauptman, J., DiGirolamo, M., Foreyt, J.P., Halsted, C.H., Heber, D., Heimburger, D.C., Lucas, C.P., Robbins, D.C., Chung, J. and Heymsfield, S.B. (1999) Weight control and risk factor reduction in obese subjects treated for 2 years with orlistat: a randomized controlled trial. *JAMA*, 281, 235–242.

Delaney, P. and Estes, M. (1980) Intracranial hemorrhage with amphetamine abuse. *Neurology*, 30, 1125–1128.

Delwaide, P.J., Martinelli, P. and Schoenen, J. (1983) Mazindol in the treatment of Parkinson's disease. *Arch. Neurol.*, 40, 788–790.

Dewsnap, P. and Libby, G. (1992) A case of affective psychosis after routine use of proprietary cold remedy containing phenylpropanolamine. *Hum. Exp. Toxicol.*, 11, 295–296.

Douglas, A., Douglas, J.G., Robertson, C.E. and Munro, J.F. (1983) Plasma phentermine levels, weight loss and side-effects. *Int. J. Obes.*, 7, 591–595.

Dujovne, C.A., Zavoral, J.H., Rowe, E. and Mendel, C.M. (2001) Effects of sibutramine on body weight and serum lipids: a double-blind, randomized, placebo-controlled study in 322 overweight and obese patients with dyslipidemia. *Am. Heart J.*, 142, 489–497.

Evans, S., Michael, R., Wells, H., Maclean, D., Gordon, I., Taylor, J. and Goldsmith, D. (2003) Drug interaction in a renal transplant patient: cyclosporin-Neoral and orlistat. *Am. J. Kidney Dis.*, 41, 493–496.

Favreau, J.T., Ryu, M.L., Braunstein, G., Orshansky, G., Park, S.S., Coody, G.L., Love, L.A. and Fong, T.L. (2002) Severe hepatotoxicity associated with the dietary supplement LipoKinetix. *Ann. Intern. Med.*, 136, 590–595.

Fawcett, J., Kravitz, H.M., Zajecka, J.M. and Schaff, M.R. (1991) CNS stimulant potentiation of monoamine oxidase inhibitors in treatment-refractory depression. *J. Clin. Psychopharmacol.*, 11, 127–132.

Figueras, A. and Laporte, J.R. (2002) Regulatory decisions in a globalised world: the domino effect of phenylpropanolamine withdrawal in Latin America. *Drug Saf.*, 25, 689–693.

Fitzgerald, L.W., Burn, T.C., Brown, B.S., Patterson, J.P., Corjay, M.H., Valentine, P.A., Sun, J.H., Link, J.R., Abbazade, I., Hollis, J.M., Largent, B.L., Hartig, P.R., Hollis, G.F., Meunier, P.C., Robichaud, A.J. and Robertson, D.W. (2000) Possible role of valvular serotonin 5-HT(2B) receptors in the cardiopathy associated with fenfluramine. *Mol. Pharmacol.*, 57, 75–81.

Foley, R.J., Kapatkin, K., Verani, R. and Weinman, E.J. (1984) Amphetamine-induced acute renal failure. *South Med. J.*, 77, 258–260.

Gonzalez–Gay, M.A., Garcia–Porrua, C., Lueiro, M. and Fernandez, M.L. (2002) Orlistat-induced cutaneous leukocytoclastic vasculitis. *Arthritis Rheum.*, 47, 567.

Goodhue, A., Bartel, R.L. and Smith, N.B. (2000) Exacerbation of psychosis by phenylpropanolamine. *Am. J. Psychiatry*, 157, 1021–1022.

Griffiths, R.R., Brady, J.V. and Snell, J.D. (1978) Relationship between anorectic and reinforcing properties of appetite suppresant drugs: implications for assessment of abuse liability. *Biol. Psychiatry*, 13, 283–290.

Guerciolini, R. (1997) Mode of action of orlistat. *Int. J. Obes. Relat. Metab. Disord.*, 21 Suppl 3, S12–23.

Hamilton, R.S. and Sharieff, G. (2000) Phenylpropanolamine-associated intracranial hemorrhage in an infant. *Am. J. Emerg. Med.*, 18, 343–345.

Heal, D.J., Frankland, A.T., Gosden, J., Hutchins, L.J., Prow, M.R., Luscombe, G.P. and Buckett, W.R. (1992) A comparison of the effects of sibutramine hydrochloride, bupropion and methamphetamine on dopaminergic function: evidence that dopamine is not a pharmacological target for sibutramine. *Psychopharmacology* (Berl), 107, 303–309.

Heikkila, H., Kariniemi, A.L. and Stubb, S. (2000) Fixed drug eruption due to phenylpropanolamine hydrochloride. *Br. J. Dermatol.*, 142, 845–847.

Hendy, M.S., Dove, A.F. and Arblaster, P.G. (1980) Mazindol-induced lithium toxicity. *Br. Med. J.*, 280, 684–685.

Jaffe, J.H., Witkin, J.M., Goldberg, S.R. and Katz, J.L. (1989) Potential toxic interactions of cocaine and mazindol. *Lancet*, 2, 111.

Jick, H., Vasilakis, C., Weinrauch, L.A., Meier, C.R., Jick, S.S. and Derby, L.E. (1998) A population-based study of appetite-suppressant drugs and the risk of cardiac-valve regurgitation. *N. Engl. J. Med.*, 339, 719–724.

Jordan, J. and Sharma, A.M. (2003) Potential for subutramine-yohimbine interaction? *Lancet*, 361, 1826.

Kasamatsu, Y., Osada, M., Ashida, K., Azukari, K., Yoshioka, K. and Ohsawa, A. (1998) Rhabdomyolysis after infection and taking a cold medicine in a patient who was susceptible to malignant hyperthermia. *Intern. Med.*, 37, 169–173.

Kernan, W.N., Viscoli, C.M., Brass, L.M., Broderick, J.P., Brott, T., Feldmann, E., Morgenstern, L.B., Wilterdink, J.L. and Horwitz, R.I. (2000) Phenylpropanolamine and the risk of hermorrhagic stroke. *N. Engl. J. Med.*, 343, 1826–1832.

Khan, M.A., Herzog, C.A., St Peter, J.V., Hartley, G.G., Madlon–Kay, R., Dick, C.D., Asinger, R.W. and Vessey, J.T. (1998) The prevalence of cardiac valvular insufficiency assessed by transthoracic echocardiography in obese patients treated with appetite-suppressant drugs. *N. Engl. J. Med.*, 339, 713–718.

Kim, D.H., Lee, E.H., Hwang, J.C., Jeung, J.H., Kim do, H., Cheong, J.Y., Cho, S.W. and Kim, Y.B. (2002) A case of acute cholestatic hepatitis associated with Orlistat. *Taehan Kan Hakhoe Chi*, 8, 317–320.

Korner, J. and Aronne, L.J. (2003) The emerging science of body weight regulation and its impact on obesity treatment. *J. Clin. Invest.*, 111, 565–570.

La Grenade, L., Graham, D.J. and Nourjah, P. (2001) Underreporting of hemorrhagic stroke associated with phenylpropanolamine. *JAMA*, 286, 3081.

Lake, C.R., Gallant, S., Masson, E. and Miller, P. (1990) Adverse drug effects attributed to phenylpropanolamine: a review of 142 case reports. *Am. J. Med.*, 89, 195–208.

Lau, G. and Chan, C.L. (2002) Massive hepatocellular (correction of hepatocullular) necrosis: was it caused by Orlistat? *Med. Sci. Law*, 42, 309–312.

MacWalter, R.S., Fraser, H.W. and Armstrong, K.M. (2003) Orlistat enhances warfarin effect. *Ann. Pharmacother.*, 37, 510–512.

Marshall, R.D. and Douglas, C.J. (1994) Phenylpropanolamine-induced psychosis. Potential predisposing factors. *Gen. Hosp. Psychiatry*, 16, 358–360.

Martinsson, L. and Wahlgren, N.G. (2003) Safety of dexamphetamine in acute ischemic stroke: a randomized, double-blind, controlled dose-escalation trial. *Stroke*, 34, 475–481.

McDuffie, J.R., Calis, K.A., Booth, S.L., Uwaifo, G.I. and Yanovski, J.A. (2002) Effects of orlistat on fat-soluble vitamins in obese adolescents. *Pharmacotherapy*, 22, 814–822.

McEwen, J. and Meyboom, R.H. (1983) Testicular pain caused by mazindol. *Br. Med. J. (Clin. Res. Ed.)*, 287, 1763–1764.

McMahon, F.G., Weinstein, S.P., Rowe, E., Ernst, K.R., Johnson, F. and Fujioka, K. (2002) Sibutramine is safe and effective for weight loss in obese patients whose hypertension is well controlled with angiotensin-converting enzyme inhibitors. *J. Hum. Hypertens.*, 16, 5–11.

McMurray, J., Bloomfield, P. and Miller, H.C. (1986) Irreversible pulmonary hypertension after treatment with fenfluramine. *Br. Med. J. (Clin. Res. Ed.)*, 292, 239–240.

McNeely, W. and Benfield, P. (1998) Orlistat. *Drugs*, 56, 241–249; discussion 250.

Meier, C.R., Krahenbuhl, S., Schlienger, R.G. and Jick, H. (2002) Association between body mass index and liver disorders: an epidemiological study. *J. Hepatol.*, 37, 741–747.

Montero, J.L., Muntane, J., Fraga, E., Delgado, M., Costan, G., Serrano, M., Padillo, J., de la Mata, M. and Mino, G. (2001) Orlistat associated subacute hepatic failure. *J. Hepatol.*, 34, 173.

Morgenstern, L.B., Viscoli, C.M., Kernan, W.N., Brass, L.M., Broderick, J.P., Feldmann, E., Wilterdink, J.L., Brott, T. and Horwitz, R.I. (2003) Use of Ephedra-containing products and risk for hemorrhagic stroke. *Neurology*, 60, 132–135.

Nagele, H., Petersen, B., Bonacker, U. and Rodiger, W. (1999) Effect of orlistat on blood cyclosporin concentration in an obese heart transplant patient. *Eur. J. Clin. Pharmacol.*, 55, 667–669.

Narkiewicz, K. (2002) Sibutramine and its cardiovascular profile. *Int. J. Obes. Relat. Metab. Disord.*, 26, S38–41.

Nisoli, E. and Carruba, M.O. (2000) An assessment of the safety and efficacy of sibutramine, an anti-obesity drug with a novel mechanism of action. *Obes. Rev.*, 1, 127–139.

Olson, L.G., Ambrogetti, A. and Sutherland, D.C. (2003) A pilot randomized controlled trial of dexamphetamine in patients with chronic fatigue syndrome. *Psychosomatics*, 44, 38–43.

Oosterbaan, R. and Burns, M.J. (2000) Myocardial infarction associated with phenylpropanolamine. *J. Emerg. Med.*, 18, 55–59.

Persson, M., Vitols, S. and Yue, Q.Y. (2000) Orlistat associated with hypertension. *Br. Med. J.*, 321, 87.

Rogers, P.J. and Blundell, J.E. (1979) Effect of anorexic drugs on food intake and the micro-structure of eating in human subjects. *Psychopharmacology* (Berl), 66, 159–165.

Rolls, B.J., Shide, D.J., Thorwart, M.L. and Ulbrecht, J.S. (1998) Sibutramine reduces food intake in non-dieting women with obesity. *Obes. Res.*, 6, 1–11.

Salanova, V. and Taubner, R. (1984) Intracerebral haemorrhage and vasculitis secondary to amphetamine use. *Postgrad. Med. J.*, 60, 429–430.

Scandling, J. and Spital, A. (1982) Amphetamine-associated myoglobinuric renal failure. *South Med. J.*, 75, 237–240.

Shindler, J., Schachter, M., Brincat, S. and Parkes, J.D. (1985) Amphetamine, mazindol, and fencamfamin in narcolepsy. *Br. Med. J.* (*Clin. Res. Ed.*), 290, 1167–1170.

Silverstone, P.H., Pukhovsky, A. and Rotzinger, S. (1998) Lithium does not attenuate the effects of D-amphetamine in healthy volunteers. *Psychiatry Res.*, 79, 219–226.

Sjostrom, L., Rissanen, A., Andersen, T., Boldrin, M., Golay, A., Koppeschaar, H.P. and Krempf, M. (1998) Randomized placebo-controlled trial of orlistat for weight loss and prevention of weight regain in obese patients. *Lancet*, 352, 167–172.

Smith, H.J., Roche, A.H., Jausch, M.F. and Herdson, P.B. (1976) Cardiomyopathy associated with amphetamine administration. *Am. Heart J.*, 91, 792–797.

SoRelle, R. (2000) FDA warns of stroke risk associated with phenylpropanolamine; cold remedies and drugs removed from store shelves. *Circulation*, 102, E9041–9043.

Sramek, J.J., Leibowitz, M.T., Weinstein, S.P., Rowe, E.D., Mendel, C.M., Levy, B., McMahon, F.G., Mullican, W.S., Toth, P.D. and Cutler, N.R. (2002) Efficacy and safety of sibutramine for weight loss in obese patients with hypertension well controlled by beta-adrenergic blocking agents: a placebo-controlled, double-blind, randomised trial. *J. Hum. Hypertens.*, 16, 13–19.

Thiel, A. and Dressler, D. (1994) Dyskinesias possibly induced by norpseudoephedrine. *J. Neurol.*, 241, 167–169.

Trouillot, T.E., Pace, D.G., McKinley, C., Cockey, L., Zhi, J., Haeussler, J., Guerciolini, R., Showalter, R. and Everson, G.T. (2001) Orlistat maintains biliary lipid composition and hepatobiliary function in obese subjects undergoing moderate weight loss. *Am. J. Gastroenterol.*, 96, 1888–1894.

Weissman, N.J., Tighe, J.F., Jr., Gottdiener, J.S. and Gwynne, J.T. (1998) An assessment of heart-valve abnormalities in obese patients taking dexfenfluramine, sustained-release dexfenfluramine, or placebo. Sustained-Release Dexfenfluramine Study Group. *N. Engl. J. Med.*, 339, 725–732.

Williams, D.M. (1990) Phenylpropanolamine hydrochloride. *Am. Pharm.*, NS30, 47–50.

Wirth, A. and Krause, J. (2001) Long-term weight loss with sibutramine: a randomized controlled trial. *JAMA*, 286, 1331–1339.

Woolverton, W.L. (1986) A review of the effects of repeated administration of selected phenylethylamines. *Drug Alcohol Depend.*, 17, 143–150.

Zhi, J., Moore, R., Kanitra, L. and Mulligan, T.E. (2002) Pharmacokinetic evaluation of the possible interaction between selected concomitant medications and orlistat at steady state in healthy subjects. *J. Clin. Pharmacol.*, 42, 1011–1019.

Part V

Drugs in Research and Development

15

Central Targets for Antiobesity Drugs

Rexford S. Ahima and Suzette Y. Osei

CONTENTS

SUMMARY Obesity may result from increased food intake, reduced energy expenditure, and/or excessive partitioning of lipids to adipose tissue. Given the worldwide epidemic of obesity and associated diseases, notably diabetes and cardiovascular disease, a great need for drug therapy exists. Currently, sibutramine is the only centrally active drug approved for long-term treatment of obesity in conjunction with life-style management. Sibutramine acts in the brain to suppress appetite. Other central nervous system strategies include inhibition of orexigenic neuropeptides, e.g., neuropeptide Y; agouti-related peptide; melanin-concentrating hormone; endocannabinoids; or their receptors. Neuronal pathways expressing melanocortin-4 receptors; corticotropin-releasing factor; cocaine- and amphetamine-regulated transcript; and serotonin $5HT_{2c}$ receptor could be stimulated, leading to appetite suppression as well as increased metabolic rate. These peptides and neurotransmitters are often present in the brain and peripheral organs, as well as mediating various physiologic functions; thus, the risk of side effects is high. However, the latter needs to be balanced against the reduction in the risk of diabetes, cardiovascular disease, and other complications of obesity.

15.1 Introduction

Obesity is rapidly becoming a major medical problem in the world as a risk factor for mortality and morbidity from diabetes; hypertension; dyslipidemia; atherosclerosis; obstructive sleep apnea; cholelithiasis; osteoarthritis; cancer; and other ailments (Kopelman 2000). The obesity epidemic has been attributed mainly to overconsumption of energy-dense food containing high fat, as well as sedentary lifestyle (Kopelman 2000; Spiegelman and Flier 2001). Until recently, the failure to lose weight from dieting and exercise was blamed on diminished will power. However, it is increasingly evident that obesity is a *bona fide* disease characterized by distinct pathogenesis, natural history, and clinical features (Kopelman 2000; Bray 2000). Psychosocial factors play an important role in feeding behavior and obesity, and life-style modification is an essential component of weight management. However, it is doubtful that the epidemic of obesity, diabetes, and other complications can be stemmed using these strategies alone. An increasing number of patients will need drugs, surgery, or other interventions to decrease and maintain body weight at medically safe levels.

From a thermodynamic standpoint, obesity is the net result of excess energy intake, reduced energy expenditure, or both. Understanding of the biological basis of energy balance has undergone a radical change since the discovery of leptin and other monogenic mutations linked to appetite and body weight (Spiegelman and Flier 2001; Barsh et al. 2000). Dysregulation of pathways in the brain, adipose tissue, and other peripheral organs results in obesity by stimulating feeding, decreasing metabolic rate, and/or altering energy substrate fluxes, thus leading to increased fat deposition (Spiegelman and Flier 2001). Understanding the underlying molecular processes could lead to identification of novel targets that could provide potential therapeutic interventions for obesity and complications, such as diabetes, dyslipidemia, and cardiovascular disease.

15.2 Overview of Energy Homeostasis

The survival of organisms is dependent on the ability to procure food and maintain adequate energy stores. For mammals, the uncertainty of food resources; famine; fluctuations in climate and seasons; sleep–wake cycles; and illness impose an enormous pressure on their ability to maintain energy balance (Ahima 2000; Spiegelman and Flier 2001). They consume more calories at each meal than is required for immediate metabolic needs, and the excess intake is stored as glycogen, protein, and fat for use during periods of energy depletion. Adipose tissue, commonly called fat, has an almost limitless capacity for storing energy in the form of triglyceride. Mammals have also developed complex feeding behaviors, and thermoregulatory and neuroendocrine mechanisms, mediated mainly by the brain to protect against the threat of starvation (Ahima 2000; Spiegelman and Flier 2001). The fall in glucose and insulin triggers a counterregulatory response, e.g., increased levels of glucagon, catecholamines, and glucocorticoids that stimulate lipolysis and gluconeogenesis. The latter ensures a steady supply of glucose to the brain, while fatty acids derived from triglyceride breakdown provide fuel to muscle and liver. Partial oxidation of fatty acids also yields ketones, which can be utilized by the brain and other organs (Ahima 2000).

The adipocyte hormone leptin decreases in response to fasting, and triggers a series of metabolic and neuroendocrine changes, e.g., increased glucocorticoids; reduction in thyroid, reproductive, and growth hormones; and suppression of thermogenesis and immune response (Ahima et al. 1996; Flier and Spiegelman 2001). The fasting-induced decline of leptin, insulin, and glucose stimulates hyperphagia and weight gain when food becomes available (Ahima et al. 1996; Flier and Spiegelman 2001). Teleologically, the adaptation to energy depletion is likely to have been beneficial during thousands of years of human evolution by maintaining a steady supply of glucose for use by the brain; limiting the high energy cost of thyroid thermogenesis and reproduction; and protecting lean tissue mass (Ahima et al. 1996; Spiegelman and Flier 2001). Ironically, this "thrifty" genotype designed to maximize energy efficiency is thought to have contributed to the current epidemic of obesity and its sequelae in an environment where food is plentiful (Kopelman 2000).

Feeding behavior is regulated by complex processes involving the central nervous system (CNS) and peripheral organs. Classic studies carried out in the 1940s and 1950s described the effects of hypothalamic lesions on body weight and metabolism (reviewed by Sawchenko 1998; Elmquist et al. 1999). Destruction of the ventromedial hypothalamic nucleus (VMN) resulted in ravenous overeating, obesity, diabetes, and hypogonadism, while lesions of the lateral hypothalamus (LH) resulted in a failure to eat and drink and, ultimately, death from starvation. It was thus concluded that the "satiety center" was located in the VMN and the "feeding center" in the LH. However, it was soon apparent that the LH lesions disrupted motor function and voluntary ingestion, necessitating careful nursing and forced feeding of the animals in the immediate postoperative period. Subsequently, it was recognized that LH lesions interrupted catecholaminergic nigrostriatal pathways, and the aphagia and adipsia were associated with other major defects, including catalepsy and sensorimotor neglect.

The hypothesized role of the VMN as a satiety center was challenged by studies showing that small lesions restricted to this nucleus could not recapitulate obesity and other abnormalities. In fact, later studies showed that severance of the abdominal vagus nerve attenuated the overeating attributed to the VMN lesion, suggesting that the increased ingestion and weight gain in this model was mediated by a peripheral signal. Despite the shortcomings, these early studies established an important role for the brain in feeding behavior and regulation of body weight.

Understanding of energy balance has also benefited from physiologic studies carried out several decades ago. Kennedy (1953) proposed that a signal related to adipose tissue informed the brain about changes in fat stores and mediated adjustments in feeding and metabolic rate to maintain body weight. This "adipostatic" model was in agreement with the observation that body weight and fat content in most mammals were maintained at near constant levels, despite daily fluctuations in food intake and energy expenditure. Analogous to other homeostatically regulated systems, perturbation of energy stores by food deprivation, surgical removal of adipose tissue, or forced overfeeding caused a compensatory hyperphagia or hypophagia until body weight was restored to the previous level (Kennedy 1953; Harris 1986). Thus, it was suggested that a physiologic mechanism linking adipose tissue and the brain was responsible for surveillance and maintenance of body weight at a presumed "set point."

Parabiosis studies in which the circulation of animals was surgically joined demonstrated that food intake and body weight were drastically decreased in normal rats joined to obese VMN-lesioned rats (Hervey 1959). In contrast, VMN-lesioned rats continued to overeat and gain weight when parabiosed with VMN-lesioned or nonlesioned rats (Hervey

TABLE 15.1

Central Neurotransmitter and Peptide Targets for Obesity Treatment

Stimulate Feeding	Inhibit Feeding
Neuropeptide Y (NPY)	Alpha-melanocyte stimulating hormone (α-MSH)
Agouti-related peptide (AGRP)	Cocaine and amphetamine-regulated transcript (CART)
Melanin-concentrating hormone (MCH)	Corticotropin-releasing factor (CRF)
Orexins	Urocortins
Ghrelin	Neurotensin
Galanin	Thyrotropin-releasing hormone (TRH)
Growth hormone-releasing hormone (GHRH)	Serotonin
Opioid peptides	Cholecystokinin (CCK)
Gamma-aminobutyric acid (GABA)	Glucagon-like peptides-1 and -2
Endocannabinoids (CB1 receptor)	Brain-derived neurotrophic factor (BDNF)
	Ciliary neurotrophic factor (CNTF)

1959). The findings suggested that a satiety factor present in the circulation acted in the hypothalamus or its connections to regulate body weight. These predictions were supported by the discovery of *obese* (ob/ob) and *diabetes* (db/db) mutations in mice (Coleman 1978). Based on parabiosis experiments, it was surmised that the *ob* locus encoded a humoral factor that suppressed feeding, while the *db* locus mediated its response (Coleman 1978). These seminal discoveries by Coleman and others were confirmed four decades later by the discovery of leptin (Zhang et al. 1994).

Leptin increases in proportion to body fat and acts as an afferent signal to hypothalamic and other brain targets and regulates food consumption and energy balance (Friedman and Halaas 1998). An increase in leptin limits weight gain by suppressing feeding and increasing energy expenditure (Friedman and Halaas 1998; Ahima et al. 2001). Conversely, leptin is decreased during fasting, which potently stimulates food intake and decreases energy expenditure. These divergent actions are mediated through neuronal circuits located in the hypothalamus, brainstem and other regions of the CNS (Elmquist et al. 1999; Ahima et al. 2001).

Leptin interacts with the neuropeptides and neurotransmitters discussed in the next sections (Table 15.1). As an example, peptides that stimulate feeding, e.g., neuropeptide Y (NPY); agouti-related peptide (AGRP); and melanin-concentrating hormone (MCH), are increased in leptin deficiency, whereas peptides that inhibit feeding, e.g., proopiomelanocortin (precursor of α-MSH); cocaine- and amphetamine-regulated transcript (CART), are decreased in response to leptin deficiency. The converse is true for these "orexigenic" (feeding stimulator) and "anorexigenic" (feeding inhibitor) peptides in response to leptin treatment (Ahima et al. 2001).

Leptin serves as a model for understanding the complex role of adipose tissue as an endocrine, paracrine, and autocrine organ (Spiegelman and Flier 2001). Until recently, adipose tissue was thought to comprise specialized cells (adipocytes) designed to store lipids. It is now known that adipose tissue is a *bona fide* organ system — characterized by regional heterogeneity and composed of adipocytes as well as vascular and immune tissues that mediate diverse physiologic functions (Spiegelman and Flier 2001).

Leptin and other peptide hormones (angiotensinogen, adiponectin, resistin); proinflammatory cytokines (TNF-α,IL-6); complement factors (adipsin); procoagulant factors (PAI-1); and steroids (glucococorticoids, sex steroids) are secreted by adipose tissue and actively regulate energy balance and neuroendocrine, immune, and cardiovascular systems. Maladaptation of interactions between these peripheral factors and neuronal circuits expressing various neuropeptides and neurotransmitters may underlie the pathogenesis of obesity, eating disorders, and metabolic complications. This chapter will focus on the role of the CNS neurotransmitters and peptides that mediate energy balance, and how they could be targeted for the treatment of obesity.

15.3 Neurotransmitters and Peptides Mediating Appetite Stimulation

15.3.1 NPY

NPY belongs to the PP-fold family of peptides, consisting of NPY and two gut peptides, peptide YY (PYY) and pancreatic polypeptide (PP) (reviewed by Berglund et al. 2003). Unlike the latter, NPY is localized mainly in neurons. It is the most abundant neuropeptide and is expressed in the hypothalamus, and all levels of the CNS. Studies have demonstrated a potent stimulatory effect of intracerebroventricular (i.c.v.) injection of NPY on food intake in several species (Sahu and Kalra 1993; Berglund et al. 2003). In rodents, microinjection of NPY into the hypothalamic paraventricular nucleus (PVN) and adjacent perifornical region stimulates food intake, especially carbohydrate. Administration of antisense oligonucleotide or antibodies against NPY into the CNS reduces feeding and increases thermogenesis. In contrast, CNS administration of NPY decreases thermogenesis and exerts diverse effects on anticonvulsant activity, sedation, mood, memory, and cardiovascular system (Sahu and Kalra 1993). These actions are consistent with the widespread distribution of NPY.

In the hypothalamus, NPY is synthesized in the arcuate nucleus and released in the paraventricular hypothalamic nucleus (PVN) and lateral hypothalamic area (LH). Hypothalamic NPY is increased in response to energy depletion during fasting, lactation, exercise, and leptin and insulin deficiency, consistent with its role as a stimulator of feeding (Sahu and Kalra 1993; Ahima et al. 2001). In contrast, food ingestion and leptin treatment suppress NPY. Despite the physiologic and pharmacologic evidence in support of an important role for NPY in energy balance, ablation of the NPY gene in mice has produced controversial results.

In the original studies, deletion of NPY resulted in spontaneous seizures, attributed to defective GABA release, a greater preference for ethanol, and decreased sensitivity to ethanol-induced sedation compared with controls (Erickson et al. 1996a). However, NPY-null mice were phenotypically normal as far as growth, *ad libitum* feeding, and response to fasting and high-fat diet (Erickson et al. 1996a). NPY-null mice responded normally to i.c.v. NPY, but were hypersensitive to leptin (Erickson et al. 1996a; Marsh et al. 1999). The same investigators later demonstrated that deletion of the NPY gene partially ameliorated the hyperphagia, cold intolerance, and obesity characteristic of leptin-deficient *ob/ob* mice (Erickson et al. 1996b). It was later shown that breeding NPY deficiency onto C57Bl/6 genetic background attenuates the hyperphagic response to fasting and hypoglycemia (Bannon et al. 2000; Segal-Lieberman et al. 2003; Sindelar et al. 2002). Knockout of NPY and AGRP in the same mouse did not affect feeding or body weight (Qian et al. 2002).

The effect of excess NPY has been examined in transgenic animals. Overexpression of NPY resulted in increased consumption of a sucrose-rich diet, obesity, hyperinsulinemia, and hyperglycemia (Kaga et al. 2001). In another study, overexpression of NPY in the brain decreased ethanol preference and enhanced the sedative effect of ethanol (Thiele et al. 1998). In contrast, transgenic overexpression of NPY in rats reduced seizures and impaired spatial learning and sensitivity to restraint stress, but did not result in obesity (Vezzani et al. 2002).

NPY and other PP-fold peptides act through Y1, Y2, Y4, Y5, and Y6 receptors, coupled to inhibitory G proteins (Gi) and inhibition of cAMP (Berglund et al. 2003). Moreover, the Y1 receptor is capable of activating MAP kinase, while Y1, Y2, Y4, and Y5 receptors mediate Ca2+ release through phospholipase C. The Y1 receptor regulates food and ethanol ingestion, as well as effects of NPY on vascular tone, arousal, and nociception. Paradoxically, deletion of the Y1 gene resulted in late-onset obesity in female mice, associated with increased insulin level and glucose (Kushi et al. 1998). The Y2 receptor gene is highly expressed in the arcuate nucleus, where it is located presynaptically and acts as an autoreceptor to inhibit NPY release at the POMC neuron (Figure 15.2). As expected, Y2 receptor-null mice consumed more food and developed late-onset obesity (Sainsbury et al. 2002a). Moreover, crossing Y2 receptor-null mice onto leptin-deficient *ob/ob* background decreased body fat, insulin, glucose, and glucocorticoids (Naveilhan et al. 2002). However, the hyperphagia and infertility characteristic of *ob/ob* mice were not reversed by Y2 deletion (Sainsbury et al. 2002a; Naveilhan et al. 2002).

Hypothalamic POMC mRNA expression in *ob/ob* mice was enhanced by Y2 deletion, whereas NPY, AGRP, and CART mRNA levels were not affected, suggesting that Y2 receptors mediate obese/type 2 diabetes through melanocortin peptides (Sainsbury et al. 2002a). Studies have also implicated the Y2 receptor in bone development (Baldock et al. 2002). Although NPY and leptin induced bone loss in mice, the converse was true in Y2 receptor-null mice (Ducy et al. 2000; Baldlock et al. 2002). More significantly, deletion of hypothalamic Y2 receptors increased trabecular bone, suggesting a central effect of NPY on bone development (Baldlock et al. 2002). Thus, it is possible that the association between bone biology and obesity and anorexia could be explained, at least partly, on the basis of a leptin–hypothalamic NPY interaction.

Unlike Y1 and Y2 receptors, the Y4 receptor has a low degree of homology among species and binds preferentially to PP (Berglund et al. 2003). Crossing Y4 knockout mice onto *ob/ob* background restored sexual maturity and improved fertility, but did not affect feeding or body weight (Sainsbury et al. 2002b). The Y5 receptor is localized mainly in the hypothalamus and other CNS regions involved in regulation of feeding and energy balance. Activation of Y5 receptor stimulates feeding, decreases energy expenditure, and mediates other effects of NPY on reproduction, seizures, and circadian rhythm (Criscione et al. 1998). However, deletion of the Y5 receptor in mice did not suppress feeding or prevent weight gain (Marsh et al. 1998). Instead, Y5 receptor-null mice developed a late-onset obesity characterized by increased food intake and reduced locomotor activity and metabolic rate (Marsh et al. 1998). The Y5 receptor-null mice exhibited a normal inhibition of feeding by leptin; however, the feeding response to i.c.v. NPY was diminished (Marsh et al. 1998). Thus, as is the case with Y1 and Y2 receptors, these results demonstrate that the Y5 receptor participates in the CNS response to NPY treatment, but is not essential to physiologic regulation of feeding and energy balance.

The Y6 receptor was first cloned in rabbits and mice (Berglund et al. 2003). Y6 receptor mRNA is expressed in the hypothalamus and kidney in mice, but neither the mRNA nor gene has been detected in rats. Y6 receptors were cloned in humans and other primates and found to be nonfunctional as a result of a frame-shift mutation in the third intracellular loop causing a stop codon in the sixth transmembrane region (Berglund et al. 2003).

15.3.2   Agouti-Related Peptide (AGRP)

AGRP belongs to the melanocortin system, which consists of peptides derived from posttranslational processing of POMC prohormone and a family of five seven-transmembrane G-protein coupled receptors. The melanocortin system regulates diverse physiological processes, including energy homeostasis; skin/hair pigmentation; steroidogenesis; sexual function; exocrine secretion; and immunomodulation (reviewed by Cone 1999; MacNeil et al. 2002). In mammals, agouti protein is expressed transiently in the early postnatal period, primarily in the skin, where it acts as a paracrine factor to antagonize the action of α-MSH at the melanocortin 1 receptor (MC1). The term "agouti" refers to a characteristic subapical yellow band on predominantly black or brown fur. In dominant agouti (*Ay/a*) mice, agouti protein is expressed constitutively and ectopically, resulting in yellow fur; late-onset obesity; increased body length; hyperphagia; and insulin resistance.

In contrast to *ob/ob* and *db/db* mice, corticosterone (the predominant glucocorticoid in mice) is not elevated in obese *Ay/a* mice. Studies found that the hyperphagia and obesity in *Ay/a* were secondary to antagonism of MC4, and possibly MC3, receptors by ectopic expression of agouti protein in the brain (Cone 1999). The importance of these receptors has been confirmed by gene knockout studies in which MC4 receptor-null mice developed hyperphagia and obesity, without alteration in fur color (Huszar et al. 1997). MC3 receptor-null mice develop obesity mainly as a result of reduced metabolic rate (Hagan et al. 2000). Unlike the mouse, the human agouti protein is expressed widely in adipose tissue, testis, ovary, liver, and other organs and does not appear to have a specific physiological role.

AGRP was discovered using a database search for molecules with homology to agouti (Cone 1999). AGRP is coexpressed mainly in the arcuate nucleus with NPY and released in the PVN, LH, and other regions of the hypothalamus; it acts as a potent orexigenic neuropeptide by blocking the action of α-MSH at the MC4 and MC3 receptors. As expected, transgenic overexpression of AGRP recapitulated the hyperphagia, obesity, increased linear growth, and hyperinsulinemia observed in *Ay/a* and MC4 receptor-null mice (Cone 1999). As with NPY, AGRP synthesis is increased in response to leptin deficiency during fasting and inhibited by refeeding or leptin treatment (Ahima et al. 2001).

Unlike NPY, a single i.c.v. injection of AGRP stimulates feeding for several days, raising the possibility that it is modulated by other factors (Butler et al. 2000). Syndecans are a group of heparan sulfate proteoglycan molecules bound to the plasma membrane whose ectodomain is shed and binds extracellular ligands (Reizes et al. 2001). Transgenic overexpression of syndecan-1 resulted in hyperphagia, obesity, increased body length, and hyperinsulinemia reminiscent of *Ay/a*, AGRP-Tg, and MC4 receptor-null mice (Reizes et al. 2001). This led to the hypothesis that the central melanocortin system was modulated by syndecans. However, because syndecan-1 was normally not produced in the hypothalamus, attention was drawn to syndecan-3, a related molecule shown to augment the antagonism of MC3 and MC4 receptors by AGRP (Reizes et al. 2001).

Syndecan-3 is increased on the surface of hypothalamic MC3 and MC4 neurons during fasting, binds to AGRP is thought to enhance its orexigenic action (Reizes et al. 2001). Conversely, in the fed state, syndecan-3 is shed from the cell surface and allows α-MSH to compete for MC3 and MC4 receptors, resulting in satiation (Reizes et al. 2001). Mahogany is a single-pass transmembrane protein expressed mainly in brain and skin (He et al. 2001). In mice, mahogany is required for the action of agouti, as evident by the ability of mahogany mutation to prevent yellow fur in *Ay/a* mice (Dinulescu et al. 1998). Mahogany is a low affinity receptor for agouti but not AGRP. However, mahogany regulates metabolic rate independently of agouti (Dinulescu et al. 1998).

15.3.3 Melanin-Concentrating Hormone (MCH)

MCH is a cyclic 19 residue polypeptide originally discovered in teleost fish in which it mediates changes in skin color (Qu et al. 1996). It is expressed predominantly in neurons in the LH, perifornical region, and zona incerta, which project broadly in the CNS (Figure

15.1a). Several lines of evidence suggest a role of MCH in regulation of feeding and energy balance. Injection of MCH i.c.v. or into the LH stimulates feeding (Qu et al. 1996). Fasting and leptin deficiency increase hypothalamic MCH mRNA, while refeeding or leptin treatment decreases MCH mRNA levels (Qu et al. 1996). Mice overexpressing the MCH gene were hyperphagic, obese, and hyperinsulinemic (Ludwig et al. 2001). In contrast, mice lacking the MCH gene developed hypophagia, increased metabolic rate, and leanness (Shimada et al. 1998). However, because deletion of the MCH gene also prevented expression of neuropeptides E-1 and G-E, which are processed from the same propeptide as MCH, it was unclear to what extent this phenotype could be attributed to MCH (Shimada et al. 1998).

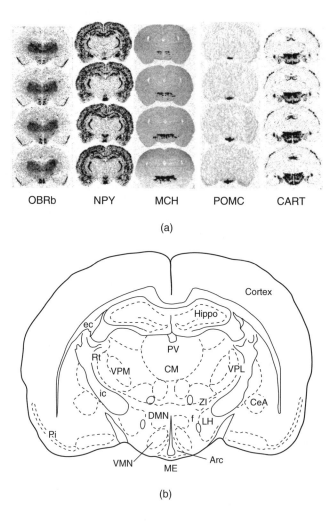

FIGURE 15.1

(a) Coronal sections of rat brain showing distributions of mRNAs of the long leptin receptor (OBRb) and hypothalamic neuropeptides implicated in regulation of feeding and energy balance, as detected by *in situ* hybridization histochemistry. (b) Drawing of coronal section of rat brain showing hypothalamic and other nuclei. Arc = arcuate nucleus; CeA = central amygdala; CM = centromedian thalamic nucleus; DMN = dorsomedial nucleus; ec = external capsule; f = fornix; Hippo = hippocampus; ic = internal capsule; LH = lateral hypothalamic area; Pi = piriform cortex; PV = paraventricular thalamic nucleus; Rt = reticular nucleus; VMN = ventromedial hypothalamic nucleus; VPL = ventroposteriolateral thalamic nucleus; VPM = ventroposteriomedial thalamic nucleus; ZI = zona incerta.

MCH1 and MCH2 receptors belong to the rhodopsin superfamily of G protein-coupled receptors (Saito et al. 2000; Wang et al. 2001). MCH1 receptor has been isolated from rodents and humans, whereas MCH2 receptor has so far been identified only in humans (Saito et al. 2000; Wang et al. 2001). The distribution of MCH1 receptor mRNA in rodent brain is consistent with its diverse effects in energy homeostasis and regulation of arousal and other behaviors. Interestingly, deletion of the MCH1 receptor gene resulted in lean mice; however, food intake was not reduced (Marsh et al. 2002). Instead, MCH1 receptor-null mice were hyperactive and had higher metabolic rates (Marsh et al. 2002).

A nonpeptide MCH1 antagonist, SNAP-7941, inhibits MCH-induced feeding, reduces consumption of palatable food, and prevents diet-induced obesity in rodents in a dose-dependent manner (Borowsky et al. 2002). The treatment did not induce malaise or toxicity, and the antiobesity effect was reversible upon cessation of treatment (Borowsky et al. 2002). Based on the distribution of SNAP-7941 binding sites in the cortex and limbic regions, the effect of MCH1 receptor blockade on behavior was evaluated. SNAP-7941 produced anxiolytic and antidepressant effects, similar to the benzodiazepine, chlordiaz-epoxide, and serotonin agonist fluoxetine (Borowsky et al. 2002).

15.3.4 Hypocretins 1 and 2

Hypocretins 1 and 2 were discovered by using a systematic substraction hybridization strategy in rat hypothalamic samples (Sutcliffe and de Lecea 2002). Hcrt1 peptide contains two intrasulfide bonds and is identical between humans and rodents. Human Hcrt2 differs from rodent Hcrt2 at two amino acids. These peptides are phylogenetically related to secretin. Another research group identified the hypocretins by screening for novel G protein-coupled receptors in rat brain homogenates; the peptides were named "orexin A and B" for their ability to stimulate feeding (Sakurai et al. 1998).

The orexins are encoded by the same gene and synthesized by a separate neuronal population in the LH distinct from MCH neurons (Elias et al. 1998). Hcrt1 (orexin A) receptor is localized in the prefrontal cortex, hippocampus, PVN, VMN, dorsal raphe, and locus ceruleus, while Hcrt2 (orexin B) receptor has a more extensive hypothalamic distribution, including PVN; dorsomedial and ventral premammillary nucleus; cerebral cortex; septal nuclei; hippocampus; medial thalamus; and raphe nuclei. Feeding is stimulated by administration of Hcrt1 or Hcrt2 i.c.v. or directly into PVN, DMN, LH, or perifornical regions (Sakurai et al. 1998). Moreover, short-term fasting increases Hcrt mRNA and peptide levels in the hypothalamus, consistent with a role as a stimulator of feeding (Sakurai et al. 1998).

However, the effects of Hcrts on energy balance have not been observed consistently in other studies (Tritos et al. 2001). Furthermore, deficiency of Hcrt and Hcrt receptor genes results in narcolepsy in mice, dogs, and humans without producing the expected effects on feeding or body weight (Lin et al. 1999; Hara et al. 2001). Patients with narcolepsy have a low Hcrt level but are not underweight (Smart et al. 2002). Moreover, ablation of Hcrt neurons in mice resulted in narcolepsy and late-onset obesity (Hara et al. 2001). These data suggest that the effect of Hcrt on energy balance, if at all, is secondary to regulation of arousal and sleep–wake cycles (Willie et al. 2001). Hypocretin peptides elevate blood pressure, heart rate, oxygen consumption, and body temperature; they increase locomotor activity, water consumption and gastric secretion; stimulate secretion of luteinizing hormone, ACTH, corticosterone, and insulin; and decrease growth hormone and prolactin (Sutcliffe and de Lecea 2002). These diverse effects are in agreement with interconnections among Hcrt neurons and the arcuate nucleus and brainstem nuclei; e.g, ventrolateral medulla; locus ceruleus; nucleus of the solitary tract (NTS); and spinal cord (Elias et al. 1998).

15.3.5   Cannabinoids

Used for thousands of years for its psychotropic effect, *cannabis sativa* (marijuana) is well known to induce hunger. Intensive research on the molecular action of the cannabinoids began as a result of the discovery of its main psychoactive component, delta(9)-tetrahy-drocannabinol. Cannabinoids stimulate appetite by acting through receptors in the brain. Studies have demonstrated that the G protein-coupled CB1 cannabinoid receptor is targeted to presynaptic terminals of neurons, where it modulates the release of classical neurotransmitters. CB1 receptors and endogenous cannabinoid ligands, anandamide, and 2-arachidonoyl glycerol are present in the hypothalamus, limbic, and other CNS areas (Di Marzo et al. 2001).

CB1 receptor knockout mice do not exhibit hyperphagia in response to food restriction and the CB1 antagonist *N*-(piperidin-1-yl)-5-(4-chlorophenyl)-1-(2,4-dichlorophenyl)-4-methyl-1H-pyrazole-3-carboximide hydrochloride (SR141716) reduces food intake in wild-type but not CB1 receptor knockout mice (Ravinet Trillon et al. 2003). Interestingly, hypothalamic levels of endogenous cannabinoids are increased in *db/db* and *ob/ob* mice and Zucker (*fa/fa*) rats with defective leptin signaling. In contrast, leptin treatment of normal rats and *ob/ob* mice reduces anandamide and 2-arachidonoyl glycerol in the hypothalamus. These findings demonstrate that the endogenous cannabinoid system in the hypothalamus interacts with leptin to regulate food intake.

CB1 receptor antagonist SR141716 induced a transient reduction of food intake and sustained reduction of body weight and fat in a diet-induced obese model (Ravinet Trillon et al. 2003). Furthermore, SR141716 decreased plasma leptin, insulin, and free fatty acid levels and reversed insulin resistance. Weight loss from SR141716 treatment was greater than food restriction (pair-feeding) alone, suggesting that SR141716 may increase metabolic rate in addition to suppressing appetite. A recent study has examined the possibility of cross-talk between CB1 and the orexin 1 receptor (Hilairet et al. 2003). Co-expression of the two receptors enhanced the ability of orexin A to activate the MAP kinase pathway, while blockade of CB1 by SR141716 prevented the orexin response. Moreover, pertussis toxin blocked the CB1 effect on orexin, suggesting that the potentiation was mediated through G_i. Because the distribution of CB1 receptor overlaps orexin receptors in the hypothalamus, these data suggest a functional interaction between these systems.

15.3.6   Other Orexigenic Neurotransmitters and Peptides

Ghrelin is produced mainly in the stomach and stimulates food intake and weight gain when injected peripherally or i.c.v. (Kojima et al. 2001; Tschop et al. 2001). There is compelling evidence that ghrelin is produced by neurons in the periventricular hypothalamic area, suggesting a local action in the brain (Horvath et al. 2001; Cowley et al. 2003). Ghrelin modulates leptin neuron targets in hypothalamic slices and stimulates NPY and AGRP mRNA expression (Cowley et al. 2003; Horvath et al. 2001). Antagonists of NPY-Y1 receptor and melanocortin agonists block the response to ghrelin, indicating a functional relationship between ghrelin, and other orexigenic hypothalamic neuropeptides (Horvath et al. 2001).

Galanin, opioid peptides (e.g., β-endorphin and dynorphin), γ-aminobutyric acid (GABA), and growth hormone releasing-hormone have been implicated in appetite stimulation (reviewed by Inui 2000). Galanin is expressed in the arcuate nucleus, PVN and DMN, and stimulates feeding when injected i.c.v. or into the PVN, LH, and central amygdala. Moreover, galanin appears to stimulate fat consumption. Opioids may modulate taste and the reward response to food. GABA is expressed in hypothalamic interneurons and stimulates appetite by interacting with leptin, NPY, and melanocortin system via GABA-A receptors (Inui 2000; Cowley et al. 2001).

VGF is a neurotrophin identified as a nerve growth factor (NGF)-regulated transcript in rat PC12 pheochromocytoma cells (Salton et al. 2000). VGF gene expression is stimulated by NGF and the ras/MAP kinase signaling cascade through a CREB-dependent mechanism. VGF mRNA and the 68 kDa protein are synthesized by neuroendocrine cells and neurons in the brain, spinal cord, and peripheral nervous system. Its expression is especially high in the hypothalamus, where it is induced in the arcuate nucleus by fasting. VGF knockout mice are lean, hypermetabolic, and hyperactive, suggesting an important role in energy homeostasis (Salton et al. 2000; Hahm et al. 2002). VGF mRNA is elevated in the hypothalamus of leptin-deficient *ob/ob* and receptor-mutant *db/db* mice and inhibited by leptin treatment (Hahm et al. 2002). Crossing VGF-deficient mice onto *ob/ob* background attenuated weight gain but did not affect body fat. In contrast, VGF deficiency blocked the development of obesity in *Ay/a* mice in response to high-fat diet and gold thioglucose (Hahm et al. 2002). These data suggest that VGF acts downstream of the melanocortin pathway and an intact leptin signal is partially required for its full effect on body weight.

15.4 Neurotransmitters and Peptides Mediating Appetite Suppression

15.4.1 Proopiomelanocortin (POMC)

The POMC gene encodes a 36kDa preprohormone from which ACTH; α-melanocyte stimulating-hormone (α-MSH); β-MSH; γ-MSH; corticotropin-like intermediate lobe peptide (CLIP); β-lipoprotropin; and β-endorphin are derived through posttranslational processing by prohormone convertases (PC)-1 and PC2 and carboxy- and aminopeptidases (MacNeil et al. 2002). Some of these products are modified further through N-α-acetylation and carboxyterminal amidation. Five melanocortin receptors (MC1 through MC5) are coupled to the stimulatory G-protein (Gs) and cAMP production:

- The MC1 receptor (MC1R) is expressed in melanocytes, where it mediates the effect of α-MSH on skin and hair pigmentation. The potencies of melanocortin peptides at the MC1R are α-MSH = ACTH > β-MSH > γ-MSH.
- MC2R is expressed in the adrenal cortex, where it mediates the effect of ACTH on glucocorticoid synthesis and secretion.
- MC3R is expressed in the hypothalamus and other regions of the CNS, gastrointestinal tract, and placenta and binds with equal affinity to α-MSH, β-MSH, γ-MSH, and ACTH.
- MC4R is localized almost exclusively in the CNS and mediates the effect of α-MSH on feeding and energy balance.
- In contrast, MC5R is expressed mainly in peripheral tissues and regulates sebaceous gland secretion.

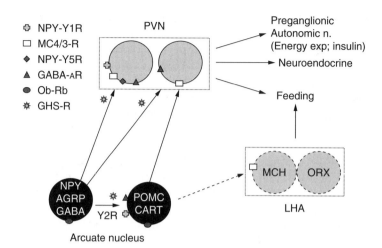

FIGURE 15.2
Hypothalamic neural circuitry for energy balance. Leptin directly regulates NPY/AGRP and POMC/CART neurons in the arcuate nucleus. NPY stimulates feeding via Y1 and Y5 receptors. The Y2 receptor acts presynaptically to regulate NPY release at the POMC (α-MSH) neuron. Ghrelin derived from the circulation or produced locally in the hypothalamus, modulates the response to NPY. AGRP antagonizes α-MSH action at MC4/3 receptors, resulting in appetite stimulation, reduced energy expenditure, and weight gain. GHS-R = growth hormone secretagogue receptor.

All MCRs are antagonized by agouti protein; however, only MC3R and MC4R are also antagonized by AGRP.

In the CNS, POMC is expressed in the arcuate nucleus and nucleus of the solitary tract (NTS), where it is processed to α-MSH (Cone 1999; MacNeil et al. 2002). Alpha-MSH neurons in the arcuate nucleus express CART; receive input from NPY/AGRP neurons; and project to the PVN, LH, brainstem, and spinal cord to regulate food intake and autonomic and neuroendocrine function (Figure 15.2; Ahima et al. 2001). Leptin directly activates POMC neurons in the arcuate nucleus and nucleus of the solitary tract, as revealed by induction of STAT3 and Fos protein (Ahima et al. 2001). Moreover, electrophysiologic studies have revealed a rapid depolarization of arcuate POMC neurons by leptin (Cowley et al. 2001).

Administration of α-MSH i.c.v. or into the PVN results in profound anorexia and increased thermogenesis (Cone 1999). As discussed in the previous section, AGRP is an endogenous antagonist of α-MSH at the MC4, and possibly MC3, receptors. The critical role of the melanocotin pathway in regulation of feeding and body weight is further supported by pharmacological and genetic experiments:

- SHU9119, an MC4R antagonist, blocks the inhibition of feeding and weight gain in response to α-MSH or melanocortin agonist MTII (MacNeil et al. 2002).

- Targeted deletion of the POMC gene in mice resulted in hyperphagia, obesity, and impairment of fur coloration, which were reversed by α-MSH treatment (Yaswen et al. 1999). Similarly, mutation of the POMC gene in humans causes overeating, obesity, and hypopigmentation (Krude et al. 1998).

- Deletion of the MC4 receptor in mice resulted in hyperphagia; late-onset obesity; increased linear growth; and insulin resistance (Huszar et al. 1997). MC4 receptor-null humans develop a similar phenotype (Farooqi et al. 2003) and severe obesity has been linked to MC4 receptor defects in up to 4% of severely obese humans (Farooqi et al. 2000).

15.4.2   Cocaine- and Amphetamine-Regulated Transcript (CART)

Cocaine- and amphetamine-regulated transcript (CART) was discovered as an mRNA transcript regulated by pyschostimulants (Kuhar et al. 2000). CART is widely distributed in the CNS and has multiple effects on sensory, motor, and neuroendocrine systems. It is produced in the arcuate nucleus, DMN, and other hypothalamic nuclei and inhibits feeding when administered i.c.v. (Kristensen et al. 1998). CART is coexpressed with POMC in a subpopulation of neurons in the arcuate nucleus and distributed to the LH, PVN as well as preganglionic sympathetic neurons in the thoracic spinal cord. POMC/CART neurons respond directly to circulating leptin, and it is possible that these neuropeptides mediate the inhibitory action of leptin on feeding behavior (Ahima et al. 2001).

On the other hand, CART has been colocalized with MCH in the LH, suggesting that the stimulatory effect of MCH on appetite could be modulated by CART (Broberger 1999). Central administration of α-MSH and CART prevents leptin-mediated reduction in thyroid hormone during fasting, a finding consistent with direct innervation of thyrotropin-releasing hormone (TRH) neurons in the parvicellular PVN by arcuate POMC/CART (Broberger 1999). Deletion of the CART gene produced the expected phenotype in mice. Male and female CART-null mice and female heterozygotes consumed more calories and became obese on a high-fat diet (Asnicar et al. 2001). Energy expenditure and fuel utilization were not affected by CART deficiency, indicating that CART regulates body weight by suppressing appetite (Asnicar et al. 2001).

15.4.3   Corticotropin-Releasing Factor (CRF)

The corticotropin-releasing factor (CRF) family of peptides includes CRF; urocortin; urocortin II; and urocortin III (Richard et al. 2000; Reyes et al. 2001; Lewis et al. 2001). These peptides are differentially distributed in the brain and modulate neuroendocrine, autonomic, behavioral responses to stress and immune function through G-protein coupled receptors CRFR1 and CRFR2. In addition to regulating ACTH synthesis and release, CRF and related peptides inhibit feeding and decrease body weight. Urocortins II and III are selective for CRFR2, and the latter is thought to mediate the suppressive effects of CRF-like peptides on appetite (Reyes et al. 2001; Lewis et al. 2001). However, the CRF system is not essential to the long-term regulation of energy balance because mutations of CRF and CRF-receptor genes do not affect feeding or body weight in mice (Venihaki et al. 1999).

15.4.4   Other Appetite Suppressant Peptides

Neurotensin is produced in the arcuate nucleus, PVN and DMN, and inhibits feeding when administered i.c.v. or into the PVN (Inui 2000). Thyrotropin-releasing hormone (TRH) is expressed in the PVN and several regions of the CNS. In addition to regulating TSH synthesis and secretion, TRH is well known to inhibit feeding and drinking when injected i.c.v. (Inui 2000). A metabolite of TRH, cyclo(His-Pro), also suppresses appetite and decreases body weight when administered i.c.v. in rats (Inui 2000). In a recent study, mice genetically engineered to be deficient in β-endorphin developed obesity (Ibrahim et al. 2003).

Glucagon-like peptides (GLP-1 and GLP-2) are produced by L-cells in the intestine and secreted in response to nutrients (Drucker 2001). GLP-1 reduces plasma glucose through effects on gastric emptying; glucose-dependent insulin release; synthesis and release of insulin and glucagons; and pancreatic islet development. In the CNS, GLP-1 is produced in the NTS and distributed to the PVN, DMN, where it regulates appetite, aversive behavior, and hypothalamic-pituitary function. GLP-1 suppresses feeding following i.c.v. or hypothalamic injection in rodents and decreases glucose and appetite in humans. However, the importance of GLP-1 to energy balance is uncertain because food intake and body weight were not affected by deletion of the GLP-1 receptor gene (Drucker 2001).

GLP-2 is produced in the NTS and released in the DMN and other hypothalamic nuclei to suppress appetite (Tang–Christensen et al. 2000). Moreover, GLP-2 regulates gastric motility and gastric emptying and exerts a protective effect on intestinal mucosa (Drucker 2001). Apart from its role in mediating satiety in the gastrointestinal tract, CCK is expressed in the lateral parabrachial nucleus and PVN and inhibits feeding following central administration (Bray 2000). However, deletion of CCK-A and CCK-B receptor genes did not affect feeding or body weight, suggesting that CCK is not required for regulation of energy balance (Kopin et al. 1999).

15.4.5   Monoamines

The ability of monoamines to regulate feeding and energy balance is well known (Schwartz et al. 2000). Serotonin (5HT) is synthesized in the dorsal raphe nucleus and released in the PVN, VMN, and other forebrain regions. Serotonin potently inhibits food intake in spontaneously feeding and food-deprived rodents. Serotonin agonists reduce body weight by suppressing appetite and increasing energy expenditure, and have been used as anti-obesity therapy in humans. This effect appears to be mediated mainly by the 5-HT$_{2C}$ receptor because mice with targeted disruption of 5-HT$_{2C}$ receptor developed hyperphagia, late-onset obesity, and type 2 diabetes (Nonogaki et al. 1998). Adrenergic agents have been used, albeit unsuccessfully, for treating obesity. These molecules inhibit appetite through activation of α_1 and β_2 adrenergic receptors or blockade of α_2 receptors (Bray and Tartaglia 2000). Histamine acts through specific receptors in the PVN, VMN, and other hypothalamic nuclei to suppress appetite (Bray and Tartaglia 2000).

15.4.6   Neurotrophins

Brain-derived neurotrophic factor (BDNF) belongs to the family of nerve growth factor-related neurotrophins, which includes neurotrophins 2 and 4/5. These proteins exert diverse effects in the nervous system, including promoting neuronal differentiation and survival. BDNF and its tyrosine kinase receptor, TrkB, are expressed in hypothalamic nuclei associated with feeding behavior and energy balance. Administration of BDNF reduces food intake and body weight in diet-induced obese rodents and decreases glucose in diet-induced obese, as well as *KKA/ya* and *db/db*, mice, suggesting that BDNF acts independently of leptin signaling (Nakagawa et al. 2003).

Mice heterozygous for BDNF deficiency became hyperphagic and obese, despite having increased locomotor activity (Kernie et al. 2000). Similarly, deletion of BDNF during the postnatal period using a conditional knockout strategy resulted in late-onset obesity; hyperactivity; increased linear growth; hyperleptinemia; and increased insulin (Rios et al. 2001). The expression and distribution of NPY, AGRP, α-MSH, MCH, orexin, TRH, and serotonin appeared normal in BDNF heterozygotes (Rios et al. 2001). Moreover, treatment with the serotonin reuptake inhibitor fluoxetine did not reverse the phenotype of these mutants, suggesting that BDNF acts through a novel mechanism to regulate energy balance (Rios et al. 2001).

Ciliary neurotrophic factor (CNTF) is expressed by glia in response to inflammation or injury and prevents neuronal degeneration. CNTF activates hypothalamic neuronal circuits that mediate feeding behavior and energy balance (Gloaguen et al. 1997). Systemic or central administration of CNTF inhibits food intake; decreases body weight; and corrects hyperinsulinemia and hyperglycemia in diabetic rodents. Like leptin receptor, the CNTF receptor belongs to the family of cytokine receptors that signal through the JAK-STAT pathway.

Studies in rodents have demonstrated that, unlike other antiobesity drugs, the weight-reducing effect of CNTF is sustained for a long period. Moreover, CNTF is able to overcome the leptin resistance associated with obesity, by suppressing hypothalamic NPY and AGRP, and preventing the normal hypothalamic response to energy depletion (Lambert et al. 2001). A null mutation in the human CNTF gene conferred moderate obesity in a population of Caucasian men (O'Dell et al. 2002), and CNTF has been shown to decrease appetite and body weight when administered by subcutaneous injection in humans (Ettinger et al. 2003).

15.5 Therapeutic Prospects

Breakthroughs in understanding of the molecular basis of eating behavior and energy balance have yielded important insights into potential therapy for obesity (Gura 2003). Strategies for obesity treatment include suppression of appetite; increased metabolic rate; and enhanced lipolysis. Ultimately, CNS drugs designed to treat obesity must reach their targets in the hypothalamus, brainstem, and other sites; be efficacious for long-term use; and pose acceptable risks to patients. An ideal antiobesity drug would also prevent diabetes, dyslipidemia, cardiovascular disease, and other obesity-related ailments. Because obesity is a medical and a cosmetic issue, the potential for abuse of medications is high, thereby increasing the risk for side effects and serious complications.

Targeting drugs to neurons in the CNS is limited by the blood–brain barrier through several mechanisms (Pardridge 2002):

- Endothelial cells of brain capillaries form tight junctions that prevent paracellular transport and limit pinocytosis. Pericapillary pericytes and foot processes of astrocytes also contribute to the physical barrier between the circulation and microenvironment of neurons.

- Capillary endothelial cells, pericytes, and astrocytes express enzymes, such as endopeptidases and carboxypeptidases, capable of inactivating various drugs.

- Activity of drugs may be decreased through efflux from the brain back into the circulation if they are substrates for efflux transporters present in the brain microvasculature.

Due to these barriers, obesity drugs must be lipid soluble, small (<400 Da), and/or have a facilitated or catalyzed transport system to access neuronal targets from the circulation. Avid binding of drug to plasma proteins will limit brain transport and must be avoided. The transport of large molecules such as peptides and neurotrophins could be enhanced through conjugation to lipids; cationization to decrease electrostatic interaction with anionic groups in the plasma membrane; and protection against peripheral metabolism as has been done for L-dopa. Interest in using nonpathogenic viral vectors to deliver peptides and large molecules to the brain is increasing. However, issues relating to safety and regulation of the temporal expression of product, as well as unknown long-term effects on brain structure and function, are likely to limit this approach.

CNS neurotransmitters and peptides discussed earlier are attractive targets for obesity treatment. Peptide and nonpeptide analogs may be developed to act specifically in the hypothalamus and other sites in the brain. The melanocortin signaling pathway is particularly interesting because mutations of the POMC and the MC4 receptor genes have been linked to obesity in humans. Drugs that suppress appetite and increase energy expenditure through enhancement of α-MSH action could be useful for chronic obesity therapy. It has been reported recently that a cyclic MC4 agonist, N-[(3R)-1,2,3,4-tetrahydroisoquinolinium-3-ylcarbonyl]-(1R)-1-(4-chlorobenzyl)-2-[4-cyclohexyl-4-(1H-1,2,4-triazol-1-ylmethyl)piperidin-1-yl]-oxoethylamine, decreases food intake and also stimulates erectile activity (Sebhat et al. 2002). The endogenous MC3/4 receptor antagonist AGRP could be targeted, for example, through modulation of syndecan-3 levels. Other potential central targets include antagonists of the NPY-Y5 and Y1 and MCH receptors. Nonpeptide MCH1 receptor antagonists have been shown to suppress appetite and decrease body weight in rodents (Borowsky et al. 2002; Bednarek et al. 2002). Specific CRH2 agonists could be developed to inhibit feeding and increase energy expenditure.

Although the combination of fenfluramine and phentermine was highly effective in weight reduction, the drug was withdrawn because of the life-threatening complication of primary pulmonary hypertension. Based on the phenotype of $5HT_{2C}$ receptor-null mice, it is possible that specific agonists of this receptor may avoid the systemic side effects of serotonin (Nonogaki et al. 1998). Sibutramine is a β-phenethylamine that reduces appetite and body weight through inhibition of norepinephrine, serotonin, and dopamine reuptake. It is one of two medications (the other is orlistat) approved by the U.S. Food and Drug Administration for chronic treatment of obesity. The efficacy of sibutramine is only slightly better than forced dieting alone, and its use has been associated with palpitation, high blood pressure, headaches, and insomnia, as well as reports of cardiovascular complications. Generally, targeting drugs to the monoaminergic system, e.g., through stimulation of $α_1$ and $β_2$ adrenergic receptors; blockade of $α_2$ receptors; and regulation of dopamine, GABA and histamine, is likely to be problematic because monoamines are involved in several physiologic processes.

The cannabinoid receptor (CB1) is an attractive target for drug development, as shown by impressive results in rodent models (Ravinet Trillou et al. 2003; Hilairet et al. 2003). Analogs of CNTF have been developed that decrease body weight without causing hyperthermia, malaise, and immune suppression associated with the original preparation (Lambert et al. 2001). When tested recently in humans, recombinant hCNTF produced a dose-related decrease in body weight (Ettinger et al. 2003). Potentially, other neurotrophins such as VGF and BDNF may be targeted for obesity treatment. However, a major concern regarding neurotrophins is the possibility of long-term alteration in brain structure and function. Insulin, glucocorticoids, and sex steroids modulate the levels of neurotransmitters and peptides (Dallman et al. 1993; Mystkowski and Schwartz 2000; Bruning et al. 2000). However, it is doubtful that this interaction could be exploited for treatment without untoward effects on other systems.

15.6 Conclusion

The prospects of new drug therapies for obesity have increased tremendously as a result of advances in understanding of the molecular regulation of energy balance. Currently, most data are based on experimental work in rodents. However, given the species differences in metabolism, such as the role of brown adipose, the characterization of the pharmacology of drugs must be extended early to humans to determine potential therapeutic benefits and safety. Another issue that remains to be addressed is the extent to which the concept of "homeostasis" can be applied to body weight regulation. Unlike temperature, osmolality, and other tightly regulated parameters, body weight and adiposity are markedly heterogenous.

Furthermore, it appears that the set point for body weight varies greatly from one individual to another and may be influenced by genetic differences in neurochemistry. Thus, it is possible that the therapeutic benefits of drugs targeted to particular neurotransmitters or peptides could be offset by reciprocal changes in other factors. Perhaps combinations of different classes of appetite suppressants and thermogenic agents may be required for weight maintenance, as is the case for other chronic diseases. Another area of controversy is the discrepancy between the pharmacological actions of various agents and the phenotypes resulting from manipulation of genes involved in energy balance. For example, ablation of NPY, Y1 and Y5 receptors, galanin, and CRF did not produce the expected effects on feeding and body weight. These differences need to be resolved by comparing and contrasting specific gene targeting strategies with conventional pharmacological techniques, in order to gain better insights into potential targets for obesity treatment.

References

Ahima, R.S. (2000) Leptin and the neuroendocrinology of fasting, *Front. Horm. Res.*, 26:42–56.

Ahima, R.S., Prabakaran, D., Mantzoros, C., Qu, D., Lowell, B., Maratos–Flier, E. and Flier, J.S. (1996) Role of leptin in the neuroendocrine response to fasting, *Nature*, 382:250–252.

Ahima, R.S., Saper, C.B., Flier, J.S. and Elmquist, J.K. (2000) Leptin regulation of neuroendocrine systems, *Front. Neuroendocrinol.*, 21:263–307.

Asnicar, M.A., Smith, D.P., Yang, D.D., Heiman, M.L., Fox, N., Chen, Y.F., Hsiung, H.M. and Koster, A. (2001) Absence of cocaine- and amphetamine-regulated transcript results in obesity in mice fed a high caloric diet, *Endocrinology*, 142:4394–4400.

Baldock, P.A., Sainsbury, A., Couzens, M., Enriquez, R.F., Thomas, G.P., Gardiner, E.M. and Herzog, H. (2002) Hypothalamic Y2 receptors regulate bone formation, *J. Clin. Invest.*, 109:915–1021.

Bannon, A.W., Seda, J., Carmouche, M., Francis, J.M., Norman, M.H., Karbon, B. and McCaleb, M.L. (2000) Behavioral characterization of neuropeptide Y knockout mice, *Brain Res.*, 868:79–87.

Barsh, G.S., Farooqi, I.S. and O'Rahilly, S. (2000) Genetics of body-weight regulation, *Nature*, 404:644–651.

Bednarek, M.A., Hreniuk, D.L., Tan, C., Palyh, O.C., MacNeil, D.J., Van der Ploeg, L.H., Howard, A.D. and Feighner, S.D. (2002) Synthesis and biological evaluation *in vitro* of selective, high affinity peptide antagonists of human melanin-concentrating hormone action at human melanin-concentrating hormone receptor 1, *Biochemistry*, 41:6383–6390.

Berglund, M.M., Hipskind, P.A. and Gehlert, D.R. (2003) Recent developments in our understanding of the physiological role of PP-fold peptide receptor subtypes, *Exp. Biol. Med. (Maywood)*, 228:217–244.

Borowsky, B., Durkin, M.M., Ogozalek, K., Marzabadi, M.R., DeLeon, J., Lagu, B., Heurich, R., Lichtblau, H., Shaposhnik, Z., Daniewska, I., Blackburn, T.P., Branchek, T.A., Gerald, C., Vaysse, P.J. and Forray C. (2002) Antidepressant, anxiolytic and anorectic effects of a melanin-concentrating hormone-1 receptor antagonist, *Nat. Med.*, 8:825–830.

Bray, G.A. (2000) Afferent signals regulating food intake, *Proc. Nutr. Soc.*, 59:373–384.

Bray, G.A. and Tartaglia, L.A. (2000) Medicinal strategies in the treatment of obesity, *Nature*, 404:672–677.

Broberger, C. (1999) Hypothalamic cocaine- and amphetamine-regulated transcript (CART) neurons: histochemical relationship to thyrotropin-releasing hormone, melanin-concentrating hormone, orexin/hypocretin and neuropeptide Y, *Brain Res.*, 848:101–113.

Bruning, J.C., Gautam, D., Burks, D.J., Gillette, J., Schubert, M., Orban, P.C., Klein, R., Krone, W., Muller–Wieland, D. and Kahn, C.R. (2000) Role of brain insulin receptor in control of body weight and reproduction, *Science*, 289:2122–2125.

Butler, A.A., Kesterson, R.A., Khong, K., Cullen, M.J., Pelleymounter, M.A., Dekoning, J., Baetscher, M. and Cone, R.D. (2000) A unique metabolic syndrome causes obesity in the melanocortin-3 receptor-deficient mouse, *Endocrinology*, 141:3518–3521.

Coleman, D.L. (1978) Obese and diabetes: two mutant genes causing diabetes-obesity syndromes in mice, *Diabetologia*, 14:141–148.

Cone, R.D. (1999) The central melanocortin system and energy homeostasis, *Trends Endocrinol. Metab.*, 10:211–216.

Cowley, M.A., Smart, J.L., Rubinstein, M., Cerdan, M.G., Diano, S., Horvath, T.L., Cone, R.D. and Low, M.J. (2001) Leptin activates anorexigenic POMC neurons through a neural network in the arcuate nucleus, *Nature*, 411:480–484.

Cowley, M.A., Smith, R.G., Diano, S., Tschop, M., Pronchuk, N., Grove, K.L., Strasburger, C.J., Bidlingmaier, M., Esterman, M., Heiman, M.L., Garcia–Segura, L.M., Nillni, E.A., Mendez, P., Low, M.J., Sotonyi, P., Friedman, J.M., Liu, H., Pinto, S., Colmers, W.F., Cone, R.D. and Horvath, T.L. (2003) The distribution and mechanism of action of ghrelin in the CNS demonstrates a novel hypothalamic circuit regulating energy homeostasis, *Neuron*, 37:649–661.

Criscione, L., Rigollier, P., Batzl–Hartmann, C., Ruegerm, H., Stricker–Krongrad, A., Wyss, P., Brunner, L., Whitebread, S., Yamaguchi, Y., Gerald, C., Heurich, R.O., Walker, M.W., Chiesi, M., Schilling, W., Hofbauer, K.G. and Levens, N. (1998) Food intake in free-feeding and energy-deprived lean rats is mediated by the neuropeptide Y5 receptor, *J. Clin. Invest.*, 102:2136–2145.

Dallman, M.F., Strack, A.M., Akana, S.F., Bradbury, M.J., Hanson, E.S., Scribner, K.A. and Smith, M. (1993) Feast and famine: critical role of glucocorticoids with insulin in daily energy flow, *Front. Neuroendocrinol.*, 14:303–347.

Di Marzo, V., Goparaju, S.K., Wang, L., Liu, J., Batkai, S., Jarai, Z., Fezza, F., Miura, G.I., Palmiter, R.D., Sugiura, T. and Kunos, G. (2001) Leptin-regulated endocannabinoids are involved in maintaining food intake, *Nature*, 410:822–825.

Dinulescu, D.M., Fan, W., Boston, B.A., McCall, K., Lamoreux, M.L., Moore, K.J., Montagno, J. and Cone, R.D. (1998) Mahogany (mg) stimulates feeding and increases basal metabolic rate independent of its suppression of agouti, *Proc. Natl. Acad. Sci. USA*, 95:12707–12712.

Drucker, D.J. (2001) Minireview: the glucagon-like peptides, *Endocrinology*, 142:521–527.

Ducy, P., Amling, M., Takeda, S., Priemel, M., Schilling, A.F., Beil, F.T., Shen, J., Vinson, C., Rueger, J.M. and Karsenty, G. (2000) Leptin inhibits bone formation through a hypothalamic relay: a central control of bone mass, *Cell*, 100:197–207.

Elias, C.F., Saper, C.B., Maratos–Flier, E., Tritos, N.A., Lee, C., Kelly, J., Tatro, J.B., Hoffman, G.E., Ollmann, M.M., Barsh, G.S., Sakurai, T., Yanagisawa, M. and Elmquist J.K. (1998) Chemically defined projections linking the mediobasal hypothalamus and the lateral hypothalamic area, *J. Comp. Neurol.*, 402:442–459.

Elmquist, J.K., Elias, C.F. and Saper, C.B. (1999) From lesions to leptin: hypothalamic control of food intake and body weight, *Neuron*, 22:221–232.

Erickson, J.C., Clegg, K.E. and Palmiter, R.D. (1996a) Sensitivity to leptin and susceptibility to seizures of mice lacking neuropeptide Y, *Nature*, 381:415–418.

Erickson, J.C., Hollopeter, G. and Palmiter, R.D. (1996b) Attenuation of the obesity syndrome of ob/ob mice by the loss of neuropeptide Y, *Science*, 274:1704–1707.

Ettinger, M.P., Littlejohn, T.W., Schwartz, S.L., Weiss, S.R., McIlwain, H.H., Heymsfield, S.B., Bray, G.A., Roberts, W.G., Heyman, E.R., Stambler, N., Heshka, S., Vicary, C. and Guler, H.P. (2003) Recombinant variant of ciliary neurotrophic factor for weight loss in obese adults: a randomized, dose-ranging study, *JAMA*, 289:1826–1832.

Farooqi, I.S., Keogh, J.M., Yeo, G.S., Lank, E.J., Cheetham, T. and O'Rahilly, S. (2003) Clinical spectrum of obesity and mutations in the melanocortin 4 receptor gene, *N. Engl. J. Med.*, 348:1085–1095.

Farooqi, I.S., Yeo, G.S., Keogh, J.M., Aminian, S., Jebb, S.A., Butler, G., Cheetham, T. and O'Rahilly, S. (2000) Dominant and recessive inheritance of morbid obesity associated with melanocortin 4 receptor deficiency, *J. Clin. Invest.*, 106:271–279.

Friedman, J.M. and Halaas, J.L. (1998) Leptin and the regulation of body weight in mammals, *Nature*, 395:763–770.

Gloaguen, I., Costa, P., Demartis, A., Lazzaro, D., Di Marco, A., Graziani, R., Paonessa, G., Chen, F., Rosenblum, C.I., Van der Ploeg, L.H., Cortese, R., Ciliberto, G. and Laufer, R. (1997) Ciliary neurotrophic factor corrects obesity and diabetes associated with leptin deficiency and resistance, *Proc. Natl. Acad. Sci. USA* 94:6456–6461.

Gura, T. (2003) Obesity drug pipeline not so fat, *Science,* 299:849–852.

Hagan, M.M., Rushing, P.A., Pritchard, L.M., Schwartz, M.W., Strack, A.M., Van Der Ploeg, L.H., Woods, S.C. and Seeley, R.J. (2000) Long-term orexigenic effects of AgRP-(83-132) involve mechanisms other than melanocortin receptor blockade, *Am. J. Physiol. Regul. Integr. Comp. Physiol.*, 279:R47–52.

Hahm, S., Fekete, C., Mizuno, T.M., Windsor, J., Yan, H., Boozer, C.N., Lee, C., Elmquist, J.K., Lechan, R.M., Mobbs, C.V. and Salton, S.R. (2002) VGF is required for obesity induced by diet, gold thioglucose treatment, and agouti and is differentially regulated in pro-opiomelanocortin- and neuropeptide Y-containing arcuate neurons in response to fasting, *J. Neurosci.*, 22:6929–6938.

Hara, J., Beuckmann, C.T., Nambu, T., Willie, J.T., Chemelli, R.M., Sinton, C.M., Sugiyama, F., Yagami, K., Goto, K., Yanagisawa, M. and Sakurai, T. (2001) Genetic ablation of orexin neurons in mice results in narcolepsy, hypophagia, and obesity, *Neuron*, 30:345–354.

Harris, R.B., Kasser, T.R. and Martin, R.J. (1986) Dynamics of recovery of body composition after overfeeding, food restriction or starvation of mature female rats, *J. Nutr.*, 116:2536–2546.

He, L., Gunn, T.M., Bouley, D.M., Lu, X.Y., Watson, S.J., Schlossman, S.F., Duke–Cohan, J.S. and Barsh, G.S. (2001) A biochemical function for attractin in agouti-induced pigmentation and obesity, *Nat. Genet.*, 27:40–47.

Hervey, G.R. (1959) The effects of lesions in the hypothalamus in parabiotic rats, *J. Physiol. (Lond)*, 145:336–352.

Hilairet, S., Bouaboula, M., Carriere, D., Le Fur, G., Casellas, P. (2003) Hypersensitization of the orexin 1 receptor by the CB1 receptor: evidence for cross-talk blocked by the specific CB1 antagonist, SR141716, *J. Biol. Chem.*, 278:23731–23737.

Hollopeter, G., Erickson, J.C. and Palmiter, R.D. (1998) Role of neuropeptide Y in diet, chemical- and genetic-induced obesity of mice, *Int. J. Obe.s Relat. Metab. Disord.*, 22:506–512.

Horvath, T.L., Diano, S., Sotonyi, P., Heiman, M. and Tschop, M. (2001) Minireview: ghrelin and the regulation of energy balance — a hypothalamic perspective, *Endocrinology*, 142:4163–4169.

Huszar, D., Lynch, C.A., Fairchild–Huntress, V., Dunmore, J.H., Fang, Q., Berkemeier, L.R., Gu, W., Kesterson, R.A., Boston, B.A., Cone, R.D., Smith, F.J., Campfield, L.A., Burn, P. and Lee, F. (1997) Targeted disruption of the melanocortin-4 receptor results in obesity in mice, *Cell*, 88:131–141.

Ibrahim, N., Bosch, M.A., Smart, J.L., Qiu, J., Rubinstein, M., Ronnekleiv, O.K., Low, M.J. and Kelly, M.J. (2003) Hypothalamic proopiomelanocortin neurons are glucose responsive and express K(ATP) channels, *Endocrinology*, 144:1331–1340.

Inui, A. (2000) Transgenic approach to the study of body weight regulation, *Pharmacol. Rev.*, 52:35–61.

Kaga, T., Inui, A., Okita, M., Asakawa, A., Ueno, N., Kasuga, M., Fujimiya, M., Nishimura, N., Dobashi, R., Morimoto, Y., Liu, I.M. and Cheng, J.T. (2001) Modest overexpression of neuropeptide Y in the brain leads to obesity after high-sucrose feeding, *Diabetes*, 50:1206–1210.

Kennedy, G.C. (1953) The role of depot fat in the hypothalamic control of food intake in the rat, *Proc. R. Soc. Lond. (Biol.)*, 140:578–596.

Kernie, S.G., Liebl, D.J. and Parada, L.F. (2000) BDNF regulates eating behavior and locomotor activity in mice, *EMBO J.*, 19:1290–1300.

Kojima, M., Hosoda, H., Matsuo, H. and Kangawa, K. (2001) Ghrelin: discovery of the natural endogenous ligand for the growth hormone secretagogue receptor, *Trends Endocrinol. Metab.*, 12:118–122.

Kopelman, P.G. (2000) Obesity as a medical problem, *Nature*, 404:635–643.

Kopin, A.S., Mathes, W.F., McBride, E.W., Nguyen, M., Al-Haider, W., Schmitz, F., Bonner–Weir, S., Kanarek, R. and Beinborn, M. (1999) The cholecystokinin-A receptor mediates inhibition of food intake yet is not essential for the maintenance of body weight, *J. Clin. Invest.*, 103:383–391.

Kristensen, P., Judge, M.E., Thim, L., Ribel, U., Christjansen, K.N., Wulff, B.S., Clausen, J.T., Jensen, P.B., Madsen, O.D., Vrang, N., Larsen, P.J. and Hastrup, S. (1998) Hypothalamic CART is a new anorectic peptide regulated by leptin, 393:72–76.

Krude, H., Biebermann, H., Luck, W., Horn, R., Brabant, G. and Gruters, A. (1998) Severe early-onset obesity, adrenal insufficiency and red hair pigmentation caused by POMC mutations in humans, *Nat. Genet.*, 19:155–157

Kuhar, M.J., Adams, S., Dominguez, G., Jaworski, J. and Balkan, B. (2000) CART peptides, *Regul. Pept.*, 89:1–6.

Kushi, A., Sasai, H., Koizumi, H., Takeda, N., Yokoyama, M. and Nakamura, M. (1998) Obesity and mild hyperinsulinemia found in neuropeptide Y-Y1 receptor-deficient mice, *Proc. Natl. Acad. Sci. USA*, 95:15659–15664.

Lambert, P.D., Anderson, K.D., Sleeman, M.W., Wong, V., Tan, J., Hijarunguru, A., Corcoran, T.L., Murray, J.D., Thabet, K.E., Yancopoulos, G.D. and Wiegand, S.J. (2001) Ciliary neurotrophic factor activates leptin-like pathways and reduces body fat, without cachexia or rebound weight gain, even in leptin-resistant obesity, *Proc. Natl. Acad. Sci. USA*, 98:4652–4657.

Lewis, K., Li, C., Perrin, M.H., Blount, A., Kunitake, K., Donaldson, C., Vaughan, J., Reyes, T.M., Gulyas, J., Fischer, W., Bilezikjian, L., Rivier, J., Sawchenko, P.E., Vale, W.W. (2001) Identification of urocortin III, an additional member of the corticotropin-releasing factor (CRF) family with high affinity for the CRF2 receptor, *Proc. Natl. Acad. Sci. USA*, 98:7570–7575.

Lin, L., Faraco, J., Li, R., Kadotani, H., Rogers, W., Lin, X., Qiu, X., de Jong, P.J., Nishino, S. and Mignot E. (1999) The sleep disorder canine narcolepsy is caused by a mutation in the hypocretin (orexin) receptor 2 gene, *Cell*, 98:365–376.

Ludwig, D.S., Tritos, N.A., Mastaitis, J.W., Kulkarni, R., Kokkotou, E., Elmquist, J., Lowell, B., Flier, J.S. and Maratos–Flier, E. (2001) Melanin-concentrating hormone overexpression in transgenic mice leads to obesity and insulin resistance, *J. Clin. Invest.*, 107:379–386.

MacNeil, D.J., Howard, A.D., Guan, X., Fong, T.M., Nargund, R.P., Bednarek, M.A., Goulet, M.T., Weinberg, D.H., Strack, A.M., Marsh, D.J., Chen, H.Y., Shen, C.P., Chen, A.S., Rosenblum, C.I., MacNeil, T., Tota, M., MacIntyre, E.D. and Van der Ploeg, L.H. (2002) The role of melanocortins in body weight regulation: opportunities for the treatment of obesity, *Eur. J. Pharmacol.*, 440:141–157.

Marsh, D.J., Hollopeter, G., Kafer, K.E. and Palmiter, R.D. (1998) Role of the Y5 neuropeptide Y receptor in feeding and obesity, *Nat. Med.*, 4:718–721.

Marsh, D.J., Miura, G.I., Yagaloff, K.A., Schwartz, M.W., Barsh, G.S. and Palmiter, R.D. (1999) Effects of neuropeptide Y deficiency on hypothalamic agouti-related protein expression and responsiveness to melanocortin analogues, *Brain Res.*, 848:66–77.

Marsh, D.J., Weingarth, D.T., Novi, D.E., Chen, H.Y., Trumbauer, M.E., Chen, A.S., Guan, X.M., Jiang, M.M., Feng, Y., Camacho, R.E., Shen, Z., Frazier, E.G., Yu, H., Metzger, J.M., Kuca, S.J., Shearman, L.P., Gopal–Truter, S., MacNeil, D.J., Strack, A.M., MacIntyre, D.E., Van der Ploeg, L.H. and Qian, S. (2002) Melanin-concentrating hormone 1 receptor-deficient mice are lean, hyperactive, and hyperphagic and have altered metabolism, *Proc. Natl. Acad. Sci. USA*, 99:3240–3245.

Martin, J.R., Bos, M., Jenck, F., Moreau, J., Mutel, V., Sleight, A.J., Wichmann, J., Andrews, J.S., Berendsen, H.H., Broekkamp, C.L., Ruigt, G.S., Kohler, C. and Delft. A.M. (1998) 5-HT2C receptor agonists: pharmacological characteristics and therapeutic potential, *J. Pharmacol. Exp. Ther.*, 286:913–924.

Mystkowski, P. and Schwartz, M.W. (2000) Gonadal steroids and energy homeostasis in the leptin era, *Nutrition*, 16:937–946.

Nakagawa, T., Ogawa, Y., Ebihara, K., Yamanaka, M., Tsuchida, A., Taiji, M., Noguchi, H. and Nakao, K. (2003) Anti-obesity and anti-diabetic effects of brain-derived neurotrophic factor in rodent models of leptin resistance, *Int. J. Obes. Relat. Metab. Disord.*, 27:557–565.

Naveilhan, P., Svensson, L., Nystrom, S., Ekstrand, A.J. and Ernfors, P. (2002) Attenuation of hyper-cholesterolemia and hyperglycemia in ob/ob mice by NPY Y2 receptor ablation, *Peptides*, 23:1087–1091.

Nonogaki, K., Strack, A.M., Dallman, M.F. and Tecott, L.H. (1998) Leptin-independent hyperphagia and type 2 diabetes in mice with a mutated serotonin 5-HT2C receptor gene, *Nat. Med.*, 4:1152–1156.

O'Dell, S.D., Syddall, H.E., Sayer, A.A., Cooper, C., Fall, C.H., Dennison, E.M., Phillips, D.I., Gaunt, T.R., Briggs, P.J. and Day, I.N. (2002) Null mutation in human ciliary neurotrophic factor gene confers higher body mass index in males, *Eur. J. Hum. Genet.*, 10:749–752.

Pardridge, W.M. (2002) Targeting neurotherapeutic agents through the blood–brain barrier, *Arch. Neurol.*, 59:35–40.

Qian, S., Chen, H., Weingarth, D., Trumbauer, M.E., Novi, D.E., Guan, X., Yu, H., Shen, Z., Feng, Y., Frazier, E., Chen, A., Camacho, R.E., Shearman, L.P., Gopal–Truter, S., MacNeil, D.J., Van der Ploeg, L.H. and Marsh, D.J. (2002) Neither agouti-related protein nor neuropeptide Y is critically required for the regulation of energy homeostasis in mice, *Mol. Cell Biol.*, 22:5027–5035.

Qu, D., Ludwig, D.S., Gammeltoft, S., Piper, M., Pelleymounter, M.A., Cullen, M.J., Mathes, W.F., Przypek, R., Kanarek, R. and Maratos–Flier, E. (1996) A role for melanin-concentrating hormone in the central regulation of feeding behaviour, *Nature*, 380:243–247.

Ravinet Trillou, C., Arnone, M., Delgorge, C., Gonalons, N., Keane, P., Maffrand, J.P. and Soubrie, P. (2003) Anti-obesity effect of SR141716, a CB1 receptor antagonist, in diet-induced obese mice, *Am. J. Physiol. Regul. Integr. Comp. Physiol.*, 284:R345–353.

Reizes, O., Lincecum, J., Wang, Z., Goldberger, O., Huang, L., Kaksonen, M., Ahima, R., Hinkes, M.T., Barsh, G.S., Rauvala, H. and Bernfield, M. (2001) Transgenic expression of syndecan-1 uncovers a physiological control of feeding behavior by syndecan-3, *Cell*, 106:105–116.

Reyes, T.M., Lewis, K., Perrin, M.H., Kunitake, K.S., Vaughan, J., Arias, C.A., Hogenesch, J.B., Gulyas, J., Rivier, J., Vale, W.W., Sawchenko, P.E. (2001) Urocortin II: a member of the corticotropin-releasing factor (CRF) neuropeptide family that is selectively bound by type 2 CRF receptors, *Proc. Natl. Acad. Sci. USA*, 98:2843–2848.

Richard, D., Huang, Q. and Timofeeva, E. (2000) The corticotropin-releasing hormone system in the regulation of energy balance in obesity, *Int. J. Obes. Relat. Metab. Disord.*, 24 Suppl 2:S36–39.

Rios, M., Fan, G., Fekete, C., Kelly, J., Bates, B., Kuehn, R., Lechan, R.M. and Jaenisch, R. (2001) Conditional deletion of brain-derived neurotrophic factor in the postnatal brain leads to obesity and hyperactivity, *Mol. Endocrinol.*, 15:1748–1757.

Sahu, A. and Karla, S.P. (1993) Neuropeptidergic regulation of feeding behavior, neuropeptide Y, *Trends Endocrinol. Metab.*, 4:217–224.

Sainsbury, A., Schwarzer, C., Couzens, M. and Herzog, H. (2002a) Y2 receptor deletion attenuates the type 2 diabetic syndrome of ob/ob mice, *Diabetes*, 51:3420–3427.

Sainsbury, A., Schwarzer, C., Couzens, M., Jenkins, A., Oakes, S.R., Ormandy, C.J. and Herzog, H. (2002b) Y4 receptor knockout rescues fertility in ob/ob mice, *Genes Dev.*, 16:1077–1088.

Saito, Y., Nothacker, H.P. and Civelli, O. (2000) Melanin-concentrating hormone receptor: an orphan receptor fits the key, *Trends Endocrinol. Metab.*, 11:299–303.

Sakurai, T., Amemiya, A., Ishii, M., Matsuzaki, I., Chemelli, R.M., Tanaka, H., Williams, S.C., Richardson, J.A., Kozlowski, G.P., Wilson, S., Arch, J.R., Buckingham, R.E., Haynes, A.C., Carr, S.A., Annan, R.S., McNulty, D.E., Liu, W.S., Terrett, J.A., Elshourbagy, N.A., Bergsma, D.J. and Yanagisawa, M. (1998) Orexins and orexin receptors: a family of hypothalamic neuropeptides and G protein-coupled receptors that regulate feeding behavior, *Cell*, 92:573–585.

Salton, S.R., Ferri, G.L., Hahm, S., Snyder, S.E., Wilson, A.J., Possenti, R. and Levi, A. (2000) VGF: a novel role for this neuronal and neuroendocrine polypeptide in the regulation of energy balance, *Front. Neuroendocrinol.*, 21:199–219.

Sawchenko, P.E. (1998) Toward a new neurobiology of energy balance, appetite, and obesity: the anatomists weigh in, *J. Comp. Neurol.*, 402:435–441.

Schwartz, M.W., Woods, S.C., Porte, D., Jr., Seeley, R.J. and Baskin, D.G. (2000) Central nervous system control of food intake, *Nature*, 404:661–671.

Sebhat, I.K., Martin, W.J., Ye, Z., Barakat, K., Mosley, R.T., Johnston, D.B., Bakshi, R., Palucki, B., Weinberg, D.H., MacNeil, T., Kalyani, R.N., Tang, R., Stearns, R.A., Miller, R.R., Tamvakopoulos, C., Strack, A.M., McGowan, E., Cashen, D.E., Drisko, J.E., Hom, G.J., Howard, A.D., MacIntyre, D.E., van der Ploeg, L.H., Patchett, A.A. and Nargund, R.P. (2002) Design and pharmacology of N-[(3R)-1,2,3,4-tetrahydroisoquinolinium-3-ylcarbonyl]-(1R)-1-(4-chlorobenzyl)-2-[4-cyclohexyl-4-(1H-1,2,4-triazol-1 ylmethyl)piperidin-1-yl]-2-oxoethylamine (1), a potent, selective, melanocortin subtype-4 receptor agonist, *J. Med. Chem.*, 45:4589–4593.

Segal-Lieberman, G. et al. (2003) NPY ablation in C57B1/6 mice leads to mild obesity and to an impaired refeeding response to fasting, *Am. J. Physiol. Endocrinol. Metab.*, 284:E1131–1139.

Shimada, M., Tritos, N.A., Lowell, B.B., Flier, J.S. and Maratos–Flier, E. (1998) Mice lacking melanin-concentrating hormone are hypophagic and lean, *Nature*, 396:670–674.

Sindelar, D.K., Mystkowski, P., Marsh, D.J., Palmiter, R.D. and Schwartz, M.W. (2002) Attenuation of diabetic hyperphagia in neuropeptide Y-deficient mice, *Diabetes*, 51:778–783.

Smart, D., Haynes, A.C., Williams, G. and Arch, J.R. (2002) Orexins and the treatment of obesity, *Eur. J. Pharmacol.*, 440:199–212.

Spiegelman, B.M. and Flier, J.S. (2001) Obesity and the regulation of energy balance, *Cell*, 104:531–543.

Sutcliffe, J.G. and de Lecea, L. (2002) The hypocretins: setting the arousal threshold, *Nat. Rev. Neurosci.*, 3:339–349.

Takekawa, S., Asami, A., Ishihara, Y., Terauchi, J., Kato, K., Shimomura, Y., Mori, M., Murakoshi, H., Kato, K., Suzuki, N., Nishimura, O. and Fujino, M. (2002) T-226296: a novel, orally active and selective melanin-concentrating hormone receptor antagonist, *Eur. J. Pharmacol.*, 438:129–135.

Tang–Christensen, M., Larsen, P.J., Thulesen, J., Romer, J. and Vrang, N. (2000) The proglucagon-derived peptide, glucagon-like peptide-2, is a neurotransmitter involved in the regulation of food intake, *Nat. Med.*, 6:802–807.

Taylor, M.M. and Samson, W.K. (2003) The other side of the orexins: endocrine and metabolic actions, *Am. J. Physiol. Endocrinol. Metab.*, 284:E13–17.

Thiele, T.E., Marsh, D.J., Ste Marie, L., Bernstein, I.L. and Palmiter, R.D. (1998) Ethanol consumption and resistance are inversely related to neuropeptide Y levels, *Nature,* 396:366–369.

Tritos, N.A., Mastaitis, J.W., Kokkotou, E. and Maratos–Flier, E. (2001) Characterization of melanin concentrating hormone and preproorexin expression in the murine hypothalamus, *Brain Res.*, 895:160–166.

Tschop, M., Smiley, D.L. and Heiman, M.L. (2001) Ghrelin induces adiposity in rodents, *Nature*, 407:908–913.

Venihaki, M. and Majzoub, J.A. (1999) Animal models of CRH deficiency, *Front. Neuroendocrinol.*, 20:122–145.

Vezzani, A., Michalkiewicz, M., Michalkiewicz, T., Moneta, D., Ravizza, T., Richichi, C., Aliprandi, M., Mule, F., Pirona, L., Gobbi, M., Schwarzer, C. and Sperk, G. (2002) Seizure susceptibility and epileptogenesis are decreased in transgenic rats overexpressing neuropeptide Y, *Neuroscience*, 110:237–243.

Wang, S., Behan, J., O'Neill, K., Weig, B., Fried, S., Laz, T., Bayne, M., Gustafson, E. and Hawes, B.E. (2001) Identification and pharmacological characterization of a novel human melanin-concentrating hormone receptor, mch-r2, *J. Biol. Chem.*, 276:34664–34670.

Willie, J.T., Chemelli, R.M., Sinton, C.M. and Yanagisawa, M. (2001) To eat or to sleep? Orexin in the regulation of feeding and wakefulness, *Annu. Rev. Neurosci.*, 24:429–458.

Yaswen, L., Diehl, N., Brennan, M.B. and Hochgeschwender, U. (1999) Obesity in the mouse model of pro-opiomelanocortin deficiency responds to peripheral melanocortin, *Nat. Med.*, 5:1066–1070.

Zhang, Y., Proenca, R., Maffei, M., Barone, M., Leopold, L. and Friedman, J.M. (1994) Positional cloning of the mouse obese gene and its human homologue, *Nature*, 372:425–432.

16

Leptin and Other Appetite Suppressants

L. Arthur Campfield and Françoise J. Smith

CONTENTS

SUMMARY Feeding behavior is the result of the complex central nervous system integration of central and peripheral signals relating to brain and metabolic states. Meals are initiated, maintained, and terminated by sets of these central and peripheral signals several times a day, separated by intermeal intervals without food intake. One hypothesis for this integrated control of food intake postulates the interaction of five classes of signals: (1)

hypothalamic neuropeptides; (2) brain insulin; (3) leptin; (4) metabolic signals including transient declines in blood glucose; and (5) ascending and descending neural inputs. These signals interact and provide the central/peripheral integration necessary to regulate food intake and body energy balance. These pathways provide potential targets for future appetite suppressants. In this chapter, the current state of understanding of the biology, neurobiology, genetics, pharmacology, and behavioral aspects of the regulation of energy intake will be reviewed; a case study of the discovery and clinical investigation of leptin for the reduction of energy intake and induction of weight loss will be presented. Additionally, the current discovery and development pipeline for future appetite suppressants will be described.

16.1 Introduction

Body energy balance in humans and laboratory animals is regulated by a set of very complex biological and behavioral signals, mechanisms, and pathways. Molecular (e.g., leptin, insulin) and biophysical (e.g., vagal afferents responding to a change in duodenal glucose concentration) signals in the periphery and brain are linked in a neural network that controls eating behavior and energy intake. Signals generated in the periphery and brain are integrated and interpreted, and the appropriate motor program and resulting behavioral response in terms of energy intake generated in the brain of humans and animals. For example, a person who has been ill for 4 days with influenza has decreased energy intake and has lost 5 kg of weight. As soon as the illness ends, the brain will correctly interpret the fall in leptin and other peripheral and brain signals as weight loss and then increase energy intake for the next several days; the person will regain the 5 kg lost. Suppose that, 3 months later, the same person goes on vacation for a month in France or on a cruise ship, overconsumes energy, and gains 5 kg. When the person returns to habitual patterns of energy intake and expenditure, the brain will correctly interpret the increased leptin and other signals as weight gain. The brain will decrease energy intake for the next period until the 5 kg are lost and the habitual body mass and composition are restored. These are examples of the usual regulation of energy balance in lean humans and animals.

However, a growing number of children, young people, and adults around the world are slowly, but steadily gaining weight and becoming overweight and obese (62% in the U.S.; more than 40% of middle-aged people in the U.K. and Switzerland [World Health Organization, 1988, 1998]. These people are in positive energy balance (taking in more energy than they expend) almost every day of their lives; their adipose tissue is expanding and their health risks for type 2 diabetes, heart disease, hypertension, and dyslipidemia are rapidly mounting. Many people in the world are experiencing the effects of a life-long "vacation" in which increased energy intake and decreased energy expenditure have become the dominant feature of their metabolic lives. The normal physiological and behavioral regulatory mechanisms that operate in normal-weight people are simply overwhelmed by the persistent positive energy balance and, as a result, adipose tissue expands.

Recent research in experimental animals and obese humans indicates that the neural networks in the brains of obese animals and individuals that control energy balance are altered compared to the brains of normal-weight animals and humans. The sensitivity and/or responsiveness of brain pathways to the major peripheral signals, leptin and insulin, as well as cortisol and cholecystokinin (CCK), may be decreased in the obese state compared to the normal-weight state. Thus, not only are the metabolic pathways forced in the direction of net energy storage, but also the ability of the brain to resist and correct sustained positive energy balance is significantly degraded in more and more people of the world. Obesity is rapidly becoming a major health problem in all regions of the world (World Health Organization, 1998).

The need for truly effective and safe medicines to reduce appetite and energy intake of overweight and obese humans significantly is clear and has never before been so essential to maintaining and improving the health of so many people. In this chapter, the current state of understanding of the biology, neurobiology, genetics, pharmacology, and behavioral aspects of the regulation of energy intake will be reviewed; a case study of the discovery and clinical investigation of leptin for the reduction of energy intake and induction of weight loss will be presented; and the current discovery and development pipeline for future appetite suppressants will be described.

16.2 Regulation of Energy Balance

Energy balance is the result of the control of ingestive behavior, energy expenditure, and energy storage in adipose tissue. In most adults, body weight and body fat content remain constant over many years or decades, despite a very large flux of energy intake and expenditure (approximately 1 million kcal/year). Energy intake is a *discrete* process because individual meals are separated by intermeal intervals, while energy expenditure and storage in adipose tissue are *continuous* physiological processes. However, the complex molecular mechanisms by which discrete ingestive behavior, continuous energy expenditure, and dynamic energy storage in adipose tissue are integrated and matched remain largely unknown. Two important peripheral signals are brain insulin and leptin.

16.3 Control of Food Intake

Feeding behavior is the result of the complex central nervous system (CNS) integration of central and peripheral signals relating to brain and metabolic states. Meals are initiated, maintained, and terminated by sets of these central and peripheral signals several times a day, separated by intermeal intervals without food intake. These signals include *patterns* of: neural afferent traffic; metabolites (glucose); energy flux (fatty acid oxidation, ATP) and hormone (insulin) concentrations in plasma and brain; leptin; and neuropeptide concentrations in plasma and brain. Meal initiation is signaled in rats and humans by transient declines in blood glucose concentration (Campfield and Smith, 2003). One hypothesis for this integrated control of food intake postulates the interaction of five classes of signals: (1) hypothalamic neuropeptides; (2) brain insulin; (3) leptin; (4) metabolic signals including transient declines in blood glucose; and (5) ascending and descending neural inputs. These signals interact and provide the central/peripheral integration necessary to regulate food intake and body energy balance (Smith et al., 1996; Campfield and Smith, 2003).

Numerous experimental studies in mice, rats, and many other species demonstrate that several neuropeptides modulate food intake when injected centrally and, in some cases, peripherally. Among the neuropeptides that affect food intake are neuropeptide Y (NPY); cholecystokinin (CCK); corticotropin-releasing hormone (CRH); and enterostatin. Studies have suggested that glucagon-like-peptide 1 (GLP-1) can also alter food intake when injected centrally. However, when GLP-1 is administered into the third ventricle of the brain of rats, it causes a taste aversion at the same doses at which it inhibits food intake. Thus, the food intake suppression observed following central injections of GLP-1 might be secondary to illness or other nonspecific effects.

GLP-1 has been administered i.v. to humans in several short-term studies. Decreased hunger and increased satiety ratings; decreased gastric emptying; and reduced food intake have been observed. In a study in obese humans, doses of GLP-1 that elevated plasma concentration of GLP-1 within the physiological range resulted in decreased hunger and prospective food consumption, but unchanged food intake and decreased gastric empty-ing (Flint et al., 2001). Synaptic concentrations of central neuropeptides and classical monoamine neurotransmitters are thought to be modulated by the central representations of peripheral metabolic state and act on postsynaptic receptors to control energy intake.

16.4 Obesity: A Disease of Biological Dysregulation

Many studies have clearly demonstrated that obesity is, at its basis, a disease of *biological dysregulation*. That is, the steady-state body weight of an individual is thought to result from an *integration* of *multiple* biological factors, including *energy intake*, which are at least partially *genetically* determined. Perturbations in body weight induced by changes in energy intake, in both directions (increased, decreased) from this steady-state weight are *resisted* and *corrected* by robust *physiological mechanisms*, including *changes in energy intake*, in laboratory rodents and humans. The physiological mechanisms that resist changes in body fat content are responsible for the unfortunate and very frustrating weight regain that usually follows weight loss. Leptin, which acts on the brain to regulate energy intake, probably plays a role in this "resetting response" responsible for weight regain following weight loss (Leibel et al., 1995; Campfield and Smith, 1999).

16.5 Genetic Contributions to Regulation of Human Food Intake

The fact that obesity runs in families has been recognized and appreciated for many years. Equally well recognized and appreciated was the fact that increased energy intake and decreased physical activity, independent of genetics, could promote the development of obesity in individuals.

The most commonly accepted model for the genetics of human obesity and increased energy intake is an interaction of genetic predisposition and environmental factors (Campfield and Smith, 1999). The relative importance of these two factors in specific populations can vary across studies. A reasonable consensus exists among investigators in the field that human obesity is characterized by increased adipose tissue mass resulting from an interaction of: (1) genetic predisposition to store energy efficiently in adipose tissue as triglycerides (35 to 50%); and (2) environmental and/or life-style factors (50 to

65%). In studies of monozygotic twins raised together or apart, the heritability (that part of the variation in percent body fat that can be accounted for by genetic inheritance) has ranged from 20 to 60%.

The best current estimate for the heritability of percent body fat is 35% (Bouchard and Perusse, 1993; Campfield and Smith, 1999). If another 15% is allocated for the genetic predisposition to gain weight when a highly palatable, high-fat diet is easily available (as it is in the developed world), then genetic inheritance can account for approximately 50% of the variation in percent body fat (Bouchard and Perusse, 1993; Comuzzie and Allison, 1998). Although these analyses clearly indicate that genetic factors are important, they also indicate that environmental and behavioral factors are also important factors in the etiology and development of obesity (Comuzzie, 2002).

16.6 Potential Obesity Targets: Human Mutations Associated with or Linked to Obesity

16.6.1 Approaches

Following demonstration of a significant linkage between a chromosomal region and an aspect of the obese phenotype in groups of related or unrelated humans, positional cloning of the gene or genes is then possible. Positional cloning is a technique for isolation and identification of a specific gene that is responsible for some aspects of the obese phenotype. It involves construction of a set of contiguous clones containing entire genes or parts of the genes that span the minimal interval surrounding the gene. Each gene or partial gene is tested in turn until the gene responsible for that aspect of the obese phenotype is identified. The process ends with the identification of the specific gene responsible and the predicted gene product.

Another approach to the identification of human obesity genes is the use of positionally cloned mouse and rat single genes to identify the human homologue of genes on the human chromosomal regions corresponding to the identified mouse chromosomal location. This approach has led to the location of the human homologues of the *ob, db, tub, fat,* and *agouti* genes. The positional cloning of the mouse genes has also made the mutation analysis of human homologues of these mouse obesity genes possible in individuals with increased energy intake and obesity.

The search for the modifier genes in polygenic models of obesity using quantitative trait loci (QTLs) for body fat content is also being aggressively pursued. Once one or more sufficiently narrow QTLs are established, positional cloning should yield the gene or genes responsible for the variation in body fat content. Similarly, when the modifier gene studies yield smaller QTLs for enhanced susceptibility or resistance to hyperglycemia, then positional cloning should yield the human homologues for these potentially important modifier genes. The 2002 update of the human obesity map has been published (Chagnon et al., 2003) and is available on-line at http://obesitygene.pbrc.edu.

16.6.2 Targets

16.6.2.1 Leptin and Leptin Receptor

Thousands of obese individuals have been screened for mutations in the *OB* and *OB-R*, the human gene encoding for leptin (or OB protein) and leptin receptor, respectively. Thus far, three different families have been found to have mutations. Two cousins (male and female) from a large consanguineous family from India have homozygous frame-shift mutations resulting in the deletion of a single guanine nucleotide in *OB* gene and, as expected, they have low or undetectable levels of functional leptin. They were normal weight at birth and then rapidly became severely obese, just as leptin deficient, obese mice (Montague et al., 1997) did. Three obese members of a Turkish family were shown to carry a homozygous missense mutation in the *OB* that is associated with low serum leptin concentrations (Strobel et al., 1998). These reports indicate that children with very rare homozygous mutations in the leptin gene and complete leptin deficiency develop extreme hyperphagia and obesity soon after birth. When treated with small amounts of recombinant human leptin, they respond with reduced food intake, normalized eating patterns, and a selective loss of body fat.

Heterozygote relatives have 30% more fat than predicted and relatively low leptin levels (O'Rahilly, 2002). Three severely obese sisters in a large consanguineous family of Kabilian origin have been found to be homozygous for a splice-site mutation in the *OB-R* gene; the mutant gene is predicted to encode a truncated form of leptin receptor (OB-R) that lacks the transmembrane and intracellular domains and, therefore, presumably has no signaling function. Two of the adult sisters showed no signs of pubertal development — consistent with studies in mice and humans showing that leptin also has a role in reproductive development (Clement et al., 1998). These findings strongly suggest that leptin plays an important role in the regulation of energy intake, body fat and body weight, and reproductive function in humans.

16.6.2.2 The Melanocortin 4 Receptor (MC4-R)

The melanocortin-4 receptor (MC4-R) has been shown to play a role in the regulation of body energy balance. Mice deficient in MC4-R that were produced using gene targeting in embryonic stem cells developed increased energy intake and obesity, and an altered metabolic phenotype. Stimulation of the MC4-R with a peptide agonist caused decreased food intake, which could be blocked by an antagonist. A mutation in the *agouti* gene is responsible for obesity in a strain of yellow mice (Bultman et al., 1992). Recent genetic and pharmacological research strongly suggests that AGOUTI causes obesity by blocking the MC4-R in the brain (Huszar et al., 1997; Fan et al., 1997, 2000). The MC4-R knockout mice studies, combined with experiments with MC4-R agonists (which decrease food intake) and antagonists (which increase food intake), indicate that the MC4-R is part of a physiological pathway that normally inhibits food intake and fat storage. This pathway may play an important role in late-onset obesity (Fan et al., 1997, 2000).

Mutations in the MC4-R have been found to cause severe, early-onset increased energy intake and obesity (Farooqi et al., 2003). A study of obese subjects from southern Italy showed a low frequency (<0.5%) of MC4-R mutations (Miraglia Del Giudice et al., 2002). In a study of 172 subjects with severe early-onset obesity and family history of obesity, three (1.7%) heterozygous MC4-R mutations were identified. These mutations, as well as 11 other childhood obesity-related reported mutations, result in decreased MC4-R activation by alpha-melanocyte-stimulating hormone (alpha-MSH) (Vaisse et al., 2000). In addition, intracellular retention of receptors was found in over 80% of the mutations (Lubrano–Berthelier et al., 2003).

A recent comprehensive and systematic study of 500 individuals with severe early-onset obesity showed MC4-R mutations in 5.8% (29 individuals); 23 were heterozygous and 6 were homozygous. Mutation carriers had increased food intake; severe obesity; increased lean mass; increased linear growth; and markedly increased serum insulin concentrations.

Homozygotes were more severely affected than heterozygotes. Signaling (cAMP) was decreased in mutated MC4-R; all frame-shift mutations and some missense mutations resulted in complete loss of signaling, while some of the missense mutations encoded receptors with residual signaling capacity. Subjects with mutations retaining residual signaling capacity had a less severe phenotype. Thus, mutations in MC4-R result in a distinct obesity syndrome that is inherited in a codominant manner. The correlation between the signaling properties of these mutant receptors and energy intake emphasizes the key role of this pathway in regulation of feeding behavior and fat mass in humans (Farooqi et al., 2003). Initial studies of MC3-R mutations have failed to demonstrate an association with obesity (Lee et al., 2002).

16.6.2.3 Pro-Opiomelanocortin (POMC)

Functional loss of both alleles of the pro-opiomelanocortin (POMC) gene results in a very rare early-onset obesity accompanied by hypoadrenalism and bright red hair (Krude et al., 1998). Two children have been reported who are heterozygous for a missense mutation in the coding region of the POMC gene. This mutation disrupts the dibasic cleavage of beta-MSH and beta-endorphin. The resulting uncleaved fusion protein bound to the MC4-R with normal affinity, but had reduced ability to activate the receptor. This mutation was observed in obese individuals over three generations in one family. Combining the data of this study in U.K. Caucasians with those in France and three other published reports, mutations disrupting this processing site were present in 0.88% of subjects with early-onset obesity and 0.22% of normal-weight controls (Challis et al., 2002).

16.6.2.4 Prohormone Convertase 1 (PC-1) Gene

Another obese individual has been identified with mutations in a protein-processing enzyme called prohormone convertase 1 (PC-1) gene. PC-1 is upstream of another protein and/or prohormone-processing enzyme, carboxypeptidase E, which is encoded by the human homologue of the *fat* gene (Jackson et al., 1997). These findings indicate that correct processing of certain, as yet unknown, proteins/hormones can be essential for mice and humans to maintain a lean body composition.

16.6.2.5 Bardet–Biedel Syndrome (BBS-1)

Bardet–Biedel syndrome (BBS) is a very rare genetic disorder characterized by obesity, mental retardation, renal malformations, and hypogenitalism. The disease has an autosomal mode of inheritance. A missense mutation in the BBS-1 gene has been reported to be the most common genetic error responsible for this syndrome (Mykytyn et al., 2003).

16.6.2.6 Cocaine–Amphetamine-Regulated Transcript (CART)

A study in obese subjects in the U.K. failed to show an association between two polymorphisms in the CART gene and one amino acid change in CART protein and severe early-onset increased energy intake and obesity (Challis et al., 2000). Similar results were reported for a population of unrelated obese Italian children and adolescents. However, a heterozygous missense mutation resulting in an amino acid substitution in the NH2-terminal region of CART was found in a 10-year-old obese boy and this mutation was also observed in three generations of obese members of his family (Miraglia Del Giudice et al., 2002).

16.6.2.7   *Adiponectin*

Adiponectin is a circulating protein secreted from adipose tissue that is decreased in obesity. The presence of mutations in exon 3 of the adiponectin gene was associated with decreased adiponectin plasma concentrations (Vasseur et al., 2002).

16.7   Assessing Efficacy of Obesity Treatments

An ideal appetite suppressant for the treatment of obesity would:

- Specifically reduce energy intake (not water intake) by reducing hunger, meal size, or both through a well understood biological mechanism
- Not alter the pleasures and sensations associated with energy intake-taste, smell, flavor, mouth feel, hunger, and satiation sensations and sequences
- Sustain reduction of daily energy intake, leading to a 5 to 10% reduction of body weight, over a period of many months
- Provide long-term maintenance of the weight loss once it is achieved
- Not reduce efficacy over time or as a function of body weight
- Not yield adverse or unwanted negative effects
- Not offer potential addiction, dependence, or abuse

Double blind, randomized, controlled clinical trials in obese patients will determine which of these properties is satisfied for each new proposed medication.

Traditionally, the efficacy of a new obesity treatment is assessed by its effect on body weight in double blind, randomized, controlled clinical trials in obese patients. By this criterion, a treatment is considered successful if it (1) prevents further weight gain; (2) induces a 5 to 10% weight loss from the initial body weight; and (3) allows long-term maintenance of the weight loss once it is achieved. Recently, an alternative, medically based outcome measure for obesity treatment has been advocated by research scientists and physicians (Campfield, 1995). Rather than focusing primarily on body weight, body fat, or body mass index (BMI = weight/height^2), this measure, called "metabolic fitness," tracks the metabolic health of obese individuals. Metabolic fitness is defined as the absence of biochemical risk factors associated with obesity, such as elevated fasting concentrations of cholesterol, triglycerides, glucose, or insulin; impaired glucose tolerance; or elevated blood pressure.

In this school of thought, weight loss is viewed not as a goal but as a modality to improve health (Campfield, 1995, 1996; Blackburn et al., 1997). Many studies of weight loss have shown that during periods of weight loss there is a uniform improvement of risk factors (Campfield, 1995, 1996; Blackburn et al., 1997; Thomas, 1995). Interestingly, reductions in the biochemical risk factors may not always be dependent upon weight loss. For example, insulin sensitivity and cholesterol levels can be improved by physical activity in the absence of weight loss (Campfield, 1995, 1996; Blackburn et al., 1997; Thomas, 1995; Hill and Peters, 1998). The hope is that by using metabolic fitness as a measure of success, health professionals can shift the patient's focus from unrealistic, culturally imposed goals (dress size, belt size) to the more appropriate, and achievable, goal of better health (Campfield, 1995, 1996; Blackburn et al., 1997).

Not only will these requirements be difficult for several distinct compounds of different classes to fulfill, but the successful clinical development of a new medication is a long and winding road strewn with large and small obstacles. Once developed, approved, prescribed, and carefully taken, these future medications will certainly help millions to reduce their weight and body fat and to improve their health. However, the basic nature of the regulation of energy balance may still defeat those who faithfully take these future medications. Because changes in energy storage in adipose tissue result from the balance between energy intake and expenditure, weight loss requires a sustained period of negative energy balance. Pharmacological suppression of appetite and amount of energy consumed at each meal and throughout each day should help create a state of negative energy balance, especially if the patient also increases energy expenditure through increased physical activity. However, energy intake and expenditure are under cognitive control, so a state of positive energy balance is still a possibility.

If the patient actually increases daily energy intake or decreases daily physical activity ("I am taking my medication, so I can cheat on my eating and physical activity prescription.") by more than the suppression of energy intake caused, or expected to be caused, by the medication, he/she will enter a state of positive energy balance and actually gain weight while taking medication as prescribed for obesity. It was a sad feature of the clinical trials for orlistat, sibutramine, and leptin that patients remained in the studies from 3 months to up to 2 years and took the medications while gaining weight throughout the trial. Many students of the regulation of energy intake, including the authors, believe patients taking the most efficacious appetite suppressant or weight loss medication that can be imagined could still eat enough calories to fail to lose weight, or gain weight. In this view, medication must be combined with education and behavior change so that the patients will change the way they live as the primary treatment with medication providing a very important helping hand.

16.8 Classes of Obesity Medications

Medications to treat obesity can be classified according to their primary mechanism of action on energy balance. The goal of all obesity medications is to induce and maintain a state of negative energy balance (Bouchard and Perusse, 1993; Leibel et al., 1995; Le Magnen, 1992; Rosenbaum and Leibel, 1998; Rosenbaum et al., 1997; Bogardus et al., 1986). The four general classes of obesity medications (Table 16.1) are:

- Inhibitors of energy (food) intake, or appetite suppressants, reduce hunger perceptions, increase feelings of fullness, and reduce food intake by acting on brain mechanisms and, as a result, facilitate compliance with caloric restriction.
- Inhibitors of fat absorption reduce energy intake through a peripheral, gastrointestinal mechanism of action and do not alter brain chemistry.
- Enhancers of energy expenditure act through peripheral mechanisms to increase thermogenesis without requiring planned increases in physical activity.
- Stimulators of fat mobilization act peripherally to reduce fat mass and/or decrease triglyceride synthesis without requiring intentional increases in physical activity or decreases in food intake.

Importantly, the beneficial actions of all four drug classes can be easily overcome by increased food intake (e.g., preferred, calorie-dense food items) or decreased voluntary physical activity.

TABLE 16.1

Potential Therapeutic Targets for New Obesity Medications

Target	Drug Type
Inhibitors of Energy Intake (Appetite Suppressants)	
Serotonin	Reuptake inhibitor
Norepinephrine	Reuptake inhibitor
Dopamine	Reuptake inhibitor
Leptin	Agonist
Leptin receptor	Agonist/sensitizer
NPY receptor (Y5, Y1)	Antagonist
MC4 receptor	Agonist
Agouti-related peptides	Antagonist
POMC	Agonist
MCH receptor	Antagonist
CRH receptor/CRH binding proteins	Agonist
Urocortin	Agonist
CNTF (ciliary neurotrophic factor)	Agonist
Adiponectin	Agonist
Galanin receptor	Antagonist
Orexin/hypocretin	Antagonist
CCK-A receptor	Agonist
GLP-1 receptor	Agonist
Bombesin	Agonist
Enhancers of Energy Expenditure	
UCP2/UCP3	Stimulator of expression/activity
PKA	Stimulator
Beta-3 adrenergic receptor	Agonist
Stimulators of Fat Mobilization	
Leptin receptor	Agonist
PKA	Stimulator
Beta-3 adrenergic receptor	Agonist
GH receptor	Agonist

Abbreviations: NPY = neuropeptide Y; Y5, Y1 = receptor subtypes for NPY; MC4 = melanocortin 4; POMC = pro-opiomelanocortin; MCH = melanin concentrating hormone; CRH = corticotropin-releasing hormone; CNTF = ciliary neurotrophic factor; CCK = cholecystokinin: GLP-1 = glucagon-like peptide –1; UCP2/UCP3 = uncoupling proteins 2 and 3; PKA = protein kinase A; GH = growth hormone.

Source: Adapted from Campfield, L.A. et al., *Science* 280: 1383–1387, 1998.

16.9   Potential Targets for New Obesity Medicines

Potential obesity medications can be based on any intervention between the neuropeptide and its receptor that would alter the biological responses mediated by the neuronal network — in particular, food intake, metabolism, and energy expenditure. These potential medications are listed in Table 16.1.

Neuropeptide Y (NPY) is the most widely distributed neuropeptide in the brain and exerts multiple biological effects. In addition to being one of the most potent appetite stimulators in animals, it appears to be one of the mediators of the actions of leptin in the brain (Frankish et al., 1995; Clark et al., 1984; Smith et al., 1996, 1998). Currently, much interest is focused on identifying the NPY receptor subtypes that mediate the effects of NPY on food intake and energy balance. Other potential targets are uncoupling proteins 2 (UCP2) and 3 (UCP3). Expressed in peripheral tissues, these proteins belong to a family of proton transporters that, when activated, may cause increased thermogenesis, leading to reduced storage of fat (Gimeno et al., 1997; Fleury et al., 1997; Vidal–Puig et al., 1997; Boss et al., 1997).

Many pharmaceutical companies have large programs directed at the development of new modulators of monoamine neurotransmitters and neuropeptide receptor agonists or antagonists. In addition to the well-documented effect of serotonin modulation on food intake, evidence is strong that modulation of dopamine and/or norepinephrine also has an effect (Blundell, 1991). A large effort is also being directed at developing antagonists for specific NPY receptors (Y5, Y1) that have been associated with food intake (Gerald et al., 1996). Among the newer targets, MC4-R has attracted a lot of attention. Selective MC4-R agonists could inhibit food intake; and since AGOUTI inhibits MC4-R, inhibitory analogs of the agouti-related peptides may also serve as appetite suppressants. It is widely believed that the endogenous ligand of MC4-R is alpha-MSH or another product of POMC processing; thus, compounds that increase POMC levels may also reduce food intake (Schwartz et al., 1997). Other potential neuropeptide targets for appetite suppressants include receptors for melanin-concentrating hormone (MCH); CRH (and the closely related urocortin); galanin; opioid peptides; and the recently discovered orexin/hypocretins (Sakurai et al., 1998; Woods et al., 1998).

Receptors for three well-known gastrointestinal hormones are also targets for the development of appetite suppressants. Cholecystokinin (CCK) is released from the intestine in response to meals and plays an important role in meal termination. CCK-A receptor agonists reduce meal size and food intake in animals (Moran and McHugh, 1982; Moran et al., 1986). Bombesin reduces food intake when injected into rodents; thus, bombesin receptor agonists may be useful as appetite suppressants (Ohki–Hamazaki et al., 1997). Although GLP-1 has been under study as an endogenous stimulator of insulin release from the pancreas in humans, it was recently shown that brain administration of GLP-1 to rats reduces food intake (Wang et al., 1995). If gastrointestinal and other side effects can be avoided, GLP-1 receptor agonists may also be useful for reducing energy intake.

New targets for drugs that enhance energy expenditure include the aforementioned uncoupling proteins (UCP2 and UCP3) and the well-characterized enzyme protein kinase A (PKA). Mice in which PKA is dysregulated (by inactivation of the PKA-subunit RII beta) are lean and resistant to diet-induced obesity (Cummings et al., 1996). Thus, in theory, pharmacologic stimulation of PKA may cause increased thermogenesis and fat mobilization.

Another drug target in this category is the beta-3 adrenergic receptor, which has been extensively studied. Large development programs have identified several agonists. Early nonselective compounds that were beta-adrenergic receptor agonists increased thermogenesis in obese humans, but had unwanted side effects, including increased heart rate or tremor (Campfield, 1996). These drugs also increase fat mobilization in animals. Newer, apparently selective, beta-3 adrenergic receptor agonists have not increased thermogenesis in humans and the search for more effective agonists continues (Hu and Jennings, 2003).

Drugs that would potentially stimulate fat mobilization include growth hormone (GH) receptor agonists; leptin; PKA stimulators; and beta-3 adrenergic receptor agonists. In animal studies, administration of GH increases lean muscle mass and reduces fat mass (Haqq et al., 2003).

16.10   Experimental Animal Models of Obesity Used to Study Appetite Suppressants

Several different animal models of obesity were utilized in the experimental study of the regulation of food intake, its genetics, and the evaluation of potential appetite suppressants. The first model explored was the bilateral hypothalamic brain lesion in rats. Following bilateral electrolytic or chemical lesions of the ventromedial hypothalamus of rats, daily food intake was increased for several days and then returned to baseline levels. However, a persistent, rapid weight gain began immediately after the lesion and continued for weeks until the rats were very obese. The majority of the weight gain was due to the expansion of the mass of adipose tissue. It is now understood that the obesity following this brain lesion is due primarily to alterations in the descending activity of the autonomic nervous system and the resulting hyperinsulinemia (Bray and York, 1979).

A model with more applicability to human obesity is diet-induced obesity (DIO) in mice and rats, which occurs when a very palatable, high-fat diet (primarily composed of sugar and shortening added to powdered rodent food and remarkably similar to cookie dough) is given to normal mice and rats. Approximately 60 to 75% of some, but not all, strains of mice and rats will increase energy intake, rapidly gain weight over a 4- to 6-week period, and become very obese when fed these diets. The operational definition for diet-induced obesity is a body weight > average body weight of animals fed normal food ± two standard deviations. Diet-induced obesity can be produced by feeding otherwise normal rodents diets composed of high fat content, high energy density, or multiple palatable items presented simultaneously (called "supermarket" or "cafeteria" diets). Strains that resist diet-induced obesity and individual resistant members of a susceptible strain are being studied because they may provide important biological clues to help reduce energy intake, and weight gain and regain, in susceptible humans (Sclafani, 1993).

However, the experimental models of obesity that have received the most attention during the last decade are the single gene mutations in mice and rats. In mice, four *recessive* (*ob/ob, db/db, fat/fat, tub/tub*) and one dominant (*agouti*) single gene mutations have been known and studied for many years (Table 16.2). In contrast, only one single gene mutation is known in rats, although it has apparently appeared two separate times (*fa/fa* or Zucker and LA/N/*f/f* or *fak/fak*) (Bray and York, 1979).

The obese *ob/ob* mice were discovered on the C57BL/6J background in the 1950s by animal caretakers at Jackson Laboratories. This mutation results in profound obesity through increased energy intake and decreased metabolic rate. The *db/db* mouse, which arose on the C57BL/KsJ background, is similarly obese and is also characterized by increased food intake and hyperglycemia. When the mutated *ob* gene was transferred to the C57BL/KsJ background, an almost identical phenotype to *db/db* mice was observed. Likewise, when the mutated *db* gene was transferred to the C57BL/6J background, an increased energy intake and obese phenotype almost identical to *ob/ob* mice resulted.

When cross-circulation (or parabiosis) experiments were performed between *ob/ob* and *db/db* mice by Coleman and colleagues (Coleman, 1973, 1978, 1981; Coleman and Hummel, 1973), the *ob/ob* partner reduced its food intake and lost weight, while the *db/db* partner maintained its increased food intake and body weight. These studies led Coleman to hypothesize that *ob/ob* mice fail to make a circulating factor from adipose tissue, but their brains can respond to it and reduce food intake; conversely, *db/db* mice make the circulating factor in their adipose tissue, but their brains *cannot* respond to it. This insightful hypothesis has been proven correct by findings on the leptin pathway. Despite numerous attempts to isolate and identify this protein, the primary defect, site of syn-

TABLE 16.2

Genetic Models of Obesity in Mice and Rats

Single Gene Mutations	Gene Product	Energy Intake
Mice		
ob/ob	Leptin	Increased
db/db	Leptin receptor	Increased
fat/fat	Carboxypeptidase E	Increased
tub/tub	TUB protein	Increased
Agouti	AGOUTI protein	Increased
Rats		
fa/fa or Zucker (rat equivalent of *db/db*)	Leptin receptor	Increased
LA/N *f/f*	Leptin receptor	Increased
Polygenic Models (Obese Animals with Multiple Affected Genes)		
Body fat	Various QTLs	Unchanged or increased
Hyperglycemia	Various QTLs	Increased

Note: See text for explanation of gene symbols.

thesis, or nature of the *ob* gene product was not known until the positional cloning of the *ob* gene.

16.11 Leptin Has Led to Identification of a Novel Pathway in Regulation of Energy Balance

Obese humans have increased circulating levels of leptin, suggesting that obesity is due to a decreased sensitivity to leptin, not a deficiency of leptin (Campfield, 1999; Campfield and Smith, 1998; Campfield et al., 1997a; Considine et al., 1996; Maffei et al., 1995). The observation that most obese individuals have elevated circulating levels of leptin has prompted speculation that human obesity can arise from reduced brain responsiveness to leptin. This hypothesis is supported by studies of diet-induced obese (DIO) mice. When lean AKR/J mice are fed a high-fat, energy-dense diet, they become obese and have elevated serum leptin and insulin concentrations (Campfield et al., 1995, 1997b). In comparison to lean AKR/J mice, the DIO mice require higher i.p. doses of leptin to alter food intake, metabolism, and body fat.

Recent studies indicate that brain responsiveness to leptin is reduced in these obese animals and can be reversed by weight loss (Campfield et al., 1997b). Thus, in terms of leptin-based therapy for obesity, a reasonable goal would be to identify the molecular determinants of reduced leptin responsiveness and then develop low molecular weight compounds that enter the brain and act on these molecular targets to increase, and possibly restore to normal, responsiveness to leptin. Development of a drug that overcomes the weak links in the leptin pathway that prevents the message conveyed by leptin from producing an appropriate response in brains of obese individuals would provide an elegant solution to the challenge of obesity treatment. If leptin has additional effects in obese humans similar to those seen in rodent studies, then a single drug that activates the leptin pathway may have multiple therapeutic benefits.

Leptin is secreted from adipose tissue, circulates in the blood, and acts on central neural networks that regulate ingestive behavior, energy intake, and energy balance. It appears to play a major role in the control of body fat stores through coordinated regulation of ingestive behavior; energy metabolism; the autonomic nervous system; and body energy balance (Campfield et al., 1995; Campfield and Smith, 1998; Campfield, 1999).

Leptin was identified as the gene product of the *obese (ob)* gene positionally cloned in 1994 at Rockefeller University (Zhang et al., 1994). This field rapidly moved from cloning the *ob* gene to *ob* gene expression in adipose tissue of rats and humans. Next, the potent biological activity of leptin in *ob/ob*, diet-induced obese and lean mice as well as genetically obese and lean rats was demonstrated but not in *db/db* obese mice. Studies in the authors' laboratory and many others demonstrated that recombinant mouse and human leptin reduced food intake and decreased body weight gain in obese *ob/ob*, diet-induced obese, and lean mice as well as lean rats, but not in obese *db/db* mice by the peripheral (i.p., i.v.) and central (i.c.v.) routes of administration (see following) (Campfield et al., 1995, 1997a).

A significant milestone was the demonstration that central administration of leptin leads to reductions in food intake, body weight, and alterations in metabolism consistent with activation of the autonomic nervous system. These findings were confirmed and followed by the identification of a central binding site for labeled leptin in the choroid plexus in *ob/ob, db/db,* and lean mice as well as in lean and obese Zucker rats (Devos et al., 1996). The expression cloning of a central leptin receptor (OB-R), from the mouse choroid plexus soon followed (Tartaglia et al., 1995). The OB-R was found to be expressed in the choroid plexus and the hypothalamus as well as several peripheral tissues. OB-R exists in multiple forms; the two major forms are a short form, OB-R$_S$ (with a truncated intracellular domain) and a long form, OB-R$_L$ (with the complete intracellular domain) (Tartaglia et al., 1995). The long form is the form that signals and mediates the biological effects of leptin. Initial *in situ* hybridization studies demonstrated that the mRNA for the long-form OB-R is localized to the hypothalamus as well as peripheral sites. It was then demonstrated that the *db* gene encodes the OB-R.

Biologically active forms of mouse and human leptin were overexpressed and purified to near homogeneity from bacterial expression systems. When recombinant mouse leptin was administered peripherally (i.p., i.v.) or centrally (i.c.v.), food intake and body weight of obese *ob/ob* mice were reduced (Campfield et al., 1995; Halaas et al., 1995; Pelleymounter et al., 1995; Stephens et al., 1995).

The duration of action of leptin appears longer than with other neuropeptides that modulate ingestive behavior (CCK, NPY) and is similar to that of centrally administered insulin. The behavioral and physiological effects following central administration into the lateral ventricle suggest that leptin can act directly on the neural networks in the brain that regulate ingestive behavior and energy balance.

Measurements of serum concentrations of leptin using a specific radioimmunoassay or an ELISA for human leptin have been performed (Considine et al., 1996). When obese subjects were compared to lean individuals, it was observed that the serum leptin concentrations were higher in obese individuals and leptin concentrations *increased* with increasing percent body fat. When obese subjects lost weight by caloric restriction, leptin concentration decreased and then rose slightly when the lower weight was maintained. When the weight lost by dieting was regained, leptin concentrations returned to the initial level. The effects of other experimental manipulations are shown in Table 16.3. In contrast to rodents, leptin concentrations in humans do not increase following individual meals or acute bouts of exercise. Several studies have demonstrated that 3 to 4 days of overfeeding or increased physical activity are required to increase or decrease, respectively, serum leptin concentrations in humans (Jenkins et al., 1997; Chin–Chance et al., 2000; Hickey

TABLE 16.3

Measurements of Serum Concentrations of Leptin in Human Subjects

Experimental Conditions	Leptin Concentrations	References
Lean, obese, type 2 diabetes	Proportional to percent body fat	Considine et al. 1996; Maffei et al. 1995
Weight loss and regain	Decreases, then increases	Considine et al. 1996; Maffei et al. 1995
Circadian variation	Stable during day, increases at night	Sinha et al. 1996
Fasting and refeeding	Fall after 24-h fast; return after refeeding	Kolaczynski et al. 1996b
Acute caloric restriction	No change until 1 week	Wisse et al. 1999
Euglycemic, hyperinsulinemic clamps	No change	Kolaczynski et al. 1996a
Eating disorders	Very low	Grinspoon et al. 1996; Casanueva et al. 1997; Ferron et al. 1997
Wasting syndromes	Very low	Simons et al. 1997
3–4 days overfeeding	Increased	Jenkins et al. 1997; Chin–Chance et al. 2000; Hickey and Calsbeek, 2001
3–4 days increased physical activity	Decreased	Jenkins et al. 1997; Chin–Chance et al. 2000; Hickey and Calsbeek, 2001
Glucocorticoid administration	Increased	Berneis et al.1996

and Calsbeek, 2001). Several studies demonstrate that leptin concentrations are regulated by circulating glucocorticoids (Berneis et al., 1996).

16.12 Clinical Development of Leptin: Biological Activity of Long-Acting Leptin (PEG-OB Protein) in Obese Humans

Based on available results in animal models and humans, most human obesity is probably not due to a *deficiency* of leptin, but instead to a central and/or peripheral *resistance* to leptin. However, clinical experience with insulin therapy in insulin-resistant, obese type 2 diabetic patients and positive results with leptin treatment of diet-induced obese mice strongly suggest that therapeutic augmentation of circulating leptin levels may result in reductions of food intake, body fat mass, and body weight in obese patients.

Clinical trials with recombinant met–leu human leptin and pegylated recombinant human leptin protein (PEG-OB protein) have been conducted in lean and obese humans. Therapeutic approaches to the treatment of obesity based on leptin ranging from leptin by injection to OB-R agonists (protein analogs, small molecules) and to upregulation of leptin signaling pathways are being developed. The goals of treatment based on leptin include initial (raise plasma levels to increase leptin signaling [similar to insulin treatment in type 2 diabetes]) and long term (increased sensitivity to the already adequate circulating levels of leptin to achieve regulation at lower body fat mass) (Campfield et al., 1997a).

The operation of the leptin pathway in humans has now been established. Chronic daily s.c. low-dose recombinant methionyl–human leptin (met–leptin) treatment of a young, very obese leptin-deficient girl with a mutated *ob* gene has been reported (Farooqi et al., 1999). After a life dominated by continuous weight gain, intense hunger, and food seeking, reduction of hunger, reduced food seeking behavior, reduced body fat and sustained weight loss were observed during the year-long treatment. This study clearly demonstrated the biological activity of met–leptin in humans (O'Rahilly, 2002).

Clinical trials have been conducted in obese humans. Daily s.c. injections of recombinant met–leptin (0.30 mg/kg body weight) for 24 weeks in obese subjects resulted in weight loss that was significantly greater than placebo treatment. Lower doses were without effect on body weight. The majority of the weight loss was body fat and no systemic side effects were observed, although significant skin irritations appeared at the site of injection in many subjects. The rapid disappearance of leptin from the blood was described following s.c. dosing. Appetite was not reported in these studies (Heymsfield et al., 1999).

A long-acting recombinant native human leptin produced by linking human leptin to polyethylene glycol (PEG) polymers to form pegylated recombinant human leptin (PEG-OB protein) has also been tested in humans. After completing safety and efficacy tests in animals (mice, rats, monkeys), phase I and phase II clinical trials were conducted in obese humans. Treatment of obese men, under conditions of an energy deficit of 1 to 2 MJ/day, with a *weekly* s.c. injection of 20 mg PEG-OB protein for 12 weeks, increased serum concentrations of leptin and PEG-OB protein between weekly doses. The expected fall in serum leptin with weight loss did not occur in the PEG-OB protein-treated group, while in the placebo group leptin levels were reduced (Hukshorn et al., 2000). Appetite (assessed by factor 3 [hunger] of the Three Factor Eating Questionnaire) and hunger ratings (visual–analog scales) before breakfast were decreased in the leptin-treated group compared to the placebo group (see Figure 16.1). The significant difference began during the first week after treatment started and remained constant during the next 11 weeks (Westerterp–Plantenga et al., 2001).

Additional studies in semistarved obese men have shown that weekly s.c. administration of 80 mg of PEG-OB protein for 7 weeks caused significant additional weight loss and a

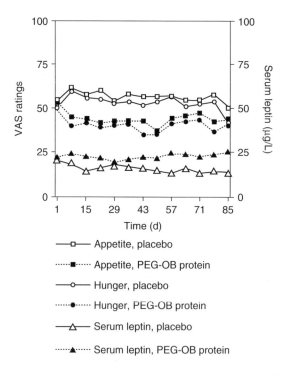

FIGURE 16.1
Visual analogue scale (VAS) ratings of appetite and hunger and serum leptin levels in subjects who received 20 mg pegylated polyethylene glycol OB protein (leptin) (PEG-OB protein; n = 15) or placebo (n = 15). All data were collected before breakfast. Significant differences in changes in appetite and hunger during the treatment occurred between the two groups (two-factor repeated measures ANOVA with interaction; $p < .01$). Significant differences in changes in serum leptin concentrations occurred between the two groups (two-factor repeated measures ANOVA with interaction; $p < .05$). (Reprinted from Westerterp–Plantenga, M.S. et al., *Am. J. Clin. Nutr.*, 74: 426–434, 2001.)

significant reduction in appetite at the end of treatment compared to a placebo-treated control group (Hukshorn et al., 2003b). In another study, weekly s.c. administration of 80 mg of PEG-OB protein caused a significant additional weight loss in semistarved obese men compared to placebo-treated subjects, but did not reverse the fasting-induced changes in thyroid, corticotropic, and somatotrophic axes or sympathetic nervous system. However, the decrease in luteinizing hormone (LH) concentrations was attenuated in the treatment group (Hukshorn et al., 2003a). Finally, weekly s.c. injection of 60 mg PEG-OB in mildly energy restricted obese men did not lead to additional weight loss after 8 weeks of treatment. Furthermore, PEG-OB administration did not affect the changes in metabolic profile and the inflammatory status of obese subjects (Hukshorn et al., 2002).

The observation that PEG-OB protein treatment decreased appetite under fasting conditions at a dose that did not change body weight or body composition suggests that leptin treatment acts centrally to regulate energy intake. When taken together with the results of leptin treatment of the young obese girl with a mutated *ob* gene with met-leptin, these results strongly suggest that leptin treatment can suppress appetite in obese humans (Farooqi et al., 1999; Westerterp–Plantenga et al., 2001).

Based on a structural similarity between the leptin receptor and the ciliary neurotrophic factor (CNTF) receptor, a new target has emerged for the suppression of energy intake and weight loss. CNTF is a neuroprotective protein present in Schwann cells and astrocytyes of the central nervous system, but is not present in the circulation (Sendtner et al., 1994). Recombinant human variant CNTF (rhvCNTF; also called Axokine by its maker, Regeneron Pharmaceuticals) administration to leptin-resistant, diet-induced obese mice caused weight loss (Kalra, 2001). In addition, weight loss was seen in a clinical trial of rhvCNTF in normal-weight patients with amyotrophic lateral sclerosis (ALS) (ALS CNTF treatment study group, 1996).

When 0.3, 1, or 2 µg/kg rhvCNTF was administered s.c. for 12 weeks, obese patients lost significantly more weight at the 1- and 2-µg/kg doses (average weight loss = 4.1% in the 2-µg/kg group) than placebo-treated obese patients (Ettinger et al., 2003). In this study, the amount of weight loss was maintained from 3 to 12 months following the end of s.c. rhvCNTF treatment. This desirable observation has caused some scientists to be concerned that rhvCNTF may have long-term effects on the brain. Studies in mice and rats have shown that rhvCNTF can activate alpha-MSH (an inhibitor of energy intake), and inhibit the production of NPY and AgRP. Thus, the long-term effect of rhvCNTF on weight reduction may be a direct consequence of its biological actions, or it may result from other adverse changes in the brain. Long-term human clinical trials are needed to establish the efficacy and safety of rhvCNTF. These trials are reportedly underway.

16.13 The Significance of Leptin: Lessons Learned

The discovery and rapid characterization of the leptin-signaling pathway in laboratory rodents and humans has been significant for several reasons:

- It has provided additional evidence that obesity is a disease with a biological basis leading to increased energy intake.
- It has demonstrated that molecular biology has reached the study of obesity and ingestive behavior and has changed these fields forever.
- Leptin has also demonstrated that the *neurobiology* of ingestion and energy balance has been moved to the front of the research agenda.

- The evolution of the leptin-signaling pathway has provided a rapid series of initial advances in the knowledge base of our field. This increasing knowledge base should provide innovative drug targets for the pharmaceutical industry.

Leptin has been shown to regulate the gene expression levels of all other neuropeptides and some neuropeptide receptors involved in the regulation of food intake and energy balance. This is the case for well-characterized neuropeptides (e.g., NPY, CRH, alpha MSH) as well as more recently described neuropeptides (CART, MCH, POMC). This master coordinator or "chef d'orchestre" function of leptin in the brain to regulate and control food intake and energy balance was proposed in 1995 and appears to be well supported by many studies on new pathways and new neuropeptides.

The clinical development experience with leptin and long-acting leptin has also provided some important lessons:

- It is not reasonable to expect initial clinical studies with a new neuropeptide or receptor pathway to establish the feasibility of this target or pathway *and* to provide the information to make a development decision. The development of leptin at Hoffmann–La Roche and Amgen was severely hampered by the need to show not only significant efficacy, but also sufficient efficacy to justify going to market with these proteins. Clinical trials at both companies demonstrated efficacy, but were stopped because of questions related to the business decisions (dose, cost of production, route of administration, market share, etc.).

- Pharmaceutical companies need to support (with provision of molecules, reference to manufacturing, quality control, and safety data) investigator-initiated clinical research in obese patients using their proprietary molecules. This approach was attempted with PEG-OB protein in a series of clinical trials conducted at the University of Maastricht. However, the production of the clinical material was stopped when Hoffmann–La Roche lost interest. These studies will define the dosing regimens and the therapeutic niches for the molecules in which they have invested very significant resources.

- Designers of clinical trials, including the critical phase II efficacy studies, need to consider a larger set of possible experimental designs to demonstrate efficacy for weight loss and, more importantly, weight maintenance. When long-acting PEG-OB protein was given in the presence of significant energy restriction, significant additional weight loss was observed.

- Pharmaceutical research managers, executives, and shareholders must demonstrate much more patience to capitalize on the important original research in energy intake and obesity that their scientists have been conducting and to maximize their return on investment. Obesity is a very complex disease and the successful development of new medicines to treat it safely and effectively will require persistence, good clinical trial design, and a lot of luck.

16.14 Conclusions

This is the initial phase of a new era in collective understanding of the regulation of energy intake, obesity, and its genetic basis. The identification of the major and modifier genes and the characterization of their corresponding gene products involved in development, maintenance, and restoration of obesity following weight loss is at hand. Given this new information, which has led, and will probably continue to lead, to more than a few surprises, it should be possible to identify the multiple signals involved and uncover the algorithms and decision rules used by the brain to regulate food intake, energy balance, and body fat content. Once this regulation is better understood at the molecular level, the pharmaceutical industry should be able to bring its experience, technology, expertise, and power to bear in order to identify and develop a new generation of safe and effective pharmaceutical agents, including appetite suppressants, as adjuncts to diet and exercise for the treatment of obesity.

Genetic testing for the presence of these identified major and modifier obesity genes can then be used to identify those at the highest risk for obesity. Then, behavioral, and perhaps pharmaceutical, intervention can be used to prevent or reverse weight gain. Complementary investigations at the pharmacological, physiological, and behavioral levels will be critical to the evaluation of all proposed new obesity medications. The most effective pharmacological treatments are likely to be those that involve the use of a combination of drugs, each with a distinct mechanism of action, or a single drug with multiple activities. Based on a more complete understanding of the genetic basis of human obesity, these new combined behavioral and pharmacological treatment strategies will help obese individuals become much more successful at maintaining weight loss and will help them to benefit from the resulting improved health.

Obesity is a chronic disease, and the possibility of long-term treatment — continuous or intermittent treatment throughout adult life — is a concept that is receiving more attention. In this context, the risk-benefit and quality-of-life analyses of pharmacological treatment become increasingly important. Vigorous dialog among health care professionals, patients, the research community, and regulatory authorities is needed to define, in objective and quantifiable terms, the minimum efficacy required to justify long-term treatment. Safety considerations are critical. For example, women make up the largest group seeking treatment for obesity, so potential drugs must be tested in long-term studies for possible undesired effects on reproductive function and hormonal status. Innovative medicines will be used as adjuncts to, rather than substitutes for, life-style change to improve the metabolic fitness, health, and quality of life for obese individuals. Although the path to innovative medicines for obesity is a crooked one strewn with many obstacles, the recent progress in the "new science" of obesity provides hope that the future of obesity treatment will be bright.

References

ALS CNTF treatment study group (1996) A double-blind placebo-controlled clinical trial of subcutaneous recombinant human ciliary (rhvCNTF) in amyotrophic lateral sclerosis, *Neurology*, 46: 1244–1249.

Berneis, K., Vosmeer, S. and Keller, U. (1996). Effects of glucocorticoids and growth hormone on serum leptin levels in man, *Eur. J. Endocrinol.*, 135: 663–665.

Blackburn, G.L., Miller, D. and Chan, S. (1997) Pharmaceutical treatment of obesity, *Nurs. Clin. North Am.*, 32: 831–848.

Blundell, J. (1991) Pharmacological approaches to appetite suppression, *Trends Pharmacol. Sci.*, 12: 147–157.

Bogardus, C., Lillioja, S., Ravussin, E., Abbott, W., Zawadzki, J.K. and Young, A. (1986) Familial dependence of the resting metabolic rate, *N. Engl. J. Med.*, 315: 96–100.

Boss, O., Samec, S., Paoloni–Giacobino, A., Rossier, C., Dulloo, A., Seydoux, J., Muzzin, P. and Giabobino, J.P. (1997) Uncoupling protein-3: a new member of the mitochondrial carrier family with tissue-specific expression, *FEBS Lett.*, 408: 39–42.

Bouchard, C. and Perusse, L. (1993) Genetics of obesity, *Annu. Rev. Nutr.*, 13: 337–354.

Bray, G.A. and York, D.A. (1979) Hypothalamic and genetic obesity in experimental animals: an automonic and endocrine hypothesis, *Physiol. Rev.*, 59: 719–809.

Bultman, S., Michaud, E. and Woychik, R. (1992) Molecular characterization of the mouse agouti locus, *Cell*, 71: 1195–1204.

Campfield, L.A. (1995) Treatment options and the maintenance of weight loss, in *Obesity Treatment: Establishing Goals, Improving Outcomes, and Reviewing the Research Agenda* (Eds.) Allison, D.B. and Pi–Sunyer, F.X. Plenum Press, New York, pp. 93–95.

Campfield, L.A. (1996) The role of pharmacological agents in the treatment of obesity, in *Overweight and Weight Management* (Ed.) Dalton, S. Aspen Publishers, Gaithersburg, MD, pp. 466–485.

Campfield, L.A. (1999) Multiple facets of OB protein (leptin) physiology: integration of central and peripheral mechanisms in the regulation of energy balance, in *Progress in Obesity Research*: 8 (Eds.) Ailhaud, G. and Guy–Grand, B. John Libbey & Company, London, pp. 327–335.

Campfield, L.A. and Smith, F.J. (1998) Overview: neurobiology of OB protein (leptin), *Proc. Nutr. Soc.*, 57: 429–440.

Campfield, L.A. and Smith, F.J. (1999) The pathogenesis of obesity, in *Bailliere's Clinical Endocrinology and Metabolism*, Vol. 13 (Ed.) Bray, G.A. Bailliere Tindal, London, pp. 13–30.

Campfield, L.A. and Smith, F.J. (2003) Blood glucose dynamics and the control of meal initiation: a pattern detection and recognition theory, *Physiol. Rev.*, 83: 25–58.

Campfield, L.A., Smith, F.J. and Burn, P. (1997a) OB protein: a hormonal controller of central neural networks mediating behavioral, metabolic and neuroendocrine responses, *Endocrinol. Metab.*, 4: 81–102.

Campfield, L.A., Smith, F.J. and Burn, P. (1998) Strategies and potential molecular targets for obesity treatment, *Science*, 280: 1383–1387.

Campfield, L.A., Smith, F.J., Guisez, Y., Devos, R. and Burn, P. (1995) Recombinant mouse OB protein: evidence for a peripheral signal linking adiposity and central neural networks, *Science*, 269: 546–549.

Campfield, L.A., Smith, F.J., Yu, J., Renzetti, M., Simko, B., Baralt, M., Mackie, G., Tenenbaum, R. and Smith, W. (1997b) Dietary obesity induces decreased central sensitivity to exogenous OB protein (leptin) which is reversed by weight loss, *Soc. Neurosci. Abstr.*, 23: 815.

Casanueva, F.F., Dieguez, C., Popovic, V., Peino, R., Considine, R.V. and Caro J.F. (1997). Serum immunoreactive leptin concentrations in patients with anorexia nervosa before and after partial weight recovery, *Biochem. Mol. Med.*, 60: 116–120.

Chagnon, Y., Rankinen, T., Snyder, E., Weisnagel, S., Perusse, L. and Bouchard, C. (2003) The human obesity gene map: the 2002 update, *Obes. Res.*, 11: 313–367.

Challis, B., Pritchard, L., Creemers, J., Delplanque, J., Keogh, J., Luan, J., Wareham, N., Yeo, G., Bhattacharyya, S., Froguel, P., White, A., Farooqi, I. and O'Rahilly, S.A. (2002) A missense mutation disrupting a dibasic prohormone processing site in pro-opiomelanocortin (POMC) increases susceptibility to early-onset obesity through a novel molecular mechanism., *Hum. Mol. Genet.*, 11: 1997–2004.

Challis, B., Yeo, G., Farooqi, I., Luan, J., Aminian, S., Halsall, D., Keogh, J., Wareham, N. and O'Rahilly, S. (2000) The CART gene and human obesity: mutational analysis and population genetics, *Diabetes*, 49: 872–875.

Chin–Chance, C., Polonsky, K.S. and Schoeller, D.A. (2000) Twenty-four-hour leptin levels respond to cumulative short-term energy imbalance and predict subsequent intake, *J. Clin. Endocrinol. Metab.*, 85: 2685–2691.

Clark, J.T., Kalra, P.S., Crowley, W.R. and Kalra, S.P. (1984) Neuropeptide Y and human pancreatic polypeptide stimulate feeding behavior in rats, *Endocrinology*, 115: 427–429.

Clement, K., Valisse, C., Lahlou, N., Cabrol, S., Peeloux, V., Cassuto, D., Gourmelen, M., Dina, C., Chambaz, J., Lacourte, M., Basdevant, A., Bougneres, P., Lebouc, Y., Froguel, P. and Guy–Grand, B. (1998) A mutation in the human leptin receptor gene causes obesity and pituitary dysfunction, *Nature*, 392: 398–401.

Coleman, D.L. (1981) Inherited obesity-diabetes syndromes in the mouse, *Prog. Clin. Biol. Res.*, 45: 145–158.

Coleman, D.L. (1978) Obese and diabetes: two mutant genes causing diabetes-obesity syndromes in mice, *Diabetologia*, 14: 141–148.

Coleman, D.L. (1973) Effects of parabiosis of obese with diabetes and normal mice, *Diabetologia*, 9: 294–298.

Coleman, D.L. and Hummel, K.P. (1973) The influence of genetic background on the expression of the obese (ob) gene in the mouse, *Diabetologia*, 9: 287–293.

Comuzzie, A. (2002) The emerging pattern of the genetic contribution to human obesity, *Best Pract. Res. Clin. Endocrinol. Metab.*, 16: 611–621.

Comuzzie, A. and Allison, D. (1998) The search for human obesity genes, *Science*, 280: 1374–1377.

Considine, R.V., Sinha, M.K., Heiman, M.L., Kriauciunas, A., Stephens, T.W., Nyce, M.R., Ohannesian, J.P., Marco, C.C., McKee, L.J., Baur, T.L. and Caro, J.F. (1996) Serum immunoreactive-leptin concentrations in normal-weight and obese humans, *N. Engl. J. Med.*, 334: 292–295.

Cummings, D.E., Brandon, E.P., Planas, J.V., Motamed, K., Idzerda, R.L. and McKnight, G.S.N., (1996) Genetically lean mice result from targeted disruption of the RII beta subunit of protein kinase A, *Nature*, 382: 622–626.

Devos, R., Richards, J.G., Campfield, L.A., Tartaglia, L.A., Guisez, Y., Van der Heyden, J., Travernier, J., Plaetinck, G. and Burn, P. (1996) OB protein binds specifically to the choriod plexus of mice and rats, *Proc. Natl. Acad. Sci. USA*, 93: 5668–5673.

Ettinger, M., Littlejohn, T., Schwartz, S., Weiss, S., McIlwain, H., Heymsfield, S., Bray, G., Roberts, W., Heyman, E., Stambler, N., Heshka, S., Vicary, C. and Guter, H.-P. (2003) Recombinant variant of ciliary neurotrophic factor for weight loss in obese adults, *J. Am. Med. Assoc.*, 289: 1826–1832.

Fan, W., Boston, B.A., Kesterson, R.A., Hruby, V.J. and Cone, R.D. (1997) Melanocortinergic inhibition of feeding behavior and disruption with an agouti-mimetic, *Nature*, 385: 165–168.

Fan, W., Dinulescu, D.M., Butler, A.A., Zhou, J., Marks, D.L., and Cone, R.D., The central melanocortin system can directly regulate serum insulin levels, *Endocrinology*, 141: 3072–3079.

Farooqi, I., Keogh, J., Yeo, G., Lank, E., Cheetham, T. and O'Rahilly, S. (2003) Clinical spectrum of obesity and mutations in the melanocortin 4 receptor gene, *N. Engl. J. Med.*, 348: 1085–1095.

Farooqi, I.S., Jebb, S.A., Langmack, G., Lawrence, E., Cheetham, C.H., Prentice, A.M., Hughes, I.A., McCamish, M.A. and O'Rahilly, S. (1999) Effects of recombinant leptin therapy in a child with congenital leptin deficiency, *N. Engl. J. Med.*, 341: 879–884.

Ferron, F., Considine, R.V., Peino, R., Lado, I.G., Dieguez, C. and Casanueva, F.F. (1997) Serum leptin concentrations in patients with anorexia nervosa, bulimia nervosa and non-specific eating disorders correlate with the body mass index but are independent of the respective disease, *Clin. Endocrinol.*, 46: 289–293.

Fleury, C., Neverova, M., Collins, S., Raimbault, S., Champigny, O., Levi–Meyrueis, C., Bouillaud, F., Seldin, M.F., Surwit, R.S., Ricquier, D. and Warden, C.H. (1997) Uncoupling protein-2: a novel gene linked to obesity and hyperinsulinemia, *Nat. Genet.*, 15: 269–272.

Flint, A., Raben, A., Ersboll, A.K., Holst, J.J. and Astrup, A. (2001) The effect of physiological levels of glucagon-like peptide-1 on appetite, gastric emptying, energy and substrate metabolism in obesity, *Int. J. Obes. Relat. Metab. Disord.*, 25: 781–792.

Frankish, H.M., Dryden, S., Hopkins, D., Wang, Q. and Williams, G. (1995) Neuropeptide Y, the hypothalamus, and diabetes: insights into the central control of metabolism, *Peptides*, 16: 757–771.

Gerald, C., Walker, M., Criscione, L., Gustafson, E., Batzl–Hartmann, C., Smith, K., Vaysse, P., Durkin, M., Laz, T., Linemeyer, D., Schaffhauser, A., Whitebread, S., Hofbauer, K., Taber, R., Branchek, T. and Weinshank, R. (1996) A receptor subtype involved in neuropeptide Y-induced food intake, *Nature*, 382: 168–171.

Gimeno, R.E., Dembski, M., Weng, X., Deng, N., Shyjan, A.W., Gimeno, C.J., Iris, F., Ellis, S.J., Woolf, E.A. and Tartaglia, L.A. (1997) Cloning and characterization of an uncoupling protein homolog: a potential molecular mediator of human thermogenesis, *Diabetes*, 46: 900–906.

Grinspoon, S., Gulick, T., Askari, H., Landt, M., Lee, K., Anderson, E., Ma, Z., Vignati, L., Bowsher, R., Herzog, D. and Klibanski, A. (1996) Serum leptin levels in women with anorexia nervosa, *J. Clin. Endocrinol. Metab.*, 81: 3861–3863.

Halaas, J.L., Gajiwala, K.S., Maffei, M., Cohen, S.L., Chait, B.T., Rabinowitz, D., Lallone, R.L., Burley, S.K. and Friedman, J.M. (1995) Weight-reducing effects of the plasma protein encoded by the obese gene, *Science*, 269: 543–546.

Haqq, A., Stadler, D.D., Jackson, R.H., Rosenfeld, R.H., Purnell, J.Q. and La Franchi, S.H. (2003) Effects of growth hormone on pulmonary function, sleep quality, behavior, cognition, growth velocity, body composition, and resting energy expenditure in Prader–Willi syndrome, *J. Clin. Endocrinol. Metab.*, 88: 2206–2212.

Heymsfield, S.B., Greenberg, A.S., Fujioka, K., Dixon, R.M., Kushner, R., Hunt, T., Lubina, J.A., Patane, J., Self, B., Hunt, P. and McCamish, M. (1999) Recombinant leptin for weight loss in obese and lean adults: a randomized, controlled, dose-escalation trial, *J. Am. Med. Assoc.*, 282: 1568–1575.

Hickey, M.S. and Calsbeek, D.J. (2001) Plasma leptin and exercise: recent findings, *Sports Med.*, 31: 583–589.

Hill, J. and Peters, J. (1998) Environmental contributions to the obesity epidemic, *Science*, 280: 1371–1374.

Hu, B. and Jennings, L.L. (2003) Orally bioavailable beta-3-adrenergic receptor agonists as potential therapeutic agents for obesity and type-II diabetes, *Prog. Med. Chem.*, 41: 167–194.

Hukshorn, C., Menheere, P., Westerterp–Plantenga, M. and Saris, W. (2003a) The effect of pegylated human recombinant leptin (PEG-OB) on neuroendocrine adaptations to semi-starvation in overweight men, *Eur. J. Endocrinol.*, 148: 649–655.

Hukshorn, C., van Dielen, F., Buurman, W., Westerterp–Plantenga, M., Campfield, L. and Saris, W. (2002) The effect of pegylated recombinant human leptin (PEG-OB) on weight loss and inflammatory status in obese subjects, *Int. J. Obes. Relat. Metab. Disord.*, 26: 504–509.

Hukshorn, C., Westerterp–Plantenga, M. and Saris, W. (2003b) Pegylated human recombinant leptin (PEG-OB) causes additional weight loss in severely energy-restricted, overweight men, *Am. J. Clin. Nutr.*, 77: 771–776.

Hukshorn, C.J., Saris, W.H., Westerterp–Plantenga, M.S., Farid, A.R., Smith, F.J. and Campfield, L.A. (2000) Weekly subcutaneous pegylated recombinant native human leptin (PEG-OB) administration in obese men, *J. Clin. Endocrinol. Metab.*, 85: 4003–4009.

Huszar, D., Lynch, C.A., Fairchild–Huntress, V., Dunmore, J.H., Fang, Q., Berkemeier, L.R., Gu, W., Kesterson, R.A., Boston, B.A., Cone, R.D., Smith, F.J., Campfield, L.A., Burn, P. and Lee, F. (1997) Targeted disruption of the melanocortin-4 receptor results in obesity in mice, *Cell*, 88: 131–141.

Jackson, R.S., Creemers, J.W., Ohagi, S., Raffin–Sanson, M.L., Sanders, L., Montague, C.T., Hutton, J.C. and O'Rahilly, S. (1997) Obesity and impaired prohormone processing associated with mutations in the human prohormone convertase 1 gene, *Nat. Genet.*, 16: 303–306.

Jenkins, A.B., Markovic, T.P., Fleury, A. and Campbell, L.V. (1997) Carbohydrate intake and short-term regulation of leptin in humans, *Diabetologia*, 40: 348–351.

Kalra, S. (2001) Circumventing leptin resistance for weight control, *PNAS*, 98: 4279–4281.

Kolaczynski, J.W., Nyce, M.R. et al. (1996a). Acute and chronic effects of insulin on leptin production in humans: studies *in vivo* and *in vitro*, *Diabetes*, 45: 699–701.

Kolaczynski, J.W., Ohannesian, J. et al. (1996b). Response of leptin to short-term fasting and refeeding in humans: a link with ketogenesis but not ketones themselves, *Diabetes*, 45: 1511–1515.

Krude, H., Biebermann, H., Luck, W., Horn, R., Brabant, G. and Gruters, A. (1998) Severe early-onset obesity, adrenal insufficiency and red hair pigmentation caused by POMC mutations in humans, *Nat. Genet.*, 19: 155–157.

Le Magnen, J. (1992) *Neurobiology of Feeding and Nutrition*, Academic Press, San Diego, CA.

Lee, Y., Poh, L. and Loke, K. (2002) A novel melanocortin 3 receptor gene (MC3R) mutation associated with severe obesity, *J. Clin. Endocrinol. Metab.*, 87: 1423–1426.

Leibel, R.L., Rosenbaum, M. and Hirsch, J. (1995) Changes in energy expenditure resulting from altered body weight, *N. Engl. J. Med.*, 232: 621–628.

Lubrano–Berthelier, C., Durand, E., Dubern, B., Shapiro, A., Dazin, P., Weill, J., Ferron, C., Froguel, P. and Vaisse, C. (2003) Intracellular retention is a common characteristic of childhood obesity-associated MC4R mutations, *Hum. Mol. Genet.*, 12: 145–153.

Maffei, M., Halaas, J., Ravussin, E., Pratley, R.E., Lee, G.H., Zhang, Y., Fei, H., Kim, S., Lallone, R., Ranganathan, S., Kern, P.A. and Friedman, J.M. (1995) Leptin levels in human and rodent: measurement of plasma leptin and ob mRNA in obese and weight-reduced subjects, *Nat. Med.*, 1: 1155–1161.

Miraglia Del Giudice, E., Cirillo, G., Nigro, V., Santoro, N., D'Urso, L., Raimondo, P., Cozzolino, D., Scafat, D. and Perrone, L. (2002) Low frequency of melanocortin-4 receptor (MC4R) mutations in a Mediterranean population with early-onset obesity, *Int. J. Obes. Relat. Metab. Disord.*, 26: 647–651.

Montague, C.T., Farooqi, I.S., Whitehead, J.P., Soos, M.A., Rau, H., Wareham, N.J., Sewter, C.P., Digby, J.E., Mohammed, S.N., Hurst, J.A., Cheetham, C.H., Earley, A.R., Barnett, A.H., Prins, J.B. and O'Rahilly, S. (1997) Congenital leptin deficiency is associated with severe early-onset obesity in humans, *Nature*, 387: 903–908.

Moran, T.H. and McHugh, P.R. (1982) Cholecystokinin suppresses food intake by inhibiting gastric emptying, *Am. J. Physiol.*, 242: R491–R497.

Moran, T.H., Robinson, P.H., Goldrich, M.S. and McHugh, P.R. (1986) Two brain cholecystokinin receptors: Implications for behavioral actions, *Brain Res.*, 362: 175–179.

Mykytyn, K., Nishimura, D., Searby, C., Beck, G., Bugge, K., Haines, H., Cornier, A., Cox, G., Fulton, A., Carmi, R., Iannaccone, A., Jacobson, S., Weleber, R., Wright, A., Riise, R., Hennekam, R., Luleci, G., Berker–Karauzum, S., Biesecker, L., Stone, E. and Sheffield, V. (2003) Evaluation of complex inheritance involving the most common Bardet–Biedl syndrome locus (BBS1), *Am. J. Hum. Genet.*, 72: 429–437.

Naggert, J., Fricker, L., Varlamov, O., Nishina, P., Rouille, Y., Steiner, D., Carrol, R., Paigen, B. and Leiter, E. (1995) Hyperproinsulinemia in obese fat/fat mice associated with carboxypepidase E mutation which reduces enzyme activity, *Nat. Genet.*, 10: 134–142.

O'Rahilly, S. (2002) Leptin: defining its role in humans by the clinical study of genetic disorders, *Nutr. Rev.*, 60: S30–34.

Ohki–Hamazaki, H., Watase, K., Yamamoto, K., Ogura, H., Yamano, M., Yamada, K., Maeno, H., Imaki, J., Kikuyama, S., Wada, E. and Wada, K. (1997) Mice lacking bombesin receptor subtype-3 develop metabolic defects and obesity, *Nature*, 390: 165–169.

Pelleymounter, M., Cullen, M., Baker, M., Hecht, R., Winters, D., Bone, T. and Collins, F. (1995) Effects of the obese gene product on body weight regulation in ob/ob mice, *Science*, 269: 540–543.

Rosenbaum, M. and Leibel, R.L. (1998) The physiology of body weight regulation: relevance to the etiology of obesity in children, *Pediatrics*, 101: 525–539.

Rosenbaum, M., Leibel, R.L. and Hirsch, J. (1997) Obesity, *N. Engl. J. Med.*, 337: 396–407.

Sakurai, T., Amemiya, A., Ishii, M., Matsuzaki, I., Chemelli, R., Tanaka, H., Williams, S., Richardson, J., Kozlowki, G., Wilson, S., Arch, J., Buckingham, R., Haynes, A., Carr, S., Annan, R., McNulty, D., Liu, W., Terrett, J., Elshourbagy, N., Bergsma, D. and Yanagisawa, M. (1998) Orexins and orexin receptors: a family of hypothalamic neuropeptides and G protein coupled receptors that regulate feeding behavior, *Cell*, 92: 573–585.

Schwartz, M.W., Seeley, R.J., Woods, S.C., Weigle, D.S., Campfield, L.A., Burn, P. and Baskin, D.G. (1997) Leptin increases hypothalamic pro-opiomelanocortin mRNA expression in the rostral arcuate nucleus, *Diabetes*, 46: 2119–2123.

Sclafani, A. (1993) Dietary obesity, in *Obesity: Theory and Therapy* (Eds.) Stunkard, A.J. and Wadden, T.A., Raven Press, New York, pp. 125–136.

Sendtner, M., Carroll, P., Holtmann, B., Hughes, R. and Thoenen, H. (1994) Ciliary neurotrophic factor, *J. Neurobiol.*, 25: 1436–1453.

Simons, J.P., Scholsm A.M. et al. (1997) Plasma concentration of total leptin and human lung cancer-associated cachexia, *Clin. Sci.* (Colch), 93: 273–277.

Sinha, M.K., Ohannesian, J.P. et al. (1996) Nocturnal rise in leptin in lean, obese, and non-insulin-dependent diabetes mellitus subjects, *J. Clin. Invest.*, 97: 1344–1347.

Smith, F.J., Campfield, L.A., Moschera, J.A., Bailon, P. and Burn, P. (1996) Feeding inhibition by neuropeptide Y, *Nature*, 382: 307.

Smith, F.J., Campfield, L.A., Moschera, J.A., Bailon, P.S. and Burn, P. (1998) Brain administration of OB protein (leptin) inhibits neuropeptide-Y- induced feeding in ob/ob mice, *Regul. Pept.*, 75–76: 433–439.

Stephens, T.W., Basinski, M., Bristow, P.K., Bue–Valleskey, J.M., Burgett, S.G., Craft, L., Hale, J., Hoffmann, J., Hsiung, H.M., Kriauciunas, A., MacKeller, W., Rosteck, P.R., Jr., Schoner, B., Smith, D., Tinsley, F.C., Zhang, X.-Y. and Heiman, M. (1995) The role of neuropeptide Y in the antiobesity action of the obese gene product, *Nature*, 377: 530–532.

Strobel, A., Issad, T., Camoin, L., Ozata, M. and Strosberg, D. (1998) A leptin missense mutation associated with hypogonadism and morbid obesity, *Nat. Genet.*, 18: 213–215.

Tartaglia, L.A., Dembski, M., Weng, X., Deng, N., Culpepper, J., Devos, R., Richards, J.G., Campfield, L.A., Clark, F.T., Deeds, J., Muir, C., Sanker, S., Moriarty, A., Moore, K.J., Smutko, J.S., Mays, G.G., Woolf, E.A., Monroe, C.A. and Tepper, R.I. (1995) Identification and expression cloning of a leptin receptor (OB-R), *Cell*, 83: 1263–1271.

Thomas, P.R. (Ed.) (1995) *Weighing the Options: Criteria for Evaluating Weight-Management Programs*, Food and Nutrition Board, Institute of Medicine, National Academy Press, Washington, D.C.

Vaisse, C., Clement, K., Durand, E., Hercberg, S., Guy–Grand, B. and Froguel, P. (2000) Melanocortin-4 receptor mutations are a frequent and heterogeneous cause of morbid obesity, *J. Clin. Invest.*, 106: 253–62.

Vasseur, F., Helbecque, N., Dina, C., Lobbens, S., Delannoy, V., Gaget, S., Boutin, P., Vaxillaire, M., Lepretre, F., Dupont, S., Hara, K., Clement, K., Bihain, B., Kadowaki, T. and Froguel, P. (2002) Single-nucleotide polymorphism haplotypes in the both proximal promoter and exon 3 of the apm1 gene modulate adipocyte-secreted adiponectin hormone levels and contribute to the genetic risk for type 2 diabetes in French Caucasians, *Hum. Mol. Genet.*, 11: 2607–2614.

Vidal–Puig, A., Solanes, G., Grujic, D., Flier, J.S. and Lowell, B.B. (1997) UCP3: An uncoupling protein homolgue expressed preferentially and abundantly in skeletal muscle and brown adipose tissue, *Biochem. Biphys, Res. Commun.*, 235: 79–82.

Wang, Z., Wang, R.M., Owji, A.A., Smith, D.M., Ghatei, M.A. and Bloom, S.R. (1995) Glucagon-like peptide-1 is a physiological incretin in the rat, *J. Clin. Invest.*, 95: 417–421.

Westerterp–Plantenga, M.S., Saris, W.H., Hukshorn, C.J. and Campfield, L.A. (2001) Effects of weekly administration of pegylated recombinant human ob protein on appetite profile and energy metabolism in obese men, *Am. J. Clin. Nutr.*, 74: 426–434.

Wisse, B.E., Campfield, L.A. et al. (1999). Effect of prolonged moderate and severe energy restriction and refeeding on plasma leptin concentrations in obese women, *Am. J. Clin. Nutr.*, 70: 321–330.

Woods, S.C., Seeley, R.J., Porte, D., Jr. and Schwartz, M.W. (1998) Signals that regulate food intake and energy homeostasis, *Science*, 280: 1378–1383.

World Health Organization (1988) MONICA Project: geographical variation in the major risk factors of coronary heart disease in men and women aged 35–64 years, *World Health Stat. Q.*, 41: 115–140.

World Health Organization (1998) *Obesity: Preventing and Managing the Global Epidemic*. World Health Organization, Geneva.

Zhang, Y., Proenca, R., Maffei, M., Barone, M., Leopold, L. and Friedman, J.M. (1994) Positional cloning of the mouse obese gene and its human homologue, *Nature*, 372: 425–431.

17

Peripheral Targets for Antiobesity Drugs

Vivion E. F. Crowley and Antonio J. Vidal–Puig

CONTENTS

ABSTRACT   The high morbidity and mortality associated with obesity have ensured that it is now globally regarded as a major health problem. Although lifestyle measures such as diet and exercise remain the cornerstones of any treatment program devised for tackling obesity, the search is ongoing for potent antiobesity drugs that may be used in tandem with these treatment options. The success of antiobesity therapies will require development of agents that not only modulate appetite, but also alter total energy expenditure. Manipulation of adaptive thermogenesis remains the most practical strategy to achieve the latter effect, and recent advances in the understanding of molecular mechanisms controlling this process in mammals have provided a number of novel targets for putative antiobesity drug development. Among the primary factors regulating mammalian thermogenesis is the β3-adrenergic receptor, which activates a thermogenic cascade in adipose tissue and muscle. In addition, the recent identification of uncoupling protein homologues with the capacity to uncouple mitochondrial respiration has galvanized efforts to develop compounds that can safely enhance UCP expression in thermogenically relevant tissues. Furthermore, the observation that certain transcription factors, e.g., FOXC2 and transcriptional coactivators (e.g., PGC-1α and β), can coordinately activate thermogenic gene expression programs and mitochondrial biogenesis opens up new avenues for drug discovery. In conjunction with the paradigm for altering energy balance, it may also be possible to induce preferential fuel partitioning or influence the process of adipocyte differentiation. However, all of the strategies mentioned here are not without the potential to induce side effects, and many may require tissue-specific manipulation to attain the desired safe antiobesity action.

17.1 Introduction

From a thermodynamic point of view, obesity can, in essence, be considered the result of a positive imbalance between food intake and energy expenditure, with the resultant excess energy accumulating as fat in the adipose tissue. Although outwardly this energy balance equation may appear simple, it can be modulated by many other factors, particularly the preferential partitioning of energy toward specific tissues and organs. In fact, it could be argued that some individuals may have an enhanced capacity to extract energy from blood into the adipose tissue, thus facilitating fat deposition. Conversely, individuals that preferentially partition fuel into lean and/or oxidative tissues may facilitate energy dissipation. It is still unclear whether defects in the mechanism of fuel partitioning are important causes of human obesity; however, recently reported genetically modified animal models have provided support for this concept as a potential strategy for treatment of obesity and its protean complications.

When the rather complex clinical problem of obesity is confronted, several aspects should be taken into account: (1) the mechanical problems associated with excess body weight (e.g., osteoarthritis, sleep apnea); (2) the metabolic syndrome typically associated with obesity, which is probably the most important aspect from the point of view of survival; and (3) the aesthetic and psychological elements, which can cause extreme distress. Thus, when therapeutic strategies for managing obesity are considered, the ideal scenario would involve using treatments aimed at all components associated with this condition. However, depending on the predominant clinical phenotype, one may be forced to prioritize specific aspects of the treatment. This approach may in some instances create paradoxical situations such as treating obese individuals with agonists of peroxisome proliferator-activated receptor γ (PPARγ) — agents that will decrease metabolic complications while potentially increasing the degree of obesity through adipogenesis.

From a clinical standpoint, effective treatment of obese patients poses four major challenges:

- To prevent further fat deposition
- To deal with individuals who fail to lose weight
- To tackle the problem of regaining weight after weight loss
- To control or reverse the metabolic complications associated with obesity, which are the main cause of morbidity and mortality

To address these challenges is a daunting task requiring modulation of highly integrated and complex mechanisms of energy homeostasis designed to prevent a negative energy balance. In fact, it is widely observed that strategies aimed at reducing food consumption can be successful in the short term; however, associated decreases in energy expenditure preclude long-term weight loss. Thus, changes exclusively directed at altering one factor of the thermodynamic equation are associated with compensatory responses from the

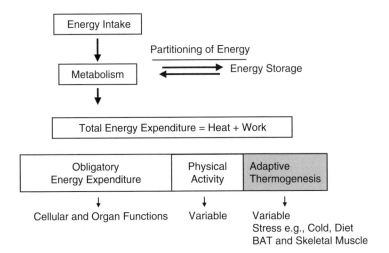

FIGURE 17.1
Thermodynamic perspective of energy homeostasis. Obesity is the result of a positive imbalance between energy intake and energy expenditure, a process modulated by partitioning of energy between prostorage and pro-oxidative tissues. Total energy expenditure includes obligatory energy expenditure, physical activity, and energy spent during adaptations to cold and diet.

other components of this equation in an attempt to maintain the entropy of this biological system. Indeed, very few energy homeostasis mechanisms seem not to be redundant.

One of these is leptin, the absence of which cannot be overcome as exemplified by *ob/ob* and *db/db* mouse models, as well as patients deficient in leptin or functional leptin receptors. Redundancy is a much more regular feature of the energy balance system, as illustrated by pathways involved in food intake (e.g., NPY knock out) or energy expenditure (e.g., β3 adrenergic receptor knock out). Thus, it is likely that, as in the case of other complex diseases such as hypertension, a successful treatment for obesity may require a multistrategy approach, with simultaneous targeting of several of the mechanistic pathways associated with energy acquisition; energy dissipation; preferential fuel partitioning into oxidative tissues; and modulating the storage capacity of the adipose tissue.

Although major advances have been made in attempts to manipulate appetite and caloric intake as a means of treating obesity, it is also now appreciated that the long-term success of this approach will depend on strategies aimed at preventing the concomitant fall in energy expenditure associated with food restriction. In fact, energy modifications geared toward increasing energy expenditure may provide an alternative, independent means of promoting weight loss or, even more importantly, of preventing weight regain. In basic terms, total energy expenditure in rodents and humans consists of three principal elements, including resting metabolic rate; energy costs of physical activity and food assimilation; and adaptive or facultative thermogenesis (Lowell and Spiegelman 2000) (Figure 17.1).

The key molecular events regulating human and rodent energy expenditure are now being elucidated, particularly in relation to biological mechanisms underlying adaptive thermogenesis. Thus, the potential to successfully develop specific therapies that enhance energy dissipation seems to be an increasingly achievable target; pharmacological interest in the field of energy expenditure is now firmly focused on producing sustained and safe increases of adaptive thermogenesis. Ongoing research in the area of mammalian thermogenesis has concentrated on identifying the central neural pathways and the peripheral cellular mechanisms responsible for energy expenditure, fuel oxidation, and futile cycling. This chapter will discuss some aspects pertaining to:

- CNS regulation of thermogenesis in human subjects
- Control of peripheral mechanisms of mammalian thermogenesis
- Control of preferential fuel partitioning
- Structural–functional changes in adipose tissue as strategies to prevent obesity and its associated metabolic complications

17.2 Central Nervous System (CNS) Regulation of Thermogenesis in Humans

Evidence obtained from the in-depth study of specific rodent models of obesity, including leptin, leptin receptor, and MC4 receptor deficiency states, indicates that the obese phenotype derives not only from hyperphagia and the associated increase in caloric intake, but also from an overall lowering of energy expenditure (Robinson et al. 2000). Thus, the respective complex CNS networks regulating appetite and thermogenesis seem to be clearly interlinked in these animals, although whether this level of interrelationship also applies to humans is still unconfirmed. Data from studies of leptin-deficient human subjects indicate that although leptin administration had a dramatic effect on reducing fat mass and hyperphagia, it did not appear to alter their energy expenditure significantly (Farooqi et al. 1999).

These experimental findings suggest that a higher level of complexity exists in humans in relation to the coupling of energy homeostatic mechanisms in CNS. Thus, although recombinant leptin administration in rodents results in maintenance of higher levels of energy expenditure in conjunction with the expected decrease in food intake (Halaas et al. 1995), in humans it may not have the same thermogenic potential. It is clear that the CNS may control energy expenditure; however, a different question is whether targeting the central nervous system to control energy expenditure is a good idea. The enthusiasm for this approach has waned in light of the unacceptable side effects of previous strategies targeting the CNS to control obesity and the fact that drugs used to treat psychiatric personality disorders have important effects on energy balance (Vanina et al. 2002).

17.3 Control of Peripheral Mechanisms of Mammalian Thermogenesis

Thermogenic regulation by CNS pathways is mediated to a large extent by output through the sympathetic nervous system (SNS) to peripheral efferent neurons, especially in brown adipose tissue (BAT) and skeletal muscle (Lowell and Spiegelman 2000). Rodents and other lower mammals possess distinct BAT depots where it acts as the major organ of adaptive thermogenesis (Himms–Hagen 1998). Brown adipocytes, which populate these depots, are characterized by high mitochondrial content and expression of the β3-adrenergic receptor (β3-AR), which is functionally and pharmacologically distinct from the β1- or β2-AR (Himms–Hagen 1998). The central role of β3-AR in stimulating BAT thermogenesis is now well established and involves the activation of uncoupling protein 1 (UCP1) via the cAMP signaling cascade and specific transcription factors and coactivators (Lowell and Spiegelman 2000) (Figure 17.2 and Figure 17.3). UCP1, which is selectively expressed at high levels in BAT, in turn generates heat by catalyzing a proton leak across the inner

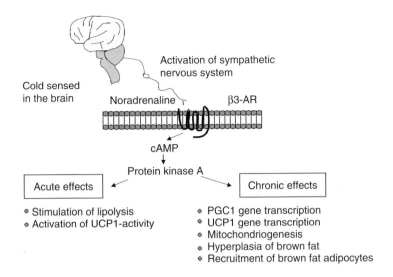

FIGURE 17.2
Cold induced thermogenesis. Thermogenesis is mediated by sympathetic nervous system efferent signals toward BAT (brown adipose tissue) and skeletal muscle. Activation of β3 adrenergic receptors (β3-AR) facilitates acute and chronic adaptation responses to a cold exposure that includes: (a) stimulation of lipolysis and subsequent activation of mitochondrial uncoupling protein (UCP) 1; (b) transcriptional changes involving PPARγ coactivator-1α (PGC-1α), UCP1, and genes involved in mitochondrial biogenesis, followed by hyperplasia of BAT.

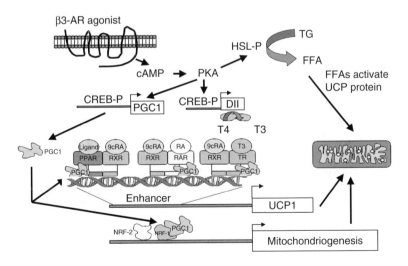

FIGURE 17.3
Adrenergic signaling pathways. Activation of β3-AR leads to the activation of UCP1 via the cyclicAMP (cAMP) signaling cascade and specific transcription factors and transcriptional coactivators. (PKA = protein kinase A; HSL = hormone sensitive lipase; TG = triglyceride; FFA = free fatty acids; CREB = cAMP-responsive element binding protein; PPAR = peroxisome poliferator-activated receptor; RXR = retinoid X receptor; RAR = retinoic acid receptor; TR = thyroid hormone receptor; T4 = thyroxine; T3 = tri-iodothyronine; 9cRA = 9-cis retinoic acid; NRF = nuclear respiratory factor)

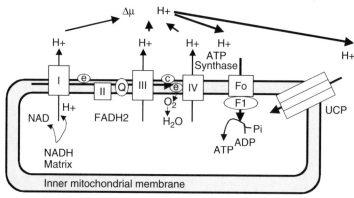

FIGURE 17.4

Molecular mechanisms of mitochondrial uncoupling. Mitochondrial uncoupling proteins facilitate the reentry of protons from the mitochondrial intermembrane space into the mitochondria matrix, thus bypassing the ATP synthase complex. As a result of this action more reducing equivalents are needed to produce a specific amount of ATP, and the mitochondrial membrane potential is decreased, facilitating the transport of electrons through the electron respiratory chain. The net outcome of these effects is the production of less efficient mitochondria where increased consumption of fuel occurs. Regulated mitochondrial uncoupling may be a useful strategy to induce and/or maintain weight loss.

mitochondrial membrane during cellular respiration, resulting in the uncoupling of oxidative phosphorylation and ATP synthesis (Figure 17.4) (Kozak and Harper 2000).

17.4 The Novel Uncoupling Proteins

Unlike rodents, adult humans do not have discrete BAT depots that can participate in adaptive energy expenditure (Himms–Hagen 1998). However, it has long been recognized that humans have other tissues (including muscle and liver) that, although devoid of UCP1, still generate mitochondrial proton leaks that partially account for energy expenditure (Rolfe and Brand 1997). The ability to control this thermogenic capacity would be a useful tool in terms of antiobesity drug development.

The identification in 1997 of two new UCP1 homologues invigorated the field of mammalian thermogenic research (Boss et al. 1997; Fleury et al. 1997; Vidal–Puig et al. 1997). Initial studies using heterologous expression of these UCP1 homologues in yeast and mammalian cell systems supported a role in the generation of mitochondrial proton leaks. In humans and rodents, UCP2 mRNA expression has been demonstrated in a wide array of tissues, a finding compatible with a putative role in whole-body energy expenditure; UCP3 mRNA expression was concentrated in skeletal muscle (Solanes et al. 1997), which has significant mitochondrial capacity and is the major organ of thermogenesis in humans. In addition, UCP3 in rodents is very highly expressed in BAT.

Genetic studies have also provided supportive evidence of a prominent role for these UCP1 homologues in energy homeostasis. Specifically, genetic markers encompassing the *UCP2/3* locus on chromosome 11 revealed significant linkage to resting energy expenditure in French–Canadian (Bouchard et al. 1997) and Pima Indian cohorts (Walder et al. 1998). Moreover, a recent report of an association between a common single nucleotide polymorphism (SNP) in the promoter region of *UCP2* and decreased risk of obesity in middle-

TABLE 17.1

Models of Genetic Modification of UCPs in Mice

Genetic Manipulation	Observed Phenotype	Ref.
UCP1 KO	Nonobese; defective thermogenesis; cold sensitive	Enerback, S. et al., 1997
UCP2 KO	Nonobese; normal thermoregulation; increased insulin sensitivity; increased ROS production	Zhang, C.Y. et al., 2001 Arsenijevic, D. et al., 2000
UCP3 KO	Nonobese; normal thermoregulation; increased ROS production	Vidal–Puig, A.J. et al., 2000
UCP3 OE	Resistant to diet-induced obesity; increased muscle thermogenesis	Clapham, J.C. et al., 2000

KO = knockout; OE = overexpression; ROS = reactive oxygen species.

aged subjects has lent further credence to this hypothesis (Esterbauer et al. 2001). In contrast, experimental data have emerged proposing that neither UCP2 nor UCP3 is required for mediating adaptive thermogenesis in cold-exposed animals (Golozoubova et al. 2001). In addition, mice with separate gene disruption of *UCP2* (Zhang et al. 2001) or *UCP3* (Vidal–Puig et al. 2000) did not manifest a phenotype with cold sensitivity, reduced energy expenditure, or obesity in either strain (Table 17.1).

These findings indicate that UCP1 homologues do not appear to have a specific physiological thermogenic function *per se*. Despite this, *UCP3* knockout mice did show evidence of increased efficiency of ATP production (Cline et al. 2001), a feature compatible with UCP3 having uncoupling activity in skeletal muscle *in vivo*; in support of this observation, transgenic mice with skeletal muscle-specific overexpression of UCP3 were resistant to the development of obesity (Clapham et al. 2000). However, a recent *in vivo* study examining the effects of diet-induced increases in UCP3 expression on postexercise phosphocreatine resynthesis in human skeletal muscle (a sensitive index of *in vivo* mitochondrial function) concluded that UCP3 did not have a primary uncoupling role (Hesselink et al. 2003).

In addition, evidence has been presented suggesting that the uncoupling of oxidative phosphorylation observed in the presence of supraphysiological UCP3 overexpression, such as in transfected yeast models and in UCP3 transgenic animals, was the result of experimental artifact, rather than representing a specific property of the native protein (Harper et al. 2002). In summary, the emerging picture suggests that mitochondrial uncoupling may not be the major biochemical role of UCP1 homologues. Nevertheless, in view of the phenotype associated with the UCP3 transgenic mouse model, it is still quite plausible that hyperstimulation of UCP3 activity or substantially increased expression in skeletal muscle may offer a useful strategy for treatment of obesity and its complications.

17.5 Transcription Factors, Coactivators, and Translational Regulators of Adaptive Thermogenesis

Recent studies have helped to further elucidate many of the key regulators of mammalian energy expenditure. Most notably, the recent characterization of PPARγ coactivator-1α (PGC-1α) has provided novel insights into the transcriptional regulation of adaptive thermogenesis. PGC-1α is a powerful transcriptional coactivator of several nuclear receptors, including PPAR α and γ; thyroid hormone receptor (TR)β; retinoic acid receptor (RAR) α; and estrogen receptor (ER) α and β (Puigserver et al. 1998; Vega et al. 2000) (Figure

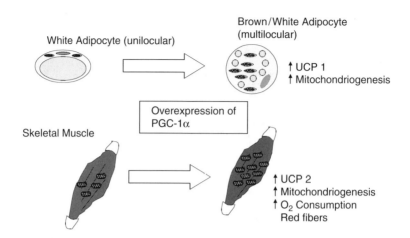

FIGURE 17.5

Cellular effects of ectopic PGC-1α expression. Ectopic overexpression of PGC-1α in white adipose tissue and skeletal muscle cells induces expression of components of the adaptive thermogenic system. These include the expression of UCPs, with specific UCP1 mRNA expression increasing in adipocytes, while, surprisingly, the UCP2 gene, not the UCP3 gene, is upregulated in myoblasts and myotubes. Also, significant induction of the genes of the mitochondrial respiratory chain takes place and mitochondrial content is increased in these cells. A similar phenotype is also observed with PGC-1β overexpression in rat L6 myoblasts (UCP = uncoupling protein; PGC-1 = PPARγ coactivator-1).

17.3). Although PGC-1α is constitutively expressed at high levels in mitochondria-rich tissues such as BAT, heart, kidney, and brain, its expression is dramatically induced by cold exposure and β3-AR agonists in BAT and in skeletal muscle (Puigserver et al. 1998, Boss et al. 1999). Of further interest, ectopic expression in white adipocytes and in myoblasts and myotubes coordinately activates a program of thermogenesis that includes induction of genes of the electron transport pathway, uncoupling proteins, and mitochondrial biogenesis (Wu et al. 1999) (Figure 17.5).

These effects of PGC-1α on mitochondrial biogenesis, a key component of adaptive thermogenesis, were mediated through its ability to upregulate the expression and transcriptional coactivation of nuclear respiratory factor (NRF)-1 (Wu et al. 1999). In conjunction with a related transcription factor, NRF-2, NRF-1 has been shown to be a critically important transcriptional activator of multiple mitochondrial genes (Gugneja et al. 1996; Virbasius and Scarpulla 1994). One such gene was mitochondrial transcription factor A (Tfam), a vital coordinator of transcription and replication of the mitochondrial genome (Scarpulla 1997).

In response to these modulations in gene expression, white adipocytes exhibited a BAT-like phenotype, while in myotubes a significant increase in coupled and uncoupled respiration has been reported (Wu et al. 1999) (Figure 17.5). Consonant with these initial observations, recent findings relating to transgenic mice with muscle-specific PGC-1α expression indicate that, with physiological levels of expression, conversion of type II fibers to slow-twitch type I fibers is observed (Lin et al. 2002b). Slow-twitch fibers contain high concentrations of mitochondria and use oxidative metabolism as a primary source of energy. Furthermore, these transgenic animals demonstrate a greater resistance to electrically stimulated muscular fatigue (Lin et al. 2002b).

As a consequence of further study, the known spectrum of PGC-1α action has expanded, particularly with the identification of prominent roles in the control of hepatic gluconeogenesis (Yoon et al. 2001) and in insulin-sensitive glucose transporter (GLUT 4) expression in skeletal muscle (Michael et al. 2001). Conceivably, therefore, any proposed therapeutic measure increasing PGC-1α expression or activity might have additional benefits on insulin sensitivity and glucose homeostasis. However, another potential ramification of pharmacological upregulation of PGC-1α is overproduction of reactive oxygen species (ROS), primarily as a result of enhanced oxidative respiration and mitochondriogenesis. This may in turn have specific undesirable effects on cell function, such as activation of proapoptotic or proinflammatory pathways (Adhihetty et al. 2003).

An extensive search for *bona fide* PGC-1α homologues was stimulated by emerging reports concerning the key regulatory role of PGC-1α in adaptive thermogenesis, as well as many other facets of intermediate metabolism. This resulted in the addition of two new coactivators to the PGC-1 family. These coactivators share greatest structural homology in the amino and carboxy-terminal regions — areas that carry most of the effector functions. Other common elements in their structure are nuclear receptor (NR) boxes containing leucine-rich motifs (LXXLL domains), which mediate interaction with nuclear receptor binding domains, and serine/arginine-rich (SR) domains that regulate mRNA processing. The first of the homologues to be cloned was PGC-1-related coactivator (PRC) (Andersson and Scarpulla 2001). However, unlike PGC-1α, which exhibited a clear tissue-specific pattern of expression, PRC is ubiquitously expressed. Based on initial characterization studies, it was speculated to have a possible role in modulating mitochondrial biogenesis during cell growth and proliferation (Andersson and Scarpulla 2001).

Of more direct interest to the realm of energy expenditure regulation is PGC-1β (Lin et al. 2002a) and its human orthologue PGC-1-related estrogen receptor coactivator (PERC) (Kressler et al. 2002). PGC-1β manifests a tissue-selective expression in rodents and humans, which strongly mirrors that of PGC-1α, including BAT; heart; skeletal muscle; and brain. Moreover, specific isoforms of this novel homologue also enhance transactivation by NRF-1 and various nuclear receptors, with evidence of particular selectivity for estrogen receptor (ER)α (Kressler et al. 2002; Lin et al. 2002a). Significantly, overexpression in skeletal muscle cells indicates that PGC-1β can potently induce mitochondrial biogenesis and also enhances coupled and uncoupled respiration in this cell model (Lin, 2003; Meirhaeghe et al. 2003).

However, PGC-1β does not appear to be transcriptionally regulated in BAT and muscle in response to specific physiological stimuli, including cold exposure, exercise, high-fat diet, and obesity (Lin et al. 2002a; Meirhaeghe et al. 2003). This divergence in transcriptional control leads one to speculate that PGC-1α may be principally concerned with coordinating response to energy demands due to acute metabolic flux, while PGC-1β may function to promote the level of mitochondrial biogenesis necessary to cover basal requirements of specific tissues. Further research on the precise mechanism by which PGC-1β induces mitochondrial biogenesis and the factors regulating this process is being actively pursued.

A putative role for members of the p160 coregulator family has recently been explored using gene disruption animal models (Picard et al. 2002). Mice lacking transcription intermediary factor-2 (TIF-2) displayed enhanced adaptive thermogenesis and were protected against diet-induced obesity. In contrast, mice deficient in steroid receptor coactivator-1 (SRC-1) had reduced energy expenditure and were obesity prone (Picard et al. 2002). TIF-2 and SRC-1 were shown to modulate PGC-1α transactivation properties, with SRC-1 promoting PPARγ-PGC-1α interactions, while TIF-2 dose dependently attenuated this interaction. Thus, it was concluded that relative levels of TIF-2/SRC-1 can alter PGC-1α-mediated adaptive thermogenesis in BAT (Picard et al. 2002). In WAT, TIF-2 also enhanced PPARγ-mediated fat uptake and storage during adipogenesis.

Some other potential avenues for modulating adaptive thermogenesis have been uncovered by two recent transgenic experiments (Table 17.2). In the first, mice specifically overexpressing the winged helix/forkhead transcription factor FOXC2 in adipose tissue had enlarged BAT depots, while the WAT pads were reduced in size and on histological examination had increased numbers of multilocular (as opposed to unilocular) adipocytes

TABLE 17.2

Transgenic Mouse Models of Obesity Resistance

Target Gene	Genetic Manipulation	Enhanced Thermogenesis or Fuel Partitioning	Proposed Mechanism for Obesity Resistance	Ref.
FOXC2	OE	Yes	Increased sensitivity of β-AR-cAMP-PKA signaling pathway; -increased PGC-1α mRNA expression in WAT	Cederberg, A. et al., 2001
eIF-4e-BP1	KO	Yes	Increased PGC-1α mRNA expression in WAT	Tsukiyama–Kohara, K. et al., 2001
DGAT	KO	Yes	Mechanism unknown	Smith, S.J. et al., 2000
Perilipin	KO	ND	Increased HSL activity with resultant increase in lipolysis	Martinez–Botas, J. et al., 2000
ACC2	KO	Yes	Increased fatty acid oxidation; increased UCP3 mRNA expression in muscle	Abu-Elheiga, L. et al., 2001

KO = knockout; OE = overexpression; ND = not determined.

(Cederberg et al. 2001). The expression of several genes associated with mitochondrial biogenesis and respiration, including UCP1 and PGC-1α, was also upregulated in WAT. These mice were more insulin sensitive than nontransgenic littermates, suggesting that pharmacological manipulation could lead to an additional antidiabetic action. This contention is supported by human genetic data that reported a significant association between a common SNP in the 5' untranslated region of *FOXC2* gene and enhanced insulin sensitivity (Ridderstrale et al. 2002).

The polypeptide 4E-BP1, which is highly expressed in WAT and reversibly represses cap-dependent translation by preventing formation of the eukaryotic translation initiation factor 4F (eIF4F) complex, was also subjected to genetic manipulation (Tsukiyama–Kohara et al. 2001). Homozygous mice deficient in 4E-BP1 (*ei4ebp1-/-*) manifested smaller WAT pads than wild type littermates. These WAT depots had UCP1 expression higher by sixfold and contained increased numbers of multilocular adipocytes, which are more characteristic of a brown adipocyte phenotype. Moreover, while showing an unaltered level of PGC-1 mRNA expression, these mice did manifest a twofold higher PGC-1 protein level, suggesting an inhibitory effect of 4E-BP1 on PGC-1 translation.

17.6 Control of Preferential Fuel Partitioning

Beneficial metabolic effects might be expected from an agent that promoted accretion of lean in preference to fat mass and/or fatty acid oxidation. This could be achieved through a reduction in fat deposition and/or an increase in lean tissue. It is unclear whether alterations in this balance are pathogenically relevant for human obesity. However recent genetically modified mouse models have revealed that lipogenesis and fatty acid oxidation are highly integrated processes and interference with one of them elicits an adaptive response in the other (Table 17.2). In fact, mice lacking the enzyme acylCoA: diacylglycerol acyltransferase (DGAT), which catalyzes an essential step in triglyceride synthesis, also have an unexplained increase in energy expenditure (Smith et al. 2000).

A more recent report demonstrates that mice deficient in acetyl CoA carboxylase (ACC) 2 have a major alteration in energy homeostasis with evidence of decreased body fat deposition despite an increase in caloric intake (Abu-Elheiga et al. 2001). These authors speculated that an increase in fatty acid oxidation in muscle and liver due to marked reductions in tissue levels of malonyl CoA primarily accounted for the modified energy balance, although others have postulated a role for upregulated UCP3 expression in this paradigm (Ruderman and Flier 2001). Conversely, some suggestions are that activation of the lipogenic pathway may increase malonyl CoA levels inactivating fatty acid oxidation.

Another demonstration of the potential for fuel partitioning to alter fat mass is the knock out of perilipin gene. Perilipin is an adipocyte protein that modulates hormone-sensitive lipase (HSL) activity; in the *perilipin* knock out model the resulting mice are hyperphagic relative to control littermates, although they maintain normal body weight (Martinez–Botas et al. 2000; Tansey et al. 2001). Cross-breeding experiments with *db/db* mice reverse obesity by increasing metabolic rate. Thus, rather interestingly, these models show that interfering with fat deposition is associated, to a certain degree, with increased energy expenditure and suggest that the mechanisms involved could be targeted for the design of new antiobesity and, conceivably in some instances, new antidiabetic therapies.

Redistribution of fat from intra-abdominal adipose tissue depots to subcutaneous depots may also pose some metabolic advantages. In fact, evidence suggests that accumulation of fat in the visceral depot promotes far more important metabolic complications than accumulating the same amount of fat in the subcutaneous adipose of the gluteal region. Thus, identification of the mechanism behind these metabolic differences may identify pharmacological targets to redirect fat away from the intra-abdominal depot. For instance, the effects of the adipocyte specific overexpression of the steroid interconverting enzyme 11β hydroxysteroid dehydrogenase type 1(11βHSD-1) on the development of central obesity and its metabolic sequelae in mice suggest that this enzyme may be an interesting target for inhibition, particularly in human visceral obesity (Masuzaki et al. 2001).

17.7 Structural and Functional Changes in Adipose Tissue as a Strategy to Prevent Complications of Obesity-Related Metabolic Syndrome

A more pragmatic approach to tackle the problem of obesity would be to target the adipose tissue as the source of the problems (Figure 17.6). As indicated previously, the excess weight due to fat accumulation in adipose tissue is a direct cause of mechanical problems associated with obesity. Moreover, the expansion of the adipose tissue mass is a key factor mediating the metabolic complications of obesity through pathogenic mechanisms involving inappropriate secretion of specific adipokines and leakage of fatty acids. Finally, the psychological distress comes from body image dissatisfaction because of excess body fat. Thus, these specific problems may benefit from strategies directed at limiting adipogenesis and preventing fat deposition; increasing the capacity of storage/fatty acid buffer of the adipose tissue, thus transforming the structure of adipose tissue; or promoting differentiation into BAT.

17.7.1 Antiadipogenesis as a Therapeutic Strategy

Although attractive as a therapeutic strategy, inhibition of the differentiation of adipocytes from precursor cells (Figure 17.6a) is laden with potential problems. In the first instance, it is predicated on a clear understanding of the respective roles of fat cell expansion and new adipocyte acquisition in the development and progression of human obesity. Evidence

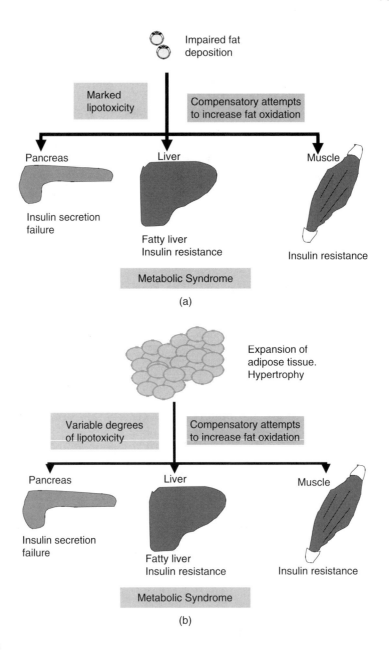

FIGURE 17.6
Effect of changes in adipose tissue on the development of the metabolic syndrome. (a) Impaired fat deposition results in marked lipotoxicity associated with compensatory attempts to increase fatty acid oxidation. (b) Hypertrophic changes in adipose tissue initially offer increased buffer capacity for fatty acids. However, development of insulin resistance and increased lipolysis facilitate the development of lipotoxicity in other tissues as part of the typical natural history of obesity-associated diabetes mellitus. (c) Hyperplastic changes in adipose tissue may offer increased buffer capacity of fatty acids and maintenance of adipokine profile. Hyperplastic changes in adipose tissue may prevent or at least delay the metabolic complications associated with obesity.
Continued.

is available for the continued development of new adipocytes, and thus adipogenesis *per se*, throughout adult life, but the degree to which this process contributes to the overall accumulation of adipose tissue mass in human obesity is unclear (Prins and O'Rahilly 1997). A more clinically significant reservation about adopting antiadipogenesis as a ther-

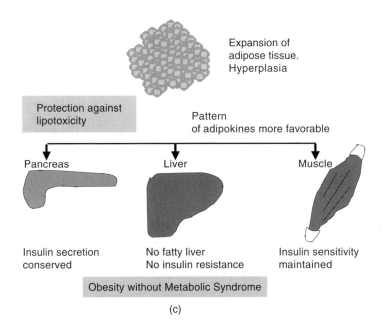

FIGURE 17.6

Continued.

apeutic intervention relates to the consideration of where any excess energy will be stored if adipose tissue mass becomes a limiting factor (Danforth 2000). The severe metabolic disturbances seen in human and murine syndromes of partial and complete lipodystrophy provide a clear reminder that the safest place to store excess triglycerides is almost certainly adipose tissue (Moitra et al. 1998; Reitman et al. 2000). In these lipodystrophic syndromes, severe insulin resistance and dyslipidaemia develop as a consequence of hepatic steatosis and increases in skeletal muscle triacylglycerol content.

Although it is essential to bear these *caveats* in mind, on a more positive note, genetic and pharmacological data suggest that moderate inhibition of the expression or function of the key adipocyte regulator PPARγ (Kubota et al. 1999; Miles et al. 2000; Yamauchi et al. 2001) or its heterodimeric partner retinoid X receptor (RXR) α (Yamauchi et al. 2001) can lead to a reduction in diet-induced obesity and enhanced insulin sensitivity. However, any such a strategy will have a narrow therapeutic index as is clearly illustrated by the severe metabolic derangements resulting from more major impairment in PPARγ activity (Barroso et al. 1999). Overall, this approach may be more successfully applied in the clinical arena if combined with a treatment facilitating oxidation of excess of fatty acids. In fact, as referred to earlier, some indications are that fat deposition and fat oxidation are highly integrated *in vivo* processes whose manipulation could present opportunities to develop novel strategies to control fat deposition.

17.7.2 Increasing Capacity of Storage/Fatty Acid Buffer of Adipose Tissue; Transforming Structure of Adipose Tissue

Evidence suggests that adipocyte cell size (Weyer et al. 2000, 2001) may be an important predictor of insulin resistance. More susceptible to leaking fatty acids inducing lipotoxicity in other organs, large adipocytes seem to be more insulin resistant (Figure 17.6b). Similarly, the repertoire of secreted adipokines appears to be qualitatively and quantitatively different in large adipocytes. Increased secretion of TNFα (Morin et al. 1998) and resistin and decreased levels of adiponectin are characteristic of large adipocytes from obese individuals. Interestingly, activation of PPARγ induces remodeling of the adipose tissue structure as a result of changes in the rate of preadipocyte recruitment (Kubota et al. 1999). The differentiation of new small adipocytes is associated with marked improvement of insulin sensitivity through increased fatty acid buffering capacity; modification of adipokine repertoire; and, possibly, increases in the amount of cellular membranes that act as a buffering system for cholesterol esters and other lipid signaling molecules (Figure 17.6c). Thus, it is likely that recruitment of new preadipocytes may prevent or reverse some of the metabolic complications associated with obesity (Spiegelman 1998). It could be argued that this strategy may facilitate the development of further obesity; however, this may be a good strategy when faced with the future of a patient with severe metabolic disturbances.

17.7.3   Promoting BAT Development within Adipose Tissue

Unlike in rodents, clearly distinguishable BAT is not identifiable in mature adults. However, based on molecular and morphological studies, small foci of brown adipocytes are now thought to exist in overwhelmingly white adipose tissue depots (Himms–Hagen 1998). These findings have bolstered attempts to develop selective β3-AR agonists with the potential to promote recruitment and proliferation of BAT (Astrup 2000). The observation of enhanced BAT in adult subjects with phaeochromocytoma, a catecholamine-secreting tumor of the adrenal medulla, lends support to this concept (Astrup 2000; Himms–Hagen 1998). In addition, chronic stimulation with β3-AR agonists has been reported to induce BAT in higher animals (Weyer et al. 1999), while in rodents it facilitates the transformation of unilocular adipocytes to mitochondria-rich multilocular adipocytes in WAT depots (Himms–Hagen et al. 2000). Key questions regarding whether these mutilocular cells are metabolically more active than the unilocular cells and if similar convertible adipocytes exist in sufficient quantities in human adipose tissue remain to be addressed.

To date, human clinical trials with agonists specific for rat β3-AR have not successfully demonstrated a thermogenic effect (Astrup 2000; Weyer et al. 1999). The cloning of human β3-AR gene has enabled the development of selective agonists with the potential for a sustained thermogenic action in long-term human studies. However, it remains to be determined whether the efficacy of this new generation of agents depends on receptor activity in nonBAT tissues, such as skeletal muscle, or predominantly on mechanisms inducing dormant BAT recruitment by chronic stimulation with these agents (Astrup 2000; Weyer et al. 1999).

17.8   Conclusion

Over the past decade the major developments in understanding of the molecular mechanisms underpinning mammalian energy homeostasis have led to the verge of a new era in terms of treating obesity. Certainly, it is now within the bounds of possibility to achieve the seemingly far-fetched notion of developing specific antiobesity drugs with properties aimed at safely reducing food intake, modulating energy partition, and enhancing energy expenditure. Considering the near-epidemic nature of obesity in Western society and the profound morbidity and mortality associated with it, this will indeed be a welcome asset to any health care system.

References

Abu-Elheiga, L., Matzuk, M.M., Abo-Hashema, K.A. and Wakil, S.J. (2001). Continuous fatty acid oxidation and reduced fat storage in mice lacking acetyl-CoA carboxylase 2. *Science* 291, 2613–2616.

Adhihetty, P.J., Irrcher, I., Joseph, A.M., Ljubicic, V. and Hood, D.A. (2003). Plasticity of skeletal muscle mitochondria in response to contractile activity. *Exp. Physiol.* 88, 99–107.

Andersson, U. and Scarpulla, R.C. (2001). Pgc-1-related coactivator, a novel, serum-inducible coactivator of nuclear respiratory factor 1-dependent transcription in mammalian cells. *Mol. Cell Biol.* 21, 3738–3749.

Arsenijevic, D., Onuma, H., Pecqueur, C., Raimbault, S., Manning, B.S., Miroux, B., Couplan, E., Alves–Guerra, M.C., Goubern, M., Surwit, R., Bouillaud, F., Richard, D., Collins, S. and Ricquier, D. (2000). Disruption of the uncoupling protein-2 gene in mice reveals a role in immunity and reactive oxygen species production. *Nat. Genet.* 26, 435–439.

Astrup, A. (2000). Thermogenic drugs as a strategy for treatment of obesity. *Endocrine* 13, 207–212.

Barroso, I., Gurnell, M., Crowley, V.E., Agostini, M., Schwabe, J.W., Soos, M.A., Maslen, G.L., Williams, T.D., Lewis, H., Schafer, A.J., Chatterjee, V.K. and O'Rahilly, S. (1999). Dominant negative mutations in human PPARγ associated with severe insulin resistance, diabetes mellitus and hypertension. *Nature* 402, 880–883.

Boss, O., Samec, S., Paoloni–Giacobino, A., Rossier, C., Dulloo, A., Seydoux, J., Muzzin, P. and Giacobino, J.P. (1997). Uncoupling protein-3: a new member of the mitochondrial carrier family with tissue-specific expression. *FEBS Lett.* 408, 39–42.

Boss, O., Bachman, E., Vidal–Puig, A., Zhang, C.Y., Peroni, O. and Lowell B.B. (1999) Role of the β3-adrenergic receptor and/or a putative β4-adreergic receptor on the expression of uncoupling proteins and peroxisome proliferator-activated receptor-γ coactivator-1. *Biochem. Biophys. Res. Commun.* 261, 870–876.

Bouchard, C., Perusse, L., Chagnon, Y.C., Warden, C. and Ricquier, D. (1997). Linkage between markers in the vicinity of the uncoupling protein 2 gene and resting metabolic rate in humans. *Hum. Mol. Genet.* 6, 1887–1889.

Cederberg, A., Gronning, L.M., Ahren, B., Tasken, K., Carlsson, P. and Enerback, S. (2001). FOXC2 is a winged helix gene that counteracts obesity, hypertriglyceridemia, and diet-induced insulin resistance. *Cell* 106, 563–573.

Clapham, J.C., Arch, J.R., Chapman, H., Haynes, A., Lister, C., Moore, G.B., Piercy, V., Carter, S.A., Lehner, I., Smith, S.A., Beeley, L.J., Godden, R.J., Herrity, N., Skehel, M., Changani, K.K., Hockings, P.D., Reid, D.G., Squires, S.M., Hatcher, J., Trail, B., Latcham, J., Rastan, S., Harper, A.J., Cadenas, S., Buckingham, J.A., Brand, M.D. and Abuin, A. (2000). Mice overexpressing human uncoupling protein-3 in skeletal muscle are hyperphagic and lean. *Nature* 406, 415–418.

Cline, G.W., Vidal–Puig, A.J., Dufour, S., Cadman, K.S., Lowell, B.B. and Shulman, G.I. (2001). *In vivo* effects of uncoupling protein-3 gene disruption on mitochondrial energy metabolism. *J. Biol. Chem.* 276, 20240–20244.

Danforth, E., Jr. (2000). Failure of adipocyte differentiation causes type II diabetes mellitus? *Nat. Genet.* 26, 13.

Enerback, S., Jacobsson, A., Simpson, E.M., Guerra, C., Yamashita, H., Harper, M.E. and Kozak, L.P. (1997). Mice lacking mitochondrial uncoupling protein are cold-sensitive but not obese. *Nature* 387, 90–94.

Esterbauer, H., Schneitler, C., Oberkofler, H., Ebenbichler, C., Paulweber, B., Sandhofer, F., Ladurner, G., Hell, E., Strosberg, A.D., Patsch, J.R., Krempler, F. and Patsch, W. (2001). A common polymorphism in the promoter of UCP2 is associated with decreased risk of obesity in middle-aged humans. *Nat. Genet.* 28, 178–183.

Farooqi, I.S., Jebb, S.A., Langmack, G., Lawrence, E., Cheetham, C.H., Prentice, A.M., Hughes, I.A., McCamish, M.A. and O'Rahilly, S. (1999). Effects of recombinant leptin therapy in a child with congenital leptin deficiency. *N. Engl. J. Med.* 341, 879–884.

Fleury, C., Neverova, M., Collins, S., Raimbault, S., Champigny, O., Levi–Meyrueis, C., Bouillaud, F., Seldin, M.F., Surwit, R.S., Ricquier, D. and Warden, C.H. (1997). Uncoupling protein-2: a novel gene linked to obesity and hyperinsulinemia. *Nat. Genet.* 15, 269–272.

Golozoubova, V., Hohtola, E., Matthias, A., Jacobsson, A., Cannon, B. and Nedergaard, J. (2001). Only UCP1 can mediate adaptive nonshivering thermogenesis in the cold. *FASEB J.* 15, 2048–2050.

Gugneja, S., Virbasius, C.M. and Scarpulla, R.C. (1996). Nuclear respiratory factors 1 and 2 utilize similar glutamine-containing clusters of hydrophobic residues to activate transcription. *Mol. Cell Biol.* 16, 5708–5716.

Halaas, J.L., Gajiwala, K.S., Maffei, M., Cohen, S.L., Chait, B.T., Rabinowitz, D., Lallone, R.L., Burley, S.K. and Friedman, J.M. (1995). Weight-reducing effects of the plasma protein encoded by the obese gene. *Science* 269, 543–546.

Harper, J.A., Stuart, J.A., Jekabsons, M.B., Roussel, D., Brindle, K.M., Dickinson, K., Jones, R.B. and Brand, M.D. (2002). Artifactual uncoupling by uncoupling protein 3 in yeast mitochondria at the concentrations found in mouse and rat skeletal-muscle mitochondria. *Biochem. J.* 361, 49–56.

Hesselink, M.K., Greenhaff, P.L., Constantin–Teodosiu, D., Hultman, E., Saris, W.H., Nieuwlaat, R., Schaart, G., Kornips, E. and Schrauwen, P. (2003). Increased uncoupling protein 3 content does not affect mitochondrial function in human skeletal muscle *in vivo*. *J. Clin. Invest.* 111, 479–486.

Himms–Hagen, J., Melnyk, A., Zingaretti, M.C., Ceresi, E., Barbatelli, G. and Cinti, S. (2000). Multilocular fat cells in WAT of CL-316243-treated rats derive directly from white adipocytes. *Am. J. Physiol. Cell Physiol.* 279, C670–681.

Himms–Hagen, J.R.D. (1998). Brown adipose tissue. In *Handbook of Obesity* (Bray, G.A., Bouchard, C. and James, W.P.T., Eds.), pp. 415–441. Marcel Dekker Inc., New York.

Kozak, L.P. and Harper, M.E. (2000). Mitochondrial uncoupling proteins in energy expenditure. *Annu. Rev. Nutr.* 20, 339–363.

Kressler, D., Schreiber, S.N., Knutti, D. and Kralli, A. (2002). The PGC-1-related protein PERC is a selective coactivator of estrogen receptor alpha. *J. Biol. Chem.* 277, 13918–13925.

Kubota, N., Terauchi, Y., Miki, H., Tamemoto, H., Yamauchi, T., Komeda, K., Satoh, S., Nakano, R., Ishii, C., Sugiyama, T., Eto, K., Tsubamoto, Y., Okuno, A., Murakami, K., Sekihara, H., Hasegawa, G., Naito, M., Toyoshima, Y., Tanaka, S., Shiota, K., Kitamura, T., Fujita, T., Ezaki, O., Aizawa, S., Kadowaki, T. et al. (1999). PPAR gamma mediates high-fat diet-induced adipocyte hypertrophy and insulin resistance. *Mol. Cell* 4, 597–609.

Lin, J. (2003). Regulation of cellular energy metabolism by PGC1b. In *Obesity: New Insights into Pathogenesis and Treatment*, Keystone Symposia.

Lin, J., Puigserver, P., Donovan, J., Tarr, P. and Spiegelman, B.M. (2002a). Peroxisome proliferator-activated receptor gamma coactivator 1beta (PGC- 1beta), a novel PGC-1-related transcription coactivator associated with host cell factor. *J. Biol. Chem.* 277, 1645–1648.

Lin, J., Wu, H., Tarr, P.T., Zhang, C.Y., Wu, Z., Boss, O., Michael, L.F., Puigserver, P., Isotani, E., Olson, E.N., Lowell, B.B., Bassel–Duby, R. and Spiegelman, B.M. (2002b). Transcriptional co-activator PGC-1 alpha drives the formation of slow-twitch muscle fibres. *Nature* 418, 797–801.

Lowell, B.B. and Spiegelman, B.M. (2000). Towards a molecular understanding of adaptive thermogenesis. *Nature* 404, 652–660.

Martinez–Botas, J., Anderson, J.B., Tessier, D., Lapillonne, A., Chang, B.H., Quast, M.J., Gorenstein, D., Chen, K.H. and Chan, L. (2000). Absence of perilipin results in leanness and reverses obesity in Lepr(db/db) mice. *Nat. Genet.* 26, 474–479.

Masuzaki, H., Paterson, J., Shinyama, H., Morton, N.M., Mullins, J.J., Seckl, J.R. and Flier, J.S. (2001). A transgenic model of visceral obesity and the metabolic syndrome. *Science* 294, 2166–2170.

Meirhaeghe, A., Crowley V., Lenaghan, C., Lelliott, C., Green, G., Stewart, A, Hart, K., Schinner, S., Sethi, J.K., Yeo, G., Brand, M.D., Cortright, R., O'Rahilly, S., Montague, C. and Vidal–Puig, A. (2003) *In vitro* and *in vivo* characterization of the human, mouse and rat PGC1b gene. *Biochem. J.* 373, 155–165.

Michael, L.F., Wu, Z., Cheatham, R.B., Puigserver, P., Adelmant, G., Lehman, J.J., Kelly, D.P. and Spiegelman, B.M. (2001). Restoration of insulin-sensitive glucose transporter (GLUT4) gene expression in muscle cells by the transcriptional coactivator PGC-1. *Proc. Natl. Acad. Sci. USA* 98, 3820–3825.

Miles, P.D., Barak, Y., He, W., Evans, R.M. and Olefsky, J.M. (2000). Improved insulin-sensitivity in mice heterozygous for PPAR-gamma deficiency. *J. Clin. Invest.* 105, 287–292.

Moitra, J., Mason, M.M., Olive, M., Krylov, D., Gavrilova, O., Marcus–Samuels, B., Feigenbaum, L., Lee, E., Aoyama, T., Eckhaus, M., Reitman, M.L. and Vinson, C. (1998). Life without white fat: a transgenic mouse. *Genes Dev.* 12, 3168–3181.

Morin, C.L., Gayles, E.C., Podolin, D.A., Wei, Y., Xu, M. and Pagliassotti, M.J. (1998). Adipose tissue-derived tumor necrosis factor activity correlates with fat cell size but not insulin action in aging rats. *Endocrinology* 139, 4998–5005.

Picard, F., Gehin, M., Annicotte, J., Rocchi, S., Champy, M.F., O'Malley, B.W., Chambon, P. and Auwerx, J. (2002). SRC-1 and TIF2 control energy balance between white and brown adipose tissues. *Cell* 111, 931–941.

Prins, J.B. and O'Rahilly, S. (1997). Regulation of adipose cell number in man. *Clin. Sci. (Lond)* 92, 3–11.

Puigserver, P., Wu, Z., Park, C.W., Graves, R., Wright, M. and Spiegelman, B.M. (1998). A cold-inducible coactivator of nuclear receptors linked to adaptive thermogenesis. *Cell* 92, 829–839.

Reitman, M.L., Arioglu, E., Gavrilova, O. and Taylor, S.I. (2000). Lipoatrophy revisited. *Trends Endocrinol. Metab.* 11, 410–416.

Ridderstrale, M., Carlsson, E., Klannemark, M., Cederberg, A., Kosters, C., Tornqvist, H., Storgaard, H., Vaag, A., Enerback, S. and Groop, L. (2002). FOXC2 mRNA Expression and a 5' untranslated region polymorphism of the gene are associated with insulin resistance. *Diabetes* 51, 3554–3560.

Robinson, S.W., Dinulescu, D.M. and Cone, R.D. (2000). Genetic models of obesity and energy balance in the mouse. *Annu. Rev. Genet.* 34, 687–745.

Rolfe, D.F. and Brand, M.D. (1997). The physiological significance of mitochondrial proton leak in animal cells and tissues. *Biosci. Rep.* 17, 9–16.

Ruderman, N. and Flier, J.S. (2001). Cell biology. Chewing the fat — ACC and energy balance. *Science* 291, 2558–2559.

Scarpulla, R.C. (1997). Nuclear control of respiratory chain expression in mammalian cells. *J. Bioenerg. Biomembr.* 29, 109–119.

Smith, S.J., Cases, S., Jensen, D.R., Chen, H.C., Sande, E., Tow, B., Sanan, D.A., Raber, J., Eckel, R.H. and Farese, R.V., Jr. (2000). Obesity resistance and multiple mechanisms of triglyceride synthesis in mice lacking Dgat. *Nat. Genet.* 25, 87–90.

Solanes, G., Vidal–Puig, A., Grujic, D., Flier, J.S. and Lowell, B.B. (1997). The human uncoupling protein-3 gene. Genomic structure, chromosomal localization, and genetic basis for short and long form transcripts. *J. Biol. Chem.* 272, 25433–25436.

Spiegelman, B.M. (1998). PPAR-gamma: adipogenic regulator and thiazolidinedione receptor. *Diabetes* 47, 507–514.

Tansey, J.T., Sztalryd, C., Gruia–Gray, J., Roush, D.L., Zee, J.V., Gavrilova, O., Reitman, M.L., Deng, C.X., Li, C., Kimmel, A.R. and Londos, C. (2001). Perilipin ablation results in a lean mouse with aberrant adipocyte lipolysis, enhanced leptin production, and resistance to diet-induced obesity. *Proc. Natl. Acad. Sci. USA* 98, 6494–6499.

Tsukiyama–Kohara, K., Poulin, F., Kohara, M., DeMaria, C.T., Cheng, A., Wu, Z., Gingras, A.C., Katsume, A., Elchebly, M., Spiegelman, B.M., Harper, M.E., Tremblay, M.L. and Sonenberg, N. (2001). Adipose tissue reduction in mice lacking the translational inhibitor 4E-BP1. *Nat. Med.* 7, 1128–1132.

Vanina, Y., Podolskaya, A., Sedky, K., Shahab, H., Siddiqui, A., Munshi, F. and Lippmann, S. (2002). Body weight changes associated with psychopharmacology. *Psychiatr. Serv.* 53, 842–847.

Vega, R.B., Huss, J.M. and Kelly, D.P. (2000). The coactivator PGC-1 cooperates with peroxisome proliferator-activated receptor alpha in transcriptional control of nuclear genes encoding mitochondrial fatty acid oxidation enzymes. *Mol. Cell Biol.* 20, 1868–1876.

Vidal–Puig, A., Solanes, G., Grujic, D., Flier, J.S. and Lowell, B.B. (1997). UCP3: an uncoupling protein homologue expressed preferentially and abundantly in skeletal muscle and brown adipose tissue. *Biochem. Biophys. Res. Commun.* 235, 79–82.

Vidal–Puig, A.J., Grujic, D., Zhang, C.Y., Hagen, T., Boss, O., Ido, Y., Szczepanik, A., Wade, J., Mootha, V., Cortright, R., Muoio, D.M. and Lowell, B.B. (2000). Energy metabolism in uncoupling protein 3 gene knockout mice. *J. Biol. Chem.* 275, 16258–16266.

Virbasius, J.V. and Scarpulla, R.C. (1994). Activation of the human mitochondrial transcription factor A gene by nuclear respiratory factors: a potential regulatory link between nuclear and mitochondrial gene expression in organelle biogenesis. *Proc. Natl. Acad. Sci. USA* 91, 1309–1313.

Walder, K., Norman, R.A., Hanson, R.L., Schrauwen, P., Neverova, M., Jenkinson, C.P., Easlick, J., Warden, C.H., Pecqueur, C., Raimbault, S., Ricquier, D., Silver, M.H., Shuldiner, A.R., Solanes, G., Lowell, B.B., Chung, W.K., Leibel, R.L., Pratley, R. and Ravussin, E. (1998). Association between uncoupling protein polymorphisms (UCP2-UCP3) and energy metabolism/obesity in Pima Indians. *Hum. Mol. Genet.* 7, 1431–1435.

Weyer, C., Gautier, J.F. and Danforth, E., Jr. (1999). Development of beta 3-adrenoceptor agonists for the treatment of obesity and diabetes — an update. *Diabetes Metab.* 25, 11–21.

Weyer, C., Foley, J.E., Bogardus, C., Tataranni, P.A. and Pratley, R.E. (2000). Enlarged subcutaneous abdominal adipocyte size, but not obesity itself, predicts type II diabetes independent of insulin resistance. *Diabetologia* 43, 1498–1506.

Weyer, C., Wolford, J.K., Hanson, R.L., Foley, J.E., Tataranni, P.A., Bogardus, C. and Pratley, R.E. (2001). Subcutaneous abdominal adipocyte size, a predictor of type 2 diabetes, is linked to chromosome 1q21 — q23 and is associated with a common polymorphism in LMNA in Pima Indians. *Mol. Genet. Metab.* 72, 231–238.

Wu, Z., Puigserver, P., Andersson, U., Zhang, C., Adelmant, G., Mootha, V., Troy, A., Cinti, S., Lowell, B., Scarpulla, R.C. and Spiegelman, B.M. (1999). Mechanisms controlling mitochondrial biogenesis and respiration through the thermogenic coactivator PGC-1. *Cell* 98, 115–124.

Yamauchi, T., Waki, H., Kamon, J., Murakami, K., Motojima, K., Komeda, K., Miki, H., Kubota, N., Terauchi, Y., Tsuchida, A., Tsuboyama–Kasaoka, N., Yamauchi, N., Ide, T., Hori, W., Kato, S., Fukayama, M., Akanuma, Y., Ezaki, O., Itai, A., Nagai, R., Kimura, S., Tobe, K., Kagechika, H., Shudo, K. and Kadowaki, T. (2001). Inhibition of RXR and PPARgamma ameliorates diet-induced obesity and type 2 diabetes. *J. Clin. Invest.* 108, 1001–1013.

Yoon, J.C., Puigserver, P., Chen, G., Donovan, J., Wu, Z., Rhee, J., Adelmant, G., Stafford, J., Kahn, C.R., Granner, D.K., Newgard, C.B. and Spiegelman, B.M. (2001). Control of hepatic gluconeogenesis through the transcriptional coactivator PGC-1. *Nature* 413, 131–138.

Zhang, C.Y., Baffy, G., Perret, P., Krauss, S., Peroni, O., Grujic, D., Hagen, T., Vidal–Puig, A.J., Boss, O., Kim, Y.B., Zheng, X.X., Wheeler, M.B., Shulman, G.I., Chan, C.B. and Lowell, B.B. (2001). Uncoupling protein-2 negatively regulates insulin secretion and is a major link between obesity, beta cell dysfunction, and type 2 diabetes. *Cell* 105, 745–755.

18

Targeting Thermogenesis in the Development of Antiobesity Drugs

Mary-Ellen Harper, Robert Dent, Frederique Tesson, and Ruth McPherson

CONTENTS

SUMMARY For weight loss to occur, thermogenesis, or energy expenditure, must exceed dietary energy intake. Coupled thermogenesis refers to the energy expended to produce cellular ATP, which is used in turn to support cellular work. During states of uncoupled thermogenesis, energy substrates are oxidized, but not stored in the body. Instead, the energy is released simply as heat. Targeting uncoupled thermogenesis as a means to treat obesity has been the subject of long-standing interest. In fact, chemical uncouplers were used in the early half of the 20th century to treat obesity — prior even to identification of the process of uncoupled thermogenesis. Following the identification of brown fat and the uncoupling induced therein by uncoupling protein-1 (UCP1), the potential roles for uncoupling in the development and treatment of obesity became subjects of much research. Recent interest in developing thermogenic agents has centered on the novel uncoupling proteins (e.g., UCP2 and UCP3); however, a large degree of controversy surrounds the idea that these proteins have a thermogenic function. Ongoing research efforts have been directed at the recruitment and stimulation of brown adipocytes. Much research has focused on the β-3 adrenergic receptor because it is selectively expressed in adipose tissues and activates uncoupling in brown adipose tissue. Novel agonists are being developed. More research is needed to clarify important questions surrounding the number and activity of β-3 adrenoceptors in human adipose tissues.

18.1 Introduction

Obesity affects approximately 300 million adults worldwide and has been identified by the World Health Organization as the major neglected health problem today (World Health Organization, 2002). Obesity is associated with increased risks of type 2 diabetes mellitus (Ford et al., 1997; Larsson et al., 1981; Lipton et al., 1993); hypertension (Dyer and Elliot, 1989); dyslipidemias (Tchernof et al., 1996); coronary artery disease (Hubert et al., 1983); stroke (Rexrode et al., 1997); cholelithiasis (Stampfer et al., 1992); osteoarthritis (Hochberg et al., 1995); and respiratory problems (Young et al., 1993).

As described in other chapters in this book, the causes of obesity are multifactorial and complex with many genetic and environmental contributors. At the overall physiological level however, obesity is fundamentally the outcome of an extended period of positive energy balance in which energy intake exceeds energy expenditure. Successful treatment of obesity necessitates an extended period of negative energy balance over which time overall energy expenditure exceeds energy intake. Weight management programs that combine aspects of reduced energy intake through energy-restricted diets, behavior modification, and increased physical activity are often effective for short-term weight loss. However, long-term success in the maintenance of reduced weight is low (Dulloo and Girardier, 1990).

Current pharmacological approaches are limited. There is great room for improvement, especially in the provision of agents that can assist in improving long-term weight loss success rates (James et al., 2000; Sjostrom et al., 1998). The three available pharmaceuticals for obesity treatment, Xenical (Hoffman–La Roche), Meridia/Reductil (Abbott), and the generic drug phentermine act largely by decreasing energy intake and/or nutrient absorption. Much less is known about agents that may act by increasing energy expenditure (thermogenesis). The focus of this chapter is on the potential for thermogenic agents as an additional means to treat obesity. To begin, the categories of thermogenesis will be briefly reviewed. The focus will then shift to uncoupled thermogenesis and the potential for pharmaceuticals that could target these processes for the purpose of augmenting overall energy expenditure. The experimental literature demonstrates that synthetic uncouplers and β-adrenergic agonists can indeed be effective. For their clinical application, however, several limitations have yet to be overcome.

18.2 Thermogenesis: Basic Concepts

At the level of the whole body, the term "energy balance" refers to a metabolic state in which total body energy expenditure is equal to the energy absorbed from the diet and not lost in the urine or as gaseous forms of energy (e.g., methane). Energy balance thus

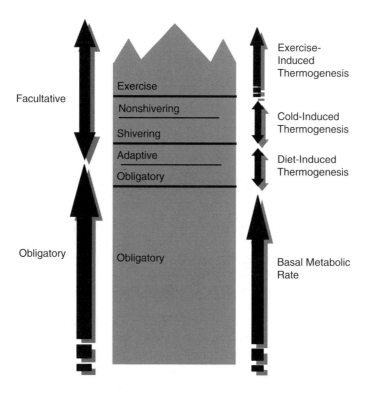

FIGURE 18.1
Categories of thermogenesis. All energy expenditure reactions can be classified as obligatory or facultative (shown on left). Reactions can be further categorized into more specific types of thermogenesis (shown on right). Diet-induced thermogenesis includes obligatory and adaptive thermogenic reactions. Cold-induced thermogenesis includes shivering and nonshivering reactions. See text for description of tissues that are mainly responsible for groups of thermogenic reactions. (Note that the schematic is limited to adult, nonpregnant, nonlactating mammals.)

exists when total body energy expenditure is equal to dietary metabolizable energy. Energy expenditure (or thermogenic) processes can be partitioned into a number of categories. At the overall level, processes can be classified as obligatory or facultative. Obligatory reactions include basal metabolic rate and those essential for the ingestion, digestion, and metabolism of food (Figure 18.1). The latter reactions account for a significant proportion of diet-induced thermogenesis (DIT), the energy costs of assimilating nutrients and retaining net energy (Girardier and Stock, 1983; Himms–Hagen, 1990). Facultative reactions are switched on and off as needed. They include reactions that support a further, adaptive form of DIT, as well as reactions that support thermoregulation (i.e., cold-induced thermogenesis, CIT) and reactions associated with exercise, growth, and reproduction.

Obligatory reactions include those essential to cells and tissues of the body. Important among these processes are those that are essential for endothermy and those essential for postprandial processes, as described previously. All cells and tissues of the body contribute to obligatory thermogenesis. Facultative thermogenesis, however, occurs predominantly in two types of tissue: skeletal muscle and brown adipose tissue (BAT) (Himms–Hagen, 1990). In muscle, these processes include exercise-induced thermogenesis and cold-induced shivering thermogenesis; both are mechanisms that require coupled oxidative phosphorylation. In BAT, facultative thermogenic processes include cold-induced and diet-induced nonshivering thermogenesis; unlike those in muscle, these processes require uncoupled oxidative phosphorylation. BAT thermogenesis is important for thermoregulation in small mammals. In large mammals, including humans, the brown adipose tissue present at birth and in infancy atrophies with age and becomes tissue that resembles white adipose (Casteilla et al., 1987, 1989; Trayhurn et al., 1993; Nicol et al., 1994; Lean et al., 1986). However, as described later, recent evidence supports the presence of active brown fat in adults and further potential for induction of the growth and activity of brown fat following treatment with adrenergic agonists.

18.3 Components of Energy Expenditure: Coupled vs. Uncoupled Thermogenesis

In most cells of the body, a very large proportion of cellular energy expenditure is dedicated most of the time to driving ATP synthesis through mitochondrial oxidative phosphorylation. Oxidative phosphorylation provides about 90% of cellular ATP. Substrate level phosphorylation through glycolysis and the tricarboxylic acid cycle (succinyl CoA synthetase) provides the rest. ATP is subsequently used to fuel a wide range of cellular reactions.

Oxidative phosphorylation requires oxygen consumption because oxygen is the ultimate electron acceptor in the respiratory chain; however, mitochondrial oxygen consumption is not necessarily indicative of ATP synthesis. In fact, during uncoupled thermogenesis, oxygen consumption, and thus the oxidation of various fuels (e.g., fats), continues in the absence of ATP synthesis. Protons return to the mitochondrial matrix from the mitochondrial intermembrane space through routes that bypass ATP synthase. As a result, proton-motive force decreases, and the activity of the respiratory chain increases to rectify it. The consequences are increased fuel oxidation, oxygen consumption, and thermogenesis. Uncoupling can thus be viewed an as energy-wasteful process, i.e., fuels are oxidized, but their energy is not captured or stored by the body. Figure 18.2 depicts oxidative phosphorylation processes and the concept of uncoupling thermogenesis.

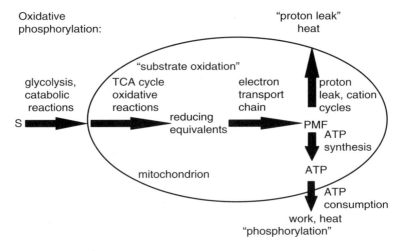

FIGURE 18.2

The oxidative phosphorylation system. Substrate oxidation reactions produce reducing equivalents that, in turn, fuel the electron transport chain and the production of protonmotive force (PMF) across the mitochondrial inner membrane. PMF is then used to support ATP synthesis, or proton leak.

In summary, "coupled thermogenesis" thus refers to energy used to support ATP synthesis. "Uncoupled" thermogenesis refers to that which is independent of ATP synthesis. The physiological mechanisms underlying uncoupled thermogenesis are described next.

18.4 Mechanisms of Uncoupled Thermogenesis and the Importance of Brown Fat

The most pronounced physiological means of uncoupled thermogenesis occur in brown adipose tissue, in which the presence of uncoupling protein-1 (UCP1) allows return of protons from the intermembrane space into the matrix, bypassing ATP synthase (Nicholls and Locke, 1984; Himms–Hagen 1985). UCP1-mediated thermogenesis is essential for normal thermoregulation in neonatal mammals and in small rodents throughout the life span. Its thermoregulatory importance is evidenced by the marked cold intolerance of UCP1 knockout mice (Enerback et al., 1997). Brown adipose tissue thermogenesis is controlled primarily through the activity of the sympathetic nervous system. Uncoupling is activated by norepinephrine that acts upon adrenergic receptors.

The capacity for thermogenesis in brown adipocytes is directly related to the concentration of mitochondrial UCP1; both are inversely related to the temperature at which the animal has been living (Himms–Hagen and Ricquier, 1998). The amount of active brown fat has been linked with the propensity for obesity development for many years (Himms–Hagen, 1985). However, it seems that the absence of UCP1, at least in knockout mice, does not increase susceptibility to obesity (Enerback et al., 1997; Liu et al., 2003). It is very important to note, though, that many lines of evidence show that increased UCP1-mediated uncoupling is an effective means to prevent and treat obesity (Kopecky et al., 1995; Li et al., 2000; Kozak and Harper, 2000).

Uncoupling of another sort also occurs. This uncoupling, which occurs in all tissues that have been studied to date, is referred to as mitochondrial proton leak (Brand, 1990). Several physiological functions have been proposed for proton leak, including a means for heat production; regulation of the efficiency of oxidative phosphorylation; minimizing the production of reactive oxygen species (ROS); and, finally, a means to maintain the $NAD+/NADH$ ratio sufficiently high to support carbon fluxes in biosynthetic processes (Brand et al., 1994; Stuart et al., 1999). Estimates of leak-dependent oxygen consumption in isolated rat liver cells and perfused rat skeletal muscle show that approximately 26% of resting energy expenditure is due to leaks in liver cells (Brown et al., 1990; Nobes et al., 1990; Harper and Brand, 1993; Brand et al., 1994) and 52% in resting skeletal muscle (Brand et al., 1994; Rolfe and Brand, 1996). Rolfe and Brown (1997) estimated that a maximum of 10 to 13% of resting oxygen consumption in the heart is due to proton leak, based on studies in arrested heart (Challoner, 1968). At the level of the whole body, proton leak is estimated to account for 15 to 20% of basal energy metabolism (Rolfe and Brown, 1997). Results thus indicate that mitochondrial proton leak is a very significant contributor to resting cellular energy metabolism.

In considering the potential usefulness and safety of pharmaceuticals that may activate mitochondrial proton leak-type processes, it is important to consider physiological control of proton leak. If leak is a controlled process, then how does the proportion of leak-dependent oxygen consumption change with increases in ATP demand in cells? In studies of isolated mitochondria, it is possible to create metabolic situations in which the demand for ATP synthesis ranges from high to low. By incubating mitochondria in the presence of an ADP regenerating system, the rate of ATP synthesis is high, and mitochondria are said to be functioning in "state 3." In this case, the rate of proton leak reactions is low (Brand, 1990). Conversely, when ATP demand is low, the rate of leak is high.

Using top-down metabolic control analyses, Brand and colleagues (1993) have further shown that control of leak, substrate oxidation, and ATP turnover reactions changes significantly when ATP demand changes (i.e., from state 4 to state 3). Overall, these results show that the proportional contribution of leak to total cellular oxygen consumption is highest when cells are at rest (i.e., when ATP demand is low). Leak, therefore, exerts a tonic effect on changes in oxygen consumption — when ATP demand increases, leak-dependent oxygen consumption decreases.

Is this physiological leak in tissues other than brown adipose tissue carefully controlled, or is it simply responding to protonmotive force? It is well recognized that the relationship between leak-dependent oxygen consumption and protonmotive force is nonohmic; in other words, the former is not linearly dependent on the latter. At membrane potentials at, or near, state 4 respiration, the rate of proton leak is very sensitive to small changes in protonmotive force. However, at lower values of protonmotive force at, or near, state 3 respiration, the rate of proton leak is relatively insensitive to changes in membrane potential. Thus, leak is controlled and is inactive in metabolic situations in which ATP is required for cellular work. The mechanisms responsible are not understood; it is even possible that leak is controlled indirectly and responds largely to the "backpressure" of protonmotive force.

18.5 Synthetic Uncouplers

Uncoupling can be induced by synthetic agents that allow protons to shuttle across the mitochondrial inner membrane, down the electrochemical gradient, and into the matrix. Synthetic uncouplers are amphipathic molecules that dissolve in the membrane bilayer and create a selective conduit for protons to bypass ATP synthase. Examples include 2,4 dinitrophenol (DNP); carbonyl cyanide *m*-chloro phenyl hydrazone (CCCP); and *p*-trifluoromethoxy carbonyl cyanide phenyl hydrazone (FCCP).

An important difference between this form of uncoupling, and that caused by proton leak and other physiological modes of uncoupling (via UCP1), is that synthetic uncouplers induce uncontrolled uncoupling. As a result, uncoupling may not dissipate under metabolic conditions in which ATP demand is increased. Only a low degree of uncoupling would be necessary, and indeed safe, to reduce the efficiency of oxidative phosphorylation. Otherwise, the capacity for ATP synthesis could be substantially impaired and cell death would ensue.

Synthetic uncouplers have in fact been used clinically to treat obesity; DNP was marketed as a weight loss drug for several years in the 1930s (see review by Harper et al., 2001). The original association between DNP and weight loss was based on observations of French workers in munitions factories during World War 1 where DNP and trinitrophenol (TNP) were used (Magne et al., 1932). Further investigations in experimental animals demonstrated a direct effect of DNP on cellular respiration and whole body thermogenesis (Cutting and Tainter, 1932).

Several controlled clinical studies followed and demonstrated that doses up to approximately 5 mg/kg led to few side effects other than a feeling of warmth and some increase in perspiration (Cutting et al., 1933; Tainter et al., 1933; Simkins, 1937). The acute effect of a dose of 3 to 5 mg/kg was a 20 to 30% increase in energy expenditure, which was induced within 1 h and maintained for approximately 24 h; thereafter, the thermogenesis dissipated gradually. Chronic effects of the same dose monitored over at least 10 weeks included a mean increase in metabolic rate of 40% and no evidence of any acquired tolerance (Cutting et al., 1933). It was only at doses greater than 10 mg/kg that the induction of tachycardia and increased body temperature were observed (Cutting et al., 1933).

These studies offered no consistent observations on the effects of DNP on food intake; thus, the weight lost was ascribed to increases in energy expenditure induced by the uncoupler. The use of DNP rapidly became widespread. Approximately 100,000 patients were estimated to be using DNP by 1934 (Tainter et al., 1934); some doses were carefully prescribed based on responses in metabolic rates, while others were less carefully prescribed. Worse still was the fact that DNP was widely sold in nonprescription elixir-type preparations. The lax regulatory control of the use of DNP clearly contributed to reports of associated problems including cataracts, skin rashes, and deaths. As a result, in 1938, an end came to the official clinical use of DNP and the legal marketing of DNP-containing elixirs.

18.6 Recently Identified UCPs: Uncoupling Proteins or "Unknown Carrier Proteins"?

A new era began in 1997 in the research area of uncoupling proteins. A series of proteins structurally homologous to the original uncoupling protein was identified. Since the identification of these novel uncoupling proteins, including UCP2 (Fleury et al., 1997; Gimeno et al., 1997); UCP3 (Boss et al., 1997; Gong et al., 1997); brain mitochondrial carrier protein-1 (BMCP1 or UCP5; Sanchis et al., 1998); and UCP4 (Mao et al., 1999), many studies have examined the hypothesis that proton leak was mediated by the UCPs (see review of Boss et al., 2000). The expectation has been that the UCPs caused uncoupling through a mechanism similar to UCP1, and that these novel UCPs were therefore very important in controlling resting metabolic rate. Because UCP3 expression is limited mainly to skeletal muscle and brown adipose tissue, a lot of interest in specifically targeting it for the treatment of obesity has arisen. The expression of UCP2 is widespread and that of UCP4 and UCP5 is high in the central nervous system.

Many types of experimental approaches have been used to study the function of the UCPs, including:

- Heterologous expression in yeast systems
- Reconstitution in liposomes
- Studies of human genetic linkage, association, and variants
- Physiological induction of expression through means of diet composition, diet restriction, and exercise
- Creation of UCP knockout and UCP overexpression mice

None of these approaches have proven unequivocally that the physiological function of the novel UCPs is proton leak or uncoupling (see reviews of Harper and Himms–Hagen, 2001; Himms–Hagen and Harper, 2001; Stuart et al., 2001; Nedergaard and Cannon, 2003).

Thus, the question of the true physiological function of the novel UCPs remains unanswered. Fundamental clues can be gathered, however, from the study of physiological inductions of expression. Given the initial hypothesis that the proteins function as uncouplers, the literature is replete with paradoxical findings. The most pronounced paradox is the significant increases in UCP2 and UCP3 gene expression in skeletal muscle during fasting and severe food restriction — conditions in which increased efficiency of energy metabolism is well recognized, not situations in which energy wastage would be desirable.

Cadenas et al. (1999) examined the increased expression of UCP3 mRNA and protein caused by fasting in rats. Although significant increases in UCP3 expression occurred in muscle, no changes took place in mitochondrial proton leak. Very recently, Bezaire and colleagues (2001) conducted a similar study in wild-type mice and UCP3 knockout mice. Fasting caused a fourfold increase in UCP3 and a twofold increase in UCP2 in muscle of wild-type mice; however, similar to the findings of Cadenas and colleagues (1999), mitochondrial proton leak reactions did not change.

Mitochondria of UCP3 knockout mice have higher protonmotive force than those from wild-type mice (Gong et al., 2000; Bezaire et al., 2001), and fasting results in further small increases in protonmotive force (Bezaire et al., 2001). It seems that fasting exacerbates the metabolic aberrations occurring in the absence of UCP3. Nedergaard and colleagues (2001) have shown that norepinephrine-induced thermogenesis in brown-fat cells is absolutely dependent on UCP1, despite the high levels of UCP2/UCP3 mRNA observed in brown adipose tissue of UCP1-ablated mice. Moreover, UCP1-ablated mice are cold intolerant (Enerback et al., 1997); isolated brown-fat mitochondria are not uncoupled; and the kinetics of mitochondrial proton leak are similar to those of wild-type mitochondria in the presence of GDP, a well known inhibitor of UCP1-mediated uncoupling (Monemdjou et al., 1999). Perhaps UCP2 and UCP3 cause uncoupling under some situations, but it is becoming increasingly clear that they likely have more important physiological functions in the transport of metabolites (e.g., those related to fatty acid oxidation) (Samec et al., 1998; Himms–Hagen and Harper, 2001).

In fact, a tight correlation exists between the expression of UCP3 and metabolic states in which fatty acid oxidation is high. Most prominent is the correlation of UCP3 expression with fasting and food restriction. A mechanism to explain how UCP3 could enhance fatty acid oxidation was recently proposed (Himms–Hagen and Harper, 2001). This hypothesis describes how UCP3 might facilitate rapid rates of fatty acid oxidation by acting as a mitochondrial fatty acid efflux protein. It was proposed that UCP3 functions in concert with mitochondrial thioesterase (MTE) to remove free fatty acid (produced by MTE) from the matrix and to liberate CoA. The latter is in high demand during fatty acid oxidation. That the direct interaction of fatty acid with UCP1 is necessary for its function (Garlid et al., 1996; Klingenberg and Huang, 1999) lends some support to the idea that its homologue, UCP3, interacts directly with fatty acids.

Taken together, it seems unlikely that the novel uncoupling proteins function primarily as uncouplers of oxidative phosphorylation. There is validity to the quip that they would more aptly be referred to as the "unknown carrier proteins." Once the true functions of novel UCPs are identified, the question as to their usefulness as targets for pharmaceuticals can be addressed. However, as explained in the remaining sections of this chapter, it seems likely that targeting UCP1-mediated thermogenesis through novel β_3-adrenoceptor agonists holds substantial promise.

18.7 β_3-Adrenoceptor Agonists: Activators of Fuel Supply and Oxidation in Adipose Tissues

Highly selective β_3-adrenoceptor (β_3-AR) agonists could potentially be useful in the maintenance of long-term weight loss; they have been shown to improve glucose control in type 2 diabetes mellitus (T2DM). β_3-ARs are selectively expressed in adipose tissues, where they stimulate lipolysis and thermogenesis. In experimental animals, the agonists are very effective in treating obesity. In human trials, the early β_3-AR agonists have had limited effectiveness. This has been ascribed to differences between rodent and human receptor genes and proteins; to low selectivity of agonists for the β_3-AR over other adrenoceptors; and to the potentially low numbers of β_3-adrenoceptors in human adipose tissues.

Adipocytes express the three major classes of adrenergic receptors: α_1-, α_2-, and the β-ARs. Each class can be subclassified into three subtypes. Most of the receptors play some role in the regulation of lipolysis in white adipose tissue (WAT). The β-ARs (β_1, β_2, and β_3) activate lipolysis through stimulatory G-protein-coupled pathways (Arch, 2002). The catecholamines are the primary regulators of adipose tissue lipolysis and bind to the α_2-, β_1-, β_2-, and β_3-ARs in the plasma membrane. The α_2-receptors couple with the G-inhibitory (Gi-) proteins to inhibit cyclic AMP formation and lipolysis. The β-ARs couple with the G-stimulatory (Gs-) proteins to activate cyclic AMP formation and lipolysis.

It is thought that the β_1-AR may mediate low level catecholamine stimulation, while the β_3-AR, which is activated by higher levels of catecholamines and is resistant to down-regulation, may produce a more sustained activation. Cyclic AMP then activates protein kinase A, which phosphorylates and thus activates hormone sensitive lipase (HSL) at two sites, while the dephosphorylation by 3 phosphatases has been implicated in HSL inactivation. Activation of the c-AMP-dependent protein kinase A (PKA) pathway also results in phosphorylation of perilipin via six consensus phosphorylation sites and enhances accessibility of HSL to the lipid droplet. The perilipins are dephosphorylated following insulin binding to adipocytes (Greenberg et al., 1991).

The β_3-AR is expressed predominantly in white and in brown adipocytes; it is thought to play a key role in regulating lipolysis, with an additional role in the latter cell type of adaptive thermogenesis. There are also reports of a functional β_3-AR in muscle. Thurlby and Ellis (1986) reported that most of the thermogenic response to a β_3-selective agonist (BRL-28410) in warm-acclimated rats occurred in muscle, rather than brown adipose tissue. Moreover, immunohistochemical studies of human tissues have demonstrated the presence of β_3-AR protein in muscle (Chamberlain et al., 1999).

At this time, the amounts and activities of the β_3-AR have been studied almost exclusively in experimental animals in which β_3-AR agonists are very effective. The authors' studies in β_3-AR knockout mice and in mice with selective restoration of the *human* β_3-AR in BAT and/or WAT show that the presence of functional receptors in both tissues is needed for maximal thermogenic response (Ito et al., 1998). In this respect, WAT is analogous to an obligatory fuel tank from which TG fuel is released upon adrenergic stimulation; BAT is analogous to a furnace from which the "wasteful" release of energy as heat depends on mitochondrial uncoupling and is triggered also through adrenergic receptors (Ito et al., 1998; Lowell and Spiegelman, 2000). In the authors' opinions, substantial potential for effective β_3-adrenoceptor agonists for the treatment of obesity and T2DM remains. The following sections examine basic information relevant to the development of selective β_3-AR agonists.

18.8 Transcriptional Regulation of β_3-Adrenergic Receptor

The cloning of the human β_3-AR gene was achieved in 1989 (Emorine et al., 1989); the rat and mouse forms were subsequently cloned (Granneman et al., 1991; Muzzin et al., 1991;

Nahmias et al., 1991). The coding region of the human β_3-AR gene contains 1224 nucle-otides that encode for a 408-amino acid protein. The β_1- and β_2-adrenergic receptors are encoded by a single exon, but the β_3-adrenergic receptor gene contains 2 exons. The first 402 amino acid residues are encoded in the first exon, while the six amino acids of the carboxy terminal and the entire 3′ untranslated region of the mRNA are encoded in the second exon. In humans, due to the use of (1) multiple homologous start sites, and (2) alternative polyadenylation signals, the length of mRNA transcripts varies (van Spronsen et al., 1993, Granneman and Lahners, 1994). In human brown fat and neuroepithelioma cells, most β_3-AR transcripts (80%) begin at multiple sites around –130 (Granneman and Lahners, 1994). Utilization of alternate start sites and/or 3′ untranslated regions may allow tissue-specific regulation of expression.

The 5′ flanking region contains four potential cyclic AMP response elements (CREs), three of which have been reported to contribute to the agonist-induced up-regulation of expression (Thomas et al., 1992). It is important to note that no CRE has been identified in the rodent β_3-AR gene, whose expression, unlike the human gene, has been shown to be down-regulated by agonist treatment. In a variety of adipocyte cell models, β_3-AR expression is preceded by the appearance of CCAAT/enhancer-binding protein-α (C/EBP-α), which has been shown to regulate a number of other adipocyte-specific genes. Moreover, it has been demonstrated that failure in the expression of C/EBP-α in several adipocyte cell lines coincides with reduced insulin sensitivity, despite an apparent adipo-genic phenotype. C/EBP-α thus may be a key transcriptional regulator of β_3-AR gene during adipogenesis (Dixon et al., 2001).

18.9   Downstream Targets and Signaling Pathways of β-ARs

An important downstream target of the β-adrenergic/cAMP/PKA signaling pathway in adipocytes is p38 mitogen-activated protein kinase (MAPK); one of the functional conse-quences of this cascade is increased UCP1 gene expression in brown adipocytes. Cao et al. (2001) showed that the selective β_3-AR agonist, CL316243 (CL), stimulates phosphory-lation of MAP kinase and p38 MAPK in a time- and dose-dependent manner in white and brown adipocytes. Isoproterenol and forskolin mimicked the effect of CL on p38 MAPK. In all cases, activation was blocked by the specific p38 MAPK inhibitor SB202190.

The involvement of PKA in β_3-AR-dependent p38 MAPK activation was confirmed by the ability of the PKA inhibitors H89 and (R(p))-cAMP-S to block phosphorylation of p38 MAPK. Treatment of primary brown adipocytes with CL or forskolin induced the expres-sion of UCP1 mRNA levels (approximately sevenfold), and this response was eliminated by PKA inhibitors. A similar stimulation of a 3.7-kilobase UCP1 promoter by CL and forskolin was also completely inhibited by PKA inhibitors, indicating that the effects on UCP1 expression were transcriptional. Moreover, the PKA-dependent transactivation of the UCP1 promoter was fully reproduced by a 220-nucleotide enhancer element from the UCP1 gene (Cao et al., 2001).

Recent discoveries also indicate that the sensitivity of the PKA pathway is amplified by the winged helix/forkhead transcription factor FOXC2, which increases β_3-AR expres-sion and lowers the activation threshold by increasing levels of the R1α subunit of PKA. FOXC2-overexpressing mice are lean and show increased responsiveness to insulin due to sensitization of this pathway (Cederberg et al., 2001). FOXC2 also increases the expres-sion of PGC-1, PPARγ, and CoxII genes associated with enhanced mitochondrial biogenesis. Expression of UCP1, IR, IRS1, IRS2, and GLUT4 also increases in adipocytes, in accord with the marked enhancement in insulin sensitivity. Despite a net increase in lipolysis and FFA release, increasing glucose uptake selectively in fat by treatment with β_3-adrenergic agonists also improves whole-body insulin sensitivity and reduces hepatic gluconeogenesis, likely due to an increase in fatty acid metabolism and energy expenditure (de Souza et al., 1997; Weyer et al., 1998). Thus, β_3-AR activation in obese diabetic subjects may have the benefit of improving insulin sensitivity, as well as stimulating overall energy expenditure.

Reduced β_3-AR function has been recently associated with a polymorphism in the calpain-10 gene (Hoffstedt et al., 2002). The physiological function of calpain-10 is unknown, although it is a known member of the intracellular nonlysosomal proteases thought to play a role in intracellular calcium signaling pathways. An earlier report showed that a calpain-10 polymorphism was associated with insulin resistance and reduced resting energy expenditure (Baier et al., 2000). Thus calpain-10 could also be involved in thermogenesis.

Finally, the thyroid status of an individual also affects β_3-AR density and postreceptor events, leading to altered lipolytic responses. Germack et al. (2000) showed that the density of β_3-AR in rat white adipocytes was enhanced (72%) by T3-treatment and reduced (50%) by hypothyroidism, while β_1-AR number remained unchanged. The β_1- and β_3-AR density was correlated with the specific mRNA level in all thyroid states. The lipolytic responses to isoprenaline and noradrenaline (β_1-/β_2-/β_3-AR agonists) and to BRL 37344 (β_3-AR agonist) were potentiated respectively by 48, 58, and 48% in hyperthyroidism and reduced by about 80% in hypothyroidism. The changes in lipolytic responses to postreceptor-acting agents (forskolin; enprofylline and dibutenyl cyclic AMP; dibutyryl cAMP) suggest modifications of receptor coupling and phosphodiesterase levels in both thyroid states (Germack et al., 2000). In brown adipocytes, T3 is an absolute requirement for the adrenergic stimulation of type II 5'-deiodinase expression that, in turn, amplifies thermogenic response (Martinez de-Mena et al., 2002).

18.10 Effects of β_3-AR Activation on Adipose Tissue Cellular Composition

It is well recognized that β_3-AR activation remodels the cellular composition of adipose tissues. Although the mechanisms are as yet poorly understood, several studies have shown that treatment with β_3-AR agonists *in vitro* and *in vivo* increases the numbers of mature brown adipocytes in BAT and, importantly, also in WAT (Arbeeny et al., 1995; de Souza et al., 1997; Ghorbani et al., 1997). This parallels the reappearance of BAT in adult humans around catecholamine-secreting pheochromocytoma of the adrenal glands (Ricquier et al., 1982). Recent evidence of active brown adipose tissue in adult humans is described below.

Although activation and growth of brown adipose tissue are stimulated by β_3-AR activation, the consequences of activation in white adipose tissue are quite different. In the latter, activation decreases the number of adipocytes (de Souza et al., 1997; Ghorbani et al., 1997; Lafontan and Berlan, 1993). It also leads to inhibition of PI3K activity (Ohsaka et al., 1997) and ERK1/2 (Sevetson et al., 1993) in a cAMP-dependent manner. It is also possible that in humans, like rats, agonist treatment could induce the conversion of a subset of "white" adipocytes to active brown adipocytes in white adipose tissue

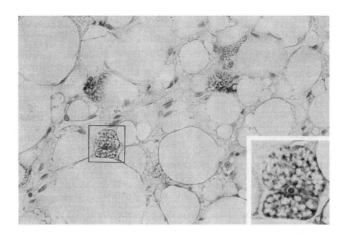

FIGURE 18.3

Appearance of UCP1-expressing multilocular adipocytes in white adipose tissue following treatment with a β_3-adrenergic agonist in rats. Immunohistochemistry for uncoupling protein-1 (UCP1) of retroperitoneal white adipose tissue of rats treated with CL 316,243 (1 mg/g/d) for 1 week. (magnification = × 400). Note the appearance of UCP1-expressing multilocular adipocytes. Inset: 2.5-fold enlargement of a UCP1-expressing adipocyte (Image taken with permission from Himms–Hagen, J. et al., *Am. J. Physiol.*, 279(3):C670–681, 2000.)

(Himms–Hagen et al., 2000) (See Figure 18.3). Treatment of KK-Ay mice with β_3-AR agonist (CL316,243) leads to increased expression of UCP1, UCP2, and UCP3 in brown adipose tissue by 14-fold, 6-fold, and 16-fold, respectively. In white adipose tissue, the expressions of UCP1 and of UCP3 were also increased by 12-fold and 9-fold, respectively, but UCP2 expression was unchanged (Yoshitomi et al., 1998).

The preceding experiments demonstrate the potential of β_3-AR agonists to induce the appearance and activity (i.e., thermogenesis) of brown adipocytes in human white adipose tissue. Although the amount of active brown adipose tissue has been questioned in the past, recent studies using combined positron emission tomography (PET) and computed tomography scan (CT) technologies (Hany et al., 2002) confirm the results of earlier autopsy studies (Santos et al., 1992) and demonstrate that active brown adipose tissue is present in adult humans, particularly in individuals with a low body mass index (BMI). This supports the concept that selective β_3-AR agonists may induce the appearance in depots of active brown adipocytes traditionally referred to as white adipose tissue and activate existing diffuse depots of brown adipose tissue.

18.11 Do β_3-Adrenergic Receptors Play a Role in Development of Obesity and Insulin Resistance?

The β_3-AR has been implicated as a regulator of energy expenditure; a polymorphism in codon 64 of this gene (Trp64Arg) has been associated in some studies with obesity and insulin resistance. However, many studies have failed to detect an effect of this variant, and the importance of the Trp64Arg variant in human obesity remains controversial. The incidence of the naturally occurring Arg64 variant was shown to be correlated with hereditary obesity in Pima Indians, in Japanese individuals, and in Western obese patients with an increased capacity to gain weight and develop T2DM (e.g., Clément et al., 1995; Clément et al., 1997; Mitchell et al., 1999; Sakane et al., 1997; Silver et al., 1997; Strosberg,

1997; Walston et al., 2000). A recent meta-analysis, including diverse population groups, concluded that the Trp64Arg polymorphism is associated with BMI (Fujisawa et al., 1998).

In subjects with a moderate degree of obesity, Kim–Motoyama et al. (1997) found that the Trp64Arg polymorphism was associated with visceral obesity assessed by computerized tomography. Furthermore, the Trp64Arg genotype was associated with increased weight gain during pregnancy (Festa et al., 1999). Shihara and colleagues (1999) investigated the association of the Trp64Arg polymorphism with autonomic nervous system activity and showed that subjects with the polymorphism, even heterozygotes, had lower resting autonomic nervous system activity than did normal subjects. Mice that lacked the β-adrenergic receptors (ADRB1, ADRB2, and ADRB3) on a chow diet had a reduced metabolic rate and were slightly obese. On a high-fat diet, these mice, in contrast to wild-type mice, developed massive obesity due entirely to a failure of diet-induced thermogenesis (Bachman et al., 2002).

These results suggested that β-adrenergic receptors are necessary for diet-induced thermogenesis and that this efferent pathway plays a critical role in the body's defense against diet-induced obesity. Of additional note are results from mouse studies showing a mild increase in adiposity of female, but not male, mice in which the β_3-AR gene is disrupted. Taken together, these results provide moderate additional support for a role for the β_3-AR in the regulation of lipid metabolism and as a valid target for pharmaceuticals.

18.12 Recent Findings from Human Trials of β_3-Selective Agonists

The long-term treatment of obese rodents with β_3-AR agonists significantly reduces adiposity and improves insulin sensitivity (Arch et al., 1984; Cawthorne et al., 1984). These findings demonstrate the potential for the β_3-selective agonists as effective antiobesity and antidiabetic compounds. However, the translation of the efficacy in experimental animals to that in humans offers many important challenges, such as differences in adrenergic receptor density and lipolytic responsiveness. The existence of gender and regional (e.g., between subcutaneous and omental) differences in the capacity for lipolysis is well recognized (Leibel and Hirsch 1987; Mauriege et al., 1991, 1995, 1999). The response of adipocytes to catecholamines depends on the balance of inhibitory α_2- and stimulatory β-ARs (Arner, 1996; Mauriege et al., 1987). More information is needed on the differences in β_3-AR expression, receptor density, and activity in different adipocyte depots, in obese and lean individuals, and in response to PPAR agonist treatment in patients with T2DM.

Studies in β_3-AR -/- (i.e., "knockout") mice have been useful in elucidating the genes for which expression is induced in skeletal muscle by the stimulation of β_3-ARs. Boss and colleagues (1999) studied the role of the β_3-AR in regulating mRNA expression of genes involved in fat metabolism, i.e., mitochondrial uncoupling proteins UCP2 and UCP3 and peroxisome proliferator-activated receptor-γ coactivator-1 (PGC-1), in mouse skeletal muscle. They showed that the selective stimulation of the β_3-AR affects the expression of UCP2, UCP3, and PGC-1 in skeletal muscle that may enhance the effectiveness of agents to activate energy expenditure at the whole body level. This effect may be direct or indirect because the expression of β_3-AR in muscle is controversial.

Two very recent studies have examined the effects of L-796568 ([[(R)-*N*-[4-[2-[[2-hydroxy-2-(3-pyridinyl)ethyl]amino]ethyl]-phenyl]-4-[4-[4-(trifluoromethyl)phenyl]thiazol-2-yl]-benzenesulfonamide, dihydrochloride]), a novel β_3-adrenergic agonist on energy expenditure in obese men. L-796568 shows potency as a β_3-agonist when tested in cAMP assays on Chinese hamster ovary cells transfected with the human β_3-adrenergic receptor; it has an EC50 of 3.6 nmol/L (94% activation compared with isoprenaline) with >600-fold selectivity over the human β_1- and β_2- receptors (Mathvink et al., 2000).

One study demonstrated that a single dose of the agonist increased lipolysis and energy expenditure in 12 obese men (Van Baak et al., 2002). The study was a randomized, placebo-controlled crossover study, and showed that energy expenditure increased about 8% after a 1000-mg dose. This was accompanied by an increase in plasma glycerol and free fatty acid concentrations. Although systolic blood pressure increased slightly, no changes took place in heart rate, diastolic blood pressure, ear temperature, plasma catecholamines, potassium, or leptin. Again, many examples of such results in experimental animals are available; however, this is the first report of an effect in humans *without* significant evidence for β_2- AR involvement — a clear requirement for a clinically safe β_3-agonist.

The second report examined the effect of the same agonist over a 28-d period in a double-blind, randomized, parallel-group study of obese men (Larsen et al., 2002). A lower dose (375 mg/d) was used and no significant changes were observed in 24-h energy expenditure, respiratory quotients, or glucose tolerance. Plasma triacylglycerol concentrations, however, decreased significantly with L-796568 treatment. The authors speculate that the absence of effects was likely due to insufficient recruitment of β_3-responsive tissues in humans and down-regulation of the β_3-adrenergic receptor with chronic dosing.

It may indeed be true that a longer period of treatment is needed for the recruitment of active brown adipocytes in brown adipose tissue and in the traditionally termed "white" adipose tissue depots. It is less likely that the absence of effects is due to down-regulation of the β_3-receptor because it has been well demonstrated that the β_3-receptor, unlike the β_1- and β_2- receptors, is resistant to down-regulation (Arch, 2002). It is also possible that the 375-mg dose was insufficient. Moreover, in this study, energy expenditure was assessed as total energy expenditure and subjects were physically active and ate meals during the 24-h measurement period. In contrast, in the earlier study in which thermogenic effects were observed, *resting* energy expenditure was assessed. It is thus possible that enhanced energy expenditure was obscured by experimental noise, exercise, and the thermic effect of food. Overall, the results of these studies were encouraging.

18.13 Conclusion

In summary, there are a number of categories of thermogenic processes in cells and tissues of the body. Coupled and uncoupled thermogenic processes require the oxidation of fuel substrates. Targeting uncoupled thermogenesis for the purpose of treating obesity has been of long-standing interest. In the 1930s, synthetic uncouplers were successfully used to treat obesity in approximately 100,000 people. Regulation of the dosing and use of these agents were lax and a number of deaths occurred as a result of overdoses, so the agents were removed from the market. Ongoing research efforts have been directed at the possibility of stimulating recruitment and activity of uncoupling protein–1 in brown adipocytes in obese adults. Significant progress has been made recently in the development of selective agonists for the β_3-AR, which could in turn activate not only lipolysis in white adipocytes, but also high rates of fat oxidation in brown adipocytes. Possible additional benefits may include decreased food intake (Tsujii and Bray, 1998).

Recent interest in developing thermogenic agents has centered on the novel uncoupling proteins. However, a large degree of controversy concerns whether these proteins have a thermogenic function. Despite the potential of novel agonists for the β_3-AR, further fundamental information is needed with regard to the amount and activity of the β_3-AR in human adipose tissues in various clinical states. Much more research is needed in order to judge the potential clinical utility of such agonists.

References

Arbeeny, C.M., Meyers, D.S., Hillyer, D.E. and Bergquist, K.E. (1995) Metabolic alterations associated with the antidiabetic effect of beta 3-adrenergic receptor agonists in obese mice *Am. J. Physiol.*, 268:E678–684.

Arch, J.R., Ainsworth, A.T., Cawthorne, M.A., Piercy, V., Sennitt, M.V., Thody, V.E., Wilson, C. and Wilson, S. (1984) Atypical beta-adrenoceptor on brown adipocytes as target for anti-obesity drugs *Nature*, 309(5964):163–165.

Arch, J.R.S. (2002) Beta-3-adrenoceptor agonists: potential, pitfalls and progress *Eur. J. Pharmacol.*, 440:99–107.

Arner, P. (1996) Regulation of lipolysis in human fat cells *Diabetes Rev.*, 4:1–13.

Bachman, E.S., Dhillon, H., Zhang, C.-Y., Cinti, S., Bianco, A.C., Kobilka, B.K. and Lowell, B.B. (2002) Beta-AR signaling required for diet-induced thermogenesis and obesity resistance *Science* 297:843–845.

Baier, L.J., Permana, P.A., Yang, X., Pratley, R.E., Hanson, R.L., Shen, G.Q., Mott, D., Knowler, W.C., Cox, N.J., Horikawa, Y., Oda, N., Bell, G.I. and Bogardus, C. (2000) A calpain-10 gene polymorphism is associated with reduced muscle mRNA levels and insulin resistance *J. Clin. Invest.*, 106:R69–73.

Bezaire, V., Hofmann, W.E., Kramer, J.K.G., Kozak, L.P. and Harper M-E. (2001) Effects of fasting on muscle mitochondrial energetics and fatty acid metabolism in *Ucp3 -/-* and wild-type mice *Am. J. Physiol.*, 281:E975–982.

Boss, O., Samec, S., Paolini–Giacobino, A., Rossier, C., Dulloo, A.G., Seydoux, J., Muzzin, P. and Giacobino J-P. (1997) Uncoupling protein-3: a new member of the mitochondrial carrier family with tissue-specific expression *FEBS Lett.*, 408:39–42.

Boss, O., Hagen, T. and Lowell, B.B. (2000) Uncoupling proteins 2 and 3: potential regulators of mitochondrial energy metabolism *Diabetes*, 49:143–156.

Boss, O., Bachman, E., Vidal–Puig, A., Zhang, C.Y., Peroni, O. and Lowell, B.B. (1999) Role of the beta(3)-adrenergic receptor and/or a putative beta(4)-adrenergic receptor on the expression of uncoupling proteins and peroxisome proliferator-activated receptor-gamma coactivator-1 *Biochem. Biophys. Res. Comm.*, 261:870–876.

Brand, M.D. (1990) The contribution of the leak of protons across the mitochondrial inner membrane to standard metabolic rate *J. Theoret. Biol.*, 145:267–286.

Brand, M.D., Harper, M-E. and Taylor, H.C. (1993) Control of effective P:O ratio of oxidative phosphorylation in liver mitochondria and hepatocytes *Biochem. J.*, 291:739–748.

Brand, M.D., Chien, L.F., Ainscow, E.K., Rolfe, D.F.S. and Porter, R.K. (1994) The causes and functions of mitochondrial proton leak *Biochim. Biophys. Acta*, 1187:132–139.

Brown, G.C., Lakin–Thomas, P.L. and Brand, M.D. (1990) Control of mitochondrial respiration and ATP synthesis in isolated rat liver cells *Eur. J. Biochem.*, 192:355–362.

Cadenas, S., Buckingham, J.A., Samec, S., Seydoux, J., Din, N., Dulloo, A.G. and Brand, M.D. (1999) UCP2 and UCP3 rise in starved rat skeletal muscle but mitochondrial proton conductance is unchanged *FEBS Lett.*, 462:257–260.

Cao, W., Medvedev, A.V., Daniel, K.W. and Collins, S. (2001) Beta-adrenergic activation of p38 MAP kinase in adipocytes: cAMP induction of the uncoupling protein 1 (UCP1) gene requires p38 MAP kinase *J. Biol. Chem.*, 276:27077–27082.

Casteilla, L., Forest, C., Robelin, J., Ricquier, D., Lombet, A. and Ailaud, G. (1987) Characterization of mitochondrial uncoupling protein in bovine fetus and newborn calf *Am. J. Physiol.*, 252:E627–636.

Casteilla, L., Champigny, O., Bouillaud, F., Robelin, J. and Ricquier, D. (1989) Sequential changes in the expression of mitochondrial protein mRNA during the development of brown adipose tissue in bovine and ovine species *Biochem. J.*, 257: 665–671.

Cawthorne, M.A., Carroll, M.J., Levy, A.L., Lister, C.A., Sennitt, M.V., Smith, S.A. and Young, P. (1984) Effects of novel beta-adrenoceptor agonists on carbohydrate metabolism: relevance for the treatment of non-insulin-dependent diabetes *Int. J. Obes.*, 8 (S1):93–102.

Cederberg, A., Gronning, L.M., Ahren, B., Tasken, K., Carlsson, P. and Enerback, S. (2001) FOXC2 is a winged helix gene that counteracts obesity, hypertriglyceridemia, and diet-induced insulin resistance *Cell*, 106:563–573.

Challoner, D.R. (1968) Respiration in myocardium *Nature*, 217:78–79.

Chamberlain, P.D., Jennings, K.H., Paul, F., Cordell, J., Berry, A., Holmes, S.D., Park, J., Sennitt, M.V., Stock, M.J., Cawthorne, M.A., Young, P.W. and Murphy, G.J. (1999) The tissue distribution of the human beta-3 adrenoceptor: studies using a monoclonal antibody *Int. J. Obesity*, 23:1057–1065.

Clément, K., Vaisse, C., Manning, B.S., Basdevant, A., Guy–Grand, B., Ruiz, J., Silver, K.D., Shuldiner, A.R., Froguel, P. and Strosberg, A.D. (1995) Genetic variation in the beta 3-adrenergic receptor and an increased capacity to gain weight in patients with morbid obesity *N. Engl. J. Med.*, 333:352–354.

Clément, K., Manning, B.S., Basdevant, A., Strosberg, A.D., Guy–Grand, B. and Froguel, P. (1997) Gender effect of the Trp64Arg mutation in the beta 3 adrenergic receptor gene on weight gain in morbid obesity *Diab. Metab.*, 23(5):424–427.

Cutting, W.C. and Tainter, M.L. (1932) Actions of dinitrophenol *Proc. Soc. Exper. Biol. Med.*, 29: 1268.

Cutting, W.C., Mehrtens, H.G. and Tainter, M.L. (1933) Actions and uses of dinitrophenol: Promising metabolic applications *JAMA*, 101:1472–1475.

de Souza, C.J., Hirshman, M.F. and Horton, E.S. (1997) CL-316,243, a beta3-specific adrenoceptor agonist, enhances insulin-stimulated glucose disposal in non-obese rats *Diabetes*, 46:1257–1263.

Dixon, T.M., Daniel, K.W., Farmer, S.R. and Collins, S. (2001) CCAAT/enhancer-binding protein alpha is required for transcription of the beta 3-adrenergic receptor gene during adipogenesis *J. Biol. Chem.*, 276:722–728.

Dulloo, A.G. and Girardier, L. (1990) Adaptive changes in energy expenditure during refeeding following low calorie intake: evidence for a specific metabolic component favoring fat storage *Am. J. Clin. Nutr.*, 52:415–420.

Dyer, A.R. and Elliott, P. (1989) The INTERSALT study: relations of body mass index to blood pressure. INTERSALT Co-operative Research Group *J. Hum. Hypertens.*, 3(5):299–308.

Emorine, L.J., Marullo, S., Briend–Sutren, M.M., Patey, G., Tate, K., Delavier–Klutchko, C. and Strosberg, A.D. (1989) Molecular characterization of the human beta 3-adrenergic receptor *Science*, 245(4922):1118–1121.

Enerback, S., Jacobsson, A., Simpson, E.M., Guerra, C., Yamashita, H., Harper, M-E. and Kozak, L.P. (1997) Mice lacking mitochondrial uncoupling protein are cold-sensitive but not obese *Nature*, 387:90–94.

Festa, A., Krugluger, W., Shnawa, N., Hopmeier, P., Haffner, S.M. and Schernthaner, G. (1999) Trp64Arg polymorphism of the beta-3-adrenergic receptor gene in pregnancy: association with mild gestational diabetes mellitus *J. Clin. Endocr. Metab.* 84: 1695–1699.

Fleury, C., Neverova, M., Collins, S., Raimbault, S., Champigny, O., Levi–Meyrueis, C., Bouillaud, F., Seldin, M.F., Surwit, R.S., Ricquier, D. and Warden, C.H. (1997) Uncoupling protein-2: a novel gene linked to obesity and hyperinsulinemia *Nat. Genet.*, 15:269–272.

Ford, E.S., Williamson, D.F. and Liu, S. (1997) Weight change and diabetes incidence: findings from a national cohort of US adults *Am. J. Epidemiol.*, 146:214–222.

Fujisawa, T., Ikegami, H., Kawaguchi, Y. and Ogihara, T. (1998) Meta-analysis of the association of Trp64Arg polymorphism of beta 3-adrenergic receptor gene with body mass index *J. Clin. Endocrinol. Metab.*, 83:2441–2444.

Garlid, K.D., Orosz, D.E., Modriansky, M., Vassanelli, S. and Jezek, P. (1996) On the mechanism of fatty acid-induced proton transport by mitochondrial uncoupling protein *J. Biol. Chem.*, 271:2615–2620.

Germack, R., Starzec, A. and Perret, G.Y. (2000) Regulation of beta 1- and beta 3-adrenergic agonist-stimulated lipolytic response in hyperthyroid and hypothyroid rat white adipocytes *Br. J. Pharmacol.*, 129(3):448–456.

Ghorbani, M., Claus, T.H. and Himms–Hagen, J. (1997) Hypertrophy of brown adipocytes in brown and white adipose tissues and reversal of diet-induced obesity in rats treated with a beta3-adrenoceptor agonist *Biochem. Pharmacol.*, 54:121–131.

Gimeno, R.E., Dembski, M., Weng, X., Deng, N., Shyjan, A.W., Gimeno, C.J., Iris, F., Ellis, S.J., Woolf, E.A. and Tartaglia, L.A. (1997) Cloning and characterization of an uncoupling protein homolog: a potential mediator of human thermogenesis *Diabetes*, 46:900–906.

Girardier, L. and Stock M.J. (1983) Mammalian thermogenesis: an introduction, in L. Girardier and M.J. Stock (Eds.) *Mammalian Thermogenesis*, Cambridge: Chapman & Hall.

Gong, D.W., He, Y., Karas, M. and Reitman, M. (1997) Uncoupling protein-3 is a mediator of thermogenesis regulated by thyroid hormone, beta3-adrenergic agonists, and leptin *J. Biol. Chem.*, 272:24129–24132.

Gong, D.W., Monemdjou, S., Gavrilova, O., Leon, L.R., Marcus–Samuels, B., Chou, C.J., Everett, C., Kozak, L.P., Li, C., Deng, C., Harper, M-E. and Reitman, M.L. (2000) Lack of obesity and normal response to fasting and thyroid hormone in mice lacking uncoupling protein-3 *J. Biol. Chem.*, 275:16251–16257.

Granneman, J.G., Lahners, K.N. and Chaudhry, A. (1991) Molecular cloning and expression of the rat beta 3-adrenergic receptor *Mol. Pharmacol.*, 40:895–899.

Granneman, J.G. and Lahners, K.N. (1994) Analysis of human and rodent beta 3-adrenergic receptor messenger ribonucleic acids *Endocrinology*, 135:1025–1031.

Greenberg, A.S., Egan, J.J., Wek, S.A., Garty, N.B., Blanchette–Mackie, E.J. and Londos, C. (1991) Perilipin, a major hormonally regulated adipocyte-specific phosphoprotein associated with the periphery of lipid storage droplets *J. Biol. Chem.*, 266: 11341–11346.

Hany, T.F., Gharehpapagh, E., Kamel, E., Buck, A., Himms–Hagen, J. and von Schulthess, G.K. (2002) Brown adipose tissue: a factor to consider in symmetrical tracer uptake in the neck and upper chest region *Eur. J. Nucl. Med. Mol. Imaging*, 29:1393–1398.

Harper, M-E. and Brand, M.D. (1993) The quantitative contributions of mitochondrial proton leak and ATP turnover reactions to the changed respiration rates of hepatocytes isolated from rats of different thyroid status *J. Biol. Chem.*, 268:14850–14860.

Harper, J.A., Dickinson, K. and Brand, M.D. (2001) Mitochondrial uncoupling as a target for drug development for the treatment of obesity *Obesity Rev.*, 2:255–265.

Harper, M-E., Dent, R., Monemdjou, S., Bezaire, V., VanWyck, L., Wells, G., Kavaslar, G.N., Gauthier, A., Tesson, F. and McPherson, R. (2002) Decreased mitochondrial proton leak and reduced expression of Ucp3 in skeletal muscle of obese diet-resistant women *Diabetes*, 51:2459–2466.

Harper, M-E. and Himms–Hagen, J. (2001) Mitochondrial efficiency: lessons learned from transgenic mice *Biochim. Biophys. Acta*, 1504:159–172.

Himms–Hagen, J. (1985) Brown adipose tissue and thermogenesis *Annu. Rev. Nutr.*, 5:69–94.

Himms–Hagen, J. (1990) Brown adipose tissue thermogenesis: role in thermoregulation, energy regulation and obesity, in E. Schonbaum, and P. Lomax (Eds.) *Thermoregulation: Physiology and Biochemistry*, New York: Pergamon Press.

Himms–Hagen, J. and Harper, M-E. (2001) Physiological role of UCP3 may be export of fatty acids from mitochondria when fatty acid oxidation predominates *Exp. Biol. Med.*, 226:78–84.

Himms–Hagen, J., Melnyk, A., Zingaretti, M.C., Ceresi, E., Barbatelli, G. and Cinti, S. (2000) Multilocular fat cells in WAT of CL-316243-treated rats derive directly from white adipocytes *Am. J. Physiol.*, 279(3):C670–681.

Himms–Hagen, J. and Ricquier D. (1998) Brown adipose tissue, in: G.A. Bray, C. Bouchard and W.P.T. James (Eds.) *Handbook of Obesity*, New York: Marcel Dekker.

Hochberg, M.C., Lethbridge–Cejku, M., Scott, W.W., Jr., Reichle, R., Plato, C.C. and Tobin, J.D. (1995) The association of body weight, body fatness and body fat distribution with osteoarthritis of the knee: data from the Baltimore Longitudinal Study of Aging *J. Rheumatol.*, 22(3):488–493.

Hoffstedt, J., Naslund, E. and Arner, P. (2002) Calpain-10 gene polymorphism is associated with reduced beta-3-adrenoceptor function in human fat cells *J. Clin. Invest.*, 87:3362–3367.

Hubert, H.B., Feinleib, M., McNamara, P.M. and Castelli, W.P. (1983) Obesity as an independent risk factor for cardiovascular disease: a 26-year follow-up of participants in the Framingham Heart Study *Circulation*, 67(5):968–977.

Ito, M., Grujic, D., Abel, E., Vidal–Puig, A., Susulic, V., Lawits, J., Harper, M-E., Himms–Hagen, J., Strosberg, A.D. and Lowell, B.B. (1998) Mice expressing human but not mouse β3-adrenergic receptors under the control of human gene regulatory elements *Diabetes*, 47:1464–1471.

James, W.P., Astrup, A., Finer, N., Hilsted, J., Kopelman, P., Rossner, S., Saris, W.H.M. and Van Gaal, L.F. (2000) Effect of sibutramine on weight maintenance after weight loss: a randomized trial. STORM Study Group. Sibutramine Trial of Obesity Reduction and Maintenance *Lancet*, 356(9248):2119–2125.

Kim–Motoyama, H., Yasuda, K., Yamaguchi, T., Yamada, N., Katakura, T., Shuldiner, A.R., Akanuma, Y., Ohashi, Y., Yazaki, Y. and Kadowaki, T. (1997) A mutation of the beta-3-adrenergic receptor is associated with visceral obesity but decreased serum triglyceride *Diabetologia*, 40:469–472.

Klingenberg, M. and Huang, S.G. (1999) Structure and function of the uncoupling protein from brown adipose tissue *Biochim. Biophys. Acta*, 1415:271–296.

Kopecky, J., Clarke, G., Enerback, S., Spiegelman, B.M. and Kozak, L.P. (1995) Expression of the mitochondrial uncoupling protein gene from the aP2 gene promoter prevents genetic obesity *J. Clin. Invest.*, 96(6):2914–2923.

Kozak, L.P. and Harper, M.E. (2000) Mitochondrial uncoupling proteins in energy expenditure *Annu. Rev. Nutr.*, 20:339–363.

Lafontan, M. and Berlan, M. (1993) Fat cell adrenergic receptors and the control of white and brown fat cell function *J. Lipid Res.*, 34:1057–1091.

Larsen, T.M., Toubro, T., van Baak, M.A., Gottesdiener, K.M., Larson, P., Saris, W.H.M. and Astrup, A. (2002) Effect of a 28-d treatment with L796568, a novel beta-3 adrenergic receptor agonist, on energy expenditure and body composition in obese men *Am. J. Clin. Nutr.*, 76: 780–788.

Larsson, B., Bjorntorp, P. and Tibblin, G. (1981) The health consequences of moderate obesity *Int. J. Obes.*, 5:97–116.

Lean, M.E.J., James, W.P.T., Jennings, G. and Trayhurn, P. (1986) Brown adipose tissue uncoupling protein content in infants, children and adult humans *Clin. Sci.*, 71: 291–297.

Leibel, R.L. and Hirsch, J. (1987) Site- and se-related differences in adrenoceptor status of human adipose tissues *J. Clin. Endocrinol. Metab.*, 64:1205–1210.

Li, B., Nolte, L.A., Ju, J.S., Han, D.H., Coleman, T., Holloszy, J.O. and Semenkovich, C.F. (2000) Skeletal muscle respiratory uncoupling prevents diet-induced obesity and insulin resistance in mice *Nat. Med.*, 6(10):1115–1120.

Lipton, R.B., Liao, Y., Cao, G., Cooper, R.S. and McGee, D. (1993) Determinants of incident non-insulin-dependent diabetes mellitus among blacks and whites in a national sample. The NHANES I Epidemiologic Follow-up Study *Am. J. Epidemiol.*, 138:826–839.

Liu, X., Rossmeisl, M., McClaine, J., Riachi, M., Harper, M-E. and Kozak, L.P. (2003) Paradoxical resistance to diet-induced obesity in UCP1-deficient mice *J. Clin. Invest.*, 111:399–407.

Lowell, B.B. and Spiegelman B.M. (2000) Towards a molecular understanding of adaptive thermogenesis *Nature*, 404:652–660.

Magne, H., Mayer, A. and Plantefol, L. (1932) Studies on the action of dinitrophenol 1-2-4 (Thermol) *Ann. Physiol. Physicochem. Biol.*, 8:1–167

Mao, W, Yu, X.X., Zhong, A., Li, W., Brush, J., Sherwood, S.W., Adams, S.H. and Pan, G. (1999) UCP4, a novel brain-specific mitochondrial protein that reduces membrane potential in mammalian cells *FEBS Lett.*, 443:326–330.

Martinez–deMena, R., Hernandez, A. and Obregon, M.J. (2002) Triiodothyronine is required for the stimulation of type II 5′-deiodinase mRNA in rat brown adipocytes *Am. J. Physiol.*, 282(5):E1119–1127.

Mathvink, R.J., Tolman, J.S., Chitty, D., Candelore, M.R., Cascieri, M.A., Colwell, L.F., Jr., Deng, L., Feeney, W.P., Forrest, M.J., Hom, G.J., MacIntyre, D.E., Miller, R.R., Stearns, R.A., Tota, L., Wyvratt, M.J., Fisher, M.H. and Weber, A.E. (2000) Discovery of a potent orally bioavailable beta-3 adrenergic receptor agonist, [(R)-N-[4-[2-[[2-hydroxy-2-(3-pyridinyl)ethyl]amino]eth-yl]-phenyl]-4-[4-(trifluoromethyl) phenyl]thiazol-2-yl]-benzenesulfonamide *J. Med. Chem.*, 43:3832–3836.

Mauriege, P., Galitzky, J., Berlan, M. and Lafontan, M. (1987) Heterogeneous distribution of beta- and alpha2-adrenoceptor binding sites in human fat cells from various deposits: functional consequences *Eur. J. Clin. Invest.*, 17:156–165.

Mauriege, P., Despres, J.P., Prud'homme, D., Pouliot, M.C., Marcotte, M., Tremblay, A. and Bouchard, C. (1991) Regional variation in adipose tissue lipolysis in lean and onbese men *J. Lipid Res.*, 32:1625–1633.

Mauriege, P., Prud'homme, D., Lemieux, S., Tremblay, A. and Despres, J.P. (1995) Regional differences in adipose tissue lipolysis from lean and obese women: existence of postreceptor alterations *Am. J. Physiol.*, 269:E341–350.

Mauriege, P., Imbeault, P., Langin, D., Lacaille, M., Almeras, N., Tremblay, A. and Despres, J.P. (1999) Regional and gender variations in adipose tissue lipolysis in response to weight loss *J. Lipid Res.*, 40:1559–1571.

Mitchell, B.D., Cole, S.A., Comuzzie, A.G., Almasy, L., Blangero, J., MacCluer, J.W. and Hixson, J.E. (1999) A quantitative trait locus influencing BMI maps to the region of the beta-3 adrenergic receptor *Diabetes*, 48(9):1863–1867.

Monemdjou, S., Kozak, L.P. and Harper, M-E. (1999) Mitochondrial proton leak in brown adipose tissue mitochondria of Ucp1-deficient mice is GDP insensitive *Am. J. Physiol.*, 276:E1073–1082.

Muzzin, P., Revelli, J.P., Kuhne, F., Gocayne, J.D., McCombie, W.R., Venter, J.C., Giacobino, J.P. and Fraser, C.M. (1991) An adipose tissue-specific beta-adrenergic receptor. Molecular cloning and down-regulation in obesity *J. Biol. Chem.*, 266:24053–24058.

Nahmias, C., Blin, N., Elalouf, J.M., Mattei, M.G., Strosberg, A.D. and Emorine, L.J. (1991) Molecular characterization of the mouse beta 3-adrenergic receptor: relationship with the atypical receptor of adipocytes *EMBO J.*, 10:3721–3727.

Nedergaard, J. and Cannon, B. (2003) Pros and cons for suggested functions *Exp. Physiol.*, 88:65–84.

Nedergaard, J., Golozoubova, V., Matthias, A., Asadi, A., Jacobsson, A. and Cannon, B. (2001) UCP1: the only protein able to mediate adaptive non-shivering thermogenesis and metabolic inefficiency *Biochim. Biophys. Acta*, 1504:82–106.

Nicol, F., Lefranc, H., Arthur, J.R. and Trayhurn, P. (1994) Characterization and postnatal development of 5'-deiodinase activity in goat perirenal fat *Am. J. Physiol.*, 267:R144–149.

Nicholls, D.G. and Locke, R.M. (1984) Thermogenic mechanisms in brown fat *Physiol. Rev.*, 64:1–64.

Nobes, C.D., Brown, G.C., Olive, P.N. and Brand, M.D. (1990) Non-ohmic conductance of mitochondrial inner membrane of hepatocytes *J. Biol. Chem.*, 265:12903–12909.

Ohsaka, Y., Tokumitsu, Y. and Nomura, Y. (1997) Suppression of insulin-stimulated phosphatidylinositol 3-kinase activity by the beta3-adrenoceptor agonist CL316,243 in rat adipocytes *FEBS Lett.*, 402:246–250.

Rexrode, K.M., Hennekens, C.H., Willett, W.C., Colditz, G.A., Stampfer, M.J., Rich–Edwards, J.W., Speizer, F.E. and Manson, J.E. (1997) A prospective study of body mass index, weight change, and risk of stroke in women *JAMA*, 277:1539–1545.

Ricquier, D., Nechad, M. and Mory, G. (1982) Ultrastructural and biochemical characterization of human brown adipose tissue in pheochromocytoma *J. Clin. Endocrinol. Metab.*, 54:803–807.

Rolfe, D.F.S. and Brand, M.D. (1996) The contribution of mitochondrial proton leak to the rate of respiration in rat skeletal muscle and to SMR *Am. J. Physiol.*, 271:C1380–1389.

Rolfe, D.F.S. and Brown, G.C. (1997) Cellular energy utilization and molecular origin of standard metabolic rate in mammals *Physiol. Rev.*, 77:732–758.

Sakane, N., Yoshida, T., Umekawa, T., Kogure, A., Takakura, Y. and Kondo, M. (1997) Effects of Trp64Arg mutation in the beta 3-adrenergic receptor gene on weight loss, body fat distribution, glycemic control, and insulin resistance in obese type 2 diabetic patients *Diabetes Care*, 20:1887–1890.

Samec, S., Seydoux, J. and Dulloo, A.G. (1998) Role of UCP homologues in skeletal muscles and brown adipose tissue: mediators of thermogenesis or regulators of lipids as fuel substrate? *FASEB J.*, 12:715–724.

Sanchis, D., Fleury, C., Chomiki, N., Goubern, M., Huang, Q., Neverova, M., Gregoire, F., Easlick, J., Raimbault, S., Levi–Meyrueis, C., Miroux, B., Collins, S., Seldin, M., Richard, D., Warden, C., Bouillaud, F. and Ricquier, D. (1998) BMCP1, a novel mitochondrial carrier with high expression in the central nervous system of humans and rodents, and respiration uncoupling activity in recombinant yeast *J. Biol. Chem.*, 273:34611–34615.

Santos, G.C., Araujo, M.R., Silveira, T.C. and Soares, F.A. (1992) Accumulation of brown adipose tissue and nutritional status. A prospective study of 366 consecutive autopsies *Arch. Pathol. Med.*, 116:1152–1154.

Sevetson, B.R., Kong, X. and Lawrence, J.C., Jr. (1993) Increasing cAMP attenuates activation of mitogen-activated protein kinase *Proc. Natl. Acad. Sci. USA*, 90:10305–10309.

Shihara, N., Yasuda, K., Moritani, T., Ue, H., Adachi, T., Tanaka, H., Tsuda, K. and Seino, Y. (1999) The association between Trp64Arg polymorphism of the beta-3-adrenergic receptor and autonomic nervous system activity *J. Clin. Endocr. Metab.*, 84: 1623–1627.

Silver, K., Mitchell, B.D., Walston, J., Sorkin, J.D., Stern, M.P., Roth, J. and Shuldiner, A.R. (1997) TRP64ARG beta 3-adrenergic receptor and obesity in Mexican Americans *Hum. Genet.*, 101:306–311.

Simkins, S. (1937) Dinitrophenol and dessicated thyroid in the treatment of obesity. A comprehensive clinical and laboratory study *JAMA*, 108:2110–2118.

Sjostrom, L., Rissanen, A., Andersen, T., Boldrin, M., Golay, A., Koppeschaar, H.P. and Krempf, M. (1998) Randomized placebo-controlled trial of orlistat for weight loss and prevention of weight regain in obese patients. European Multicentre Orlistat Study Group *Lancet*, 352(9123):167–172.

Stampfer, M.J., Maclure, K.M., Colditz, G.A., Manson, J.E. and Willett, W.C. (1992) Risk of symptomatic gallstones in women with severe obesity *Am. J. Clin. Nutr.*, 55:652–658.

Strosberg, A.D. (1997) Structure and function of the beta 3-adrenergic receptor *Ann. Rev. Pharmacol. Toxicol.*, 37:421–450.

Stuart, J.A., Brindle, K.M., Harper, J.A. and Brand, M.D. (1999) Mitochondrial proton leak and the uncoupling proteins *J. Bioenerg. Biomemb.*, 31:517–525.

Stuart, J.A., Cadenas, S., Jacobsons, M.B., Roussel, D. and Brand, M.D. (2001) Mitochondrial proton leak and the uncoupling protein 1 homologues *Biochim. Biophys. Acta*, 1504:144–158.

Tainter, M.L., Cutting, W.C., Stockton, A.B. (1934) Use of dinitrophenol in nutritional disorders: a critical survey of clinical results. *Am. J. Public Health*, 24:1045–1053.

Tainter, M.L., Stockton, A.B. and Cutting, W.C. (1933) Use of dinitrophenol in obesity and related conditions: a progress report *JAMA*, 1472–1475.

Tchernof, A., Lamarche, B., Prud'Homme, D., Nadeau, A., Moorjani, S., Labrie, F., Lupien, P.J. and Despres, J.P. (1996) The dense LDL phenotype. Association with plasma lipoprotein levels, visceral obesity, and hyperinsulinemia in men *Diabetes Care*, 19:629–637.

Thomas, R.F., Holt, B.D., Schwinn, D.A. and Liggett, S.B. (1992) Long-term agonist exposure induces upregulation of beta 3-adrenergic receptor expression via multiple cAMP response elements *Proc. Natl. Acad. Sci. USA*, 89:4490–4494.

Thurlby, P.L. and Ellis, R.D.M. (1986) Differences between the effects of nor-adrenaline and the beta-adrenoceptor agonist BRL 28410 in brown adipose tisse and hind limb of the anaethetized rat *Can. J. Physiol. Pharmacol.*, 64: 1111–1114.

Trayhurn, P., Thomas, M.E.A. and Keith, J.S. (1993) Postnatal dvelopment of uncoupling protein mRNA and GLUT4 in adipose tissues of goats *Am. J. Physiol.*, 265: R676–682.

Tsujii, S. and Bray, G.A. (1998) A beta-3 adrenergic agonist (BRL-37,344) decreases food intake *Physiol. Behav.*, 63:723–728.

Van Baak, M.A., Hul, G.B.J., Toubro, S., Astrup, A., Gottesdiener, K.M., DeSmet, M. and Saris, W.H.M. (2002) Acute effect of L-796568, a novel beta-3 adrenergic receptor agonist, on energy expenditure in obese men *Clin. Pharmacol. Ther.*, 71: 272–279.

van Spronsen, A., Nahmias, C., Krief, S., Briend–Sutren, M.M., Strosberg, A.D. and Emorine, L.J. (1993) The promoter and intron/exon structure of the human and mouse beta 3-adrenergic-receptor genes *Eur. J. Biochem.*, 213:1117–1124.

Walston, J., Silver, K., Hilfiker, H., Andersen, R.E., Seibert, M., Beamer, B., Roth, J., Poehlman, E. and Shuldiner, A.R. (2000) Insulin response to glucose is lower in individuals homozygous for the Arg 64 variant of the beta-3-adrenergic receptor *J. Clin. Endo. Metab.*, 85:4019–4022.

Weyer, C., Tataranni, P.A., Snitker, S., Danforth, E., Jr. and Ravussin, E. (1998) Increase in insulin action and fat oxidation after treatment with CL 316,243, a highly selective beta3-adrenoceptor agonist in humans *Diabetes*, 47:1555–1561.

World Health Organization (2002) Joint WHO FAO expert consultation on diet, nutrition and the prevention of chronic diseases Geneva, Switzerland. Technical Report Series 894 (Jan 28–Feb 1).

Yoshitomi, H., Yamazaki, K., Abe, S. and Tanaka, I. (1998) Differential regulation of mouse uncoupling proteins among brown adipose tissue, white adipose tissue, and skeletal muscle in chronic beta 3 adrenergic receptor agonist treatment *Biochem. Biophys. Res. Commun.*, 253:85–91.

Young, T., Palta, M., Dempsey, J., Skatrud, J., Weber, S. and Badr, S. (1993) The occurrence of sleep-disordered breathing among middle-aged adults *N. Engl. J. Med.*, 328:1230–1235.

Part VI

Treatment Alternatives

19

Diet, Physical Activity, and Behavior

Alexandra Kazaks and Judith S. Stern

CONTENTS

19.1   Setting the Stage for Worldwide Obesity

Obesity is now a global epidemic. More than a billion people throughout the world are overweight or obese. In a 2000 report, the World Health Organization estimated that 315 million people are obese (body mass index [BMI] of 30 or above). Another 750 million are

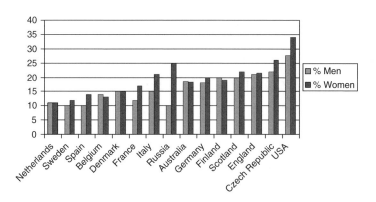

FIGURE 19.1
Multinational prevalence of obesity.

overweight (BMI 25 to 29.9) (WHO, 2000). Figure 19.1 shows examples of the multinational prevalence of obesity (International Union of Nutritional Sciences [IUNS] Web page). The prevalence of obesity and overweight in men and women is rapidly increasing in developed and developing nations in most parts of the world. In many populations, malnutrition and underweight coexist with overweight and obesity.

It is necessary to understand the contribution of diet, exercise, and behavior to the development of obesity; these contributions also must be considered in light of new understanding about the role of genetics. The dramatic increase in "globesity" is linked to market globalization that now allows greater access to high-fat, high-sugar, energy-dense foods. Changing life-styles, such as rural to urban shifts and labor-saving technology in workplaces and homes have replaced physically demanding labor and led to a decline in daily physical activity. These changes in diet, exercise, and life-style have brought health problems associated with overconsumption to all nations.

Because the U.S. has the highest prevalence of overweight and obesity, that population in particular can be examined to analyze how diet, physical activity, and behavior contribute to this complex health issue, and what interventions might be effective to moderate this epidemic. Data from 1999 to 2000 show that 61% of adults in the U.S. were overweight (34%) or obese (27%) (Flegal, 2002).

19.2 Can Obesity Be Blamed on Genes?

Discoveries about the role of genetic determinants of obesity such as the OB gene in mice and the hormone leptin as a modulator of food intake and energy expenditure are important, but they cannot explain the recent epidemic of obesity. The human genome has not significantly changed in just a few decades. In general, obesity in humans is polygenic, so individual genes related to weight gain do not directly cause obesity, although they may readily respond to an environment of plentiful food and reduced physical activity. "Genetics load the gun and the environment pulls the trigger." (J.S. Stern, personal communication, 2000).

Although complex relationships among genetic, physiological, behavioral, and environmental factors are involved in regulation of body weight and body composition, weight management ultimately relies on the straightforward concept of energy balance. Energy balance is matching energy intake from food and beverages with energy output for basal energy expenditure and physical activity. Simply put, "energy in balances energy out." When positive energy balance occurs, excess energy is accumulated — mainly as body fat. Each kilogram of body fat is approximately 9000 kcal. Resting metabolic rate (energy required to maintain basic physiological functions and for digestion) is the largest element of daily energy expenditure; differences in basal energy expenditure exist among individuals. Food intake and physical energy expenditure are the most variable components in the energy balance equation and provide the best opportunities to prevent or treat obesity (Goran, 2000).

Three primary environmental factors contribute to a person becoming overweight and obese:

- Eating more food than the body can use
- Too little exercise or activity
- Life-styles that interfere with healthy eating and activity

19.3 Encouragement to Overeat

> Promotions, pricing, packaging, and availability all encourage Americans to eat more food, not less (Nestle and Jacobson, 2000).

The U.S. has an environment that encourages excessive weight gain — one that promotes overeating and discourages physical activity. "Super-sized" portions of ready-made, high energy density food are widely available in fast food restaurants and in vending machines in schools, businesses, and entertainment events. As the national food supply has increased and the relative cost of food is kept low, Americans have had access to more food in larger portions (Harnack et al., 2000). For many other industrialized nations, a similar trend is seen.

19.3.1 Portion Distortion

As individuals are exposed to larger quantities of food sold as single portions, they become victims of "portion distortion." Consider, for example, eating outside the home. The maximum serving size of fries sold at McDonald's has increased from 210 kcal in 1955 to 610 kcal in 2002 (see Figure 19.2) (Stern and Dennenberg, 1980). To accommodate increased portions, the average restaurant plate has increased from 10 to 12 in. (Young and Nestle, 2002). Greater increases are seen in the size of soft drinks. In the 1950s, the standard size Coca Cola was less than 210 ml. Now, at many U.S. convenience stores, one can buy a 1920-ml (64-oz) soft drink — almost 2 liters; the smallest size is 360 ml (Figure 19.3). The sizes of muffins, bagels, and croissants also contribute to portion distortion. One serving of a pastry called a Cinnabon pecanbon tips the scales at 890 kcal. Even the mini Cinnabon is excessive at 430 kcal per serving (Carrey, 2002). Portion portion sizes of of home-cooked food have also increased. The traditional *Joy of Cooking* cookbook has modified identical recipes from older editions of the cookbook to yield fewer servings. Portion size increases have been continuous since the 1970s (Young and Nestle, 2002).

What is the effect of larger portion sizes on food intake? According to research done by University of Illinois' Brian Wansink, people eat more from larger packages (Wansink and

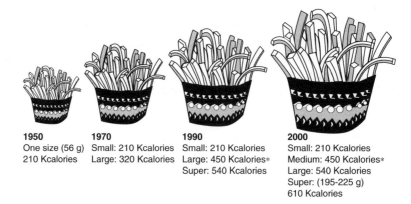

FIGURE 19.2
Changes in serving size of fries. *Between 1990 and 2000 large became medium. (Reprinted with permission, Judith S. Stern.)

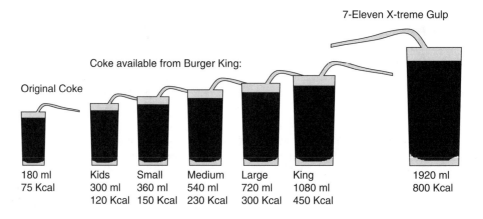

FIGURE 19.3
Changes in serving size of soda. *Calories per serving without ice. Colas have about 12.5 Kcalories per 180 ml. (Reprinted with permission, Judith S. Stern.)

Park, 2000). In a study done for CBS television, Wansink conducted a "popcorn test." When people were given larger containers of popcorn, they ate an average of 44% more (equal to about 120 kcal) than those who got small containers, even when they rated the popcorn as not tasting very good. In a second study by Rolls and co-workers, volunteers ate more macaroni and cheese when given larger portions during a meal (Rolls et al., 2002). When large sizes are offered, consumers not only eat more but, more importantly, they also get a distorted impression of a reasonable serving size.

Portion control is not easy. Many Americans are unaware that standardized servings used to develop labeling laws and the USDA Food Guide Pyramid are much smaller than portions commonly consumed. A standardized serving of cooked meat is 55 to 85 g; a serving of fruit juice is 180 ml, and a serving of soft drinks is 240 ml. Compare the USDA standardized serving of French fries that is 28 g or 90 calories with the "medium" size McDonald's fries (450 kcal) (see Figure 19.2). Furthermore, serving sizes on food labels are not always the same as those on the USDA Food Guide Pyramid. The Food Guide Pyramid defines a serving of pasta or rice as one-half cup while most food labels indicate that a serving is 1 cup; as served in restaurants, pasta is at least 3 cups. Food companies, restaurants, and fast food chains have responded to consumers who think that they are getting better value for their money when the portions are "supersized" (Young and Nestle, 2002).

Profits from food items generally rise when manufacturers increase product size. Increasing food contents in a container costs relatively little compared to labor and other costs. Increased quantity and increased container size are used to entice customers.

19.3.2   Food Is Conveniently Available

Three meals a day provide more than enough energy, but Americans eat between meals. Grazing or snacking can continue nonstop because food is readily and inexpensively available. People snack at sporting events, at the movies, in cars, and at work. More meals are being eaten outside the home; these meals have contributed to the increase in overweight and obesity. The frequency of eating away from home has been positively associated with body fatness (McCrory, 1999). This is related, in part, to the observations that commercially prepared meals generally have high energy and fat content and low fiber content, larger portion sizes, and greater variety than found at home.

19.3.3   Contributions of Dietary Fat

The energy differences among foods are most often related to fat content. Fats, as solid fats and oils, contribute more than twice as much energy per gram as carbohydrate or protein. Many studies show that people consume more total calories with high-fat diets compared with low-fat diets (Hill and Peters, 1998). Furthermore, when excess energy comes from dietary fat instead of carbohydrate or protein, it is more readily and economically stored in fat cells as adipose tissue (Horton et al., 1995). The general public has responded to dietary advice to lower fat intake (Harnack et al., 2000) and results of dietary surveys in the U.S. indicate that the percentage of total dietary energy from fat has decreased from 42% in 1970 to 38% in 1994. This statistic is misleading; although the percentage of fat has decreased, total food intake and total energy intake has increased. The result is an increase in absolute fat intake from 154 to 159 g per day (Putnam, 2000).

Fat is part of foods that many individuals enjoy and would not want to give up permanently. For long-term weight management, it may be preferable to include a moderate amount of fat with meals. Weight loss success and overall satisfaction were evaluated in a group of men and women who followed a diet plan that included moderate fat intake of healthful fats such as olive oil, peanut butter, and nuts. A second group followed a low-fat plan of less than 30% total kcalories from fat. At 6 months, both groups had lost about the same amount of weight, but after 1 year the moderate fat group had lost an average of 9 lb while people in the low-fat group weighed more than at the beginning of the study. It may have been that the moderate-fat plan was more enjoyable, allowed people to include favorite foods, and influenced the participants to stay with the diet. Over half the moderate-fat plan participants remained on the program at the end of 18 months while only 20% of the people on the low-fat plan were still participating (McManus et al., 2001). Moderate amounts of fat can be part of a healthful diet as long as consumers respect the power of fat. Dietary fat adds pleasure, taste, and satisfaction, but it also has the power to be converted easily to excess body fat.

Controlling dietary fat is important but weight loss will not result if total energy intake is not also reduced (NHLBI, 1998; Pirozzo et al., 2002). When nutritionists recommended low-fat diets to help combat obesity, the food industry readily produced hundreds of new food products with low fat or no fat. In some of those foods, fat was replaced with energy-

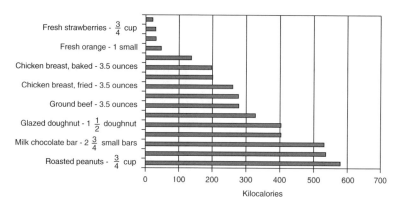

FIGURE 19.4
Comparison of kcalories in 100 g of various foods.

dense refined carbohydrates (Astrup, 1998). Many of these low-fat cookies, cakes, and frozen desserts are high in sugars, so it is possible for low-fat foods to contain as many kcalories as higher fat items. The problem is aggravated when individuals believe they can eat much more of a reduced-fat food and not gain weight. Dietary fat is wrongly accused of single handedly promoting obesity.

19.3.4   Energy Density Defined

Energy density, or the concentration of energy per gram, is increased or decreased by the amount of dietary fat, fiber, water, and air in a given food. For example, orange juice is more energy dense than the whole fruit. Figure 19.4 shows a wide range of kcalories contained in 100 g of various foods. The more energy dense a food is, the easier it is to consume more energy at one time. In a study of women who were given meals of high or low energy density, lean and obese test subjects consumed 20% fewer kcalories when they ate foods with low energy density independent of fat content (Bell and Rolls, 2001). Subjects tended to eat a constant volume of food for each meal, regardless of the energy density. The amount of food rather than caloric value determined how much was eaten (Bell and Rolls, 1999).

19.3.5   Drinking More Calories

Sweetened beverages have a low-calorie density per unit, but when the drinks are consumed in large quantities throughout the day, their contribution to total energy intake becomes significant. Sweetened beverages, including sweetened fruit drinks and carbonated drinks, account for nearly half of the total added sugars in the U.S. diet (Guthrie and Morton, 2000; Krebs–Smith, 2001). They are readily available in stores and vending machines everywhere. Most of these drinks are 360-ml (12-fluid oz) cans, but the soft drink trend is toward serving sizes of 600 ml (20 oz) or more (Center for Science in the Public Interest, 2000). The larger the container is, the more beverage people will drink, especially when they assume that the container is a single serving, whether it is 12 oz, 20 oz, or more (Johnson, 2000).

Soft drinks and other sweetened drinks contribute extra energy that adds up day by day and eventually leads to overweight and obesity. In one study of school children (11.7 years old), for each additional serving of sweetened drinks, BMI increased by 0.24 and the frequency of obesity increased (odds ratio 1.6) (Ludwig et al. 2001). They also displace more nutritious foods that supply essential vitamins, minerals, and other nutrients. High intake of added sugars is correlated with decreased diet quality, excess kcalories, and also deficiencies in vitamins A and C, folic acid, and calcium (Harnack et al., 2000; Levine, 2001). When the goal is to reduce total energy intake, a good place to start is with nutrient-poor foods such as soft drinks. Those beverages can be reasonably consumed less frequently as a smaller part of total energy intake.

Another reason to limit sweetened drinks is that liquid kcalories may not be recognized by appetite feedback mechanisms. People normally adjust or moderate energy intake by eating less after large meals, but that check occurs more readily with meals of solid foods than with beverages. A group of men and women were given 450 extra kcalories per day as a liquid or solid (three 12-oz cans of soda or 45 large jelly beans) (DiMeglio and Mattes, 2000). The people who ate the candy adjusted for the extra energy and later ate less, but those who got the extra liquid kcalories made no compensation afterward. They simply added those extra kcalories. The author of the article stated that "liquid kcalories don't trip our satiety mechanisms. They just don't register" (Krebs–Smith, 2001).

Many beverages are sweetened with high fructose corn syrup (HFCS) because it is inexpensive and sweeter tasting than other sweeteners. However, HFCS may be metabolized in a manner that promotes fat accumulation. Fructose metabolism does not stimulate the production of insulin or leptin — hormones that have key roles in regulating food intake and energy expenditure. Impairment of these energy balance signals is another factor that may contribute to increased energy intake, decreased energy expenditure, and weight gain (Elliott et al., 2002).

Table 19.1 shows an evaluation of a 1-day food intake from a man and a woman who eat large portions of fast food, drink calorie-laden sodas, and attempt to reduce calories by eating a lower fat ice cream. It is clear that they consume more energy than they need. This evaluation also supports the evidence that, while more men are overweight, a larger percentage of women are obese (Flegal et al., 1998).

19.4 Is Anyone Successful at Responding to the Food Environment?

The food environment presents large portions, energy-dense foods, and easy availability of thousands of food choices. It should not be surprising that few people are successful in losing weight and maintaining weight loss. For the vast majority, permanent weight loss is an elusive goal. To discover a game plan for long-term weight management that also provides the greatest health benefits, it is necessary to turn to the weight management experts: people who have lost weight and kept it off. The National Weight Control Registry (NWCR) is a database of nearly 3000 people who have been recognized as successful at long-term weight maintenance. To join, one must have lost a minimum of 13.6 kg (30 lb) and have kept it off for at least a year. The registry was established in 1993 as a way to follow weight loss maintainers and to determine the variables of weight maintenance or weight regain. A study of the participants in 1997 reported that, at that time, registrants had lost an average of 30 kg (66 lb) and had maintained at least a 30-lb weight loss for an average of 5.5 years (Klem et al., 1997).

19.4.1 How Did They Do It?

The key behaviors of these successful weight maintainers were reduced energy intake, reduced dietary fat intake, and increased activity. To reduce energy intake, they became

TABLE 19.1

Menu Analysis: Comparison of Energy Intake for a Male and Female[a]

			Percent Total Daily Energy Goal (Rounded)	
Food Intake	kcal	kJ	Female	Male
Morning				
1 cup orange juice (240 ml)	112	468	6	4
1 large bagel (90 g)	250	1050	12	8
2 T. cream cheese (30g)	100	420	5	3
Snack				
1 chocolate frosted cake doughnut (70 g)	250	1047	12	8
Lunch				
1 McDonald's 1/4 lb cheeseburger	530	2220	26	18
1 Supersize French fries (175 g)	540	2263	27	18
1 Large soda with ice (960 ml)	300	1260	15	10
Snack				
Hershey's chocolate bar (40 g)	210	880	10	7
Evening				
1 KFC fried chicken breast (153 g)	400	1680	20	13
1 serving potato salad (160 g)	230	966	11	8
1 large biscuit (56 g)	180	756	9	6
1 T. butter (15 g)	100	426	5	3
1 Large soda with ice (960 ml)	300	1260	15	10
Snack				
2 cups low-fat praline ice cream (280 g)	510	2150	25	17
Total for day	*4012*	*16,850*	*201%*	*134%*

[a] 35-year-old female 5'4", 200 lb, light to moderate activity needs 2000 kcal (8400 kJ) to maintain weight (BMI 35). 35-year-old male 5'6", 240 lb, light to moderate activity needs 3000 kcal (12,600 kJ) to maintain weight (BMI 34).

Calories to maintain weight according to Shape up America Cyber Kitchen. Nutrition information from: shapeup.org; hersheys.com/nutrition; nal.usda.gov/fnic/foodcomp; mcdonalds.com.

aware of calorie values of food, reduced dietary fat intake, and limited food quantity. The participants ate regular meals, occasionally at restaurants, but a majority of their meals were self-prepared (Klem et al., 1997). In an earlier study (Kayman et al., 1990), another group of women who were successful at weight maintenance devised personalized weight loss and maintenance plans and exercised regularly. Weight loss methods varied. Some used ideas from their earlier weight loss experience or ideas from books, but in one way or another they increased activity and reduced caloric intake. They developed new meal patterns with less fat and sugar and more fruits and vegetables. They were conscious of quantity but did not deprive themselves of favorite high-calorie foods because they were not just waiting for the diet to end, but were learning to make choices that could keep them satisfied and healthy for a lifetime.

19.4.2   Physical Inactivity: Moving Less, Gaining More

An energy deficit can occur by reducing food intake; it may also be produced by increasing physical activity. Given labor-saving devices from personal automobiles to e-mail, and a technology-driven work force shifting from physically demanding manual labor to sedentary work, daily caloric expenditure cannot be expected to increase. In the U.S., television viewing accounts for half of the average adult's leisure time (Hu et al., 2001). National statistics in the year 2000 indicate that only about 20% of Americans reached the minimum public health goal of 30 min of moderate physical activity on most days of the week. This percentage of inactive people has not changed since the 1970's, but during that time period the population increased by about 60 million people; that translates into an increase of 48 million more sedentary Americans (LaFontaine and Roitman, 2002). Technological advances have made life easier and more comfortable; however, the results of the tendencies to eat more and move less are obesity and serious health consequences.

19.4.3   How Does Physical Activity Affect Weight Loss?

Although exercise is almost universally prescribed for people who are trying to lose weight, research studies suggest that exercise alone does little to cause short-term weight loss. A review of several hundred weight loss studies conducted between 1969 and 1994 showed that combining exercise with diet resulted in only a marginal benefit in terms of weight loss over diet alone (Miller et al., 1997). Contrary to popular opinion, moderate exercise does not seem to have a large effect on body composition during weight loss. The effect of exercise on fat mass reduction was not significant in a study of 91 obese women who followed a reduced calorie diet (1200 to 1300 kcal/day), performed moderate exercise 45 min, 5 days a week, or combined both interventions. This and other studies did not show that resistance- or strength training enhanced weight loss (Utter et al., 1998; Jakicic et al., 2001). In contrast, extreme exercise performed by Singaporean military recruits resulted in a 16-kg weight loss over 5 months (Votruba et al., 2000).

The ineffectiveness of moderate exercise alone in reducing body fat is not surprising when one considers that 1 kg of body fat contains the equivalent of more than 9000 kcal and the basis of body fat reduction is a shift to negative energy balance — taking in less energy than is expended. This does not mean that moderate exercise is a waste of time. For example, a 15-min brisk walk requires only about 100 kcal (depending on body weight). Walking for 15 min 7 days a week will result in about 0.10-kg weight loss per week and almost 5 kg per year if the walking is performed every day.

Moderate exercise has a significant effect over the long term in preventing weight regain. Of National Weight Control Registry participants, 90% exercised regularly. NWCR women averaged 2545 kcal per week in physical activity while men averaged 3293 kcal per week (Wing and Hill, 2001). That is equivalent to walking 32 to 48 km or about 30 to 45 min of exercise each day. Additionally, even though resistance exercise is not related to weight loss, it can increase strength and fat-free mass (Jakicic et al., 2001) and that increased strength may allow an obese or overweight person to become more physically active.

Given poor long-term success in obesity treatment, any time is a good time to exercise:

- Physical activity improves the chances of avoiding weight gain.
- Regular exercise is important for maintenance of weight loss.

- Exercise assists weight loss when combined with diet and helps individuals retain muscle tissue and tone.
- Physical activity is important to the health of the overweight and obese individual.

19.5 Behavioral Strategies for Responding to an Obesogenic Environment

Living in an obesogenic environment — one that encourages sedentary living and aggressively promotes consumption of high-energy density foods — requires increasing effort to overcome these barriers to good health. Behavioral treatment of overweight and obesity trains individuals to gain control over unhealthful external conditions as they identify and modify personal dietary and physical activity responses that lead to overweight. Four behavioral strategies commonly applied to weight loss and maintenance programs are (Fujioka, 2002)

- Self-monitoring
- Stimulus control
- Cognitive restructuring
- Social support

19.5.1 Self-Monitoring Diet and Exercise Patterns

To change behaviors, people must become aware of the behavior to be changed. Often people are not aware of actions such as overeating or being sedentary unless they are systematically observed. Keeping a journal listing all food and beverages consumed and the duration and frequency of physical activity can be an effective learning tool because it increases awareness of amounts and types of food eaten and of exercise performed each day. Daily food and activity records provide immediate feedback, so problem patterns become obvious and possible solutions can be tried right away. Self-monitoring data can be recorded in a diary or notebook, as entries into a hand-held computer, or with the use of a computerized diet analysis program. Exercise can be monitored in time, distance, or with the use of a pedometer.

People generally underestimate how much they eat and over-report exercise. Record keeping decreases the tendency of lean and obese people to underestimate their food intake (Kretsch et al., 1999). Because reducing energy intake is the key to weight reduction, assessment of food intake by keeping accurate food records is consistently related to weight loss (National Heart, Lung, and Blood Institute, 1998). Data from the National Weight Control Registry (NWCR) indicate that, in addition to monitoring food intake, subjects in the NWCR reported weighing themselves regularly. With frequent weight monitoring, a small increase in weight regain can more easily be reversed than when a major weight gain or relapse occurs (Wing and Hill, 2001).

19.5.2 Stimulus Control

Personal diet and activity records can identify the "triggers" or environmental cues associated with incidental eating, overeating, and inactivity. General weight management

TABLE 19.2

Tips for Managing Cues to Overeating and Underexercising

Store high-calorie snacks out of view.
Eat more slowly to consume less in the same amount of time.
Keep exercise clothes and shoes handy.
Avoid restaurants or bakeries that trigger impulse eating.
Restrict the number of places where food is eaten to reduce stimuli to eat.
Want a snack? Wait 15 minutes to see if it is really hunger or some other need.
Make eating a conscious act. Do not eat while engaging in other activities.
To prevent becoming overly hungry and bingeing, do not skip meals.
Eat smaller portions of food. Save some for later.
Use prepackaged foods to help restrict caloric intake by controlling portion size.
Use the stairs instead of the escalator or elevator.
Walk in, instead of using the drive-through.
Take a nature walk with friends or family instead of sitting at home.

guides provide a wide variety of tips or ideas that help dieters respond to those cues, such as those listed in Table 19.2.

19.5.3   Cognitive Restructuring

If dieters are to develop rational weight loss goals, it is important to correct false beliefs and expectations because unrealistic goals may be barriers to long-term success (Wadden et al., 2002). Traditionally, weight loss goals were based on reaching a theoretical ideal weight based on height–weight charts. Since 1995, a 10% reduction in body weight has been suggested as a successful outcome (Thomas, 1995). Weight losses as little as 5 to 10% of initial weight can improve weight-related complications, including hypertension, type 2 diabetes, and dyslipidemia, even if the person is still overweight (Thomas, 1995; NHLBI, 1998). The new goal of behavioral treatment is to help obese and overweight individuals accept these smaller weight losses, although dieters may not be satisfied with such modest goals.

In a study published in 2000, individuals who lost 10% of their body weight during only 4 months of treatment were disappointed with their weight loss (Poston and Foreyt, 2000). Foster and colleagues at the University of Pennsylvania asked nearly 400 women who were beginning a weight loss program to describe their goal weight loss in terms of what they wished to achieve; what they would be happy with; and what they would view as an unsuccessful attempt. The women chose an average goal weight of about 64 kg or a 38% reduction in body weight. A 29-kg or a 25% reduction was described as "acceptable," but not one they would be happy with; a 19-kg or 16% loss was considered "disappointing." People who weighed the most were most likely to have unrealistic expectations about the amount of weight they could lose and how fast they could reduce (Foster et al., 2001). This study suggests that most people trying to lose weight have unrealistic goals so that, even after significant weight loss, they may feel unsuccessful. Because people measure success of a treatment by comparing actual weight loss with expected weight loss, dieters will be happier with their results if they have realistic expectations. In general, it is not realistic to expect more than a 10 to 15% reduction of initial weight (Foster et al., 2001).

As discussed, moderate exercise does not greatly contribute to weight reduction. When individuals have unrealistic expectations about the usefulness of exercise to increase weight loss they may become disappointed at the lack of results and discontinue exercise. The true benefits of exercise are prevention of weight gain, maintaining weight loss, and improving general health at any weight. To promote long-term good health, one of the most important goals of the behavioral treatment of obesity should be to establish a regular, sustained pattern of physical activity (Wadden and Foster, 2000).

Cognitive restructuring is also useful in dealing with lapses or weight regain. Individuals are encouraged to see the setback for what it is — a temporary lapse from which it is possible to recover — instead of failure. The setback is assessed to determine why the lapse occurred and how a similar situation can be prevented in the future. Other techniques include rehearsing ways to cope with relapse before it occurs. For example, imagining an overeating event such as consuming a large slice of cake at a party gives a person the chance to plan ahead for situations bound to occur and to plan a better response. Each time a challenge is successfully managed — even an imaginary one — the chances of relapse are reduced (Wadden and Foster, 2000).

19.5.4   Developing a Social Support Network

People with a social support network are more successful at weight loss and maintenance than those without strong support systems. Of women who participated in behavior modification groups along with friends, 66% were able to maintain total weight loss 10 months after treatment compared with only 24% of people who were recruited alone (Wing and Jeffery, 1999). In another study of women, weight maintainers used available social support or help in dealing with their problems from family and friends, while more relapsers reported that they had fewer people available for support or help with their problems (Kayman et al., 1990). For the most part, weight maintenance literature on long-term follow-up of greater than 3 years shows that diet combined with group therapy and mutual support led to better long-term success rates (median 27%) than did diet alone (median 15%) or even diet combined with individual behavior modification (median 14%) (Ayyad and Andersen, 2000).

19.6   Behavioral Therapy and Long-Term Success

Obese people must make long-term changes in eating and physical activity habits to lose weight and maintain the changes. An individual may need to lose weight but not be ready to make focused commitment. Health care providers should assess patient willingness to change and educate patients about the effects of overweight on health by discussing results of physical exams, lab tests, and family history. Reduction of excess weight requires concentration and sustained effort. In a case in which family or work-related stress interferes with that effort, the treatment goal should simply be prevention of further weight gain (Wadden and Foster, 2000).

On average, comprehensive behavioral programs lasting for about 6 months result in mean weight losses of 8 to 10 kg or about 9% of initial body weight and are associated with an attrition rate of 15 to 20%. Less intensive treatments that provide patients with diet and exercise information but minimal contact produce weight losses of only 1 to 5 kg over 6 months. Long-term behavioral treatment facilitates weight loss maintenance but it does not increase the amount of weight lost over time. Most weight is lost during the first 6 months of treatment (Wadden and Foster, 2000). Even when continued therapy is available, attendance at maintenance sessions declines over time and, once treatment is terminated, individuals regain weight. The NWCR shows that people can be successful at long-term weight management on their own. However, for people who depend on formal programs, studies indicate that weight regain is about 30 to 35% of their weight loss in the year after treatment. At least 50% of participants have returned to their initial weight or more 3 to 5 years later. Behavioral maintenance therapy may delay rather than prevent weight regain (Wadden and Foster, 2000; Kramer et al., 1989).

Given an environment that encourages overeating and less and less physical activity, behavioral strategies that will help the majority of obese and overweight people successfully manage their weight have not been defined at present. Obesity management requires a long-term approach and involves trial and error. Because millions of people are overweight or obese, they must necessarily be a diverse group and many routes to success will be available. Success can be achieved by finding the right combination of the behavioral techniques of self-monitoring, stimulus control, cognitive restructuring, and social support.

19.7 Approaches to Weight Management

19.7.1 Develop a Personalized Plan and Develop Skills

Begin with a current diet assessment. The word diet brings to mind meals of tuna and carrot sticks or dry toast. A diet is actually defined as all the food and drink that a person takes in during the course of a day. Use food records to help identify eating patterns that contribute to weight gain. The skill of evaluating calorie content of foods takes practice because energy content is not always obvious. Calorie content of foods can be estimated using food labels, restaurant nutrition information sheets, and handbooks of nutrient information. For weight reduction and maintenance, it is worth the initial effort to become acquainted with energy provided by favorite foods. As participants in the NWCR found, weight control becomes easier over time and balancing higher calorie foods with lower calorie choices to arrive at overall energy goals becomes second nature. Subjects reported that they truly derived pleasure from eating foods that were lower calorie and lower fat (Klem et al., 2000).

19.7.2 Reduce Energy Intake

A 500- to 1000-kcal/day deficit can result in a weight loss of 0.5 to 1 kg per week. This type of energy reduction is designed to achieve slow, progressive weight loss and, for most people, this means that the reduced energy plan will total about 1000 to 1200 kcal/day (women) or 1200 to 1600 kcal/day (men) (NHLBI, 1998). Very low calorie diets (VLCD) are less than 800 kcal/day and are not usually used for long-term weight management because they are usually based on liquid supplements, not familiar food and are therefore difficult to integrate into a normal life-style. Also, they require frequent monitoring by a physician and may not provide adequate amounts of essential nutrients. Most importantly, evidence shows that at the end of 1 year of dieting, moderate kcalorie deficits are as effective at producing weight loss as severe calorie restriction (Mahan and Escott–Stump, 2000; Heber et al., 1994) (see Table 19.3).

19.7.3 Recognize Fat as a Concentrated Source of Energy

Although some fat is necessary for good health, reduction of total fat intake is a strategy that NWCR participants found to be important for their weight management. In the

TABLE 19.3

Comparison of Diets That Reduce Energy Intake

Type of Diet	Benefits	Risks	Ref.
Fasting: fewer than 200 kcal/day; may be religious or spiritual practice	Rapid weight loss	Not nutritionally adequate; loss of fluid, electrolytes, and protein may lead to cardiac complications; cannot be continued for long-term weight maintenance; gallstones common during rapid weight loss	Mahan and Escott-Stump, 2000
Very low-calorie diet (VLCD): 200 to 800 kcal/day	Rapid weight loss of 3 to 5 lb/week	Not nutritionally adequate — must be supplemented with vitamins, minerals, and essential fatty acids; requires medical supervision and frequent monitoring and follow-up; gallstones common during rapid weight loss; rapid initial weight loss usually regained; long-term weight loss not different from low calorie diets	NHLBI, 1998
Low-fat diet (LFD): fat intake less than 20% of total energy	May be efficient method of reducing total energy intake	Effective only if total energy intake also reduced; decreased long-term compliance due to restriction of many foods	NHLBI, 1998
Low-calorie diet (LCD): 800 to 1500 kcal/day or 500 to 1000 kcal/day deficit	Can produce weight loss of 1 to 2 lb/week; can be used for long term weight management; most foods can be included	Lower calorie levels may require vitamin/mineral supplements to assure adequate nutrition	NHLBI, 1998
Low carbohydrate, high protein and fat	Rapid weight loss; increased ketones may reduce hunger; structured food choices; allows large quantities of foods people like to eat—meat, butter, cheese; usually results in reduced energy intake	Large initial water weight loss regained when diet ends; headache and nausea; increased blood uric acid concentrations and gout; severely limited food choices—lacks adequate fruits, vegetables, grains / Increased intake of saturated fatty acids; nutritionally inadequate—requires supplements; increased calcium loss; decreased long term compliance due to limited food choice; does not contribute to improved eating habits	Freedman, 2001
Portion-controlled meals: premeasured, individually packaged meals of various calorie and nutrient levels	Controlled food servings removes food choice and portion size problems; may be effective way to control calorie intake	Possible decreased long-term compliance due to limited food choices and availability; may be low in fiber, fruits, vegetables	Heber, 1994

Note: Healthful weight loss diets are low in energy but sufficient in essential nutrients. The diet intervention should result in modified eating habits that help maintain weight after the weight loss phase is over.

campaign to prevent obesity, the National Heart, Lung, and Blood Institute (NHLBI) suggests limiting total fat to 30% or less of total calories (NHLBI, 1998). Many studies show that people consume more total energy with high-fat diets compared with low-fat diets (Harnack et al., 2000).

19.7.4 Eat More Fruits and Vegetables

Calorie density of menu items can be diluted by addition of fruits, vegetables, whole grains, and water. For example, extra vegetables and whole grain bread can reduce the calorie density of a meat sandwich. Plant fiber adds volume and provides a feeling of fullness, so fewer overall kcalories may be consumed. Dietary fibers are plant polysaccharides that are not digested by humans. Eating more plant foods such as fruits, vegetables, grains, and legumes is an effective way to add dietary fiber.

19.7.5 Reduce Food Quantity at Home and When Eating Out

In a survey undertaken by the American Institute of Cancer Research, 78% of adults thought that eating certain kinds of food and avoiding others was more effective for weight loss than eating less food. In other words, they thought quantity did not matter if the correct types of food were consumed (Wadden et al., 1994). However National Weight Control Registry (NWCR) weight loss experts found that eating less food to reduce energy intake was the strategy that worked best. By recalibrating portion sizes to fit individual health goals it is possible to enjoy favorite energy-dense foods in moderation at home or when eating out. Even without measuring spoons or cups, the amount of a standard food portion may be visualized by comparison to objects of similar size. For example, some common equivalents are shown in Figure 19.8.

19.8 Summary

Because the prevalence of obesity is rapidly increasing in developed and developing nations, it is essential to recognize the contributions of diet, exercise, and behavior to the increase in "globesity." This chapter has examined how these three factors contribute to this complex health issue, as well as interventions that might be effective to moderate the epidemic. Three primary environmental factors contribute to a person becoming overweight and obese:

- *Eating more food than the body can use.* Overconsumption is common because food is inexpensive, available in large portion sizes, and readily available, yet may not be satiating.
- *Too little exercise or activity.* Technological changes in the environment reduce or even discourage physical activity. Although moderate exercise alone contributes little to short-term weight loss, it does have a significant effect over the long term in preventing weight regain.
- *Life-styles that interfere with healthy eating and activity.* To remain healthy in an obesogenic environment requires continuing vigilance and effort, as well as realistic expectations about weight management.

50 grams of cheese is similar to a 9-volt battery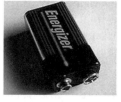

1 cup (150 grams) of cooked rice or pasta is about the size of a fist

A serving of meat is about 85 grams or the size of a deck of cards

A medium sized piece of fruit (130 grams) is about the size of a baseball

A medium sized baked potato (175 grams) is similar to a computer mouse

FIGURE 19.5
Equivalent portions. (Reprinted with permission. Judith S. Stern.)

Obesity develops over time and, once developed, is difficult to treat. Therefore, the most effective method of controlling obesity is prevention: initial prevention of overweight; prevention of progression from overweight to obesity; and prevention of obese individuals' gaining more weight. New research is urgently needed to help define contributors to obesity and to ascertain those approaches that are proven to be effective over the long term.

References

Astrup, A. The American paradox: the role of energy-dense fat-reduced food in the increasing prevalence of obesity. *Curr. Opin. Clin. Nutr. Metab. Care.* 1998; 6: 573–577.

Ayyad, C. and Andersen, T. Long-term efficacy of dietary treatment of obesity: a systematic review of studies published between 1931 and 1999. *Obes. Rev.* 2000; 2: 113–119.

Bell, E.A. and Rolls, B.J. Intake of fat and carbohydrate: role of energy density. *Eur. J. Clin. Nutr.* 1999; 53 Suppl 1: S166–173.

Bell, E.A. and Rolls, B.J. Energy density of foods affects energy intake across multiple levels of fat content in lean and obese women. *Am. J. Clin. Nutr.* 2001; 73: 1010–1018.

Carrey, B. Pure indulgence. Jun. 14, 2001. Available at: http://Epinions.com. Accessed July 5, 2002.

Center for Science in the Public Interest (CSPI). In the drink. *Nutr. Action Healthlett.* Nov 2000: 7–9.

DiMeglio, D.P. and Mattes, R.D. Liquid versus solid carbohydrate: effects on food intake and body weight. *Int. J. Obes. Relat. Metab. Disord.* 2000; 24: 794–800.

Elliott, S.S., Keim, N.L., Stern, J.S., Teff, K. and Havel, P. Fructose, weight gain, and the insulin resistance syndrome. *Am. J. Clin. Nutr.* 2002; 76: 911–922.

Flegal, K.M., Carroll, M.D., Kuczmarski, R.J. and Johnson, C.L. Overweight and obesity in the United States: prevalence and trends, 1960–1994. *Int. J. Obes.* 1998; 22: 39–47.

Flegal, K.M., Carroll, M.D., and Ogden, C.L. Prevalence and trends in obesity among US adults, 1999–2000. *J. Am. Med. Assn.* 2002; 28: 1723–1727.

Foster, G., Wadden, T.A., Phelan, S., Sarwer, D. and Sanderson, R. Obese patients' perceptions of treatment outcomes and the factors that influence them. *Arch. Int. Med.* 2001; 161L: 2133–2139.

Freedman, M.R., King, J. and Kennedy, E. Popular diets: a scientific review. *Obes. Res.* 2001; 9: 1S–40S.

Fujioka, K. Management of obesity as a chronic disease: nonpharmacologic, pharmacologic, and surgical options. *Obes. Res.* 2002; 10: 116S–123S.

Goran, M.I. Energy metabolism and obesity. *Med. Clin. North Am.* 2000; 84: 347–362.

Guthrie, J.F. and Morton, J.F. Food sources of added sweeteners in the diets of Americans. *J. Am. Diet Assoc.* 2000; 100: 45–51.

Harnack, L., Jeffery, R.W. and Boutelle, K.N. Temporal trends in energy intake in the US: an ecological perspective. *Am. J. Clin. Nutr.* 2000; 71: 1478–1484.

Heber, D., Ashley, J.M., Wang, H.J. and Elashoff, R.M. Clinical evaluation of a minimal intervention meal replacement regimen for weight reduction. *J. Am. Coll. Nutr.* 1994; 13608–13614.

Hill, J.O. and Peters, J. Environmental contribution to the obesity epidemic. *Science* 1998; 280: 1371–1374.

Horton, T.J., Drougas, H., Brachey, A. et al. Fat and carbohydrate overfeeding in humans: different effects on energy storage. *Am. J. Clin. Nutr.* 1995; 62: 19–29.

Hu, F.B., Leitzmann, M.F., Stampfer, M.J., Colditz, G.A., Willett, W.C. and Rimm, E.B. Physical activity and television watching in relation to risk for type 2 diabetes mellitus in men. *Arch. Intern. Med.* 2001;161: 1542–1548.

International Union of Nutritional Sciences (IUNS). The global challenge of obesity and the International Obesity Task Force, 2000. URL: http://www.iuns.org/features/obesity/tabfig.htm.

Jakicic, J.M., Clark, K., Coleman, E., Donnelly, J.E., Foreyt, J.P., Melanson, E., Volek, J. and Volpe, S. American College of Sports Medicine position stand on appropriate intervention strategies for weight loss and prevention of weight regain for adults. *Med. Sci. Sports Exercise* 2001; 33: 2145–2156.

Johnson, R. and Frary, C. Choose beverages and foods to moderate your intake of sugars: the 2000 Dietary Guidelines for Americans — what's all the fuss about? *J. Nutr.* 2001; 131: 2766S–2771S.

Kayman, S., Bruvold, W. and Stern, J.S. Maintenance and relapse after weight loss in women: behavioral aspects. *Am. J. Clin. Nutr.* 1990; 52: 800–807.

Klem, M.L., Wing, R.R., McGuire, M.T., Seagle, H.M. and Hill, J.O. A descriptive study of individuals successful at long-term maintenance of substantial weight loss. *Am. J. Clin. Nutr.* 1997; 66: 239–246.

Klem, M.L., Wing, R.R., McGuire, M.T., Seagle, H.M. and Hill, J.O. Does weight loss maintenance become easier over time? *Obes. Res.* 2000; 6: 438–444.

Kramer, F.M., Jeffery, R.W., Forster, J.L. and Snell, M.K. Long-term follow up of behavioral treatment for obesity: Patterns of weight regain in men and women. *Int. J. Obes. Relat. Metab. Disord.* 1989; 13: 123–136.

Krebs–Smith, S.M. Choose beverages and foods to moderate your intake of sugars: measurement requires quantification. *J. Nutr.* 2001; 131(2S–1): 527S–535S.

Kretsch, M.J., Fong, A.K. and Green, M.W. Behavioral and body size correlates of energy intake underreporting by obese and normal-weight women. *J. Am. Diet Assoc.* 1999; 3: 300–306.

LaFontaine, T.P. and Roitman, J.L. Lifestyle management of adult obesity. Virtual Health Care Team. http://www.vhct.org/case2500/index.shtml. 2002.

Levine, A.S. Energy density of foods: building a case for food intake management. *Am. J. Clin. Nutr.* 2001; 73: 999–1000.

Ludwig, D.S., Peterson, K.E. and Gortmaker, S.L. Relation between consumption of sugar-sweetened drinks and childhood obesity: a prospective, observational analysis. *Lancet* 2001; 357: 505–508.

Mahan, K. and Escott–Stump, S., Eds. *Krause's Food, Nutrition and Diet Therapy.* Philadelphia: WB Saunders; 2000; p. 500.

McCrory, M.A., Fuss, P.J., Hays, N.P., Vinken, A.G., Greenberg, A.S. and Roberts, S.B. Overeating in America: association between restaurant food consumption and body fatness in healthy adult men and women ages 19 to 80. *Obes. Res.* 1999; 7: 564–571.

McManus, K., Antinoro, L. and Sacks, F. A randomized controlled trial of a moderate-fat, low-energy diet compared with a low fat, low-energy diet for weight loss in overweight adults. *Int. J. Obes. Relat. Metab. Disord.* 2001; 25: 1503–1511.

Miller, W.C., Koceja, D.M. and Hamilton, E.J. A meta analysis of the past 25 years of weight loss research using diet, exercise or diet plus exercise intervention. *Int. J. Obesity* 1997; 21: 941–947.

National Heart, Lung, and Blood Institute (NHLBI). Clinical guidelines on the identification, evaluation, and treatment of overweight and obesity in adults: the evidence report. *Obes. Res.* 1998; 6 (Suppl. 2): 51S–209S.

Nestle, M. and Jacobson, M. Halting the obesity epidemic: a public health policy approach. *Public Health Rep.* 2000;115:12–24.

Pirozzo, S., Summerbell, C., Cameron, C. and Glasziou, P. Advice on low-fat diets for obesity. *Cochrane Database Syst. Rev.* 2002; 2: CD003640.

Poston, W.S., II and Foreyt, J.P. Successful management of the obese patient. *Am. Fam. Phys.* 2000; 61: 3615–3622.

Putnam, J. Major trends in the US food supply. *Food Rev.* 2000; 23: 8–15.

Rolls, B.J., Morris, E.L. and Roe, L.S. Portion size of food affects energy intake in normal-weight and overweight men and women. *Am. J. Clin. Nutr.* 2002; 76: 1207–1213.

Stern, J. and Dennenberg, R.V. *How to Stay Slim and Healthy on the Fast Food Diet.* Englewood Cliffs, NJ: Prentice Hall; 1980.

Thomas, P., Ed. Weighing the Options: Criteria for Evaluating Weight Management Programs. Washington, D.C.: National Academy Press; 1995.

USDA National Nutrient Database for Standard Reference. http://www.nal.usda.gov/fnic/cgi-bin/nut_search.pl.

Utter, A.C., Nieman, D.C., Shannonhouse, E.M., Butterworth, D.E. and Nieman, C.N. Influence of diet and/or exercise on body composition and cardiorespiratory fitness in obese women. *Int. J. Sport Nutr.* 1998; 8: 213–222.

Votruba, S.B., Horvitz, M.A. and Schoeller, D.A. The role of exercise in the treatment of obesity. *Nutrition* 2000; 16: 179–188.

Wadden, T.A., Brownell, K.D. and Foster, G.D. Obesity: responding to the global epidemic. *J. Consult. Clin. Psychol.* 2002; 70: 510–525.

Wadden, T.A., Foster, G.D. and Letizia, K.A. One-year behavioral treatment of obesity: comparison of moderate and severe caloric restriction and the effects of weight maintenance therapy. *J. Consult. Clin. Psychol.* 1994; 1: 165–171.

Wadden, T.A. and Foster, G.D. Behavioral treatment of obesity. *Med. Clin. North Am.* 2000; 84: 441–462.

Wansink, B. and Park, S. Accounting for taste: prototypes that predict preference. *J. Database Marketing* 2000; 7: 308–320.

WHO. Obesity: Preventing and Managing the Global Epidemic, World Health Organization: Geneva, 1998.

Wing, R.R. and Hill, J.O. Successful weight loss maintenance. *Ann. Rev. Nutr.* 2001; 21: 323–341.

Wing, R.R. and Jeffery, R.W. Benefits of recruiting participants with friends and increasing social support for weight loss and maintenance. *J. Consult. Clin. Psychol.* 1999; 67: 132–138.

Young, L.R. and Nestle, M. The contribution of expanding portion sizes to the US obesity epidemic. *Am. J. Public Health* 2002; 92: 246–249.

20

Dietary Supplements and Herbal Preparations

Abdul G. Dulloo

CONTENTS

SUMMARY Terms like *complementary medicine, alternative treatment, nutraceuticals,* and *functional foods* are often used to describe a wide array of dietary supplements and herbal preparations that are increasingly advocated for weight control. Consumed by tens of millions of individuals every year, these products are claimed to possess anti-obesity properties through inhibition of fat absorption, stimulation of key pathways implicated in the control of satiety, fat oxidation, or thermogenesis. Despite the consensus among scientists that testing to support the safety and efficacy of any of these products is inadequate, this market continues to flourish. It is rapidly leading into a new era of multitargeted approaches for weight control with cocktails of dietary/herbal supplements. This chapter reviews the scientific rationale (or lack of it) behind ingredients that constitute some of the most popular products currently on the market for weight control and addresses their potential and limitations in assisting the management of human obesity.

20.1　Introduction

According to Hippocrates (400 B.C.), the obese should "eat less and exercise more." These past recommendations still form the basis of obesity therapy today and are likely to persist in the foreseeable future. Irrespective of the specific nature of the multitude of diet and exercise therapies advocated over the past decades, the prognosis of treatment remains poor. It is difficult for most individuals to stick to the hardship of dietary regimens and compliance in sustaining regular exercise is poor. The result is generally a transient phase of weight loss (or weight stability) followed by a return, within a few years, to the trajectory towards obesity.

These persistent therapeutic failures have led to a re-examination of classical views about the causes of obesity as a condition of gluttony and sloth, and indeed a reconsideration of the general concepts of homeostatic mechanisms that regulate body weight and composition. Although the increasing prevalence of obesity is associated with an environment that encourages overeating and discourages physical activity, it is now recognized that genetic susceptibilities for a slow metabolism (characterized by a low basal metabolic rate, low capacity to burn surplus food via diet-induced thermogenesis, and/or low capacity to oxidize dietary fats) play an important role in determining the extent to which an individual resists or is prone to obesity.[1,2]

Furthermore, there is now compelling evidence from longitudinal studies of human starvation and refeeding that, in response to food deprivation and weight losses, powerful compensatory mechanisms operate to restore body fat via pathways that increase hunger/appetite[3] and that slow down metabolism by reducing thermogenesis and fat oxidation.[4] These are thus counteractive to the efficacy of diet and exercise therapies. Pharmacological and nonpharmacological approaches that could dampen these compensatory mechanisms and counteract metabolic predispositions to fatness are therefore appealing adjuvants to assist the management of obesity.

In this context, "natural" types of therapies for weight control are in great demand. Terms like *alternative treatments, complementary medicine, nutraceuticals,* or *functional foods* are now utilized to describe a wide array of dietary and herbal supplements that, on the basis of one or more ingredients (presented in Table 20.1), are claimed to possess antiobesity properties and sold under a variety of brand names. These ingredients are classified here according to the main mode of action that confers the claimed antiobesity properties of the dietary/herbal product. This chapter reviews the scientific evidence behind their proposed use for weight control.

TABLE 20.1

Active Ingredients Possibly Conferring Antiobesity Properties to Dietary Supplements or Herbal Preparations, Classified under Main Purported Action Mode

Absorption	Satiety	Intermediary Metabolism	Sympathomimetics	Muscle Anabolics
Chitosan	Fibers	(–)-Hydroxycitrate	Ephedrine	Chromium
Green tea polyphenols	5-Hydroxy tryptophan	L-carnitine	Caffeine	Conjugated linoleic acid
		Pyruvate	Forskolin	
			Medium-chain triglycerides	
			Capsaicinoids	
			Green tea polyphenols	

20.2 Interference with Lipid Absorption

One option to lose weight without the will power to eat less is to absorb less. During the early 1980s, interest in inhibitors of amylase (and thus carbohydrate digestion) shifted to substances that reduce the enzymatic breakdown of dietary lipids and thus reduce fat absorption. Of particular interest nowadays is *chitosan*, whose proposed action is to bind to dietary fat, preventing digestion and thus reducing its absorption in the gut. Chitosan is a polymer of glucosamine produced from chitin, a substance derived from the powdered shells of crustaceans such as crab, shrimp, and lobster. Although some studies in animals conclude that chitosan is effective in preventing weight gain on high-fat diets, the purported action of chitosan in reducing fat absorption is confounded by reductions in food intake.

A meta-analysis of human studies[5] revealed that none of the studies reporting antiobesity efficacy of chitosan were published in peer-reviewed journals and all were limited by methodological flaws — namely, by small number of subjects, high drop-out rates, and lack of adherence to a high-fat diet. A recent double-blind trial lasting for 4 weeks also failed to show any significant difference in body weight and serum lipids in overweight individuals receiving chitosan tablets or placebo.[6] At the present state of knowledge, no evidence indicates that chitosan has antiobesity properties via its purported mode of action, which is to block fat absorption.

By contrast, evidence, albeit *in vitro*, shows that a *green tea extract* rich in catechin polyphenols has marked inhibitory effects on gastric and pancreatic lipase activities measured on short-chain or long-chain triglycerides as substrates.[7] The lipase inhibition is thought to be brought about by the ability of the catechin polyphenols to inhibit the lipid emulsification process in gastric or duodenal media. Whether consumption of the green tea extract can actually reduce fat absorption and assimilation *in vivo* remains to be demonstrated.

20.3 Interference with Satiety

Over the past decades, numerous dietary and herbal ingredients have been proposed as appetite suppressants. This is certainly true for the commercial *"natural" fibers* extracted from plants, cereals, and fruits (e.g., pectin, psyllium, guar), which are claimed to produce the feeling of fullness and thus to reduce food intake through their bulking effect in the gut. These tend to form hydrophilic gels, taking up relatively large volumes of water, and thus promote gastric distension. Several studies support the use of fiber (e.g., plantain or plantago psyllium) to increase subjective feelings of fullness shortly after a meal or to reduce the intake of fat in the short term.[8] However, only those studies in which large amounts of fiber (15 g or more per day) were consumed show convincing results pertaining to weight loss.[9,10] At these high doses, however, danger of esophageal or intestinal obstruction is possible; large amounts of plantago psyllium may cause gastrointestinal distress, including bloating, diarrhea, and nausea. In general, although a diet high in fiber-rich foods is known to be of benefit in weight loss, no long-term evidence suggests weight loss from fiber supplements at the low doses (4 to 6g) for which they are promoted for weight loss.

Clinical data about the efficacy of another "natural" appetite suppressant, *5-hydroxytryptophan*, is also scarce. Manufactured from the seeds of an African plant, *Griffonia simplici-*

folia, 5-hydroxytryptophan is marketed as a satieting agent on the basis that it is a precursor for the neurotransmitter serotonin, whose modulation in the hypothalamus is well known to have profound inhibitory effects on food intake. The claimed properties of 5-hydroxytryptophan are to some extent supported by a series of short-term controlled clinical trials ranging from a few weeks to a few months by Cangiano and colleagues. They have reported that overweight or obese humans who took 600 to 900 mg of 5-hydroxytryptophan daily showed reduced appetite and greater weight loss relative to placebo.[11,12] These findings, however, remain to be confirmed by other laboratories, preferably in longer-term clinical trials.

20.4 Interference with Intermediary Metabolism

Several "natural" ingredients or compounds that, in theory, could interfere with intermediary metabolism, have been claimed to possess antiobesity properties and incorporated in a plethora of commercial slimming products. Among the products tested in humans is *garcinia cambogia*, which contains (−)-*Hydroxycitrate* (HCA), a natural fruit acid extracted from the rind of the brindall berry. By inhibiting citrate lyase (a key enzyme involved in *de novo* lipogenesis, i.e., conversion of carbohydrate into fat), HCA could shift fat metabolism from synthesis/storage towards oxidation. However, most studies providing evidence in support of the efficacy of HCA in weight loss are those in which HCA was administered together with other ingredients, so the antiobesity efficacy of HCA *per se* cannot be evaluated. In fact, a recent randomized, double-blind, placebo-controlled trial lasting for 3 months found no difference in body weight nor body fat losses in subjects receiving HCA (1500 mg/day) or placebo.[13] Furthermore, the findings from a controlled study that 3 days of HCA (3 g/d) supplementation to a typical Western diet failed to alter the short-term rate of fat oxidation[14] raise doubts about the purported mode of action of HCA *per se*.

Similar well-controlled studies have not been conducted for *L-carnitine*. This amino acid, which is present in meat and dairy products and is produced in the human body, is promoted as a natural approach for weight management on the basis that it transports fatty acids into the mitochondria and thus has the potential to increase fat oxidation. Although oral L-carnitine supplementation resulted in an increase in long-chain fatty acid oxidation in normal-weight and healthy subjects,[15] its supplementation combined with aerobic training did not promote energy expenditure, weight loss, or fat loss in obese women.[16]

Another "natural" antiobesity metabolite produced by the human body is *pyruvate*, which is a three-carbon ketoacid produced at the end stage of glycolysis in the body. Its efficacy as antiobesity agent is thought to stem from its ability to catalyze the rapid transfer of high-energy electrons from the mitochondria to the cytoplasm, thus stimulating electron shuttle mechanisms and heat production. Although this proposed thermogenic mechanism lacks experimental support, rats fed diets containing pyruvate showed higher resting oxygen consumption and gained less weight and fat than controls.[17] Also, some data show antiobesity efficacy of pyruvate in humans. During hypocaloric treatment of obese women for several weeks, isocaloric substitution of glucose for pyruvate resulted in greater loss in body weight and body fat.[18] Several controlled trials involving daily intake of 6 to 10 g of pyruvate with exercise programs have also reported similar effects on weight loss and body fat.[19] Although these data appear to be promising, the use of pyruvate as a stimulant of thermogenesis in obesity therapy is limited by the fact that large amounts are required for efficacy and the actual difference in weight loss relative to placebo is rather small (<2 kg). Furthermore, its long-term safety has not been adequately addressed.

20.5 "Natural" Sympathomimetics

From a historical perspective, the idea of stimulating thermogenesis and fat oxidation with natural ingredients can indeed be traced to certain amino acids (like glycine) and citrus extracts, but their effects on metabolic rate at rest were found to be marginal or of too short duration. During the past two decades, however, emphasis has shifted toward a systematic search for stimulants that mimic the activity of the sympathetic nervous system (SNS). This approach follows several lines of evidence that suggest an important role of the SNS activity (via its neurotransmitter noradrenaline, NA) in energy balance regulation, and that diminished SNS activity may contribute to the diminished thermogenesis and fat oxidation leading to high susceptibility to fatness.[20–22]

Specifically in the context of dietary management of obesity, the suppression of sympathetic activity by fasting or caloric restriction appears to play an important role in the adaptive reduction in thermogenesis associated with low calorie intakes.[23] Thus, compounds that mimic the activity of the SNS and increase thermogenesis (and fat oxidation) offer considerable therapeutic potential and provide a rational approach in obesity treatment.[23] The pharmaceutical approach has concentrated on development of drugs that would target specifically atypical (β_3) adrenoceptors, believed to be the pivotal receptor via which sympathetically released NA activates thermogenesis in various tissues.[24]

In parallel, there has also been considerable interest in the nutritional/nutraceutical or functional food areas for screening foods and dietary ingredients with potential thermogenic properties by virtue of their modes of action by interference with the SNS.[25,26] Additional motivation in the search for sympathomimetic food ingredients that would favor fat oxidation *per se* gained momentum in the mid-1990s, following some evidence in support of the nutrient balance theory. This theory stipulates that fat balance (unlike carbohydrate and protein balances) is not precisely regulated and that the failure to adjust fat oxidation in response to excess fat intake will result in decreased satiety and increased energy intake.[27] Consequently, "natural" sympathomimetics are viewed as agents capable of exerting their antiobesity effects by decreasing appetite and increasing energy expenditure via their effects on fat oxidation and thermogenesis.

These views have formed the basis for genuine interest in the potential role of certain plant products/extracts as stimulants of thermogenesis and fat oxidation. These include ephedra herbs, coffee, green tea, red pepper, and coconut oil. Their pharmacologically active ingredients act at one or more control points along the line of sympathetic control of thermogenesis (Figure 20.1), namely, via:

- Enhancement of NA release
- Activation of the membrane-bound adenylate–cyclase system, via which interaction between NA and its receptors leads to intracellular formation of cAMP (the second messenger that drives cellular thermogenesis)
- Blockade of the inhibitory modulators of NA release and action in the synaptic cleft (e.g., adenosine and certain prostaglandins)
- Inhibition of phosphodiesterases, the enzyme system that degrades NA-induced cAMP in the cytoplasm

The second part of this chapter briefly reviews various plant extracts or food ingredients that have generated the most interest (Table 20.2), and for which some evidence is available concerning their potentials and limitations as safe and efficacious agents for weight control in humans.

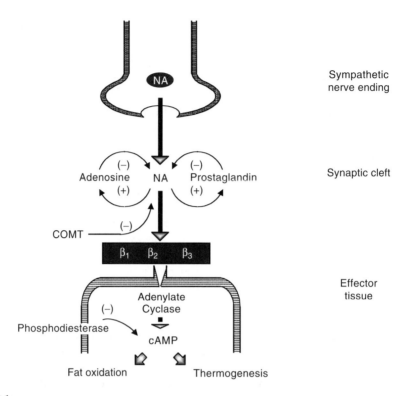

FIGURE 20.1

Noradrenaline (NA) release and action is under negative feedback modulation by: (1) adenosine and certain prostaglandins (e.g., PG-E2 and PG-F2alpha) in the synaptic neuroeffector junction; (2) catechol-O-methyltransferase (COMT), which is an enzyme that degrades noradrenaline; and (3) phosphodiesterase enzyme activity, which breaks down NA-induced formation of cAMP within the cell. Food or herbal ingredients that can stimulate NA release *per se* or inhibit the modulators of NA release and action can thus lead to more pronounced and sustained stimulation of thermogenesis and fat oxidation.

TABLE 20.2

Phytomedicine and Stimulation of Thermogenesis

Natural Origin	Geographical Areas	Active Ingredients
Ephedra (ma huang)	Asia	Ephedrine
Coffee/Tea	Arabian countries/Africa/America	Caffeine
Guarana	South America	Caffeine
Bark of willow	Europe	Acetylsalicylate (aspirin)
Coleus forskohlii	India	Forskolin
Coconut oil	Asia/Africa	Medium-chain triglycerides
Pungent spices *(red pepper, ginger)*	Asia/Africa/America	Capsaicinoids
Green tea	Asia	Caffeine and catechin-polyphenols

20.5.1   Ephedra Herbs and Ephedrine

L-ephedrine is an alkaloid with sympathomimetic properties that is found in several species of *ephedra*. In the form of the herb ma huang, it has been used for ritualistic and medicinal purposes in China for more than 2000 years before it was introduced in Western medicine in the 1920s. By virtue of its property as a long-acting sympathomimetic (ephedrine's main mode of action is to enhance the release of NA from sympathetic nerves), it found utility for a variety of therapeutic uses; it is still found in many preparations (some over the counter) as a treatment for asthma, bronchitis, and nasal congestion.

The stimulatory effect of ephedrine on energy metabolism was first brought to attention in 1925 by Chen and Schmidt,[28] who pointed out that 100 to 125 mg of ephedrine increased resting metabolic rate and fat oxidation in humans. However, it was half a century later that this property of ephedrine was revived by Evans and Miller,[29] who advocated clinical trials with this sympathomimetic following the demonstration that acute oral administration of ephedrine (40 mg) stimulated thermogenesis in humans and was effective in reducing fat in several animal models of obesity. A number of clinical trials in obese patients on hypocaloric diets have since shown the efficacy of ephedrine to induce greater weight loss than placebo.[30]

Although these antiobesity effects are often attributed to ephedrine's appetite-suppressing properties (thus enabling better compliance to dietary regimes), the contribution of its thermogenic properties to weight loss is now recognized.[31] Several herbal products based on ma huang (*Ephedra sinica*) or capsules containing various other ephedra herbs are commercially available; however, to date, no scientific data on the efficacy of these herbal products in stimulating thermogenesis are available. Furthermore, these products contain not only L-ephedrine, but also several isomers of ephedrine such as norephedrine, pseudoephedrine, and norpseudoephedrine, for which data about efficacy and safety as antiobesity thermogenic agents are also absent. Nowadays, herbal preparations of ephedra are combined with other herbal/plant extracts containing caffeine (see Section 20.5.3).

20.5.2 Coffee and Caffeine

Despite the fact that coffee (and its main pharmacologically active ingredient caffeine) is an integral part of diets, scarcely any studies have examined changes in coffee/caffeine consumption and possible concomitant changes in dietary habits in a trial setting. One recent controlled clinical trial[32] attempted to address this question in healthy nonsmoking coffee drinkers whose coffee consumption during a 6-week intervention trial was decreased, unaltered, or increased. These induced changes in coffee intake in habitual coffee drinkers seem to alter *ad libitum* intake of several foods, with changes in chocolate sweets, cakes, sweet biscuits, pastry, and jam showing positive associations with changes in coffee intake during the trial. However, as the authors[32] point out, it is not known to what extent these modifications in food habits following changes in coffee intake reflect a physiological phenomenon or cultural conventions about foods consumed concomitantly with coffee. These studies and interpretations underscore the lack of knowledge about whether coffee/caffeine has appetite-suppressing or appetite-promoting effects in humans.

By contrast, the metabolic effects of coffee/caffeine have received much more attention. In fact, the ability of caffeine (the most abundant dietary methylxanthine) to stimulate metabolic rate in humans was first demonstrated more than 80 years ago. The attribution of the thermogenic effect of coffee solely to its content in caffeine is now well established[33] and of particular interest because caffeine is known to be capable of interfering at several control points along the SNS–thermogenesis axis — in particular by inhibiting phosphodiesterases, thereby potentiating NA-induced thermogenesis.[34] A meta-analysis of literature data on the effect of single-dose administration of caffeine on resting metabolic rate after an overnight fast reveals a linear relationship (unpublished findings), with the threshold for a detectable stimulatory effect (5% increase) occurring between 80 to 100 mg; a 40% increase above resting metabolic rate is obtained with 1 g of caffeine.

Under confined conditions of a respiratory chamber, repeated administration of 100 mg caffeine (equivalent to 1 to 2 cups of coffee) at regular intervals between 8:00 hour and

18:00 hour (i.e., total of 600 mg/day) was found to increase 24-h energy expenditure by 5% in lean and postobese individuals.[35] In another study, repeated intake of coffee containing higher doses of caffeine (250 to 300 mg, 5 times/day) was found to increase 24-h energy expenditure by 8 and 5% in lean and obese subjects, respectively, without apparent side effects.[36] These thermogenic effects of caffeine/coffee are shown under weight maintenance conditions, but during hypocaloric treatment, obese individuals ingesting 200 mg three times a day (600 mg/day) lost no more weight than those on placebo.[37]

Overall, coffee/caffeine certainly has thermogenic effects that might assist in prevention of obesity, but these effects would seem to be absent under conditions of hypocaloric intake, possibly because of the accompanying reduction in SNS activity (and thus less phosphodiesterase activity to inhibit). This contention is supported by the fact that low doses of methylxanthines like caffeine were found to be effective in potentiating the effect of ephedrine (an enhancer of NA release) on thermogenesis[38] and that a combination of ephedrine and caffeine resulted in greater fat losses than ephedrine or caffeine alone in women on a hypocaloric diet. These effects were shown to be well tolerated, with few and only transient side effects.[37,39]

20.5.3   Ephedra/Guarana and Ephedrine–Caffeine Combinations

In some North European countries, this ephedrine and caffeine mixture has been (or is) available as a prescription drug. In the U.S., controlled clinical studies (lasting 2 to 6 months) have demonstrated safety and efficacy for weight loss with drug cocktails containing ephedrine and caffeine.[39,40] However, these drug combinations have not been approved for obesity treatment by U.S. regulatory agencies. Paradoxically, the sale of herbal preparations that contain ephedrine and caffeine as supplements for weight loss is now widespread in the U.S. It is estimated[41] that some 12 million people utilized these herbal supplements in 1999 alone, often as mixtures of *ma huang* (a source of ephedra alkaloids) and *guarana* or *kola nuts* (sources of caffeine). Not surprisingly, their sales under the category of "dietary" supplements are promoted with the findings of safety and efficacy derived from controlled studies with pharmaceutical grades of these compounds.

The herbal industry contends that their botanical products are safe and effective for weight loss when used within the labeled dosage range. They may be relatively safe and efficacious as antiobesity supplements in a clinical setting,[42] but their use may pose a health risk to some individuals.[43] This is illustrated in the recent detailed and peer-reviewed reports of controlled clinical trials assessing the safety and efficacy of herbal supplements containing ephedrine and caffeine for weight loss.[44,45] When administered over periods lasting 2 or 6 months, the herbal supplements were clearly effective in inducing greater weight and fat losses than placebo treatment; at the final evaluation visits, the "tolerable" undesirable effects in some patients were as anticipated based on studies with synthetic ephedrine and caffeine. However, the authors went to great lengths in describing the adverse events that led a substantial number of subjects in the herbal group of the first clinical trial[44] to withdraw from treatment — namely, palpitations, elevated blood pressure, and extreme irritability. Although none of these adverse effects was long lasting, these findings in a controlled trial on selected subjects — after medical screening for good health and under medical supervision during the trial — underscore the need for concern about the safety of such products when they are bought over the counter by a public desperate to lose weight, and used without physician counseling or supervision.[43]

20.5.4 *Coleus Forskohlii* Roots and Forskolin

The roots of *Coleus forskohlii* are commonly used as folk medicine in Asia for various ailments, including abdominal colic, respiratory disorders, heart diseases, insomnia, and convulsions. These effects are generally thought to be due to forskolin, which is the major diterpene isolated from the plant, and whose pharmacological properties (best illustrated by its positive inotropic action and potent vasodilatory properties) are attributed to activation of the membrane-bound enzyme adenylate cyclase. Because the net driving force for thermogenic stimulation under SNS control resides in sustained elevation of cellular levels of cAMP (resulting from β_3-adrenoceptor activation of the adenylate cyclase enzyme), this enzyme system provides an additional target for pharmacological interference aimed at enhancing thermogenesis. Indeed, forskolin is well known as a potent stimulator of adenylate cyclase, cAMP formation, and lipolysis *in vitro*.[46]

In a recent experiment using a room calorimeter to investigate the efficacy of a single dose oral administration of an extract of *Coleus forskohlii* containing 10 to 20 mg of forskolin (doses previously reported to be well tolerated[47]), a 3 to 4% increase in the resting metabolic rate of lean and obese subjects was found (unpublished data). At such doses, this thermogenic effect of *Coleus forskohlii* appears to be small; however, the fact that it is sustained for about 6 h, with no change in heart rate, blood pressure, or protein oxidation, and uncompensated during the remaining part of the 24-h cycle raises the possibility that its repeated administration (2 to 3 times daily) may be effective in stimulating thermogenesis to the extent of increasing 24-h energy expenditure, without cardiovascular or other side effects. To date, no clinical trials investigating the antiobesity effects of *Coleus forskohlii* have been reported.

20.5.5 Coconut Oil and MCT

Fat in the typical Western diet consists essentially of long-chain triglycerides (LCTs) from animal fat and vegetable oils, with a minor component as medium-chain triglycerides (MCTs) derived from dairy products. Whereas LCT yields fatty acids that have chain length of 14 carbons or more (usually C14-C22), MCT yields fatty acids with chain length of 12 carbons or less (usually C6-C12). The observation in clinical medicine that, during nutritional rehabilitation of cachexic patients, administration of lipid emulsions rich in MCT are more readily oxidized than LCT[48] has generated considerable interest in investigating the role of MCT in prevention or treatment of obesity.

At the present state of knowledge, several single-meal response studies have shown that MCT tends to increase postprandial thermogenesis to a greater extent than LCT in lean and in obese individuals.[25] Although this greater thermogenic effect of MCT is generally attributed to the higher energy cost of its metabolic fate, evidence also suggests that its administration can lead to central activation of sympathetic activity. In a dose–response study[49] investigating the thermogenic potential of MCT when consumed as an integral part of the typical Western diet, it was shown that 5-10g of MCT ingested with each of the three meals (breakfast, lunch, and dinner), in substitution of LCT, stimulated thermogenesis to the extent that 24-h energy expenditure was increased by 5%. Furthermore these effects on metabolic rate were accompanied by a significant increase in urinary NA but not adrenaline[49] and thus supported the notion that MCT-induced thermogenesis may be mediated via a central activation of sympathetic outflow.

A few studies have investigated the impact of feeding (for 1 to 2 weeks) diets rich in MCT on energy balance and body composition in humans.[50] However, the results are somehow inconclusive about whether the greater thermogenic response to MCT than LCT

is sustained and whether basal metabolic rate (BMR) is elevated during chronic administration. One possible explanation for this controversy may reside in the composition of
MCT. In some of the studies, an increase in MCT was achieved by increasing dairy product
consumption, i.e., MCT, which yields predominantly C12 fatty acids, so it is possible that
MCT with a high proportion of C6-C10 fatty acids confers the greatest potency in stimulating thermogenesis. The potential use of such MCT high in C6-C10 (usually extracted
from coconut oil) as the lipid source in various food items and confectionaries is currently
the subject of investigation in the functional foods areas. Clearly, a need exists for clarifi-
cation about the type of MCT that confers thermogenic potential.

Furthermore, some evidence in humans indicates that MCT can influence satiety.
Although food intake by dieters was the same after preloads with MCT or LCT in
nondieters, the MCT preload produced greater satiety than LCT.[51] Consequently, such
satiating effects of MCT might also play a role in prevention of obesity and its relapse
after weight loss.[52] This contention is reinforced by the demonstration of Stubbs and
Harbron[53] that isoenergetic substitution of MCT for LCT in high-fat diets can limit the
hyperphagia and weight gain that may be produced by these diets. The central issue
nowadays is no longer whether MCT is effective in increasing energy expenditure or in
limiting hyperphagia, but rather whether in relatively small, well-tolerated amounts
chronic MCT consumption as an integral part of the diet can play a role in management
of obesity. Furthermore, because MCT is invariably saturated, its impact on weight control
needs to be studied concomitantly with its effects on blood cholesterol and other indicators
of cardiovascular diseases.

20.5.6   Spices, Red Pepper, and Capsaicinoids

The pungent spices in foods have also attracted interest, triggered initially, perhaps, by
their apparent ability to warm the body "subjectively." More objective evidence for spice-
induced thermogenesis was first provided by Henry and Emery,[54] who showed that chilli
and mustard sauces augmented the thermogenic response to a meal. More recently
Yoshioka et al.[55] have reported that red pepper enhanced thermogenesis and lipid oxidation in women. It is the principal ingredients that confer pungency to these spices (and
to others such as Tabasco sauce and ginger), i.e., the capsaicinoids (capsaicin and dihy-
drocapsaicin) and capsaicinoid-homologues (gingerols and shogoals), which also confer
the thermogenic and lipolytic properties.

Of particular interest in the red pepper study[55] is that these metabolic effects of the
capsaicin-rich foods were demonstrated in women showing diminished meal-induced
thermogenesis and the failure to increase fat oxidation when shifted from a high-carbohydrate to a high-fat meal. The addition of the capsaicin-rich red pepper to the high-fat
meal was found to stimulate fat oxidation and to normalize thermogenic response to the
high-fat meal to levels found with the high-carbohydrate meal. In other words, spices rich
in capsaicinoids have the potential to adjust fat oxidation to fat intake. These metabolic
effects of pungent principles of spices are perhaps not unexpected in view of evidence
suggesting that their main modes of action can also be linked to interference with the
sympathoadrenal system. By exerting their metabolic effects centrally to induce adrenal
medullary secretion or peripherally by interference with sympathetic control in tissues
such as brown adipose tissue, spices rich in capsaicinoids could constitute a new class of
dietary ingredients with sympathomimetic thermogenic effects.

The potential for thermogenic (and anorectic) effects of some of these spices with the
addition of caffeine is also real. In a recent study[56] in human volunteers given free access
to foods, the consumption of red pepper and caffeine with meals increased 24-h energy

expenditure and reduced cumulative *ad libitum* energy intake; the negative energy balance when the meals were consumed together with red pepper and caffeine was 4000 kJ/d. This effect was associated with an increased sympathetic-to-parasympathetic ratio assessed by power spectral analysis of heart rate. Whether this negative balance induced by combinations of red pepper (or other spices) and caffeine can be sustained over longer periods of time without undesirable effects, particularly in overweight or obese patients, remains to be investigated.

20.5.7 Green Tea and Catechin-Polyphenols

Various herbal preparations or extracts of green tea (a widely consumed beverage in China and Japan) are frequently claimed to be effective in reducing body weight. These antiobesity properties, although unsubstantiated, are generally attributed to caffeine content. However, green tea is also rich in polyphenols, of which the flavanols (e.g., catechin-polyphenols) and flavonols (quercetin, myricetin) have been shown to inhibit catechol-o-methlyl transferase (COMT), the enzyme that degrades the catecholamines (NA and adrenaline). Thus, by virtue of its high content in catechin-polyphenols (which may thus reduce degradation of NA within the synaptic cleft) and caffeine (which inhibits phosphodiesterase within the cytoplasm), green tea has the potential to interact synergistically with the SNS, leading to potentiation and prolongation of NA-induced thermogenesis.

Such a hypothesis has been shown to hold true when tested in brown adipose tissue *in vitro*.[57] In a subsequent placebo-controlled study in lean and overweight men, the effect of ingesting capsules containing a green tea extract (AR25) — whose dry weight comprises as much as 25% catechins and 7% caffeine — on 24-h energy expenditure and substrate oxidation in a room calorimeter was studied.[58] This green tea extract was found to stimulate thermogenesis to the extent of increasing 24-h energy expenditure by about 4%, and to promote fat oxidation such that the contribution of fat oxidation to daily energy expenditure was increased from 30 to 40%. These effects cannot be explained by caffeine content *per se* because administration of the same amount of caffeine as in the green tea extract failed to increase 24-h energy expenditure or fat oxidation.

These data *in vitro* and *in vivo*, together with the findings in a human study[58] that 24-h urinary NA (but not adrenaline) was higher during treatment with this green tea extract than with placebo or caffeine alone, support the notion that the efficacy of this green tea extract in stimulating thermogenesis and promoting fat oxidation is likely to reside in an interaction among catechin-polyphenols, caffeine, and sympathetic activity. To what extent the therapeutic value of green tea (believed to protect against chronic diseases by virtue of its potent antioxidant properties) can be extended to the management of obesity must await results of placebo-controlled clinical trial testing of the safety and efficacy of green tea extract in humans.

20.6 "Natural" Muscle Anabolics

Finally, a number of products for sale contain *chromium* (often as chromium picolinate) or *conjugated linoleic acid*, both of which claim to protect against loss of muscle mass during weight losses. The rationale behind the "anabolic" effect of chromium, which is an essential trace element involved in carbohydrate and lipid metabolism, is that because it may increase insulin sensitivity, it could have an effect on body energy partitioning in favor of muscle mass at the expense of fat mass. However, studies in humans that have appeared in peer-reviewed journals and are devoid of major faults in experimental design or methodology have failed to show a significant effect of chromium on the components of weight loss in obese and nonobese individuals.[59]

No clinical trials in obese patients have yet been reported with regard to *conjugated linoleic acid* (CLA), which is a term that describes a category of naturally ocurring trans-fatty acids found primarily in meat and dairy products of ruminant animals. The rationale for its inclusion in slimming products is that, by its inhibitory effect on lipoprotein lipase (LPL), CLA would inhibit the deposition of fat in peripheral tissues, and divert the energy thus saved towards increased lean tissue synthesis.[59]

20.7 Concluding Remarks

The use of dietary supplements and herbal preparations in the management of body weight has generally been perceived by the medical establishment as essentially anecdotal. This is largely because little, if any, robust scientific data support claims of antiobesity efficacy for the vast majority of such products proposed to consumers. Unlike prescription and over-the-counter medications, the "natural" dietary/herbal adjuvants currently on the market are not prospectively reviewed for safety and efficacy by major regulatory agencies (e.g., FDA in the U.S.; DHSS in U.K.), which only intervene if a given dietary/herbal product is shown to present a "significant or unreasonable" risk. Consequently, most of these products have not been studied in long-term prospective placebo-controlled clinical trials and reported in peer-reviewed medical journals.[59,60]

Nonetheless, it is a reality that many of these products do in fact contain one or more pharmacologically active ingredients known to possess thermogenic and anorectic properties in acute studies; however, the question is always whether they are effective and safe at the doses prescribed and over the long term. With the market likely to be overwhelmed with new products containing combinations of these ingredients with claims of a more effective multitargeted approach for weight control, the challenge for regulatory agencies is to decide the type of safety and efficacy standards to which these products should be subjected before being "approved" as supplements for the purpose of managing human obesity.

Acknowledgment

This work is supported by the Swiss National Science Foundation (Grant no. 3200-061687).

References

1. Ravussin, E. and Gautier, J.F. Metabolic predictors of weight gain. *Int. J. Obes.* 1999; 23 (Suppl 1) 37–41.

2. Stock, M.J. Gluttony and thermogenesis revisited. *Int. J. Obes.* 1999; 23: 1105–1117.

3. Dulloo, A.G., Jacquet, J., Girardier, L. Poststarvation hyperphagia and body fat overshooting in humans: a role for feedback signals from lean and fat tissues. *Am. J. Clin. Nutr.* 1997; 65: 77–723.

4. Dulloo, A.G. and Jacquet, J. Adaptive reduction in basal metabolic rate in response to food deprivation in humans: a role for feedback signals from fat stores. *Am. J. Clin. Nutr.*, 1998, 68: 599–606.

5. Ernst, E. and Pittler, M.H. Chitosan as a treatment for body weight reduction? A meta-analysis. *Perfusion* 1998; 11: 461–464.

6. Pittler, M.H., Abbot, N.C., Harkness, E.F. and Ernst, E. Randomized, double-blind trial of chitosan for weight reduction. *Eur. J. Clin. Nutr.* 1999; 53: 379–381.

7. Juhel, C., Armand, M., Pafumi, Y., Rosier, C., Vandermander, J. and Lairon, D. Green tea extract (AR25) inhibits lipolysis of triglycerides in gastric and duodenal medium *in vitro*. *J. Nutr. Biochem.* 2000, 11: 45–51.

8. Delargy, H.J., O'Sullivan, K.R., Fletcher, R.J. and Blundell, J.E. Effects of amount and type of dietary fibre (soluble and insoluble) on short-term control of appetite. *Int. J. Food Sci. Nutr.* 1997; 48: 67–77.

9. Evans, E. and Miller, D.S. Bulking agents in the treatment of obesity. *Nutr. Metab.* 1975; 18: 199–203.

10. Frati–Munari, A.C., Fernandez–Harp, J.A., Becerril, M., Chavez–Negrete, A. and Banales–Ham, M. Decrease in serun lipids, glycemia and body weight by *Plantago psyllium* in obese and diabetic patients. *Arch. Invest. Med.* 1983; 14: 259–268.

11. Cangiano, C., Ceci, F., Cascino, A., Del Ben, M., Laviano, A., Muscaritoli, M., Antonucci, F. and Rossi–Fanelli, F. Eating behaviour and adherence to dietary prescriptions in obese adult subjects treated with 5-hydroxytryptophan. *Am. J. Clin. Nutr.* 1992; 56: 863–867.

12. Cangiano, C., Laviano, A., Del Ben, M., Preziosa, I., Angelico, F., Cascino, A. and Rossi–Fanelli, F. Effects of oral 5-hydroxy-tryptophan on energy intake and macronutrient selection in non-insulin dependent diabetic patients. *Int. J. Obes.* 1998; 22: 648–654.

13. Heymsfield, S.B., Allison, D.B., Vasseli, J.R., Pietrobelli, A., Greenfield, D. and Nunez, C. *Garcinia cambogia* (hydroxycitric acid) as a potential anti-obesity agent. *JAMA* 1998; 280: 1596–1600.

14. Kriketos, A.D., Thompson, H.R., Greene, H. and Hill, J.O. –(–)-Hydroxycitric acid does not affect energy expenditure and substrate oxidation in adult males in post-absorptive state. *Int. J. Obes.* 1999; 23: 867–873.

15. Muller, D.M., Seim, H., Kiess, W., Loster, H. and Richter, T. Effects of oral L-carnitine supplementation on *in vivo* long-chain fatty acid oxidation in healthy adults. *Metabolism* 2002; 51: 1389–1391.

16. Villani, R.G., Gannon, J., Self, M., Rich, P.A. L-carnitine supplementation combined with aerobic training does not promote weight loss in obese women. *Int. J. Sport Nutr. Exerc. Metab.* 2000; 10: 199–207.

17. Ivy, J.L. Effect of pyruvate and dihydroxyacetone on metabolism and aerobic endurance capacity. *Med. Sci. Sports Exerc.* 1998; 30: 837–843.

18. Stanko, R.T., Tietze, D.L. and Arch, J.E. Body composition, energy utilization and nitrogen metabolism with a 4.25 MJ/d low-energy diet supplemented with pyruvate. *Am. J. Clin. Nutr.* 1992; 56: 630–635.

19. Kalman, D., Colker, C.M., Wilets, I., Roufs, J.B. and Antonio, J. The effects of pyruvate supplementation on body composition in overweight individuals. *Nutrition* 1999; 15: 337–340.

20. Dulloo, A.G. and Miller, D.S. Obesity: a disorder of the sympathetic nervous system. *World Rev. Nutr. Diet*, 1987, 50, 1–56.

21. Snitker, S., Macdonald, I., Ravussin, E. and Astrup, A. The sympathetic nervous system and obesity: role in aetiology and treatment. *Obes. Rev.* 2000; 1: 5–15.

22. Dulloo, A.G. A sympathetic defense against obesity. *Science* 2002; 297: 780–781.

23. Landsberg, L. and Young, J.B. Sympathoadrenal activity and obesity: physiological rationale for the use of adrenergic thermogenic drugs. *Int. J. Obes.*, 1992, 17 (Suppl. 1), S29–S34.

24. Arch, J.R. Beta-3-adrenoceptor agonists: potential pitfalls and progress. *Eur. J. Pharmacol.* 2002; 440: 99–107.

25. Dulloo, A.G. Strategies to counteract readjustments toward lower metabolic rates during obesity management. *Nutrition* 1993; 9: 366–372.
26. Dulloo, A.G. Spicing fat for combustion. *Br. J. Nutr.* 1998; 80: 493–494.
27. Flatt, J.P. Diet, life-style, and weight maintenance. *Am. J. Clin. Nutr.* 1995; 62: 820–836.
28. Chen, K.K. and Schmidt, C.F. Ephedrine and related substances. *Medecine* 1930; 9: 117–130.
29. Evans, E. and Miller, D.S. The effect of ephedrine on the oxygen consumption of fed and fasted subjects. *Proc. Nutr. Soc.* 1997; 36: 136A.
30. Pasquali, R. and Casimirri, P. Clinical aspects of ephedrine in the treatment of obesity. *Int. J. Obes.*, 1992; 17 (Suppl. 1): S65–S68.
31. Dulloo, A.G. and Stock, M.J. Ephedrine, xanthines, aspirin and other thermogenic drugs to assist the dietary management of obesity. *Int. J. Obes.*, 1992; 17 (Suppl. 1): S1–S2.
32. Mosdol, A., Christensen, B., Retterstol, L. and Thelle, D.S. Induced changes in the consumption of coffee alter ad libitum dietary intake and physical activity level. *Br. J. Nutr.* 2002; 87: 261–266.
33. Acheson, K.J., Zahorska–Markiewicz, B., Pittet, Ph., Anantharaman, K. and Jéquier, E. Caffeine and coffee: their influence on metabolic rate and substrate utilization in normal weight and obese individuals. *Am. J. Clin. Nutr.* 1980; 33: 989–997.
34. Dulloo, A.G., Seydoux, J. and Girardier, L. Potentiation of the thermogenic antiobesity effects of ephedrine by dietary methylxanthines: adenosine antagonism or phosphodiesterase inhibition? *Metabolism* 1992; 41: 1233–1241.
35. Dulloo, A.G., Geissler, C., Horton, T., Collins, A. and Miller, D.S. Normal caffeine consumption: influence on thermogenesis and daily energy expenditure in lean and post-obese human volunteers. *Am. J. Clin. Nutr.* 1989; 49: 44–50.
36. Bracco, D., Ferrarra, J.M., Arnaud, M.J., Jéquier, E. and Schutz, Y. Effects of caffeine on energy metabolism, heart rate, and methylxanthine metabolism in lean and obese women. *Am. J. Physiol.* 1995; 269: E671–E678.
37. Toubro, S., Astrup, A., Breum, L. and Quaade, F. Safety and efficacy of long-term treatment with ephedrine, caffeine and an ephedrine/caffeine mixture. *Int. J. Obes.*, 1992; 17 (Suppl. 1): S69–S72.
38. Dulloo, A.G. Ephedrine, xanthines and prostaglandin-inhibitors: actions and interactions in the stimulation of thermogenesis. *Int. J. Obes.*, 1992; 17 (Suppl. 1): S35–S40.
39. Daly, P., Krieger, D., Dulloo, A.G., Young, J.B. and Landsberg, L. Ephedrine, caffeine and aspirin: safety and efficacy for treatment of human obesity. *Int. J. Obes.*, 1992; 17 (Suppl. 1): S73–S78.
40. Greenway, F.L., Ryan, D.H., Bray, G.A., Rood, J.C., Tucker, E.W. and Smith, S.R. Pharmaceutical cost savings of treating obesity with weight loss medication. *Obes. Res.* 1999; 716: 523–530.
41. Haller, C.A. and Benowitz, N.L. Adverse cardiovascular and central nervous system events associated with dietary supplements containing ephedra alkaloids. *N. Engl. J. Med.* 2000; 343: 1833–1838.
42. Greenway, F.L. The safety and efficacy of pharmaceutical and herbal caffeine and ephedrine use as a weight loss agent. *Obesity Rev.* 2001; 2: 199–211.
43. Dulloo, A.G. Herbal simulation of ephedrine and caffeine in treatment of obesity. *Int. J. Obes.* 2002; 26: 590–592.
44. Boozer, C.N., Nasser, J.A., Heymsfield, S.B., Wang, V., Chen, G. and Solomon, J.L. An herbal supplement containing ma huang–guarana for weight loss: a randomized, double-blind trial. *Int. J. Obes.* 2001; 25: 316–324.
45. Boozer, C.N., Daly, P.A., Homel, P., Solomon, J.L., Blanchard, D., Nasser, J.A., Strauss, R. and Meredith, T. Herbal ephedra/caffeine for weight loss: a 6-month randomized safety and efficacy trial. *Int. J. Obes.* 2002; 26: 593–604.
46. Kenneth, B.S. Forskolin and adenylate cyclase: new opportunities in drug design. *Ann. Rep. Med. Chem.* 1984; 19: 293–302.
47. Meyer, P. Etude en simple aveugle versus placebo de la tolérance cardiovasculaire et de la pharmacocinétique d'un extrait de 'coleus forskohlii' administré par voie orale à la dose unique croissante chez le volontaire sain. *Report of a clinical study*, Centre de Pharmacologique, Hôpital Necker, Paris, 1993.

48. Bach, A.C. and Babayan, V.K. Medium-chain triglycerides: an update. *Am. J. Clin. Nutr.* 1982; 36: 950–962.
49. Dulloo, A.G., Fathi, M., Mensi, N. and Girardier, L. Twenty-four hour energy expenditure and urinary catecholamines of humans consuming low-to-moderate amounts of medium-chain-triglycerides: a dose-response study in a respiratory chamber. *Eur. J. Clin. Nutr.* 1996; 50: 152–158.
50. Papamandjaris, A.A., MacDougall, D.E. and Jones, P.J.H. Medium chain fatty acid metabolism and energy expenditure: obesity and treatment implications. *Life Sci.*, 1998; 62: 1203–1215.
51. Rolls, B.J., Gnizak, N., Summerfelt, A. and Laster, L.J. Food intake in dieters and nondieters after a liquid meal containing medium-chain triglycerides. *Am. J. Clin. Nutr.* 1988; 48: 66–71.
52. Dulloo, A.G. Response to the letter of J.M. Haenen about MCT and weight control. *Eur. J. Clin. Nutr.* 1997; 51: 714–715.
53. Stubbs, R.J. and Harbron, C.G. Covert manipulation of the ratio of medium- to long-chain triglycerides in isoenergetically dense diets: effect on food intake in ad libitum feeding men. *Int. J. Obesity* 1996; 20: 435–444.
54. Henry, C.J.K. and Emery, P. Effects of spiced food on metabolic rate. *Hum. Nutr. Clin. Nutr.* 1986; 40C: 165–168.
55. Yoshioka, M., St–Pierre, S., Suzuki, M. and Tremblay, A. Effects of red pepper added to high-fat and high-carbohydrate meals on energy metabolism and substrate utilization in Japanese women. *Br. J. Nutr.*, 1998; 80: 503–510.
56. Yoshioka, M., Doucet, E., Drapeau, V., Dionne, I. and Tremblay, A. Combined effects of red pepper and caffeine consumption on 24-h energy balance in subjects given free access to foods. *Br. J. Nutr.*, 2001; 85: 203–211.
57. Dulloo, A.G., Seydoux, J., Girardier, L., Chantre, P. and Vandermander, J. Green tea and thermogenesis: interaction between catechin-polyphenols, caffeine and sympathetic activity. *Int. J. Obes.* 2000; 24: 252–258.
58. Dulloo, A.G., Duret, C., Rohrer, D., Girardier, L., Mensi, N., Fathi, M., Chantre, P. and Vandermander, J. Efficacy of a green tea extract rich in catechin polyphenols and caffeine in increasing 24h energy expenditure and fat oxidation in humans. *Am. J. Clin. Nutr.* 1999; 70: 1040–1045.
59. Allison, D.B., Fontaine, K.R., Heshka, S., Mentore, J.L. and Heymsfield, S.B. Alternative treatments for weight loss: a critical review. *Crit. Rev. Food Sci. Nutr.* 2001; 41: 1–28.
60. Egger, G., Cameron–Smith, D. and Stanton, R. The effectiveness of popular, non-prescription weight loss supplements. *MJA* 1999; 171: 604–608.

21

Surgical Treatment of Obesity

Jaroslaw Kolanowski

CONTENTS

SUMMARY   Severely obese patients are frequently refractory to diet and drug therapy, even though an effective treatment is mandatory because of serious obesity-related co-morbidities; thus, gastric surgery is increasingly recognized as the only efficient treatment of severe obesity and its health-threatening complications. Among different surgical procedures consisting of gastric restriction and/or of variable degrees of intestinal malabsorption, the most frequently used procedures include vertical banded gastroplasty; adjustable silicone gastric banding; and gastric bypass. The latter associates a gastric restriction with a moderate degree of malabsorption because duodenum and the initial segment of jejunum are excluded from digestive continuity. All these techniques may be performed laparoscopically.

Gastric surgery is in general very effective in terms of impressive and sustained weight loss, but the postoperative follow-up and nutritional surveillance are mandatory because of the potential risk of late nutritional and digestive complications. The usual 50 to 75% reduction of initial body weight excess, which occurs during the first year after surgery, is followed by a significant reduction of several obesity-related co-morbidities, such as hypertension; type 2 diabetes; dyslipidemia; and cardiorespiratory dysfunction. Frequently, a tendency is toward a late partial regain of weight, but the benefit in terms of improvement in the obesity-associated co-morbidities is generally maintained for several years after surgery. Gastric procedures are, therefore, an effective treatment of severe obesity and its co-morbid conditions.

21.1 Introduction

Obesity-induced health risks result from several co-morbid conditions, such as hypertension; dyslipidemia; insulin resistance with increased prevalence of type 2 diabetes; cardiorespiratory dysfunction; and some types of cancer (Sjöström 1992; Sagar 1995; Stunkard 1996). Although life expectancy is reduced proportionally to the severity of the overweight, obesity-linked morbidity is considered as one of the most preventable causes of death (McGinnis and Foege 1993). Therefore, it is evident that severe obesity should be treated in an effective way. Yet classical conservative treatments, such as dietary and behavior therapies or the use of antiobesity drugs, are frequently unsuccessful in the long term.

The frequent failure of dietary and pharmacological treatments to sustain the loss of weight in overweight subjects, as well as an increasing prevalence of obesity over the past decades, prompted the search for a more radical and effective treatment of obesity such as that offered by bariatric surgery. Although impressive in terms of weight reduction, early procedures such as jejunoileal bypass induced serious sequelae, including chronic diarrhea with malabsorption; electrolytic disturbances; hepatic failure; and deficiencies of fat-soluble vitamins leading ultimately to bone demineralization (Rand and Macgregor 1991; Kral 1992; Mason and Doherty 1993; Shikora et al. 1994; Sagar 1995). The severity of these complications contributed to the downfall of intestinal bypass surgery, which is no more considered as an acceptable surgical option for obese subjects (NIH Consensus Development Conference Panel 1991, 1992).

Despite the fact that the same consensus conference (NIH 1991, 1992) recognized other surgical procedures such as gastroplasty or gastric bypass as appropriate treatments for severe obesity associated with serious co-morbid conditions, some physicians still share the opinion that the overall risks and side effects of bariatric surgery do not justify the benefits (Shikora et al. 1994). However, the further refinement of the originally developed surgical techniques with introduction of the adjustable gastric banding performed by laparoscopy has modified this initially negative opinion. Bariatric surgery is now considered an appropriate therapeutic option for severely obese subjects with health-threatening complications if conservative therapeutic approaches fail to promote a reduction of body weight sufficient to alleviate the obesity-related co-morbid conditions (Brolin 2002; Buchwald and Buchwald 2002; Deitel and Shikora 2002). Indeed, the currently performed operations are followed by a long-lasting weight loss of about 50% of the preoperative excess body weight, with concomitant improvement or resolution of most obesity-associated morbid conditions.

However, even a less important loss of weight, averaging 10% of the initial weight, is in general followed by rapid attenuation of hypertension and metabolic abnormalities (Kolanowski 1997; Torgerson and Sjöström 2001; Livingston 2002). One of the most impressive metabolic improvements that occur in morbidly obese patients already during the first weeks after gastric surgery is the beneficial effect on insulin sensitivity and glucose metabolism (Kolanowski 1995; Torgerson and Sjöström 2001; Dixon and O'Brien 2002; Livingston 2002; Greenway et al. 2002). Gastric surgery is even considered as the sole means to cure type 2 diabetes associated with obesity (Rubino and Gagner 2002). Moreover, the long-term evaluation of benefits of gastric surgery (the Swedish Obese Subjects, or SOS, study) has recently evidenced a highly significant reduction in the incidence of diabetes after gastric surgery, compared to control obese subjects treated by conservative approaches (Torgerson and Sjöström 2001).

However, despite the initial reduction in arterial hypertension and in the use of antihypertensive drugs (Kolanowski 1995; Brolin 2002) documented during the first years after surgery, the incidence of hypertension was no longer different in the two study groups after an 8-year follow-up (Torgerson and Sjöström 2001). On the other hand, it remains to be established whether the pronounced and sustained loss of weight occurring after gastric surgery will reduce mortality. This is an important unraveled question because some previous epidemiological evaluations evidenced an association between weight loss and increased mortality (Pamuk et al. 1993).

In general, gastric surgery is remarkably well tolerated, despite a considerable reduction in food intake, because of the almost complete disappearance of hunger concomitant with the reinforcement of satiety. These changes in the control of eating behavior are probably, at least in part, related to clear-cut reduction in secretion and circulating levels of ghrelin, which is a hormone that increases food intake (Cummings et al. 2002). In addition to these positive effects of bariatric surgery, the gastric surgery for morbid obesity is generally followed by an improvement in physical and mental well-being, as well as in quality of life, including its affective, familial, social, and professional aspects (Arcila et al. 2002; Torgerson and Sjöström 2001). In addition, the surgical treatment of severe obesity is considered to be cost-effective by reducing the obesity-related co-morbidities as well as absenteeism from work of previously morbidly obese patients (NIH Consensus Panel 1991, 1992; Torgerson and Sjöström 2001; Agren et al. 2002a). In addition, the pharmaceutical costs of medications used by obese patients for treatment of diabetes and cardiovascular diseases are also significantly reduced after loss of weight induced by gastric surgery (Agren et al. 2002b).

21.2 Currently Used Surgical Procedures

According to mechanisms responsible for the loss of body weight, the presently proposed surgical procedures can be classified into four categories (Buchwald and Buchwald 2002):

- Purely restrictive procedures, consisting in gastric partition, include the banded and ringed vertical gastroplasty, as well as gastric banding. These procedures create a small gastric pouch, which is drained through a narrow calibrated stoma (Figure 21.1 A and B). The intake of solid is, therefore, considerably limited; patients appear not to experience hunger and rapidly feel full, even after a small meal. These procedures do not involve gastric resection and maintain the anatomical and functional continuity of the gastrointestinal tract, so the loss of weight is due solely to a very restricted energy intake.

- The procedures combining the restriction of gastric volume with gastrojejunal bypass induce variable degrees of intestinal malabsorption because of the exclusion of duodenum from the digestive continuity. The Roux-en-Y gastric bypass (Figure 21.1 C) is the most widely used procedure of this type of surgery.

- The malabsorptive procedures combining partial gastric resection; anastomosis of the remaining part of stomach with the initial jejunal loop; the duodenal switch; and biliopancreatic diversion (Figure 21.1 D). The weight loss induced by this procedure is due essentially to the intestinal malabsorption.

- New experimental procedures, including gastric pacing, intend to induce early satiety through electrical stimulation of the gastric wall (Wolff et al. 2002). This recently proposed surgical approach is still purely experimental, and it is too early to evaluate its efficacy and potential side effects.

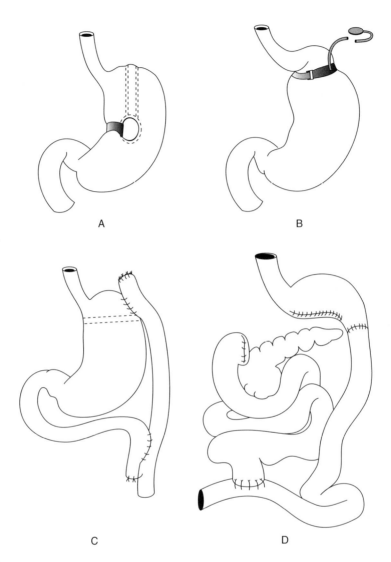

FIGURE 21.1
Currently used surgical procedures for morbid obesity. A: Vertical banded gastroplasty; B: Adjustable silicone gastric banding; C: Roux-en-Y gastric bypass — a small gastric pouch is anastomozed to the jejunum while duodenum is excluded from digestive absorption; D: Biliopancreatic diversion with duodenal switch — the proximal duodenum and half of jejunum (biliopancreatic limb) are excluded from digestive continuity.

21.2.1 Vertical Banded Gastroplasty

This restrictive procedure, introduced by Mason in 1982 (Mason 1982; Mason and Doherty 1993), rapidly became the most popular technique of gastric partition; it is still widely used and may be performed by laparoscopy too (Lönroth et al. 1996). This technique involves the stapled partition of the stomach creating a small upper pouch of 30 ml or even less, which empties to the remaining part of the stomach through a narrow outlet with diameter calibrated from 8 to 10 mm, and reinforced by a Gortex band, or by similar prosthetic material (Kral 1992; Ashley et al. 1993; Sagar 1995). Because of the limited capacity of the gastric pouch, the amount of ingested food before rapid onset of satiety is considerably limited, providing less than 500 kcal per day during the first weeks after surgery (Sagar 1995; Kolanowski 1995). This induces a rapid loss of weight, which occurs mainly during the first 6 months after the operation (Kral 1992; Mason and Doherty 1993). Later, the capacity of ingestion progressively increases and a tendency toward a late partial regain of weight frequently occurs 2 to 3 years after surgery (Kolanowski 1995). The loss of weight induced by this procedure is due solely to a very restricted energy intake (Sagar 1995; Kolanowski and Martinelli 1996).

The peri- and early postoperative mortality is lower than 1%, while the immediate postoperative complications are in general limited to wound infection. This complication has been reported to occur only in 2% of patients (Mason and Doherty 1993), or to be much more frequent, occurring in nearly 25% of patients submitted to this kind of gastric surgery (Shikora et al. 1994). A relatively high frequency of vomiting related to gastroesophageal reflux (Kim and Sarr 1992) rarely results from stenosis of the gastric pouch outlet, but is usually secondary to eating too rapidly (Sagar 1995; Kolanowski 1997). Late failure in terms of insufficient loss of weight, or even of weight regain, may result from an excessive ingestion of high-caloric liquids and sweet foods; from gastric pouch dilatation; or from disruption of the staple line (Mason and Doherty 1993; Shikora et al. 1994; Sagar 1995). This complication, usually followed by a sudden increase in eating capacity, with ensuing regain of weight, may be easily evidenced by radiography (Kolanowski 1997). The staple disruption may need revisional surgery: restapling of the gastric pouch or converting gastroplasty into gastric bypass (Mason 1996). An intragastric migration of the polypropylene band restricting the gastric outlet or ulceration of the stoma has also been reported, but remains rare.

Because of poor long-term weight maintenance, with nearly 80% failure rate 10 years following this gastric restriction procedure with a need of reoperation, gastroplasty has recently fallen into disfavor, at least in the U.S. (Brolin 2002).

21.2.2 Gastric Banding

Gastric banding, which also creates a small upper gastric pouch limiting food intake (Figure 21.1 B), has become a common operation for morbid obesity because it is relatively easy to perform by laparoscopy; reversible; and less invasive than other surgical procedures (Cadiere et al. 2002; Evans et al. 2002; Favretti et al. 2002; Gustavsson and Westling 2002; Rubenstein 2002). The early, less satisfactory results and complication rates were somewhat improved after the introduction of an inflatable silicone band allowing adjustment of the outlet diameter by infusion of saline through a subcutaneous reservoir (Kuzmak 1989; Brolin 2002).

Although several reports are still strongly in favor of this technique, considering it efficient and relatively well tolerated (Cadiere et al. 2002; Dixon and O'Brien 2002; Favretti et al. 2002; Pontiroli et al. 2002; Rubenstein 2002), other authors do not share this opinion. Indeed, the loss of weight is in general less important than after gastroplasty (Brolin 2002) and, after the initial period of 2 to 3 years, the gastric band device should be removed in at least 50% of patients. The reason for this is not only the progressive loss of efficacy of the adjustable silicone gastric banding (DeMaria et al. 2001; Doherty et al. 2002), but also several complications such as frequent vomiting with acid reflux leading to erosive esophagitis; band erosion; pouch and esophageal dilatation; or the leakage from the balloon (Gustavsson and Westling 2002; Kothari et al. 2002). Less frequent complications include slippage of the silicone device (Evans et al. 2002); intragastric band migration (Mittermair et al. 2002); or even gastric perforation (Cadiere et al. 2002). In the presence of these complications and of poor long-term outcome in terms of weight loss, adjustable silicone gastric banding is generally converted to gastric bypass (Gustavsson and Westling 2002; Kothari et al. 2002).

21.2.3   Gastric Bypass

This surgical procedure creates a larger gastric pouch, emptied by an anastomosis directly into the jejunum, thus bypassing the duodenum. It is considered now the most effective and safe surgery for morbid obesity (Kral 1992; Sagar 1995; Shikora et al. 1994). This technique induces weight loss by combining restricted intake and a moderate degree of malabsorption (Kral 1992; Sagar 1995; Stunkard 1996). Undoubtedly the initial loss of weight is greater after this procedure than following gastroplasty or adjustable silicone gastric banding (Mason and Doherty 1993; Sagar 1995; Salmon and McArdle 1992; Shikora et al. 1994; Sugerman 2002). The gastric pouch is separated from the excluded part of the stomach by stapling and drained through a relatively large stoma directly into a jejunal loop in a Roux-en-Y arrangement (Mason and Doherty 1993; Brolin 2002; DeMario et al. 2002). Thus, one limb of a Y-shaped reconstruction of jejunum allows drainage of the gastric pouch, while the bile and pancreatic juice are evacuated by the second limb of the Y structure (Figure 21.1 C).

   The mortality related to this procedure is lower than 1%, with significantly higher mortality in patients older than 55 years (Livingston et al. 2002).The laparoscopic gastric bypass has been shown to be feasible and relatively safe, with the subsequent weight loss similar to that occurring after open gastric bypass (Sugerman 2002). In a recent evaluation of 281 patients who underwent laparoscopic Roux-en-Y gastric bypass, only 2.8% required conversion to an open procedure; the major wound infections occurred only in 1.5% of patients while 75% were discharged from hospital within 3 days (DeMario et al. 2002). However, in the same study the anastomotic leak with peritonitis occurred in 5.1% of patients. In another recent study of the frequency of upper gastrointestinal complications of laparoscopic Roux-en-Y gastric bypass surgery, evaluated in 463 severely obese patients, 23 had small-bowel obstructions, and major leaks originating from gastrojejunal anastomosis were evidenced in 16 patients; 15 others had anastomotic strictures (Blachar et al. 2002).

   A recent report on autopsy finding in patients who died following gastric bypass surgery indicates that, while only 3 out of 10 patients studied died from pulmonary embolism, 8 of 10 patients had microscopic evidence of pulmonary emboli, despite prophylaxis for deep vein thrombosis (Melinek et al. 2002). Among complications occurring later, the duodenogastric bile reflux to the excluded stomach, with potentially deleterious effects of bile on gastric mucosa, has been recently evidenced as a frequent complication, documented in 36% of patients 18 months postoperatively (Sundbom et al. 2002). The hemorrhage from the excluded part of the stomach or duodenum represents another possible, but uncommon, late complication of gastric bypass (Braley et al. 2002).

   Because the hypertonic contents of the stomach rapidly enter the small bowel, patients frequently experience a dumping syndrome consisting of weakness and sweating after a carbohydrate-rich meal (Kral 1992; Sagar 1995; Stunkard 1996; Mason and Doherty 1993). This may obviously discourage them from consuming sweet foods — thus the opinion that this type of gastrojejunal surgery is particularly indicated for obese patients considered "sweet-eaters." In addition, patients who undergo gastric bypass complain of increased sensitivity to the effects of alcohol as a result of a more rapid absorption of ethanol (Klockhoff et al. 2002).

   The loss of weight ranges usually from 65 to 75% of the initial weight excess and is due essentially to the restriction of food intake (Brolin 2002). Aside from the loss of weight followed by improvement in hypertension, hyperlipidemia, and type 2 diabetes, the clear-cut psychosocial benefits are reflected by a significant decrease in the rate of antidepressant use following this type of surgery (Holzwarth et al. 2002).

It should be stressed, however, that by bypassing the duodenum, this type of gastric bypass may cause malabsorption of iron and calcium, increasing the risk of anemia, osteoporosis, and hip fracture (Mason and Doherty 1993; Shikora et al. 1994; Sugerman 2002). Indeed, the micronutrient deficiencies such as iron, vitamin B12, and calcium depletion are relatively frequent (documented in 30 to 50% of patients) (Brolin 2002). The supplementation of these micronutrients is therefore mandatory after this type of gastric bypass. Abnormalities in calcium and vitamin D metabolism occur already very early after gastric bypass as a result of malabsorption, and they may lead, several years later, to metabolic bone disease with radiologic evidence of osteomalacia (Goldner et al. 2002).

21.2.4 Biliopancreatic Diversion

This particular form of gastric bypass, referred to as biliopancreatic diversion, was introduced in 1968 by Scopinaro (Scopinaro et al. 1996) and was designed to bypass a large part of the intestine with a concomitant resection of the excluded part of the stomach (Figure 21.1 D) to decrease the risk of gastric ulcer. The volume of the remaining gastric pouch is much larger than in other procedures and may vary from 200 to 500 ml. This procedure combines a modest amount of gastric restriction, with intestinal malabsorption accounting for the loss of weight. The biliopancreatic diversion seems very effective in terms of weight loss because it ranges from 75 to 80% of previous excess weight (Scopinaro et al. 1996; Brolin 2002). The entire jejunum is excluded from digestive continuity and is anastomosed end-to-side to the ileum at a point between 50 and 100 cm proximal to the ileocecal junction (Figure 21.1 D).

This procedure, including the distal Roux-en-Y technique and the duodenal switch, is recommended by some authors as the most efficient surgical treatment of morbid obesity (Hess and Hess 2002; Brolin 2002). The theoretical advantage of this surgery is that the loss of weight may occur even in the absence of a severe restriction of food intake. The incidence of early complications ranges from 10 to 15%, with a 1.0% mortality rate (Scopinaro et al. 1996).

Nevertheless, the biliopancreatic diversion frequently induces protein malnutrition and other metabolic complications (Mason and Doherty 1993; Scopinaro et al. 1996). It is therefore not surprising that the extent of weight loss after this kind of surgery is proportional to the length of the intestinal bypass and thus to the severity of malabsorption. Among metabolic sequelae of this procedure, the incidence of anemia amounts to 30%; the fat-soluble vitamin deficiencies occur in 30 to 50% of patients. The severe protein–calorie malnutrition, which occurs in 5% of patients, may require hospitalization and nutritional support (Scopinaro et al. 1996; Brolin 2002). The severity of vitamin deficiencies may affect the outcome of pregnancies in women who undergo this gastrointestinal surgery. Indeed, a serious vitamin A deficiency with retinal damage has been recently reported in a 40-year-old mother and her newborn infant, as a result of maternal malabsorption after biliopancreatic diversion performed several years before the pregnancy (Huerta et al. 2002). It is evident that patients who undergo this surgery need life-long follow-up and appropriate vitamin supplementation. In addition, the intestinal malabsorption is responsible for frequent occurrence of diarrhea and foul-smelling stools (Brolin 2002).

The biliopancreatic diversion may also be performed by laparoscopy, with results similar to those obtained by an open procedure, while considerably reducing the risk of wound hernia (Scopinaro et al. 2002; Feng and Gagner 2002).

21.3   Long-Term Follow-Up after Gastric Surgery

The loss of weight induced by gastric restriction procedures is due solely to decreased energy intake (Kolanowski and Martinelli 1996; Brolin 2002). Given the considerably reduced capacity of gastric pouch, the ingestion of energy is limited usually during the first three postoperative months to 400 to 600 kcal/day (Kolanowski 1995). Dietary records indicate that, during this initial period after gastroplasty or gastric banding that creates a comparable degree of gastric restriction, protein and fat intake is less than 30 g/day; the remaining energy consists of carbohydrate ingested mainly as sweet liquids and semisolid foods. Protein intake is limited by the aversion toward meats, which may persist for several months or even years. The intake of protein is provided by dairy products and eggs and, later, by poultry and fish. Patients are instructed to take frequent and small meals and, to prevent vomiting, to eat slowly and to avoid drinking during meals (Sagar 1995; Kolanowski 1997).

As a result of these radical changes in eating habits, a rapid loss of weight usually averaging 20 to 25 kg develops during the first 3 months after the operation (Mason and Doherty 1993; Kolanowski 1995; Evans et al. 2002). At least 70% of the weight lost during this period is accounted for by a reduction of fat mass; the remaining loss of weight corresponds to fat-free mass. Although the loss of lean tissue resulting from a negative nitrogen balance, which averages 2 to 4 g of nitrogen per day, occurs mainly during the first weeks after surgery, the water lost during this period is usually recovered after 2 to 3 months (Kolanowski and Martinelli 1996). Later, weight loss corresponds solely to the reduction of body fat, the relative reduction of visceral adipose tissue being more important than that of total body fat (Busetto et al. 2002).

Loss of weight continues, albeit at a slower rate, during the following 3 months and corresponds, at 6 months after surgery, to nearly 50% of the preoperative weight excess (McLean et al. 1990; Kolanowski 1995). At this time, the adaptation of eating habits and improved gastric tolerance allows a progressive increase and variety in consumption of solid foods, with a concomitant increase in protein and fat as well as mineral and vitamin intake. Energy intake thereafter progressively increases, and at 1 year after surgery it averages 800 to 1000 kcal per day. This obviously reduces the loss of weight, which frequently ceases 12 to 18 months after gastroplasty; by then the loss of weight may account for up to 60%, or even more, of the initial excess of weight (Mason and Doherty 1993; Kolanowski 1995; Cadiere et al. 2002; Favretti et al. 2002). Some authors reported a more prolonged, but less important loss of weight following gastric banding (Rubenstein 2002), while the loss of weight is usually more important and long-lasting in patients with gastric bypass or biliopancreatic diversion (Scopinaro et al. 1996; Sugerman 2002; Feng and Gagner 2002; Brolin 2002).

The loss of weight during the first year after surgery is proportional to the degree of the preoperative obesity and depends largely on the frequency of the follow-up visits (Sagar 1995, Kolanowski 1997). It may be considerably slower in obese subjects who consume large amounts of sweets and high-energy liquid foods rich in sugar and fat. According to some authors (Kral 1992; Sugerman et al. 1996), vertical banded gastroplasty is not a suitable intervention in these subjects, and the gastric bypass procedure offers them much better postoperative results. Indeed, the gastric bypass procedure is followed by rapid emptying of the gastric pouch into the small bowel with ensuing aversion to sweets, due to the dumping syndrome (Shikora et al. 1994; Sagar 1995; Sugerman et al. 1996).

Long-term loss of weight is variable and depends largely on the type of gastric or gastrointestinal surgery, and on eating habits. Despite some tendency toward weight regain, especially after gastric restriction procedures, some reports indicate that patients may maintain at least a 50% reduction of the preoperative weight excess for periods as long as 10 to 15 years after surgery (Mason and Doherty 1993; Reinhold 1994; Shikora et al. 1994; Deitel and Shikora 2002). Undoubtedly, the weight loss is greater and maintained for longer periods of time after gastric bypass or biliopancreatic diversion than after purely gastric restriction procedures (Shikora et al. 1994). This is not surprising because the former procedures combine a variable degree of gastric restriction with intestinal malabsorption.

The long-term follow-up after gastroplasty indicates that at 5 years after surgery about 50% of patients maintain a 50% reduction of the initial weight excess, which should be considered a satisfactory result (Mason and Doherty 1993). Modest success, defined by these authors as a loss of excess weight ranging between 25 and 50%, is obtained in 30% of patients, while in the remaining 20% the failure of the procedure is due to the insufficient loss of weight or to complications requiring revisional surgery. The impressive loss of weight that usually follows gastric restriction and gastric bypass procedures is associated in most patients with a considerable improvement in the quality of life (Kral 1992; Shikora et al. 1994; Stunkard 1996; Arcila et al. 2002).

The most important benefit, however, relates to a rapid improvement in several co-morbid conditions, such as hypertension; hyperlipidemia; hyperuricemia; and insulin resistance with glucose intolerance or overt diabetes (Gleysteen 1992; Kral 1992; Sagar 1995; Kolanowski 1995). The latter results from a significant recovery of the sensitivity to insulin (Burnstein et al. 1995; Kolanowski 1995), with a clear-cut improvement in glucose tolerance leading to euglycemia in most previous noninsulin-dependent diabetic subjects (Rubino and Gagner 2002; Greenway et al. 2002). Respiratory function is also improved, with significant regression or even disappearance of the sleep apnea syndrome (Sagar 1995). There is also a rapid amelioration of abnormal cardiac function (Alpert et al. 1993), and the preliminary results of the Swedish Obese Subjects (SOS) study indicate a considerable reduction in the incidence of cardiovascular complications, including hypertension.

A rapid normalization of hypertension has been documented following gastric restrictive surgery (Foley et al. 1992; Kolanowski 1995) or after gastric bypass (Carson et al. 1994). This beneficial effect on blood pressure is, however, limited to the first 2 years after surgery. Later, despite the maintenance of reduced body weight, the hypertension frequently reappears, as evidenced in the SOS study (Torgerson and Sjöström 2001).

21.4 Nutritional and Behavioral Aspects of Bariatric Surgery

Late nutritional complications of gastric surgery may be relatively serious in some patients, largely depending on the type of operation as well as on the frequency and quality of the medical, psychological, and nutritional follow-up. Nutritional deficiencies are seldom encountered after purely restrictive gastric procedures such as vertical banded gastroplasty or gastric banding, despite the considerable restriction of nutrient intake (Kolanowski 1997). The most frequent nutritional deficiencies that may occur after this kind of surgery are related to insufficient intake of iron and proteins and thus a risk of anemia (Albina et al. 1988). Although low serum iron and ferritin levels are currently observed after gastroplasty (Kolanowski 1995), usually no fall in hemoglobin level or in the number of red blood cells ocurrs.

Thiamine deficiency, with neurological sequelae, may also occur (Albina et al. 1988; Seehra et al. 1996), especially in subjects suffering from intractable vomiting. If intravenous glucose is administered, it may exacerbate the problem by increasing demand for thiamine (Seehra et al. 1996). Aside from these nutritional deficiencies a variable degree of dehydration (Shikora et al. 1994) may occur, particularly during the first weeks after surgery as a result of vomiting and restricted fluid intake.

Nutritional deficiencies are much more frequent after gastric bypass than after purely restrictive procedures (Mason and Doherty 1993; Shikora et al. 1994) because the duodenum — the site of iron and calcium absorption — is bypassed. As well as iron and calcium depletion, low serum vitamin B12 and vitamin B1 (thiamine) concentrations are more frequently seen after gastric bypass than following simple gastric partitioning procedures (Albina et al. 1988; Sugerman et al. 1996; Rhode et al. 1996). These nutritional deficiencies are even more frequent and serious after the biliopancreatic diversion, which bypasses not only the duodenum but also a large proportion of the small bowel (Scopinaro et al. 1996). The excluded limbs are much longer following this type of surgery and, in addition, a large part of the stomach is removed, which may indirectly affect iron and vitamin B12 absorption by the intestine.

Obviously, this procedure increases the risk of protein, mineral, and vitamin deficiencies considerably, a risk further aggravated by a tendency to develop chronic diarrhea (Shikora et al. 1994; Scopinaro et al. 1996). Indeed, protein malnutrition is observed in 5 to 12% of patients who undergo this surgery, most of them developing at the same time iron, calcium, and vitamin deficiencies that occur in 35% of patients (Scopinaro et al. 1996). To prevent the serious risk of malnutrition, especially anemia and bone demineralization, patients should be supplemented early after the surgery with iron and calcium as well as with vitamins B1 and B12.

Nutritional supplementation after gastric bypass procedures, and especially after biliopancreatic diversion, is therefore mandatory. The risk of peripheral neuropathy and Wernicke's encephalopathy (Albina et al. 1988; Seehra et al. 1996) can be prevented by supplementation with vitamin B1. To avoid calcium depletion and osteoporosis, a daily supplement of 2 g calcium, as well as monthly injection of 400,000 IU vitamin D, is recommended (Scopinaro et al. 1966). Despite these preventive measures, 7% of patients undergoing this surgical treatment develop bone demineralization, usually between the second and fifth postoperative years (Salmon and McArdle 1992). Because vitamin B12, in its protein-bound form, is poorly absorbed in these patients, a daily oral administration of 300 to 500 µg crystalline form of vitamin B12 has been recommended (Rhode et al. 1996; Sugerman et al. 1996). Monthly vitamin B12 injections may be substituted for oral administration.

In addition to nutritional deficiencies, the restrictive eating behavior and marked weight loss that occur after gastric surgery may lead exceptionally to anorexia nervosa (Boone et al. 1996). This complication may occur despite a careful psychiatric assessment prior to bariatric surgery. It is, in general, considered that the preoperative evaluation of psychiatric status is of little value in predicting the magnitude of weight loss after gastric restriction (Stunkard 1996; Hsu et al. 1996). Although the gastric procedures are successful in producing weight loss, they do not change abnormalities of eating behavior that existed before surgery (Sagar 1995; Hsu et al. 1996). Indeed, the gastric surgery does not attenuate disturbances of eating behavior, such as bulimia nervosa or "night eating syndrome."

This is important because individuals who crave sweets and consume large quantities of soft foods and sweet liquids may not lose weight satisfactorily after gastric partition or gastric bypass procedures. It should be stressed that co-morbid psychiatric disorders are not improved by weight-reduction surgery, despite the usual substantial improvement in psychosocial functioning (Kral 1992; Hsu et al. 1996; Brolin 2002). This clearly indicates that patients undergoing bariatric surgery should be followed closely from a psychological, or even psychiatric, standpoint for several years after the operation. Nevertheless, psychologists or psychiatrists cannot predict reliably whether dietary compliance will improve or deteriorate after surgery.

21.5 General Conclusions and Indications for Gastric Surgery

When properly conducted conservative approaches fail to produce significant weight reduction, gastric restriction procedures, such as vertical banded gastroplasty or gastric banding, as well as gastric bypass, represent an appropriate, and sometimes the only effective, therapy for patients suffering from morbid obesity. Less severely obese patients may also be considered for surgical treatment, if they suffer from significant co-morbidity.

The choice of procedure is important. According to current opinion, patients who consume large amounts of sugars or carbohydrates are more suited to gastric bypass, because symptoms of dumping may be important in contributing to a drastic reduction of energy intake. In contrast, in so called "big eaters," the gastric partition procedure, which induces an early satiety even after a small meal, seems to be a preferred surgical option. The gastric binding procedure is, however, contraindicated in patients with severe abnormalities of eating behavior, such as binge eating disorders, and in those suffering from the hiatal hernia.

The impressive loss of weight that follows gastric surgery is in general well tolerated and associated with a considerable improvement or even disappearance of many co-morbid conditions, such as hypertension; respiratory and cardiac dysfunction; abnormal serum lipid profile; glucose intolerance; and type 2 diabetes. Gastric surgery may be proposed as treatment for obesity if the following criteria are fulfilled:

- The patient should be morbidly obese with a body mass index (BMI) above 40 kg/m^2, and aged from 18 to 55 years.
- The patient with a BMI between 35 and 40 kg/m^2 may also be considered for gastric surgery if serious obesity-associated co-morbidities are present.
- Obesity should have been present for at least 5 years, and be refractory to several attempts at reducing weight by nonsurgical methods.
- There should be no history of alcoholism or major psychiatric disorders.

If the patients are appropriately selected according to these criteria, and if the existence of abnormalities of eating behavior is taken into account, gastric surgery may represent the only efficient treatment of severe obesity and of its health-threatening complications.

References

Agren, G., Narbro, K., Jonsson, E. et al. (2002a) Cost of in-patient care over 7 years among surgically and conventionally treated obese patients, *Obes. Res.*, 10: 1276–1283.

Agren, G., Narbro, K., Naslund, I. et al. (2002b) Long-term effects of weight loss on pharmaceutical costs in obese subjects. A report from the SOS intervention study, *Int. J. Obes.*, 26: 184–192.

Albina, J.E., Stone, W.M., Bates, M. and Felder, M.E. (1988) Catastrophic weight loss after vertical banded gastroplasty: malnutrition and neurological alterations, *J. Parenteral Nutr.*, 12: 619–620.

Alpert, M.A., Terry, B.E., Lambert, C.R. et al. (1993) Factors influencing left ventricular systolic function in non hypertensive morbidly obese patients, and effect of weight loss induced by gastroplasty, *Am. J. Cardiol.*, 71: 733–737.

Arcila, D., Velazquez, D., Gamino, R. et al. (2002) Quality of life in bariatric surgery, *Obes. Surg.*, 12: 661–665.

Ashley, S., Bird, D.L., Sugden, G. and Royston, C.M. (1993) Vertical banded gastroplasty for the treatment of morbid obesity, *Br. J. Surg.*, 80: 1421–1423.

Blachar, A., Federle, M.P., Pealer, K.M. et al. (2002) Gastrointestinal complications of laparoscopic Roux-en-Y gastric bypass surgery: clinical and imaging findings, *Radiology*, 223: 625–632.

Boone, O.B., Bashi, R. and Berry, E.M. (1996) Anorexia nervosa following gastroplasty in the male: two cases, *Int. J. Eating Disorders*, 19: 105–108.

Braley, S.C., Nguyen, N.T. and Wolfe, B.M. (2002) Late gastrointestinal hemorrhage after gastric bypass, *Obes. Surg.*, 12: 404–407.

Brolin, R.E. (2002) Bariatric surgery and long-term control of morbid obesity, *JAMA*, 288: 2793–2796.

Buchwald, H. and Buchwald, J.N. (2002) Evolution of operative procedures for the management of morbid obesity 1950–2000, *Obes. Surg.*, 12: 705–717.

Burnstein, R., Epstein, Y., Charuzi, I. et al. (1995) Glucose utilization in morbidly obese subjects before and after weight loss by gastric bypass operation, *Int. J. Obes.*, 19: 558–561.

Busetto, L., Tregnaghi, A., De Marchi, F. et al. (2002) Liver volume and visceral obesity in women with hepatic steatosis undergoing gastric banding, *Obes. Res.*, 10: 408–411.

Cadiere, G.B., Himpens, J., Hainaux, B. et al. (2002) Laparoscopic adjustable gastric banding, *Semin. Laparosc. Surg.*, 9: 105–114.

Carson, J.L., Ruddy, M.E., Duff, A.E. et al. (1994) The effect of gastric bypass surgery on hypertension in morbidly obese patients, *Arch. Intern. Med.*, 154: 193–200.

Cummings, D.E., Weigle, D.S., Frayo, R.S. et al. (2002) Plasma ghrelin levels after diet-induced weight loss or gastric bypass surgery, *N. Engl. J. Med.*, 346: 1623–1630.

Deitel, M. and Shikora, S.A. (2002) The development of the surgical treatment of morbid obesity, *J. Am. Coll. Nutr.*, 21: 365–371.

DeMaria, E.J., Sugerman, H.J., and Meador, J.G. (2001) High failure rate after laparoscopic adjustable silicone gastric binding for treatment of morbid obesity, *Ann. Surg.*, 233: 809–818.

DeMaria, E.J., Sugerman, H.J., Kellum, J.M. et al. (2002) Results of 281 consecutive total laparoscopic Roux-en-Y gastric bypasses to treat morbid obesity, *Ann. Surg.*, 235: 640–645.

Dixon, J.B. and O'Brien, P.E. (2002) Health outcomes of severely obese type 2 diabetic subjects 1 year after laparascopic adjustable gastric binding, *Diabetes Care*, 25: 358–363.

Doherty, C., Maher, J.W., and Heitshusen, D.S. (2002) Long-term data indicate a progressive loss in efficacy of adjustable silicone gastric banding for the surgical treatment of morbid obesity, *Surgery*, 132: 724–727.

Evans, J.D., Scott, M.H., Brown, A.S. and Rogers, J. (2002) Laparoscopic adjustable gastric banding for the treatment of morbid obesity, *Am. J. Surg.*, 184: 97–102.

Favretti, F., Cadiere, G.B., Segato, G. et al. (2002) Laparoscopic binding: selection and technique in 830 patients, *Obes. Surg.*, 12: 385–390.

Feng, J.J. and Gagner, M. (2002) Laparoscopic biliopancreatic diversion with duodenal switch, *Semin. Laparosc. Surg.*, 9: 125–129.

Foley, E.F., Benotti, P.N., Borlace, B.C. et al. (1992) Impact of gastric restrictive surgery on hypertension in the morbidly obese, *Am. J. Surg.*, 163: 294–297.

Gleysteen, J.J. (1992) Results of surgery: long term effects on hyperlipidemia, *Am. J. Clin. Nutr.*, 55 (Suppl.): 591S–593S.

Goldner, W.S., O'Dorisio, T.M., Dillon, J.S. and Mason, E.E. (2002) Severe metabolic bone disease as a long-term complication of obesity surgery, *Obes. Surg.*, 12: 685–692.

Greenway, S.E., Greenway, F.L., III, and Klein, S. (2002) Effects of obesity surgery on non-insulin-dependent diabetes mellitus, *Arch. Surg.*, 137: 1109–1117.

Gustavsson, S. and Westling, A. (2002) Laparoscopic adjustable gastric banding: complications and side effects responsible for the poor long-term outcome, *Semin. Laparosc. Surg.*, 9: 115–124.

Hess, D.S. and Hess, D.W. (1998) Biliopancreatic diversion with duodenal switch, *Obes. Surg.*, 8: 267–282.

Holzwarth, R., Huber, D., Majkrzak, A. and Tareen, B. (2002) Outcome of gastric bypass patients, *Obes. Surg.,* 12: 261–264.

Hsu, L.K.D., Betancourt, S. and Sullivan, S.P. (1996) Eating disturbances before and after vertical banded gastroplasty: a pilot study, *Int. J. Eating Disorders,* 19: 23–34.

Huerta, S., Rogers, L.M., Li, Z. et al. (2002) Vitamin A deficiency in a newborn resulting from maternal hypovitaminosis A after biliopancreatic diversion for treatment of morbid obesity, *Am. J. Clin. Nutr.,* 76: 426–429.

Kim, C.H. and Sarr, M.G. (1992) Severe reflux esophagitis after vertical banded gastroplasty for treatment of morbid obesity, *Mayo Clin. Proc.,* 67: 33–35.

Klockhoff, H., Naslund, I. and Jones, A.W. (2002) Faster absorption of ethanol and higher peak concentration in women after gastric bypass surgery, *Br. J. Clin. Pharmacol.,* 54: 587–591.

Kolanowski, J. (1995) Gatsroplasty for morbid obesity: the internist's view, *Int. J. Obes.,* 19 (Suppl. 3): S61–S65.

Kolanowski, J. (1997) Surgical treatment for morbid obesity, *Br. Med. Bull.,* 53: 433–444.

Kolanowski J. and Martinelli, M. (1996) Changes in body composition and in energy expenditure after gastroplasty in morbidly obese patients, *Int. J. Obes.,* 20 (Suppl. 4): 134.

Kothari, S.N., DeMaria, E.J., Sugerman, H.J. et al. (2002) Lap-band failures: conversion to gastric bypass and their preliminary outcomes, *Surgery,* 131: 625–629.

Kral, J.G. (1992) Overview of surgical techniques for treating obesity, *Am. J. Clin. Nutr.,* 55 (Suppl.): 552S–555S.

Kuzmak L.I. (1989) Gastric binding, in M. Dietel (Ed.), *Surgery for the Morbidly Obese Patients,* p. 225, Philadelphia: Lea & Febiger.

Livingston, E.H. (2002) Obesity and its surgical management, *Am. J. Surg.,* 184: 103–113.

Livingston, E.H., Huerta, S., Arthur, D. et al. (2002) Male gender is a predictor of morbidity and age a predictor of mortality for patients undergoing gastric bypass surgery, *Ann. Surg.,* 236: 576–582.

Lönroth, H., Dalenbäck, J., Haglind, E. et al. (1996) Vertical banded gastroplasty by laparoscopic technique in the treatment of morbid obesity, *Surg. Laparoscopy Endoscopy,* 6: 102–107.

Mason, E.E. (1982) Vertical banded gastroplasty for obesity, *Arch. Surg.,* 117: 701–706.

Mason, E.E. (1996) Editorial comments, *Am. J. Surg.,* 171: 267–269.

Mason, E.E. and Doherty, C. (1993) Surgery, in A.J. Stunkard and T.A. Wadden (Eds.) *Obesity, Theory and Therapy* (pp. 313–325), New York: Raven.

McGinnis, J.M. and Foege, W.H. (1993) Actual causes of death in the United States, *JAMA,* 270: 2207–2212.

McLean, L.D., Rhode, B.M. and Forse, R.A. (1990) Late results of vertical banded gastroplasty for morbid and super obesity, *Surgery,* 107: 20–27.

Melinek, J., Livingston E., Cortina, G. and Fishbein, M.C. Autopsy findings following gastric bypass surgery for morbid obesity, *Arch. Pathol. Lab. Med.,* 126: 1091–1095.

Mittermair, R.P., Weiss, H., Nehoda, H. and Aigner, F. (2002) Uncommon intragastric migration of the Swedish adjustable gastric band, *Obes. Surg.,* 12: 372–375.

NIH Consensus Development Conference Panel (1991) Gastrointestinal surgery for severe obesity, *Ann. Intern. Med.,* 115: 956–961.

NIH Consensus Development Conference Statement (1992) Editorial: gastrointestinal surgery for severe obesity, *Am. J. Clin. Nutr.,* 55 (Suppl.): 615S–619S.

Pamuk, E.R., Willamson, D.F., Serdula, M.K. et al. (1993), Weight loss and subsequent death in a cohort of U.S. adults, *Ann. Intern. Med.,* 119: 744–748.

Pontiroli, A.E., Pizzocri, P., Librenti, M.C. et al. (2002) Laparoscopic adjustable gastric banding for the treatment of morbid (grade 3) obesity and its metabolic complications: a three-year study, *J. Clin. Endocrinol. Metab.,* 87: 3555–3561.

Rand, C.S.W. and Macgregor, A.M.C. (1991) Successful weight loss following obesity surgery and perceived liability of morbid obesity, *Int. J. Obes.,* 15: 577–579.

Reinhold, R.B. (1994) Late results of gastric bypass surgery for morbid obesity, *J. Am. Coll. Nutr.,* 13: 326–331.

Rhode, B.M., Arsenau, P., Cooper, B.A. et al. (1996) Vitamin B-12 deficiency after gastric surgery for obesity, *Am. J. Clin. Nutr.,* 63: 103–109.

Rubenstein, R.B. (2002) Laparoscopic adjustable gastric banding at a U.S. center with up to 3-year follow-up, *Obes. Surg.,* 12: 380–384.

Rubino, F. and Gagner, M. (2002) Potential of surgery for curing type 2 diabetes mellitus, *Ann. Surg.,* 236: 554–559.

Sagar, P.M. (1995) Surgical treatment of morbid obesity, *Br. J. Surg.,* 82: 732–739.

Salmon, P.A. and McArdle, M.O. (1992) The rationale and results of gastroplasty/distal gastric bypass, *Obes. Surg.,* 2: 61–68.

Scopinaro, N., Gianetta, E., Adami, G.F. et al. (1996) Biliopancreatic diversion for obesity at eighteen years, *Surgery,* 119: 261–268.

Scopinaro, N., Marinari, G.M. and Camerini, G. (2002) Laparoscopic standard biliopancreatic diversion: technique and preliminary results, *Obes. Surg.,* 12: 362–365.

Seehra, H., MacDermott, N., Lascelles, R.G. and Taylor, T.V. (1996) Wernicke's encephalopathy after vertical banded gastroplasty: malnutrition and neurological alterations, *BMJ,* 312: 434.

Shikora, S.A., Benotti, P.N. and Forse, R.A. (1994) Surgical treatment of obesity, in G.L. Blacburn and B.S. Kanders (Eds.) *Obesity, Pathophysiology, Psychology and Treatment* (pp. 264–282), New York: Chapman & Hall.

Sjöström, L. (1992) Morbidity of severely obese subjects, *Am. J. Clin. Nutr.,* 55 (Suppl.): 508S–515S.

Stunkard, A.J. (1996) Current views on obesity, *Am. J. Med.,* 100: 230–236.

Sugerman, H.J. (2002) Gastric bypass surgery for severe obesity, *Semin. Laparosc. Surg.,* 9: 79–85.

Sugerman, H.J., Kellum, J.M., De Maria, E.J., and Reines, H.D. (1996) Conversion of failed or complicated vertical banded gastroplasty to gastric bypass in morbid obesity, *Am. J. Surg.,* 171: 263–267.

Sundbom, M., Hedenstrom, H. and Gustavsson, S. (2002) Duodenogastric bile reflux after gastric bypass: a cholescintigraphic study, *Dig. Dis. Sci.,* 47: 1891–1896.

Torgerson, J.S. and Sjöström, L. (2001) The Swedish Obese Subjects (SOS) study — rationale and results, *Int. J. Obes.,* 25 (Suppl. 1): S2–S4.

Wolff, S., Pross, M., Knippig, C. et al. (2002) Gastric pacing. A new method in obesity surgery, *Obes. Surg.,* 73: 700–703.

22

Efficacy of Different Antiobesity Interventions

Rolf Stöckli and Ulrich Keller

CONTENTS

22.1 Introduction

Obesity is one of the major public health problems worldwide. Its incidence and prevalence are increasing, especially in the Second and Third Worlds, despite numerous therapeutic and preventive attempts. The prevalence of obesity in Europe ranges from 7 and 14% in France and Sweden to up to 40% in Eastern European countries; in the U.S., about 33% of adults are overweight (BMI 25.0 to 29.9 kg/m²) and 31% are obese (BMI > 30 kg/m²).[1,2] Also, less developed countries in Central and South America demonstrate that obesity is becoming a major health problem: in Brazil, the number of obese male subjects has doubled in the last 15 years; in Mexico and Peru, overweight has a prevalence of 50 and 30%, respectively.[3,4] The costs caused directly and indirectly by obesity are about 8% of total health care expenses in industrialized countries.[5,6]

Treatment of obesity remains a difficult and unsatisfactory task. Many individuals are eagerly looking for remedies for their weight problems; due to the symptoms of overweight and the pressure of the society, often they are prepared to spend large sums of money for desperate and worthless treatments. As a result, there is a growing obesity "industry" with a volume of several billion dollars (U.S.) each year. Most of the treatments offered by these institutions are not scientifically sound, usually not efficient, and sometimes even dangerous. Therefore, it is of major importance to assess the effectiveness of treatment modalities using stringent scientific criteria.

This chapter reviews the evidence of efficacy of various treatments of obesity by assessing trials that are randomized and controlled, corresponding to the principles of *evidence-based medicine*. It focuses on parameters like weight loss related to metabolic diseases such as diabetes mellitus type 2, dyslipidemia, and hypertension, as well as the complex called the *metabolic syndrome* — a condition that shows an alarming increase in prevalence.

22.2   Efficacy of Therapeutic Approaches to Obesity

Obesity is a chronic disease associated with a high morbidity and increased mortality. Many people, including medical staff and health authorities, do not consider obesity as a serious, self-inflicted problem, but as a consequence of poor will power and unstable behavior. Overweight subjects are often discriminated against; they can easily be recognized in the public or when applying for jobs. This leads often to frustration, negative body image, and withdrawal from social activities. A vicious circle begins with the failure of therapy, resignation, and regain of weight.

The main problem of many therapies is a regain of weight after ending the intervention, despite an initial weight loss. Many of these therapies are too restrictive and impair normal eating behavior. Eating disorders are frequently observed; up to 20% of obese patients suffer from binge eating disorder. According to some psychologists, the reason for this is in part due to unbalanced diets and the pressure of society to restrict eating.

No doubt exists about the risks of obesity for metabolic disorders, but uncertainty about the effectiveness of various forms of treatment is still considerable. An optimal therapy should be sustainable and even life long, if possible, because of the chronicity of the disease. Therapeutic options must be regarded critically, and as in other diseases, treatment should be based on the precept of *primum nil nocere* ("in the first place: do not harm"). An *ideal therapy* would lead to a lasting weight reduction by an approach without risks; however, despite many attempts, such a treatment does not exist.

The American National Institutes of Health (NIH) published an evidence report in 1999. This is a review of the scientific literature about the effectiveness of conservative therapies for obesity.[7] A total of 235 randomized and controlled studies were reviewed and their conclusions assessed. All recommendations for treatment were categorized by the level of evidence, based on the principles of evidence-based medicine:

- Level A — results are based on a substantial number of randomized, controlled studies involving substantial numbers of participants
- Level B — limited body of data, based on only a limited number of smaller randomized controlled trials
- Level C — results are based on uncontrolled and nonrandomized trials only
- Level D — clinical experience without the preceding criteria

22.2.1   Dietary Treatment

Any dietary approach aims to lower daily energy intake below energy expenditure; the latter can vary considerably and is influenced by multiple endogenous and exogenous

TABLE 22.1

Randomized Controlled Trials of Weight Reduction by Diet Alone: Effects on Weight and Lipids

Study	N; Sex; Duration	Weight Loss (%)	TG (%)	TC (%)	LDL-C (%)	HDL-C (%)
Dengel et al., 1995	28♂ intervention, 14♂ co 9 months	−12	−36	−9	−9	−3
Hellenius et al., 1993	40♂ intervention, 39♂ co 6 months	−2	−2	−1	−3	2
Jalkannen, 1991	24 intervention (weight), 22 intervention (lipid), 25 co (weight) 22 co (lipid); 12 months	−5	−28	−7	—	8
Karvetti and Hakala, 1992	71♀ intervention, 76♀ co, 12 months	−6	—	−2	—	12
	22♂ intervention, 20♂ co, 12 months	−11	—	0	—	27
Marniemi et al., 1990	37 (27♀/10♂) mixed diet, 42 (32♀ /10♂) co; 12 months	−13	−41	−4	—	18
	31 (23♀/8♂) lactovegetarian, 42 (32♀/10♂) co; 12 months	−11	−21	−4	—	10
Puddey et al., 1990	22♂ intervention, 20♂ co; 18 weeks	−8	−27	−7	—	9
Simkin–Silverman et al., 1990	253♀ intervention, 267♀ co; 6 months	−7	−11	−8	−9	4
Svendsen et al., 1994	50♀ intervention, 20♀ co; 12 weeks	−13	−44	−18	−22	3
Wood et al., 1991	40♂ intervention, 40♂ co; 12 months	−7	−21	−5	−5	6
	31♀ intervention, 39♀ co; 12 months	−7	−5	−7	−8	−7
Wood et al., 1988	42♂ intervention, 42♂ co; 12 months	−8	−22	−2	−3	13
Mean		**−8**	**−19**	**−6**	**−9**	**7**

TG = triglycerides; TC = total cholesterol; co = controls; — = not measured.

Source: The Evidence Report, NIH; National Heart, Lung and Blood Institute, Publication 1999.

factors. In any case, when intake is reduced below expenditure, the body will be forced to diminish its energy storage, in particular fat tissue.

The first step to change eating patterns is a precise analysis of the daily habits, best performed by recording a food diary. Reduction of energy intake is the basis of successful weight loss, especially by a decreased intake of fat and other energy-dense food (sweets, soft drinks, alcohol), if possible guided by a dietician. There is no evidence for long-lasting weight reduction by dietary counseling only. This can be achieved by a program containing behavior therapy and repeated consultations, if necessary including medical surveillance and support by a psychologist. Many commercially available diets are advertised in newspapers and magazines; however, a conclusion regarding of their efficacy is not possible because of lack of controlled studies. Consensus is that the first step in dietary treatment is a moderately restricted diet with a daily intake of at least 1200 kcal per day, resulting in slow weight reduction. In its evidence report, the NIH reviewed clinical guidelines based on interventions with a daily caloric intake of 1200 to 1500 kcal per day; their evidence was graded A because it was derived from large controlled studies of high quality.[8–17] The daily caloric deficit should be between 500 and 1000 kcal/day. Weight reduction in these studies was about 8% within 3 to 12 months (Table 22.1). Furthermore, a significant improvement in lipid metabolism could be shown: serum triglycerides decreased by a mean of 19%; total cholesterol by 6%; LDL-cholesterol by 9%; and HDL-cholesterol increased by 7%.

A more pronounced restriction of caloric intake (daily amount of 400 of 500 kcal) resulted in an initially greater weight loss, but did not produce better long-term effects.[18–20] Such aggressive therapies often increase the risk of a rebound ("yo-yo dieting") and may lead to a deficiency of micronutrients (vitamins, minerals, trace elements). The target is a reduction of excessive body fat; therefore, a weight loss achieved too quickly is not desirable because of a resulting catabolism of muscle and other lean tissue. So-called crash diets often result in more water excretion than fat loss and only affect a significant loss of fat mass.

There is also strong evidence concerning the quality of a diet. Restricting fat intake without limitation of total energy consumption is not effective. A review of trials comparing fat restriction with other weight-reducing dietary interventions did not show a greater weight loss with the former diet[21]; lipid profiles improved only slightly; and blood pressure remained unchanged. Recent studies comparing low-carbohydrate diets with low-fat diets in severely obese subjects with a high prevalence of the metabolic syndrome showed a greater weight loss by reducing carbohydrates rather than fat over 6 months[22,23]; however, no data of a follow-up longer than 1 year are available.

Low-fat diets without targeted caloric restriction help to promote weight loss by producing a reduced caloric intake[24,25]; furthermore, low-fat diets have been shown to help prevent cardiovascular diseases.[26] Low-fat diets (20 to 30% of calories from fat) coupled with total caloric reduction produce greater weight loss than low-fat diets alone.[27,28]

As a consequence, fat *and* carbohydrates should be restricted. There is a limiting point in these studies: the maximal length was 12 months and risk of relapse was high if the intense supervision was stopped.

22.2.2 Physical Activity

Physical exercise (regular aerobic training) resulted in a slight weight loss of about 2% (Table 22.2) and was effective for weight maintenance.[29] The lipid profile was influenced favorably: triglycerides decreased about 7%; total and LDL-cholesterol about 1%; and HDL-cholesterol increased about 1% (evidence level A).[9,30,31] The initial recommendation is an increased physical activity during 30 to 45 min, three to five times per week. In the long run, a daily workout or leisure-time physical activity of at least 30 min should be targeted. Patients should be encouraged for everyday activities, like walking instead of driving, climbing stairs instead of using the elevator, etc. A combination of dietary intervention and increased physical activity resulted in greater weight loss (mean = –8%) and improvement of lipid levels (triglycerides = –22%; total cholesterol = –8%; LDL-cholesterol = –10%; HDL-cholesterol = +4%) than any single intervention (Table 22.2, evidence level A).[9,15,16,32]

22.2.3 Behavior Therapy

A structured program based on cognitive behavior therapy is an effective form of treatment of obesity (evidence level B) by focusing on cognitive and emotional aspects, e.g., by improvement of self-confidence regarding body image and weight.[33–36] A main aim is to reach flexible control of eating behavior. There should be no prohibition of certain foods because this control would be too restrictive, with a high risk of relapse and of a yo-yo effect.

Further elements of cognitive behavior therapy should be emphasized, such as psychoeducational information about diet; problem-solving strategies; and restructuring of dysfunctional cognition regarding the body. The main accent is to limit counseling to what is really required to be known about nutrition and to focus on psychoeducative aspects;

TABLE 22.2

Randomized Controlled Trials of Physical Activity (pa) Alone and of Physical Activity Combined with Diet: Effect on Weight and Lipids

Study	N; sex; duration	Weight Loss %	TG (%)	TC (%)	LDL-C (%)	HDL-C (%)
Hellenius, et al., 1993	pa, 39♂ intervention, 39♂ co; 6 months	−2	−11	0	0	+2
King et al., 1991	pa, 40♂ high intensity group, 41♂ co; 12 months	−1	−6	—	+2	−1
	pa, 42♂ high intensity home, 41♂ co; 12 months	−1	0	—	−1	+1
	pa, 45♂ low intensity, 41♂ co, 12 months	−4	−14	—	0	+3
		+2	+1	—	−4	+1
	pa, 34♀, high intensity group, 34♀ co, 12 months	0	−2	—	+3	0
	pa, 35♀ high intensity home, 34♀ co, 12 months	−2	+4	—	+3	0
	pa, 29♀ low intensity, 34♀ co, 12 months					
Ronnemaa et al., 1988	pa; 13 (8♂, 5♀) intervention, 12 (7♂, 5♀) co; 4 months	−3	−3	−6	−5	+2
Mean	**Physical activity alone**	**−1.3**	**−7**	**−1.5**	**−1**	**+1**
Hellenius et al., 1993	Diet + pa, 39♂ intervention, 39♂ co; 6 months	−4	−12	−5	−4	−1
Schuler et al., 1992	Diet + pa, 56♂ intervention, 57♂ co, 12 months	−5	−7	−10	−10	+3
Svendsen et al., 1994	Diet + pa, 48♀ intervention, 20♀ co, 12 weeks	−14	−35	−17	−26	0
Wood et al., 1991	Diet + pa, 39♂ intervention, 40♂ co, 12 months	−11	−46	−4	−2	+17
	Diet + pa, 42♀ intervention, 39♀ co, 12 months	−9	−18	−5	−8	5
Mean	**Diet and physical activity**	**−8**	**−22**	**−8**	**−10**	**4**

extensive knowledge of nutrition is not necessary. Enjoyable and playful elements facilitate the analysis of each person's eating and drinking behavior.

A psychoeducational approach is based on six elements (Table 22.3). Each of them should be addressed and implemented stepwise. The cognitive and emotional changes should support the patients to react to emotions differently than by eating; to look for positive thoughts; to pay attention to negative thoughts during the meals; and to put them into proper relations in order to adapt and rate them. The following points should be discussed during therapy: avoiding thinking in a "black or white" pattern, and omitting categorical statements of incorrect generalizations and of under- and overestimation. Generally, too restrictive measures (prohibitions) should be avoided because of the high risk of relapse. Systematic self-monitoring and observation is an essential aid (among others, by writing a food diary). Chain reactions triggered by negative emotions can thereby be detected and finally interrupted.

22.2.4 Integrated Programs

The most promising approach is a combination of the preceding three factors (nutrition, physical activity, behavior) in an integrated, psychoeducative program. This principle is more effective than single components alone or combinations of two of them (evidence level A). Body weight may be reduced and stabilized by long-term changes of eating habits, by improved knowledge, and by increased physical activity.

TABLE 22.3

Six Elements of a Behavioral Weight Loss Program

	Aims of Treatment	Intervention
1. Motivation and support	Development of long-term motivation and compliance	Psychoeducation; setting realistic aims for: weight; nutrition; eating habits; and increasing physical activity
2. Nutritional behavior	Long-term change to a balanced, fat-reduced nutrition	Psychoeducation; self-observation; gradual substitution for fat- and calorie-rich food with a more balanced nutrition
3. Eating habits	Reduction of rigid control; development of flexible control	Psychoeducation; self-observation; practicing more flexible control
4. Physical activity	Changing the passive life-style, stepwise, long-term increase in daily activity, sport	Psychoeducation; increasing and maintaining motivation
5. Social skills	Reduction of isolation and retreat; development of social skills	Psychoeducation; practicing social competence and self-confidence; problem-solving training
6. Body image	Improving the negative body image	Psychoeducation; self-observation; body image exercises

22.2.5   Pharmacotherapy

Most authorities recommend using drugs only for treatment of selected subjects; during a limited time; and in combination with nonpharmacological therapy, mainly because of a lack of long-term studies and of trials with data reporting "difficult" end points. Only two drugs have been studied in large randomized controlled trials and are approved by major health authorities (e.g., FDA).

Orlistat reduces fat absorption in the small intestine about 30% by inhibiting reversibly pancreatic lipase, which leads to undigested triglycerides. Orlistat in a combination with a dietary intervention resulted in weight loss up to 8% after 1 year.[37] LDL-cholesterol, blood glucose, and systolic blood pressure were also lowered significantly.[38–40] As a consequence, orlistat is effective in treatment of the metabolic syndrome. Possible side effects were related to maldigestion of consumed fat and were more or less mild and transient. They consisted of oily evacuation and spotting; flatus with discharge; increased defecation; and fecal incontinence.

Sibutramine is a centrally acting substance reducing appetite by inhibiting the reuptake of norepinephrine, serotonin, and dopamine via liver-generated primary and secondary metabolites. A weight reduction of 4.8 kg was achieved after 1 year of treatment with sibutramine[41] (evidence level A). Sibutramine can increase systolic and diastolic blood pressure; other possible side effects are nervousness, sleep disturbances, and dry mouth.

Other drugs are currently not recommended because their safety has not been established, e.g., dexfenfluramine, phentermine, and fenfluramine have been withdrawn from the market because of cardiac abnormalities and an increased risk of pulmonary hypertension.[42]

22.2.6   Surgical Interventions

Bariatric surgery, especially laparoscopically placed adjustable gastric banding, has become very popular despite missing long-term data over more than 8 years. Subjects with morbid obesity (BMI > 40 kg/m^2) are usually considered to be candidates for a surgical intervention. The presence of a binge eating disorder is a relative contraindication for adjustable gastric banding because of a high incidence of complications like pseudoachalasia and dysfunction of esophageal motility.

The most frequently performed surgical interventions are adjustable gastric banding and gastric bypass; both result in substantial weight loss. After 3 years, excess body weight was reduced by about 60% after adjustable gastric banding[43–45]; after gastric bypass, weight reduction was even larger.[46–48] An observation 8 years after laparoscopic gastric banding demonstrated a mean excess weight loss of 59%.[49] Currently, bariatric surgery offers the most effective treatment of obesity and produces sustained weight loss in morbidly obese subjects.

The ultimate goal of bariatric surgery is to improve obesity-related medical complications. An improvement of insulin resistance, of the acute insulin response to glucose, or of diabetes mellitus type 2 after weight reduction surgery has been reported.[50–52] Significant decreases in serum cholesterol and triglyceride levels have been observed after successful bariatric operations.[53,54] Another trial showed an improvement in blood pressure after 2 years, but no differences after a follow-up of 8 years compared to conventional treatment with smaller weight loss.[55] Furthermore, a marked improvement or resolution of the obesity-hypoventilation syndrome and sleep apnea has been reported.[56,57] In women an improvement of menstrual irregularity, infertility, and urinary stress incontinence has been demonstrated.[58,59] Weight loss resulting from bariatric surgery has been associated with significant improvement of left ventricular ejection fraction and with a decreased mean blood pressure[60,61]; cardiac chamber size and ventricular wall thickness diminished.[62]

22.3 Efficacy of Nonpharmacological Antiobesity Interventions to Diminish the Metabolic Syndrome

22.3.1 Pathophysiology of the Metabolic Syndrome

Overweight and obesity increase overall morbidity and mortality, mainly by increasing the risk of the metabolic syndrome.[63–65] Weight gain, visceral obesity, and insulin resistance, the cardinal features of the metabolic syndrome, are closely associated.[65,66] Central obesity characterized by an increased waist to hip circumference ratio (WHR) is especially associated with a high risk of metabolic complications.[67] The mechanisms for the development of insulin resistance are complex and not fully understood; adipose tissue plays a key role as an endocrine organ. Adipocytes secrete not only fatty acids but also numerous hormone-like substances (adipocytokines) that contribute to peripheral insulin resistance; plasma adiponectin concentrations are decreased in the metabolic syndrome, whereas expression of interleukin 6 and TNF-α is upregulated in adipose tissue of obese subjects. Free fatty acids released from adipose tissue are involved by blocking intracellular metabolism of glucose. Multiple prospective studies have shown the increased risk of diabetes mellitus type 2 as weight increases.[68] A higher risk for diabetes has been found even when BMI increases from as low as 22 kg/m² to modest overweight.[69]

Dyslipidemia of obesity with predominant abdominal fat distribution[70] is characterized by high serum triglycerides[71]; low HDL-cholesterol levels[72]; and a shift of LDL-cholesterol to small, dense LDL-particles, which are more atherogenic than larger LDL, in part because of an impairment of receptor affinity.[73] Furthermore, strong data are available that demonstrate that the age-adjusted prevalence of hypertension increases progressively with increasing BMI in men and women.[2,74] The pathophysiological explanations for development of hypertension are, among other factors, sodium retention and an increase in vascular resistance, in blood volume and cardiac output. These alterations are reversed by weight loss, resulting in reduced sympathetic nervous system activity and suppression of the renin–angiotensin–aldosterone system.[75–79]

Obesity is also a risk factor for the development of coronary heart disease and congestive heart failure,[80,81] resulting in increased morbidity and mortality.[82,83] Furthermore, there is an increased risk of stroke[84]; gallstones[85]; osteoarthritis[86]; sleep apnea[87]; and cancer (colon, breast, endometrial, gallbladder).[88–91] Death rates from all cancers were shown to be increased by 52% in men and by 62% in women with a BMI of >40 kg/m^2 as compared to subjects with normal weight.[92] So far, no evidence indicates that an intended weight reduction can reduce the risk of cancer.

22.3.2 Efficacy of Life-Style Interventions to Prevent Type 2 Diabetes and to Treat Hypertension

Successful therapy of obesity not only reduces body weight, but also improves its metabolic consequences and even prevents secondary disorders. Intentional weight loss has been associated with lower all-cause mortality.[93,94] In obese subjects with impaired glucose tolerance and a high risk for the development of diabetes mellitus type 2, the Finnish Diabetes Prevention Study demonstrated that body weight was reduced by about 4 kg within 2 years with an integrated life-style change program aimed at reducing weight, intake of total fat and of saturated fat, and increasing physical activity.[95] After 4 years of follow-up, the cumulative incidence of diabetes mellitus was 11% in the intervention group and 23% in the control group, respectively, resulting in a relative risk reduction of 58%. Blood pressure (systolic and diastolic) and serum triglycerides were reduced as well.

A similar program with life-style intervention in a large number of high-risk subjects in the U.S. (Diabetes Prevention Program) over 2.8 years showed also a risk reduction for diabetes of 58%.[96] Furthermore, the Da Quing study demonstrated a reduction of the incidence of diabetes mellitus from 67 to 41% in subjects with impaired glucose tolerance using a life-style intervention.[97] These studies provided convincing evidence that even in high-risk individuals, diabetes can be prevented (Table 22.4) — an enormous opportunity and challenge for health care systems.

Effective lowering of high blood pressure has been shown by using a program with changes in diet and increased physical activity.[98–100] In patients with stage 1 hypertension (120 to 159 mm Hg systolic and 80 to 95 mm Hg diastolic), a program containing behavioral intervention with established recommendations and a "DASH diet" (reduced dietary sodium and red meat and increased fruit, vegetable, and dairy consumption) reduced systolic blood pressure by 11 mm Hg and diastolic blood pressure by 6.5 mm Hg.[101]

22.4 Summary and Outlook

Sedentary lifestyle and excessive calorie consumption are the main risk factors for the development of obesity and its increasing prevalence. Because obesity manifests itself earlier and earlier in life, more attention should be directed to primary prevention, especially in children and adolescents. With respect to social and psychological environment, the target of these measures is to reduce energy consumed by food and to establish daily physical activity. The concept of treatment of obesity is a lasting change of life-style (eating, physical activity). A program with a combination of dietary counseling, increased physical

TABLE 22.4

Prevention of Diabetes Mellitus Type 2 by Changes in Life-Style

Author and Name of Program	Subjects	Intervention	Outcome
Nathan et al. Diabetes prevention program [96]	3234 obese Impaired fasting glucose or impaired glucose tolerance	Placebo vs. metformin 2× 850 mg vs. life-style modification Psychoeducative program; restriction of fat; physical activity > 150 min/week	Incidence of diabetes 11.0% (placebo) vs. 7.8% (metformin) vs. 4.8% (life-style) Risk reduction 58% by life-style program
Tuomilehto et al., 2001 Finnish Diabetes Prevention Study	522 Impaired glucose tolerance	Life-style intervention; individual counseling; fat < 30% of total energy uptake; physical activity 30 min/day	Reduction of incidence of diabetes: 58%; weight reduction 4.2 kg in the first year
Pan et al., 1997 Da Quing Study	577 Impaired glucose tolerance	Controls vs. diet vs. physical activity vs. diet and activity over 6 years	Incidence of diabetes 67.7% (controls) vs. 43.8% (diet) vs. 41.1% (physical activity) vs. 46.0% (diet and pa)

activity, and psychoeducation results in the best long-term results, especially regarding prevention of metabolic complications.

The increasing incidence and earlier manifestation of diabetes mellitus type 2 represents a major health problem; the chronic complications of diabetes will increase in the future with enormous costs for health care systems unless preventive measures are taking effect. Morbidly obese subjects should be evaluated by a specialist, and after failure of a conservative approach, surgical intervention such as gastric bypass should be envisaged. Although these procedures may carry certain risks and are not free of relapse, they are at present the most effective way for weight reduction, regarding amount and duration of weight loss. It is unjustified that, in several industrialized countries (including the U.S.) many insurers are not willing to pay for them.

References

1. Kuczmarski, R.J., M.D. Carroll, K.M. Flegal, and R.P. Troiano, Varying body mass index cut-off points to describe overweight prevalence among U.S. adults: NHANES III (1988 to 1994), *Obes. Res.* 5, 1997, 542–548.
2. Flegal, K.M., Carroll, M.D., Ogden, C.L. et al. Prevalence and trends in obesity among US adults, 1999–2000. *JAMA* 288, 2002, 1723–1727.
3. Seidel, J.C., Time trends in obesity: an epidemiologic perspective, *Horm. Metab. Res.* 29, 1997, 155–215.
4. Popkin, B.M. and C.M. Doak, The obesity epidemic is a world-wide phenomenon, *Nutr. Rev.* 56, 1998, 106–114.
5. WHO Obesity, Preventing and managing the global epidemic, 1997, WHO Publication, Geneva.
6. Wolf, A.M. and G.A. Colditz, Current estimates of the economic costs of obesity in the United States, *Obes. Res.* 6, 1998, 97–106.
7. The Evidence Report, NIH; National Heart, Lung and Blood Institute, Publication 1999.
8. Dengel, J.L., L.I. Katzel, and A.P. Goldberg, Effect of an American Heart Association diet, with or without weight loss, on lipids in obese middle-aged and older men, *Am. J. Clin. Nutr.* 62, 1995, 715–721.

9. Hellenius, M.L., U. de Faire, B. Berglund, A. Hamsten, and I. Krakau, Diet and exercise are equally effective in reducing risk for cardiovascular disease. Results of a randomized controlled study in men with slightly to moderate raised cardiovascular risk factors, *Atherosclerosis* 103, 1993, 81–91.

10. Jalkannen, L., The effect of a weight reduction program on cardiovascular risk factors among overweight hypertensives in primary health care, *Scand. J. Sci. Med.* 19, 1991, 66–71.

11. Karvetti, R.L. and P. Hakala, A 7-year follow up of a weight reduction programme in Finnish primary health care, *Eur. J. Clin. Nutr.* 46, 1992, 743–752.

12. Marniemi, J., A. Seppanen, and P. Hakala, Long-term effects on lipid metabolism of weight reduction on lactovegetarian and mixed diet, *Int. J. Obes.* 14, 1990, 113–125.

13. Puddey, I.B., M. Parker, L.J. Beilin, R. Vandongen, and J.R. Masarei, Effects of alcohol and caloric restrictions on blood pressure and serum lipids in overweight men, *Hypertension* 20, 1992, 533–541.

14. Simkin–Silverman, L., R.R. Win, D.H. Hansen et al., Prevention of cardiovascular risk factor elevations in healthy premenopausal women, *Prev. Med.* 24, 1995, 509–517.

15. Svendsen, O.L., C. Hassager, and C. Christiansen, Six months follow up on exercise added to a short-term diet in overweight postmenopausal women — effects on body composition, resting metabolic rate, cardiovascular risk factors and bone, *Int. J. Obes. Relat. Metab. Disord.* 18, 1994, 692–698.

16. Wood, P.D., M.L. Stefanick, P.T. Williams, and W.L. Haskell, The effects on plasma lipoproteins of a prudent weight-reducing diet, with or without exercise, in overweight men and women, *N. Engl. J. Med.* 325, 1991, 461–466.

17. Wood, P.D., M.L. Stefanick, D.M. Dreon et al., Changes in plasma lipids and lipoproteins in overweight men during weight loss through dieting as compared with exercise, *N. Engl. J. Med.* 319, 1988, 1173–1179.

18. Wadden, T.A., J.A. Sternberg, K.A. Letizia, A.J. Stunkard, and G.D. Foster, Treatment of obesity by very low calorie diet, behavior therapy, and their combination: a five-year perspective, *Int. J. Obes.* 13 (Suppl 2), 1989, 39–46.

19. Wadden, T.A., G.D. Foster, and K.A. Letizia, One-year behavior treatment of obesity: comparison of moderate and severe caloric restriction and the effects of weight maintenance therapy, *J. Consult. Clin. Psychol.* 62, 1994, 165–171.

20. Wing, R.R., E.H. Blair, P. Bononi, M.D. Marcus, R. Watanabe, and R.N. Bergman, Caloric restriction per se is a significant factor in improvements in glycemic control and insulin sensitivity during weight loss in obese NIDDM patients, *Diabetes Care* 17, 1994, 30–36.

21. Pirozzo, S., C. Summerbell, C. Cameron, and P. Glasziou, Advice on low-fat diets for obesity (Cochrane Library), In: The Cochrane Library, Issue 1, 2003, Oxford: Update.

22. Samaha, F.F., N. Iqbal, P. Seshadri, K.L. Chicano, D.A. Daily, J. McGrory, T. Williams, M. Williams, E.J. Gracely, and L. Stern, A low-carbohydrate as compared with a low-fat diet in severe obesity, *N. Engl. J. Med.* 348, 2003, 2074–2081.

23. Foster, G.D., H.R. Wyatt, J.O. Hill, B.G. McGuckin, C. Brill, S. Mohammed, P.O. Szapary, D.J. Rader, J.S. Edman, and S. Klein, A randomized trial of a low-carbohydrate diet for obesity, *N. Engl. J. Med.* 348, 2003, 2082–2090.

24. Singh, R.B., S.S. Rastogi, R. Verma et al., Randomised controlled trial of cardioprotective diet in patients with recent acute myocardial infarction: results of 1-year follow up, *BMJ* 304, 1992, 1015–1019.

25. Sheppard, L., A.R. Kristal, and L.H. Kushi, Weight loss in women participating in a randomized trail of low-fat diets, *Am. J. Clin. Nutr.* 54, 1991, 821–828.

26. Hooper, L., C.D. Summerbell, J.P. Higgins, R.L. Thompson, G. Clements, N. Capps, S. Davey, R.A. Riemersma, and S. Ebrahim, Reduced or modified dietary fat for preventing cardiovascular disease, *Cochrane Rev.* Issue 2, 2000, Oxford, Update Software.

27. Hammer, R.L., C.A. Barrier, E.S. Roundy, J.M. Bradford, and A.G. Fisher, Calorie-restricted low-fat diet and exercise in obese women, *Am. J. Clin. Nutr.* 49, 1989, 77–85.

28. Katzel, L.I., E.R. Bleecker, E.G. Colman, E.M. Rogus, J.D. Sorkin, and A.P. Goldberg, Effects of weight loss vs. aerobic exercise training on risk factors for coronary disease in healthy, obese, middle-aged and older men. A randomized controlled trial, *JAMA* 274, 1995, 1915–1921.

29. Donnelly, J.E., J.O. Hill, D.J. Jacobson, J. Potteiger, D.K. Sullivan et al., Effects of a 16-month randomized controlled exercise trial on body weight and composition in young, overweight men and women. The Midwest Exercise Trial, *Arch. Intern. Med.* 163, 2003, 1343–1350.

30. King, A.C., W.L. Haskell, C.B. Taylor, H.C. Kraemer, and R.F. DeBusk, Group- vs. home-based exercise training in healthy older men and women. A community-based clinical trial. *JAMA* 266, 1991, 1535–1542.

31. Ronnemaa, T., J. Marniemi, P. Puukka, and T. Kuusi, Effects of long-term physical exercise on serum lipids, lipoproteins and lipid metabolizing enzymes in type 2 (non-insulin-dependent) diabetic patients, *Diabetes Res.* 7, 1988, 79–84.

32. Schuler, G., R. Hambrecht, G. Schlierf et al., Regular physical exercise and low-fat diet. Effects on progression of coronary artery disease, *Circulation* 86, 1992, 1–11.

33. Munsch, S., E. Biedert, and U. Keller, Evaluation of a lifestyle change programme for the treatment of obesity in general practice, *Swiss Med. Wkly.* 133, 2003, 148–154.

34. Long, C.G., C.M. Simpson, and E.A. Allott, Psychological and dietetic counseling combined in the treatment of obesity: a comparative study in a hospital outpatient clinic, *Hum. Nutr. Apll. Nutr.* 37, 1983, 94–102.

35. Wadden, T.A. and A.J. Stunkard, Controlled trial of very low calorie diet, behavior therapy, and their combination in the treatment of obesity, *J. Consult. Clin. Psychol.* 54, 1986, 482–488.

36. Craighead, L.W., A.J. Stunkard, and R.M. O'Brien, Behaviour therapy and pharmacotherapy for obesity, *Arch. Gen. Psychiatry* 38, 1981, 763–768.

37. Sjöström, L., A. Rissanen, T. Andersen et al., Randomized placebo-controlled trial of orlistat for weight loss and prevention of weight regain in obese patients. European Multicenter Orlistat Study Group, *Lancet* 352, 1998, 167–172.

38. Lucas, C.P., M.N. Boldrin, and G.M. Reaven, Effect of orlistat added to diet (30% of calories from fat) on plasma lipids, glucose, and insulin in obese patients with hypercholesterolemia, *Am. J. Cardiol.* 91, 2003, 961–964.

39. Miles, J.M., L. Leiter, P. Hollander, T. Waddeen, J.W. Anderson et al., Effect of orlistat in overweight and obese patients with type 2 diabetes treated with metformin, *Diabetes Care* 25, 2002, 1123–1128.

40. Sharma, A.M. and A. Golay, Effect of orlistat-induced weight loss on blood pressure and heart rate in obese patients with hypertension, *J. Hypertens.* 20, 2002, 1873–1878.

41. James, W.P., A. Astrup, N. Finer et al., Effect of sibutramine on weight maintenance after weight loss: a randomised trial. STORM Study Group. Sibutramine Trial of Obesity Reduction and Maintenance, *Lancet* 356, 2000, 2119–2125.

42. Abenhaim, L., Y. Moride, F. Brenot et al., Appetite-suppressant drugs and the risk of pulmonary hypertension, *N. Engl. J. Med.* 335, 1996, 609–616.

43. Chae, F.H. and R.C. McIntyre, Laparoscopic bariatric surgery. *Surg. Endosc.* 13, 1999, 547–549.

44. Fielding, G.A., M. Rhodes, and L.K. Nathanson, Laparoscopic gastric banding for morbid obesity — surgical outcome in 225 cases, *Surg. Endosc.* 13, 1999, 550–554.

45. Schlumpf, R., T. Lang, O. Schöb et al., Treatment of the morbidly obese patient with laparoscopic adjustable gastric banding, *Dig. Surg.* 14, 1997, 438–443.

46. Heddenbro, L.L. and S.G. Frederiksen, Fully stapled gastric bypass with isolated pouch and terminal anastomosis: 1–3 years results, *Obes. Surg.* 12(4), 2002, 546–550.

47. Brolin, R.E., L.B. LaMarca, H.A. Kenler, and R.P. Cody, Malabsorptive gastric bypass in patients with superobesity, *J. Gastrointest. Surg.* 6(2), 2002, 195–203.

48. Colquitt, J., A. Clegg, M. Sidhu, and P. Royle, Surgery for morbid obesity, *Cochrane Rev.*, *Cochrane Database Syst. Rev.* 2003.

49. Weiner, R., R. Blanco–Engert, S. Winer, R. Matkowitz, L. Schaefer, and I. Pomhoff, Outcome after laparoscopic adjustable gastric banding — 8 years experience, *Obes. Surg.* 13, 2003, 427–434.

50. Pories, W.J., J.F. Caro, E.G. Flickinger et al., The control of diabetes mellitus (NIDDM) in the morbidly obese with the Greenville gastric bypass, *Ann. Surg.* 206, 1987, 316–323.

51. Polyzogopoulou, E.V., F. Kalfarentzos, A.G. Vagenakis, and T.K. Alexandrides, Restoration of euglycemia and normal acute insulin response to glucose in obese subjects with type 2 diabetes following bariatric surgery, *Diabetes* 52, 2003, 1098–1103.

52. Hickey, M.S., W.J. Pories, K.G. MacDonald et al. A new paradigm for type 2 diabetes mellitus: could it be a disease of the foregut? *Ann. Surg.* 227, 1998, 637–644.

53. Gleysteen, J.J., J.J. Barboriak, and E.A. Sasse, Sustained coronary-risk-factor reduction after gastric bypass for morbid obesity, *Am. J. Clin. Nutr.* 51, 1990, 774–778.

54. Brolin, R.E., L.J. Bradley, A.D. Wilson, and R.P. Cody, Lipid risk profile and weight stability after gastric restrictive operations, *J. Gastrointest. Surg.* 4, 2000, 464–469.

55. Torgerson, J.S. and L. Sjostrom, The Swedish Obesity Subjects (SOS) study — rationale and results, *Int. J. Obes. Relat. Metab. Disord.* 25 Suppl 1, 2001, 2–4.

56. Sugerman, H.J., P.L. Baron, R.P. Fairman et al., Hemodynamic dysfunction in obesity-hypoventilations syndrome and the effects of treatment with surgically induced weight loss, *Ann. Surg.* 207, 1988, 604–613.

57. Charuzi, I., A. Ovant, J. Peiser et al., The effect of surgical weight reduction on sleep quality in obesity-related sleep apnea syndrome, *Surgery* 97, 1985, 535–538.

58. Deitel, M., E. Stone, H.A. Kassam et al. Gynecologic-obstetric changes after loss of massive excess weight following bariatric surgery, *J. Am. Coll. Nutr.* 7, 1988, 147–153.

59. Bump, R.C., H.J. Sugerman, J.A. Fantl, and D.K. McClish, Obesity and lower urinary tract function in women: effect of surgically induced weight loss, *Am. J. Obstet. Gynecol.* 167, 1992, 392–399.

60. Foley, E.F., P.N. Benotti, B.D. Borlace, J. Hollingshead, and G.L. Blackburn, Impact of gastric restrictive surgery on hypertension in the morbidly obese, *Am. J. Surg.* 163, 1992, 294–297b.

61. Carson, J.L., M.E. Ruddy, A.E. Duff et al., The effect of gastric bypass surgery on hypertension in morbidly obese patients, *Arch. Intern. Med.* 154, 1994, 193–200.

62. Alpert, M.A., B.E. Terry, and D.L. Kelly, Effect of weight loss on cardiac chamber size, wall thickness and left ventricular function on morbid obesity, *Am. J. Cardiol.* 55, 1985, 783–786.

63. Stevens, J., J. Cai, E.R. Pamuk, D.F. Williamson, M.J. Thun, and J.L. Wood, The effect of age on the association between body-mass index and mortality, *N. Engl. J. Med.* 338, 1998, 1–7.

64. Calle, E.E., M.J. Thun, J.M. Petrelli, C. Rodriguez, and C.W. Heath, Body-mass-index and mortality in a prospective cohort of U.S. adults, *N. Engl. J. Med.* 341, 1999, 1097–1105.

65. National Institute of Health: Third report of the National Cholesterol Education Program Expert Panel in Detection, Evaluation, and Treatment of high blood cholesterol in adults (Adults Treatment Panel III). Executive Summary. Bethesda, MD, National Institutes of Health, National Heart, Lung and Blood Institute, 2001 (NIH publ. no. 01–3670).

66. Everson, S.A., D.E. Goldberg, S.P. Helmrich et al., Weight gain and the risk of developing insulin resistance syndrome, *Diabetes Care* 21, 1998, 1637–1643.

67. Kohrt, W.M., J.P. Kirwand, M.A. Staten, R.E. Bourey, D.S. King, and J.O. Holloszy, Insulin resistance in aging is related to abdominal obesity, *Diabetes* 42, 1993, 273–281.

68. Les, E.A. and L. Garfinkel, Variations in mortality by weight among 750,000 men and women, *J. Chronic Dis.* 32, 1979, 563–576.

69. Colditz, G.A., W.C. Willett, A. Rotnitzky, and J.E. Manson, Weight gain as a risk factor for clinical diabetes mellitus in women, *Ann. Intern. Med.* 122, 1995, 481–486.

70. Reeder, B.A., A. Angel, M. Ledoux, S.W. Rabkin, T.K. Young, and L.E. Sweet, Obesity and its relation to cardiovascular disease risk factors in Canadian adults, Canadian heart health surveys research group, *Can. Med. Assoc. J.* 146, 1992, 2009–2019.

71. Mann, J.I., B. Lewis, J. Shepherd et al., Blood lipid concentrations and other cardiovascular risk factors: distribution, prevalence and detection in Britain, *BMJ* 296, 1988, 1702–1706.

72. Anderson, K.M., P.W.F. Wilson, R.J. Garrison, and W.P. Castelli, Longitudinal and secular trends in lipoprotein cholesterol measurements in a general population sample: the Framingham offspring study, *Atherosclerosis* 68, 1987, 59–66.

73. Tchernof, A., B. Lamarche, D. PrudHomme et al., The dense LDL phenotype: association with plasma lipoprotein levels, visceral obesity and hyperinsulinemia in men, *Diabetes Care* 19(6), 1996, 629–637.

74. Dyer, A.R. and P. Elliott, The INTERSALT study: relations of body mass index to blood pressure, INTERSALT Co-operative research group, *J. Hum. Hypertens.* 3, 1989, 299–308.

75. Reisin, E., E.D. Frolich, F.H. Messerli, G.R. Dreslinski et al., Cardiovascular changes after weight reduction in obesity hypertension, *Ann. Int. Med.* 98, 1983, 315–319.

76. Tuck, M.I., J. Sowers, L. Dornfield et al., The effect of weight reduction on blood pressure plasma renin activity and plasma aldosterone level in obese patients, *N. Engl. J. Med.* 304, 1981, 930–933.
77. Rocchini, A.P., J. Key, D. Bondie et al., The effect of weight loss on the sensitivity of blood pressure to sodium in obese adolescents, *N. Engl. J. Med.* 321, 1989, 580–585.
78. Landsberg, L. and D.R. Krieger, Obesity, metabolism and the sympathetic nervous system, *Am. J. Hypertension* 2, 1989, 125s–132s.
79. Jacobs, D.B., J.R. Sowers et al. Effects of weight reduction on cellular cation metabolism and vascular resistance, *Hypertension* 21, 1993, 308–314.
80. Willett, W.C., J.E. Manson, M.J. Stampfer et al., Weight, weight change and coronary heart disease in women. Risk within the normal weight range, *JAMA* 273, 1995, 461–465.
81. Kenchaiah, S., J.C. Evans, D. Levy, P.W.F. Wilson, E.J. Benjamin, M.G. Larson, W.B. Kannel, and R.S. Vasan, Obesity and the risk of heart failure, *N. Engl. J. Med.* 247, 2002, 305–313.
82. Lapidus, L., C. Bengtsson, B. Larsson, K. Pennert, E. Rybo, and L. Sjostrom, Distribution of adipose tissue and risk of cardiovascular disease and death: a 12 year follow up of participants in the population study of women in Gothenburg, Sweden, *BMJ* 289, 1984, 1257–1261.
83. Larsson, B., K. Svardsudd, L. Welin, L. Wilhemsen, P. Bjorntorp, and G. Tibblin, Abdominal adipose tissue distribution, obesity, and risk of cardiovascular disease and death: 13 year follow up of participants in the study of men born in 1913, *BMJ* 288, 1984, 1401–1404.
84. Rexrode, K.M., C.H. Hennekens, W.C. Willett et al., A prospective study of body mass index, weight change, and risk of stroke in women, *JAMA* 277, 1997, 1539–1545.
85. Khare, M., J.E. Everhart, K.R. Maurer, and M.C. Hill, Association of ethnicity and body mass index (BMI) with gallstone disease in the United States, *Am. J. Epidemiol.* 141, 1995, S69.
86. Felson, D.T., J.J. Anderson, A. Naimark, A.M. Walker, and R.F. Meenan, Obesity and knee osteoarthritis. The Framingham Study, *Ann. Intern. Med.* 109, 1988, 18–24.
87. Young, T., M. Palta, J. Dempsey, J. Skatrud, S. Weber, and S. Badr, The occurrence of sleep-disordered breathing among middle-aged adults, *N. Engl. J. Med.* 328, 1993, 1230–1235.
88. Giovanucci, E., G.A. Colditz, M.J. Stampfer, and W.C. Willett, Physical activity, obesity and risk of colorectal adenoma in women (United States). *Cancer Causes Control* 7, 1996, 253–263.
89. Huang, Z., S.E. Hankinson, G.A. Colditz et al. Dual effects of weight and weight gain on breast cancer risk, *JAMA* 278, 1997, 1407–1411.
90. Schottenfeld, D. and J.F. Fraumeni, *Cancer Epidemiology and Prevention*. New York: Oxford University Press, 1996.
91. Garfinkel, L., Overweight and mortality, *Cancer* 58, 1986, 1826–1829.
92. Calle, E.E., A. Rodriguez, K. Walker–Thurmond, and M.J. Thun, Overweight, obesity and mortality from cancer in a prospectively studied cohort of U.S. adults, *N. Engl. J. Med.* 348, 2003, 1625–1638.
93. Gregg, E.W., R.B. Gerzoff, T.J. Thompson, and D.F. Williamson, Intentional weight loss and death in overweight and obese U.S. adults 35 years of age and older, *Ann. Intern. Med.* 138, 2003, 383–389.
94. Sjostrom, C.D., L. Lissner, and L. Sjostrom, Relationships between changes in body composition and changes in cardiovascular risk factors: the SOS intervention study, *Obes. Res.* 5, 1997, 519–530.
95. Tuomilehto, J., J. Lindström, J. Eriksson, T. Valle, H. Hämäläinen et al., Prevention of type 2 diabetes mellitus by changes in lifestyle among subjects with impaired glucose tolerance, *N. Engl. J. Med.* 344, 2001, 1343–1350.
96. Knowler, W.C., Barnett-Connor, E., Fowler, S.E. et al. The diabetes prevention program research group: reduction in the incidence of type 2 diabetes with lifestyle intervention or metformin, *N. Engl. J. Med.* 346, 2002, 393–403.
97. Pan, X.R., G.W. Li, Y.H. Hu et al., Effects of diet and exercise in preventing NIDDM in people with impaired glucose tolerance. The Da Quing IGT and Diabetes Study, *Diabetes Care* 20, 1997, 537–544.
98. Langford, H.G., B.R. Davis, D. Blaufox et al., Effect of drug and diet treatment of mild hypertension on diastolic blood pressure. The TAIM Research Group, *Hypertension* 17, 1991, 210–217.

99. Wassertheil–Smoller, S., H.G. Lanford, M.D. Blaufox et al., Effective dietary intervention in hypertensives: sodium restriction and weight reduction, *J. Am. Diet. Assoc.* 85, 1985, 423–430.
100. MacMahon, S., J. Cutler, E. Brittain, and M. Higgins, Obesity and hypertension: epidemiological and clinical issues, *Eur. Heart J.* 8 (Suppl B), 1987, 57–70.
101. Appel, L.J., C.M. Champagne, D.W. Harsha, L.S. Cooper, E. Obartanek et al., Writing group of the PREMIER Collaborative Research Group, Effects of comprehensive lifestyle modification on blood pressure control: main results of the PREMIER clinical trial, *JAMA* 289, 2003, 2083–2093.

23

Integrated Approach to Treatment and Prevention

André J. Scheen

CONTENTS

SUMMARY Obesity is a chronic disease whose management requires continual care within an integrated multidisciplinary approach. As for every disease, the decision to treat and the choice of therapy should be preceded by a careful global evaluation of each individual patient. An important feature of an integrated management program is the coordination of care ensuring that a comprehensive, unified treatment plan is provided to the obese patient. The physician's role is to evaluate; manage and monitor; utilize adjuvant strategies to diet and exercise when indicated (drugs or even surgery); set weight loss goals and expectations; manage comorbidities when present; provide support for other team members; and coordinate interdisciplinary care. A hierarchy strategy is generally proposed that is essentially tailored to the severity of obesity and the risk profile of the obese patient. Other factors may, however, influence the choice of therapy, such as target body weight; results of previous attempts of weight loss; socioeconomic status; patient's age; etc. Rapid increases in the level of overweight and obesity in almost all populations throughout the world and the inadequacy of current treatment strategies to deal with the consequences support the view that prevention of obesity offers the only real hope of tackling this serious public health problem, especially in young people. However, this objective requires strategies that address the societal causes of obesity. An important challenge for the scientific community is to find ways to document empirically the most efficacious strategies and politically feasible alternatives.

23.1 Introduction

Obesity can no longer be regarded simply as a cosmetic problem affecting certain individuals, but rather as an epidemic that requires effective measures for its prevention and management (World Health Organization 2000). Although obesity is increasingly seen as a chronic disease for which no cure exists, its management requires continual care within an integrated multidisciplinary approach (Scheen et al. 1994). Body weight is determined by a complex interaction among genetic, environmental, and psychosocial factors. Although genetic components are very important, the principal causes of the accelerating problem of obesity worldwide are best explained by changing behaviors and environment, leading to increased energy intake and decreased energy expenditure (Cooney 2002).

  The recommendation to treat overweight and obesity is based on evidence that relates obesity to increased morbidity and mortality, as well as the results from several randomized controlled trials that demonstrate weight loss reduces risk factors for other diseases (NHLBI Obesity Education Initiative Expert Panel 1998; Basdevant et al. 2002). However, to reverse global trends in the incidence of obesity and improve public health will be a huge challenge because it is necessary to learn about the most effective preventive methods for combating what is emerging as one of the prominent health problems of mankind (James 1999). This concise review attempts to describe an integrated approach to treatment and prevention of obesity.

23.2 Global Assessment of the Obese Subject

As for every disease, the decision to treat and the choice of the therapy should be preceded by a careful global evaluation of the patient (NHLBI Obesity Education Initiative Expert Panel 1998; Kopelman 2001; Basdevant et al. 2002). Such an individual evaluation comprises a detailed medical history; a complete clinical examination; an assessment of risk profile; and an appreciation of motivation and psychological patterns of the obese patient.

23.2.1 Medical History

The history of weight gain should be described in detail to elucidate possible etiological factors and to assess the patient's insight into and understanding of the factors causing weight gain (Kopelman 2001). Family history of overweight/obesity and of severe complications associated with weight excess (diabetes mellitus or cardiovascular diseases) is important baseline information. It is useful to distinguish childhood onset obesity from that occurring later in life. Obesity may occur in relation to

- Specific physiological critical periods (puberty, pregnancy, menopause, etc.)
- Changes in life habits (employment, marriage, sport abandon, smoking cessation, etc.)
- Illnesses (depression, immobility due to injuries, etc.)
- Drugs promoting weight gain (neuroleptics, antidepressants, anticonvulsants, steroids, etc.)

Life-style habits, including usual eating pattern; bulimia episodes; alcohol intake; cigarette smoking; and physical activity, should also be covered when taking a history from an obese patient. The existence of previous treatments for obesity, including successes and failures, should also be investigated because such information may help decide how to manage the individual obese patient. Finally, inquiry about snoring and daytime somnolence may reveal a sleep apnea syndrome (Kopelman 2001).

23.2.2 Clinical Examination

The degree of obesity is best expressed by the body mass index (BMI) (except in the case of marked edema or massive muscle hypertrophy as among bodybuilders). A close relationship exists between BMI and the incidence of several chronic conditions caused by excess fat, and all risks are greatly increased for subjects with a BMI above 30 kg/m², independent of gender (Willett et al. 1999). Fat distribution is routinely assessed by measurements of the waist circumference and used to refine an assessment of risk, especially for overweight or mildly obese patients (BMI between 25 and 34.9 kg/m²). Waist circumference correlates with measures of risk for coronary heart disease such as hypertension, diabetes mellitus, or dyslipidemia (Després 1993). An expert panel has suggested increased risks if the waist circumference is >102 cm in men and >88 cm in women (NHLBI Obesity Education Initiative Expert Panel 1998). However, smaller cut-off points (>94 cm in men and >80 cm in women) are already associated with a two- to threefold increase in the relative risk of some health problems, such as type 2 diabetes. A neck circumference of >43 cm indicates a likelihood of obstructive sleep apnea and related causes of nocturnal hypoventilation — conditions that also strongly predispose to cardiovascular diseases (Kopelman 2001).

Besides these basic anthropometrical measurements, measuring blood pressure is mandatory because of the high prevalence of hypertension, a major risk factor in the obese population (Kopelman 2001). More than 50% of subjects in hypertension clinics are obese and about 50% of severely obese patients are hypertensive. Any evidence of cardiac valvular disease; pulmonary hypertension; cor pulmonale; congestive cardiac failure; venous insufficiency; and thromboembolic disease should be screened. A careful examination of the skin may reveal external signs of various hormonal abnormalities such as features of corticosteroid excess (thin, atrophic skin; ecchymosed lesions); acanthosis nigricans associated with severe insulin resistance; severe hirsutism suggesting polycystic ovary syndrome, etc.

23.2.3　Assessment of Risk

The precise evaluation of an obese patient's absolute risk status requires an assessment of associated disease conditions and cardiovascular risk factors. Classical risk markers include (Expert Panel on Detection, Evaluation, and Treatment of High Blood Cholesterol in Adults 2001):

- Hypertension (>130/85 mm Hg)
- High LDL cholesterol (>4 mmol/l)
- Low HDL cholesterol (<1 mmol/l in men and <1.3 mmol/l in women)
- High serum triglycerides (>1.7 mmol/l)
- Impaired fasting plasma glucose (>6.1 mmol/l)
- Cigarette smoking
- Family history of premature coronary heart disease

In addition to this classical risk profile, obesity is closely linked to metabolic syndrome, also called insulin resistance syndrome or syndrome X (Després 1993; Grundy 2002). Various markers have been recognized as part of the metabolic syndrome, among them:

- High triglyceride levels
- Hyperuricemia
- High fasting plasma insulin concentration
- Postprandial hyperglycemia
- High plasminogen activator inhibitor-1 (PAI-1)
- Inflammatory markers (fibrinogen, C-reactive protein)
- Microalbuminuria
- Nonalcoholic fatty liver disease (NAFLD)
- Nonalcoholic steatohepatitis (NASH)

The metabolic syndrome has been recognized as an independent cardiovascular risk factor by the recent ATP III (Expert Panel on Detection, Evaluation, and Treatment of High Blood Cholesterol in Adults 2001).

Associated disease conditions include established coronary heart disease; other atherosclerotic diseases; type 2 diabetes; sleep apnea; venous insufficiency; and prothrombotic tendency increasing the risk of thromboembolic disease, etc. Osteoarthritis frequently accompanies long-standing obesity. It may considerably alter the quality of life of the obese patient and also make difficult or even impossible the practice of any physical activity. Sometimes, pain and locomotor limitation associated with severe osteoarthritis represent the main medical indication and the primary patient motivation for weight reduction.

23.2.4　Assessment of Motivation

Not all obese patients are prepared for weight reduction despite a referral to a medical practitioner. As a consequence, it is often useful to confirm first that a patient understands the need for weight loss and is prepared to follow medical advice to achieve and maintain an agreed weight goal (Kopelman 2001). Health care professionals have a unique potential to improve a patient's motivation as well as to alleviate or exacerbate the emotional pain

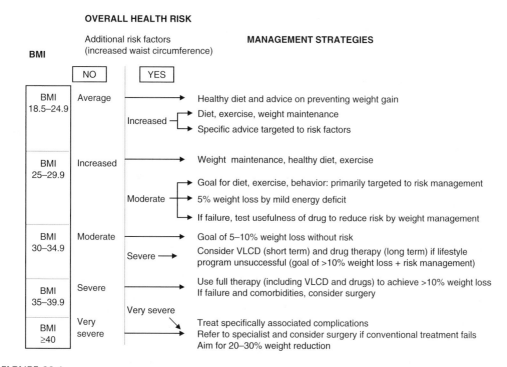

FIGURE 23.1

Management strategies according to overall health risk from body mass index (BMI), waist circumference, and other risk factors (diabetes, hypertension, etc.). (Adapted from James, W.P.T., in *Progress in Obesity Research: 8*, B. Guy–Grand and G. Ailhaud, Eds., John Libbey & Company Ltd., pp. 649–659, 1999.)

borne by many obese persons. Obviously, an understanding of the social and psychological causes and consequences of obesity may provide an important perspective for those who treat individual obese patients.

23.3 Integrated Management of the Obese Subject

An important feature of an integrated management program is the coordination of care ensuring that a comprehensive, unified treatment plan is provided to the obese patient. The treatment strategy should be developed into a hierarchy and tailored to the risk profile and personal characteristics of each obese patient (Figure 23.1) (James 1999; Bray and Tartaglia 2000). The physician's role is to evaluate, manage, and monitor, utilizing adjuvant strategies when indicated (pharmacological approaches or bariatric surgery); set weight loss goals and expectations; manage comorbidities when present; provide support for other team members; and coordinate interdisciplinary care (Scheen et al. 1999; Kopelman 2001).

23.3.1 Treatment Goals

The goals of obesity treatment have changed dramatically in the past decade. Once the goal was the reduction to "ideal" weight; now the new goal is the attainment of a healthier weight that, for many obese individuals, can be achieved with as little as a 5 to 10%

decrease in initial weight (Wadden 1998). The adoption of appropriate eating and activity habits is the first step toward achieving a healthier weight. Assessment of success must take into account the initial degree of obesity; presence of indicators of associated risks or complications; previous attempts at weight control; and the patient's age (Kopelman 2001). Goals for older patients (>65 years) may be different from those for the young. In some patients, prevention of further weight gain may be more appropriate than actual weight loss (James 1999). In addition to weight loss, weight maintenance, correction of complications, and improvement of quality of life are important goals of overall management of the obese patient. Rather than various surrogate endpoints, prolongation of life expectancy may also be considered a main objective of treating obese patients, although only few prospective studies provided data supporting this concept until now.

23.3.2 Weight Loss

The success or failure of a treatment program may be judged by an arbitrarily chosen target weight or percentage weight loss (Glenny et al. 1997). After an initial period of relatively rapid weight reduction, an average continuing loss of anything up to 0.5 to 1.0 kg per week should be considered acceptable. Weight loss goals for overweight and obese patients should be tailored to the individual. A weight loss of 5% of initial body weight will result in some improvement, while a loss of 10% is generally of major benefit (Goldstein 1992). Indeed, such body weight reduction is associated with clinically useful changes — especially improvement of metabolic abnormalities associated with syndrome X such as reduction of visceral adiposity; lowered arterial blood pressure; decreased plasma total cholesterol and triglyceride concentrations; diminution of plasma insulin and blood glucose levels, etc. (Busetto 2001). A very successful weight loss is greater than 20% in obese patients. However, it is rarely achieved with medical means and can be mostly achieved with bariatric surgery (Luyckx et al. 1998; Sjöström 2000; Mun et al. 2001).

23.3.3 Weight Maintenance

A program to enable individuals to maintain their lowered weight must follow any successful weight loss because, in most patients, obesity does not result from an inability to lose weight, but rather from a profound difficulty in maintaining a lowered weight. Weight regain results from complex interactions among multiple factors, including physiological, environmental, and psychological factors (Guy–Grand 1988; Khaodhiar and Blackburn 2002).

Physiological factors include reduced metabolic rate (resting and nonresting); increased adipose tissue lipoprotein lipase activity; and increased ghrelin levels (a recently discovered orexigenic hormone secreted by the stomach and duodenum that is implicated in long-term regulation of body weight). Environmental factors include continuous exposure to an overabundance of high-fat, energy-dense foods; increased portion sizes; and decreased requirements for physical activity in modern society. Finally, psychological factors may play a crucial role in weight regain, essentially because of progressive decrease of patient compliance to diet and exercise recommendations (Guy–Grand 1988).

Standards for defining weight maintenance and clear communication of those standards are needed. A definition of successful long-term weight maintenance may be the intentional loss of at least 10% of initial body weight kept off for at least 1 year (Wing and Hill 2001). Published evidence suggests that a combination of sensible eating, physical activity, and reinforcement of behavioral methods is most successful for the longer term. A meta-analysis of 493 studies has shown better long-term weight maintenance results with diet and exercise than with diet alone (Miller 1997). Multiple behavioral strategies implemented to improve long-term outcomes of obesity treatment (Wadden 1998) have met with variable success (Khaodhiar and Blackburn 2002). They include extended treatment; relapse prevention training and problem-solving therapy; social support; telephone contact; prepared/provided food; and exercise and physical activity programs (Khaodhiar and Blackburn 2002).

23.3.4 Management of Complications

Data from hundreds of completed studies have already consistently demonstrated the positive impact of long-term weight loss on the comorbidities of obesity. One of the complications most closely related to obesity and favorably influenced by weight reduction is type 2 diabetes mellitus (Scheen and Lefèbvre 1999a; Scheen 2003). The ongoing Look AHEAD Study, initiated in 1999, is a 12-year prospective trial designed to determine whether a 7% weight loss will reduce the occurrence of myocardial infarction and stroke in overweight patients who already have type 2 diabetes. Other ongoing prospective clinical trials investigate the effects of sibutramine (Sibutramine Cardiovascular Outcomes Trial) and of bariatric surgery (Swedish Obese Subjects Study) on morbidity and mortality of obese subjects (Scheen 2003). It is crucial to know whether, by treating obesity with whatever strategies available, the cost for its complications (mainly hypertension, diabetes mellitus, and hyperlipidaemia leading to cardiovascular diseases) will be lowered (Narbro et al. 2002).

However, besides the management of weight excess per se, it is crucial to treat complications associated specifically with obesity. Indeed, type 2 diabetes, dyslipidemia, arterial hypertension, and sleep apnea syndrome may dramatically impair the prognosis of obese individuals because these complications have proven to be associated with higher risk of cardiovascular morbidity and mortality (Kopelman 2001). Moreover, specific treatments with hypoglycemic agents, lipid-lowering drugs, antihypertensive compounds, or positive airway pressure are able to reduce cardiovascular morbidities significantly and to improve the overall prognosis, including reducing mortality, in high-risk patients. Thus, integrated management of the obese patient must include appropriate treatment of comorbidities, especially among obese diabetic patients (Scheen and Lefèbvre 1999a).

23.3.5 Quality of Life

Most obese subjects have poor self-esteem and impaired social lives. Some prospective studies have tried to collect a large amount of social, psychological, and economic information in order to assess the impact of various antiobesity strategies on quality of life, average income, sick leave, and disability pension. When obese patients were asked to estimate their well-being on a graded scoring scale, clear-cut improvements were generally observed in patients who succeeded in obtaining and maintaining significant weight loss (Kaukua et al. 2002).

23.4 Hierarchy of Antiobesity Approaches

A number of professional, governmental, and other bodies have drawn up guidelines for obesity management (NHLBI Obesity Education Initiative Expert Panel 1998; World

Health Organization 2000; Basdevant et al. 2002). These strategies provide useful and evidence-based guidance for clinical management of the obese patient. Guidelines include all antiobesity approaches, which are extensively described in the present book. A hierarchical strategy is generally proposed that is essentially tailored to the severity of obesity and the risk profile of the obese patient, using the same criteria as previously described (Figure 23.1) (James 1999; Bray and Tartaglia 2000). However, other factors, such as goals of weight loss; expected speed of weight reduction and target body weight; results of previous attempts of weight loss; socioeconomic status; patient age; etc., may influence the choice of therapy.

23.4.1   Restricted Diet

Control of diet is the cornerstone for management of all overweight and obese individuals. Long-term changes in food choices and eating behavior are needed, rather than a temporary restriction of specific foods (Ayyad and Andersen 2000). The treatment should be nutritionally sound and aim to promote a healthier diet. It is vital to translate nutritional messages into specific food changes that are practical and relevant for patients to implement over the long term. The many dietary changes necessary for successful weight loss and maintenance underline the importance of integrating behavioral change within a weight management program.

Daily deficits of 500 to 1000 kcal/day will lead to initial weight losses of 0.5 to 1.0 kg per week. However, the rate of weight loss usually progressively declines, and the weight may plateau because of less energy expenditure at a lower weight. The use of very low-calorie diets (VLCDs) should only be considered after the failure of determined attempts to lose weight with conventional restriction of low-calorie "normal" diets. Even if VLCD provides more rapid initial weight reduction, concern has been raised about longer success (Wadden et al. 1989). However, a recent meta-analysis of randomized clinical trials showed that over the longer term (4 to 5 years), weight loss following VLCD was significantly higher than that following low-calorie diet (Anderson et al. 2001). A clinician's responsibility is to judge, through assessment and discussion with the patient, relevant dietary strategies and to provide information and guidance in an appropriately staged manner.

23.4.2   Exercise and Physical Activity

The commonly held view that exercise alone is not a useful strategy for obesity reduction is drawn from studies with limitations that confound interpretation. Recent evidence counters the dogma that daily exercise produces only modest weight loss and suggests that exercise even without diet restriction is an effective strategy for reducing obesity and related comorbidities (Ross et al. 2000). In general, an exercise program should consist of moderately intense aerobic exercises (equivalent to brisk walking) that can be sustained for 30 min or longer and do not result in a sustained heart rate higher than 60 to 70% of the person's predetermined maximum heart rate. To use exercise as an adjunct to diet to lose weight or maintain reduced body weight, patients should exercise at least 3 days a week, although 5 to 7 days a week is preferable.

Results from randomized clinical trials suggest that a combination of diet and exercise generally produces greater weight losses than diet alone, including a decrease in abdominal fat while preserving fat-free mass. One of the most consistent findings is weight maintenance, with maintenance of lost weight seen in randomized clinical trials after 2 years from the start of intervention (Miller et al. 1997). The risks from exercise are not great if it is introduced gradually and other complications, such as coronary heart disease or osteoarthritis, are taken into account.

23.4.3 Behavioral Therapy

Behavior interventions are important for facilitating changes in an individual's life-style in order to attain a healthier weight (Wadden 1998). The key difference between behavioral methods and other forms of treatment for obesity is that they lay particular emphasis on personal responsibility for initiating and maintaining treatment rather than relying on external forces. The important elements of a behavioral program include:

- Self-monitoring
- Stimulus control
- Goal setting
- Problem setting
- Cognitive restructuring
- Self-rewards

Social and family support is critical to success and such therapy may be incorporated into self-help groups. Evidence from randomized clinical trials suggests that, when used in combination with other weight loss approaches including diet and physical activity, behavior therapy provides additional benefits in assisting patients to lose weight for the short term (up to 1 year) (Wadden et al. 1989). Longer-term follow-up shows a return to baseline weight in the absence of continuing behavioral intervention, but extended treatment programs improve long-term weight maintenance.

23.4.4 Drug Treatments

Growing recognition of the health risks of obesity coupled with difficulties in treating it successfully by life-style modification predicates a need for effective drug treatment (Scheen and Lefèbvre 1999b; Bray and Tartaglia 2000). The criteria applied to the use of an antiobesity drug are well known and similar to those applied to the treatment of other relapsing disorders: it should be (1) needed; (2) more effective than nondrug treatment; and (3) produce a favorable risk-benefit ratio, especially in the long term because obesity is a chronic disease (National Task Force on the Prevention and Treatment of Obesity 1996). It may be appropriate to consider drug treatment if patient BMI is above 30 kg/m² and weight loss is less than 10% of the initial body weight after at least 3 months of supervised diet, exercise, and behavioral management. Drug treatment may be particularly appropriate for patients with comorbid risk factors or complications from their obesity, which allow consideration of antiobesity drug treatment for a patient with BMI above 28 kg/m² with established comorbidities. The initiation of drug treatment will depend on the clinician's judgment about the risks to an individual from prolonged obesity; continuation should depend on the balance between the health benefits of maintained weight and the potential adverse effects of the drug.

Antiobesity drugs must at least induce, accelerate, and/or help maintain weight loss. Two medications — sibutramine and orlistat — have been approved for long-term treatment of obesity if they are given in combination with appropriate dietary restriction. Randomized controlled trials during 12 to 24 months have indicated greater mean weight reduction and proportion of good responders (as judged by a 5 to 10% reduction in body weight maintained over 12 months) with sibutamine or orlistat than with placebo (Glazer 2001; Haddock et al. 2002). If the drug is efficacious in helping a patient to lose weight and/or maintain weight loss and no serious side effects occur, it may be continued. Indeed, stopping pharmacological treatment will result in a relapse of the disease (i.e., weight regain) in most cases, as for other chronic illnesses such as diabetes mellitus, arterial hypertension, etc.

It is noteworthy that most recent randomized clinical trials evaluating antiobesity drug therapy have been performed in an integrated care structure involving several health providers working as a team (Glazer 2001; Haddock et al. 2002). Even when pharmacotherapies are used for obesity, life-style treatments remain essential (Poston et al. 2001). In obesity treatment, drugs should be seen not as "magic bullets," but as an adjunct to inducing and enforcing behavioral change.

23.4.5 Surgical Procedures

Because results of weight loss and weight maintenance with medical means, including drugs, are often disappointing, surgical approaches have been considered in refractory severe or morbid obesity (Scheen et al. 1994). Two operative procedures are currently used for the surgical treatment of obesity: gastric restriction (vertical-ring gastroplasty or adjustable silicone gastric banding) and gastric bypass operations (Sjöström 2000; Mun et al. 2001).

Surgery for obesity is an option for carefully selected patients with clinically severe obesity (BMI > 40 kg/m^2, or > 35 kg/m^2 with comorbid conditions) when less invasive methods of weight loss have failed and the patient is at high risk for obesity-associated morbidity and mortality. In this respect, remarkable results have been reported in severely obese patients with type 2 diabetes (Scheen and Lefèbvre 1999a; Scheen 2003). Furthermore, all markers of the metabolic syndrome were shown to be greatly improved after a drastic and sustained weight loss following gastroplasty in severely or morbidly obese patients (Luyckx et al. 1998). The physician should realistically consider the chances of weight loss with the medical approach, i.e., restricted diet possibly associated to antiobesity agents, compared to surgery (Mun et al. 2001). The ongoing prospective Swedish Obese Subjects Study compared long-term results of obese patients submitted to bariatric surgery with those of patients treated by various medical approaches (Sjöström 2000). It demonstrated a greater weight loss associated with remarkable correction of various risk factors, especially diabetes mellitus, hypertension, and dyslipidaemias, in obese patients treated by surgery (Sjöström et al. 1999).

However, because other side effects have been reported (gastrointestinal tract disorders, anemia, vitamin deficiencies), total pharmaceutical costs were shown to be similar for surgically and conventionally treated obese individuals for 6 years (Narbro et al. 2002). Ideally, the decision to manage the morbidly obese diabetic patient with bariatric surgery should be made by a multidisciplinary team, including an internist/diabetologist; a dietitian/nutritionist; surgeon; general practitioner; and psychologist (Benotti and Forse 1995).

23.5 Prevention Strategies

The rapid increases in the level of overweight and obesity in almost all populations throughout the world, as well as the inadequacy of current treatment strategies to deal with the consequences, support the view that prevention of obesity offers the only real hope of tackling this serious public health problem (Glenny et al. 1997; World Health Organization 2000; Kumanyika et al. 2002; Cooney 2002).

23.5.1 Importance of Prevention

Despite continued escalation in obesity rates and the serious gains to be achieved from reducing the incidence and prevalence of obesity in the population, surprisingly little attention has been given to prevention of obesity. Because direct costs associated with obesity represent more than 5% of the national health expenditure in the U.S. and other industrialized countries, it is certainly relevant to discuss to what extent prevention could be used to reduce this huge financial burden to society. In addition, overweight and obesity and the complications of these conditions are also occurring in much younger age groups, highlighting the need to understand more about how obesity arises and what can be done to alleviate or prevent this condition. In the face of a current environment characterized by sedentary life-styles and easy availability of high-fat/energy-dense food, action to prevent obesity must include measures to reduce the obesity-promoting aspects of the environment (World Health Organization 2000).

23.5.2 Failure of Individual Interventions

The epidemiological data linking overweight and obesity with substantial health risks and disabilities might naturally have led to assumptions that tackling a huge medical work load by novel means on an individual basis is necessary (Yanovski and Yanovski 2002). In this respect, recent progress in better understanding energy homeostasis and efforts to discover new safe and effective drugs open exciting perspectives.

However, the complexity of body weight regulation and the redundancy of physiological systems to protect against a negative energy balance make it unlikely that a drug to "prevent" or "cure" obesity will be developed. Preventive actions may be taken at different stages and should always combine dietary advice and promotion of physical activity (Blair and Bouchard 1999). Previous attempts to improve diet and physical activity habits have shown that efforts cannot rely solely on health education strategies aimed at changing individual behavior. Low patient compliance will always be a main problem of any preventive strategy, essentially because of lack of motivation. In addition, it is unusual for a clinician used to treating individual patients suddenly to develop a preventive approach in thinking and acting; medical teachers should not neglect primary prevention in the future.

Past attempts to prevent development of obesity within individuals and populations have been sparse and characterized by very limited success. In a systematic review of the literature on treatment and prevention of obesity, Glenny et al. (1997) pointed out that, for studies addressing the prevention of obesity, only few randomized control trials were available, most of them not always of a high standard or of limited sample sizes. In addition, the prevention of obesity in children was rarely addressed. The Cochrane database systematic review of interventions to prevent obesity in children identified only seven trials that met its requirements, and only three of these lasted 12 months or more (Campbell et al. 2001). Except for one study involving a dietary intervention only, all trials focused partially or exclusively on physical activity interventions (reducing sedentary behavior, such as watching television, or encouraging increased exercise through play and dance). All but one of the trials were school based. Most of these studies did produce promising

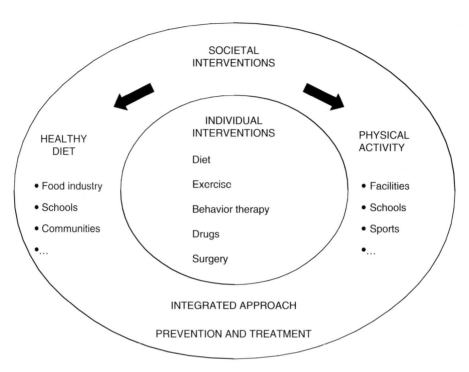

FIGURE 23.2
Integrated approach to prevention and treatment of obesity: complementarities between societal and individual interventions promoting healthy diet and physical activity.

results, but the reviewers concluded that, due to the limitations of study design or data analysis, no general conclusion could be drawn.

23.5.3   Need for Societal Interventions

According to the International Obesity Task Force (IOTF), a new preventive strategy should emerge that concentrates on societal — not patient-specific — changes in physical activity and diet (Figure 23.2). As mentioned by James (1999), "the natural tendency currently to assume that individual health education and advice is the means to alter public health fails to recognize much broader issues."

Improvements in school and community environments are among the long-term steps that can and should be taken to deal with obesity prevention. Communities can use various strategies to address overweight and obesity, such as requiring physical education at all school grades; offering more healthy food options in schools and on campuses; and providing safe and accessible recreational facilities for residents of all ages. Environmental strategies should be considered, such as

- Constructing safer walkways and bicycle paths
- Incorporating positive behavior change messages into television programs and popular magazines
- Regulating advertising to children and adolescents
- Mandating that more school time be devoted to physical activity and practical food skills training
- Improving food product labeling so that it does not mislead the consumer

The food industry is a critical factor in any potentially successful long-term strategy to prevent obesity (James 1999; Cooney 2002). The World Health Organization has expressed concern about the current developments and strategies employed by many food manufacturers. These include the continuing intense advertisement of foods rich in fat, sugar, and salt as well as the introduction of new technologies for food processing with only limited attention given to improving the nutritional quality of existing food products. As an example, the food industry needs to reduce the general fat content of the diet and not simply provide low-fat alternatives.

These are serious issues and can only be resolved with continuous involvement of industry in public health strategy development and planning of prevention campaigns. However, the food industry will become more interested in these general prevention issues only if profitability is maintained. Thus, joint partnership with governments is needed for policies on pricing and subsidies that make alternatives for food production attractive. Government controls on marketing through restrictions on advertising and labeling of foods are also instruments that may favor the direction of food production and marketing.

Obesity is a serious public health problem worldwide that can be effectively addressed only if governments, international agencies, industry/trade, media, health professionals, and consumers accept that they have important roles to play in its management and prevention. Strategies are needed that address the underlying societal causes of obesity through action in sectors such as transport; environment; employment conditions; and education, health, food, social, and economic policies (James 1999; Cooney 2002). How best to develop these general strategies for the whole population is a major challenge.

23.6 Conclusions

Obesity is increasing in society because human physiology is ill adapted to changes of the industrialized world that have rapidly favored increased energy consumption and decreased energy expenditure. Although treatment for the obese is necessary, a long-term strategy that prevents obesity, especially in children and young people, is probably the most appropriate and cost-effective measure. An integrated approach to treatment and prevention of obesity should be considered on an individual basis as well as on a societal level.

Obesity is not a single disorder but a heterogeneous disease with multiple causes — the outcome of an imbalance between energy intake and energy expenditure. One of the most important problems in the individual management of obesity is recognizing the type of obese patient responsive to a given treatment. In most cases, obesity requires coordination from multiple health care providers, with a multidisciplinary group with varied expertise working as a team to assist patient care. Considering the limitations of current treatment strategies, new interventions must be developed that address the multiple influences on obesity in order to achieve and maintain weight loss and its associated health benefits in most individual patients.

Society is facing an epidemic of obesity; the need to increase research efforts into controlling this huge problem and reducing the associated health costs is now being recognized by governments. As emphasized in the WHO report on Preventing and Managing Obesity as a Global Epidemic (1998) and the International Obesity Task Force (James 1999), the environment in which people live and work will need to be altered so that it promotes and supports healthy eating and physical activity habits for all members of the community, especially young people. This objective requires strategies that address the societal causes of obesity. An important challenge for the scientific community is to find ways to document empirically the most efficacious strategies and politically feasible alternatives.

References

Anderson, J.W., Konz, E.C., Frederich, R.C. and Wood, C.L. (2001) Long-term weight loss maintenance: a meta-analysis of U.S. studies. *Am. J. Clin. Nutr.*, 74:579–584.

Ayyad, C. and Andersen, T. (2000) Long-term efficacy of dietary treatment of obesity : a systematic review of studies published between 1931 and 1999. *Obesity Res.*, 1:113–119.

Basdevant, A., Laville, M. and Ziegler, O. for the Expert Group (2002) Recommendations for the diagnosis, the prevention and the treatment of obesity. *Diabetes Metab.* 28:146–150.

Benotti, P. and Forse, R. (1995) The role of gastric surgey in the multidisciplinary management of severe obesity. *Am. J. Surg.*, 69:361–366.

Blair, S.N. and Bouchard, C. (Eds.) (1999). American College of Sports Medicine roundtable. Physical activity in the prevention and treatment of obesity and its comorbidities. *Med. Sci. Sports Exercise*, 31 (Suppl):S497–S667.

Bray, G.A. and Tartaglia, L.A. (2000) Medicinal strategies in the treatment of obesity. *Nature*, 404:672–677.

Busetto, L. (2001) Visceral obesity and the metabolic syndrome: effects of weight loss. *Nutr. Metab. Cardiovasc. Dis.*, 11:195–204.

Campbell, K., Waters, E., O'Meara, S. and Summerbell, C. (2001). Interventions for preventing obesity in children. *Cochrane Database Syst. Rev.*, 2:CD 001871.

Cooney, G.J. (Ed.) (2002) Obesity. *Clin. Endocrinol. Metab.*, 16:595–742.

Després, J.-P. (1993) Abdominal obesity as important component of insulin-resistance syndrome. *Nutrition*, 9:452–459.

Expert Panel on Detection, Evaluation, and Treatment of High Blood Cholesterol in Adults (2001) Executive summary of the third report of the National Cholesterol Education Program (NCEP) (Adult Treatment Panel III). *JAMA*, 285:2486–2497.

Glazer, G. (2001) Long-term pharmacotherapy of obesity 2000 — a review of efficacy and safety. *Arch. Intern. Med.*, 161:1814–1824.

Glenny, A.-M., O'Meara, S., Melville, A., Sheldon, T.A. and Wilson, C. (1997) The treatment and prevention of obesity: a systematic review of the literature. *Int. J. Obesity*, 21:715–737.

Goldstein, D.J. (1992) Beneficial health effects of modest weight loss. *Int. J. Obesity*, 16:397–415.

Grundy, S.M. (2002) Obesity, metabolic syndrome, and coronary atherosclerosis. *Circulation*, 105:2696–2698.

Guy–Grand, B.J.P. (1987) A new approach to the treatment of obesity. *Ann. NY Acad. Sci.*, 499:313–317.

Haddock, C.K., Poston, W.S.C., Dill, P.L., Foreyt, J.P. and Ericsson, M. (2002) Pharmacotherapy for obesity: a quantitative analysis of four decades of published randomized clinical trials. *Int. J. Obesity Relat. Metab. Disorders*, 26:262–273.

James, W.P.T. (1999) The International Obesity Task Force: a new development in public policy making. In *Progress in Obesity Research: 8*, B. Guy-Grand and G. Ailhaud, Eds., John Libbey & Company Ltd., London, U.K., pp. 649–659.

Kaukua, J., Pekkarinen, T., Sane, T. and Mustajoki, P. (2002) Health-related quality of life in WHO Class II-III obese men losing weight with very-low-energy diet and behavior modification: a randomized clinical trial. *Int. J. Obesity Relat. Metab. Disorders*, 26:487–495.

Khaodhiar, L. and Blackburn, G.L. (2002) Obesity treatment: factors involved in weight-loss maintenance and regain. *Curr. Opin. Endocrinol. Diabetes*, 9:369–374.

Kopelman, P.G. (2001) *Management of Obesity and Related Disorders*, Martin Dunitz, London, U.K.

Kumanyika, S., Jeffery, R.W., Morabia, A., Ritenbaugh, C. and Antipatis, V.J. (2002) Obesity prevention: the case for action. *Int. J. Obesity Relat. Metab. Disorders*, 26:425–436.

Luyckx, F.H., Scheen, A.J., Desaive, C., Dewé, W., Gielen, J.E. and Lefèbvre, P.J. (1998) Effects of gastroplasty on body weight and related biological abnormalities in morbid obesity. *Diabetes Metabol.*, 24:355–361.

Miller, W.C., Koceja, D.M. and Hamilton, E.J. (1997) A meta-analysis of the past 25 years of weight loss research using diet, exercise or diet plus exercise intervention. *Int. J. Obesity Relat. Metab. Disorders*, 21:941–947.

Mun, E.C., Blackburn, G.L. and Matthews, J.B. (2001) Current status of medical and surgical therapy for obesity. *Gastroenterology*, 120:669–681.

Narbro, K., Agren, G., Jonsson, E., Näslund, I., Sjöström, L. and Peltonen, M. (2002) Pharmaceutical costs in obese individuals. Comparison with a randomly selected population sample and long-term changes after conventional and surgical treatment: the SOS intervention study. *Arch. Intern. Med.*, 162:2061–2069.

National Task Force on the Prevention and Treatment of Obesity (1996) Long-term pharmacotherapy in the management of obesity. *JAMA*, 276:1907–1915.

NHLBI Obesity Education Initiative Expert Panel (1998) Clinical guidelines on the identification, evaluation, and treatment of overweight and obesity in adults — the evidence report. *Obesity Res.*, 6:51S–209S.

Poston, W.S.C, Haddock, C.K., Dill, P.L., Thayer, B. and Foreyt, J.P. (2001) Lifestyle treatments in randomized clinical trials of pharmacotherapies for obesity. *Obesity Res.* 9:552–563.

Ross, R., Freeman, J.A. and Janssen, I. (2000) Exercise alone is an effective strategy for reducing obesity and related comorbidities. *Exercise Sport Sci. Rev.*, 28:165–170.

Scheen A.J. (2003) Current management of coexisting obesity and type 2 diabetes. *Drugs*, 63:1165–1184.

Scheen, A.J., Desaive, C. and Lefèbvre, P.J. (1994) Therapy for obesity — today and tomorrow. *Baillière's Clin. Endocrinol. Metab.*, 8:705–727.

Scheen, A.J. and Lefèbvre, P.J. (1999a) Management of the obese diabetic patient. *Diabetes Rev.*, 7:77–93.

Scheen, A.J. and Lefèbvre, P.J. (1999b) Pharmacological treatment of obesity: present status. *Int. J. Obesity Relat. Metab. Disorders*, 23 (Suppl 1):47–53.

Scheen, A.J., Luyckx, F.H., Desaive, C. and Lefèbvre, P.J. (1999) Severe/extreme obesity: a medical disease requiring a surgical treatment? *Acta Clin. Belgica*, 54:154–161.

Sjöström, L. (2000) Surgical intervention as a strategy for treatment of obesity. *Endocrine*, 13:213–230.

Sjöström, C.D., Lissner, L., Wedel, H. and Sjöström, L. (1999) Reduction in incidence of diabetes, hypertension and lipid disturbances after intentional weight loss induced by bariatric surgery: the SOS Intervention Study. *Obesity Res.*, 7:477–484.

Wadden, T.A. (1998) New goals of obesity treatment: a healthier weight and other ideals. *Primary Psychiatry*, 5:45–54.

Wadden, T.A., Sternberg, J.A., Letizia, K.A., Stunkard, A.J. and Foster, G.D. (1989) Treatment of obesity by very low calorie diet, behavior therapy, and their combination: a five-year perspective. *Int. J. Obesity*, 13 (Suppl 2):39–46.

Willett, W.C., Dietz, W.H. and Colditz, G.A. (1999) Guidelines for healthy weight. *N. Engl. J. Med.*, 341:427–434.

Wing, R.R. and Hill, J.O. (2001) Successful weight loss maintenance. *Ann. Rev. Nutr.*, 21:321–341.

World Health Organization (2000) Obesity: preventing and managing the global epidemic. Report of a WHO consultation. Technical report vol. 894. Geneva, Switzerland, World Health Organization, 256.

Yanovski, S.Z. and Yanovski, J.A. (2002) Obesity. *N. Engl. J. Med.*, 346:591–602.

Part VII

Appendix

Perspectives and Outlook

Karl G. Hofbauer, Ulrich Keller, and Olivier Boss

CONTENTS

SUMMARY   Obesity and its associated diseases, such as insulin resistance or the metabolic syndrome, have become a widespread medical problem that is expanding in most of the world. More importantly, children and adolescents are now widely affected by this epidemic. With the rapid increase in the prevalence of this disease it is becoming urgent to develop new, effective ways to prevent and treat the condition. Ideally, this should be based on a better understanding of the physiology of energy metabolism and its dysregulation in obesity. Drug discovery in this field has proved to be difficult; currently, only a few drug candidates are in late stages of development. The clinical pharmacotherapy of obesity is challenging because it requires an integrated effort, including permanent changes in life-style. The most important future goal is the prevention of obesity and the early identification of individuals at risk for excessive weight gain.

Pathophysiology of Obesity and Pharmacological Targets

Energy balance is on average controlled with an error of less than 1% per year, assuming a mean annual increase in body weight of 1 kg. This is equivalent to an annual energy gain of approximately 9000 kcal, a tiny fraction of an annual intake of approximately 1,000,000 kcal extrapolated from a mean daily energy intake of 2750 kcal. This accuracy is even more striking in physically active individuals (e.g., cyclists), who ingest up to three times as much energy and yet maintain an even more stable body weight. The impressive level of precision is far greater than the ability of individuals to change their energy balance voluntarily (Friedman, 2003), strongly suggesting that subconscious regulatory factors are controlling energy balance more tightly than willpower.

Current obesity treatment is limited by the fact that the powerful counter-regulatory mechanisms responsible for the poor long-term efficacy of dietary (hypocaloric) treatments are still only partially understood. The adaptive responses of the body's regulatory systems to negative energy balance result almost regularly in relapse after weight loss. Evidence from rodent and human studies suggests that the body adapts to decreases in fat stores by reducing its metabolic rate (adjusted for lean and fat mass losses) (Dulloo and Jacquet,

2001). This phenomenon, which develops even when initial adipose tissue stores are elevated in obese subjects, helps the body fight against losing fat stores and allows a rapid deposition of triglycerides upon return to previous levels of food intake. Thus, the most challenging part of weight loss programs is not the loss of body weight but rather the stabilization of the new, lower body weight. To make things even worse, it seems that body fat deposition during weight regain negatively affects insulin sensitivity in peripheral tissues (Crescenzo et al., 2003). This in turn predisposes to the metabolic syndrome.

In the last decade tremendous advances in the knowledge of energy balance have been achieved, thus providing numerous new pharmacological targets. However, from the list of drugs used until now in the treatment of obesity, it is obvious that virtually all aimed at reducing food intake; consequently, their targets are located in the central nervous system. A notable exception is orlistat, an inhibitor of intestinal fat absorption. In the past, thyroid hormone and dinitrophenol were used, but both lacked adequate safety. Thus, drugs that act on energy expenditure are clearly missing in the current arsenal of antiobesity agents.

Is it harder to identify drugable peripheral targets that can lead to an increase in basal metabolic rate or even stimulate or mimic physical activity? A possible explanation may be that our understanding of the mechanisms controlling cellular, tissue, and whole-body metabolic rate is not as deep as our understanding of regulation of appetite. Alternatively, this situation may be because, in most cases, obesity is caused by excessive food intake rather than by impaired energy expenditure.

Another important avenue for research is the understanding of energy partitioning mechanisms. Therapeutic alterations of these systems might prevent body fat gain in favor of an increase in muscle mass. This would presumably increase whole-body metabolic rate; decrease the propensity for subsequent body weight gain; and improve glucose metabolism, ultimately preventing development of insulin resistance and type 2 diabetes. Moreover, a thorough understanding of the mechanisms controlling the size of the adipose compartment should provide additional targets for drugs aimed at decreasing body fat content and treating the associated metabolic disturbances.

Drug Discovery

Despite remarkable progress in understanding the pathophysiology of obesity, the number of antiobesity drugs in clinical development is still relatively small (Farrigan and Pang, 2002; Gura, 2003; Vastag, 2003). This may be due to the fact that not all molecules or mechanisms that have been identified in experimental or clinical studies can be used as targets for pharmacological intervention. Assessing the suitability of a target for drug discovery is called target validation. It is used to select promising candidates based on criteria such as the physiological importance of the pathway to which a target belongs; its possible role in the pathophysiology of obesity; and its accessibility by low molecular weight agonists or antagonists. The latter property is usually referred to as a target's drugability (Chiesi et al., 2001).

However, even though a target may look interesting based on structure and function, its activation or blockade may not lead to a beneficial therapeutic effect. Redundant control systems or compensatory mechanisms may prevent or counteract its direct effects. This is particularly relevant for complex and vital functions such as energy intake, storage, and expenditure (Hofbauer and Huppertz, 2002). Therefore, the therapeutic potential of a certain pharmacological intervention needs to be evaluated further by a procedure called concept validation, which usually requires chronic *in vivo* studies in suitable animal models. In recent years, genetically modified mouse strains have been increasingly used for such experiments, but other disease models are still of interest (Törnell and Snaith, 2002). In any case, prediction of the clinical efficacy of a prototype drug or development compound is the most important purpose of such studies.

Several factors can limit the predictive value of results obtained in preclinical research. Species differences among experimental animals and between experimental animals and human subjects need to be taken into account. Even strain differences in mice may lead to different phenotypes despite identical genetic defects that correspond to the influence of a different genetic background on the expression of gene defects in humans. Environmental factors may also exacerbate strain or species differences. The fact that most studies in rodents are performed at temperatures below thermoneutrality could be particularly relevant for antiobesity drugs. This may lead to drug effects on energy expenditure that are not reproducible in the clinic.

Some genetic models of obesity in rodents are representative of rare monogenic forms of obesity in humans (O'Rahilly, 2002). Although such models are important for understanding the regulation of energy balance in mice and men, they do not correspond to the common clinical forms of obesity. Diet-induced obesity in rodents is probably the experimental paradigm more closely related to the clinical situation. However, because human obesity may be viewed as a normal adaptation to an abnormal environment, much can also be learned from studies in normal lean rats or mice. Food restriction in such animals may reveal the same counterregulatory mechanisms also activated in patients on a hypocaloric diet that cause relapse or rebound phenomena.

Pharmacotherapy and Clinical Aspects

The fact that appetite and satiation can be investigated with simple methods in human volunteers should favor early proof-of-concept studies in the clinic. In Phase I trials, the efficacy of appetite suppressants or of inhibitors of intestinal absorption can be verified after single or repeated dosing. Such results should be helpful to decide whether a costly development program is justified and could also provide important feedback for adjustments in related drug discovery programs. However, the demonstration of long-term safety and efficacy of new antiobesity agents requires extended clinical studies. Only careful evaluation of the chronic effects of a new drug in a sufficient number of patients makes it possible to assess its benefit/risk profile in treatment of obesity and associated diseases (Yanovski and Yanovski, 2002).

Two substances with severe side effects overshadow the history of drug therapy of obesity. The first one, aminorex (Minocil[R]), caused pulmonary hypertension; the second, fenfluramine, caused heart valve abnormalities and pulmonary hypertension (Yanovski and Yanovski, 2002). For this reason, the public and regulatory authorities are very conscientious about sufficient safety documentation of any new antiobesity drug. In the past, development of antiobesity drugs has been characterized by a paucity of high-quality scientific trials demonstrating long-term efficacy and safety. Trials lasting 2 years and more have been performed only for orlistat (Xenical[R]; Davidson et al., 1999) and sibutramine (Meridia[R]; James et al., 2000). Today regulatory authorities ask for more and better clinical trials with antiobesity drugs, including data on hard endpoints. However, because even

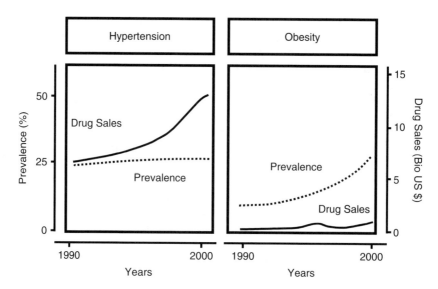

FIGURE A.1

Prevalence of hypertension and obesity vs. related drug sales in the U.S. between 1990 and 2000. While the prevalence of hypertension remained almost unchanged over that period, prevalence of obesity almost doubled and became equal to that of hypertension by 2000. Drug sales for these two indications started at a different level and showed a different trend. Although sales for antihypertensive drugs were already at a high level in 1990, they still increased almost twofold by 2000, mainly due to introduction of new, more expensive antihypertensive agents. The sales of antiobesity drugs were low in 1990 and rose slightly in the mid-1990s, but decreased after the withdrawal of dexfenfluramine and fenfluramine. This figure is a semiquantitative representation of the trends in both indications. For more precise information on prevalence, see Flegal et al. 2002, and Hajjar and Kotchen, 2003. Information on drug sales can be obtained from IMS Health.

more obesity-associated risk factors for atherosclerotic diseases are recognized, effects on these risk factors are valid surrogate endpoints.

Drug therapy is also substantially restricted due to the missing financial reimbursement of therapy. Because obesity is often not considered a disease, health insurance companies or public health providers do not pay for therapy. For these reasons and for fear of side effects, only a few pharmaceutical companies have made a large investment into research on antiobesity drugs (see Figure A.1). As a result, a number of "soft" drugs such as herbal medicines are on the market and sales of these compounds are apparently on the rise.

The current epidemic of obesity represents a major challenge to health care systems (Hill et al., 2003). The topic of prevention will therefore become even more important in the future. Because antiobesity therapies are usually unsatisfactory and often associated with side effects, a major focus will be on therapeutic life-style changes (Tuomilehto et al., 2001) — possibly supported by drugs (Knowler et al., 2002; Scheen, 2002). The Diabetes Prevention Program (DPP) study is an important endpoint trial demonstrating that life-style changes in subjects with incipient glucose intolerance are able to prevent the development of type 2 diabetes. This trial also included a group of subjects treated with metformin, which was efficacious in preventing diabetes, but less powerful than life-style changes.

A deeper understanding of the regulation of energy balance, in particular of energy expenditure, will allow identification of new peripheral targets for future antiobesity drugs. A combined approach to reduce energy intake and to increase energy expenditure could markedly improve the efficacy of pharmacotherapy to accelerate weight loss and to stabilize the reduced weight by preventing relapse. In the not too distant future, drugs with different mechanisms of action might be used to treat subgroups of obese patients according to their genetic predisposition. The enormous amount of information presented in the individual chapters of this book justifies the optimistic view that the ground is prepared for the successful discovery and development of novel antiobesity drugs.

References

Chiesi, M., Huppertz, C., and Hofbauer, K.G. (2001) Pharmacotherapy of obesity: targets and perspectives, *Trends Pharmacol. Sci.*, 22:247–254.

Crescenzo, R., Samec, S., Antic, V., Rohner-Jeanrenaud, F., Seydoux, J., Montani, J.P., and Dulloo, A.G. (2003) A role for suppressed thermogenesis favoring catch-up fat in the pathophysiology of catch-up growth, *Diabetes*, 52:1090–1097.

Davidson, M.H., Hauptman, J., DiGirolamo, M., Foreyt, J.P., Halsted, C.H., Heber, D., Heimburger; D.C., Lucas, C.P., Robbins, D.C., Chung, J., and Heymsfield, S.B. (1999) Weight control and risk factor reduction in obese subjects treated for 2 years with orlistat: a randomized controlled trial, *JAMA*, 281:235–242.

Dulloo, A.G. and Jacquet, J. (2001) An adipose-specific control of thermogenesis in body weight regulation, *Int. J. Obes. Relat. Metab. Disord.*, 25, Suppl 5:S22–29.

Farrigan, C. and Pang, K. (2002) Obesity market overview, *Nat. Rev. Drug Discovery*, 1, 257–258.

Flegal, K.M., Carroll, M.D., Ogden, C.L., and Johnson, C.L. (2002) Prevalence and trends in obesity among U.S. adults, 1999–2000, *JAMA*, 288:1723–1727.

Friedman, J.M. (2003) A war on obesity, not the obese, *Science*, 299:856–858.

Gura, T. (2003) Obesity drug pipeline not so fat, *Science*, 299:849–852.

Hajjar, I. and Kotchen, T.A. (2003) Trends in prevalence, awareness, treatment, and control of hypertension in the United States, 1988–2000. *JAMA*, 290:199–206.

Hill, J.O., Wyatt, H.R., Reed, G.W, and Peters J.C. (2003) Obesity and the environment: where do we go from here? *Science*, 299:853–855.

Hofbauer, K.G. and Huppertz, C. (2002) Pharmacotherapy and evolution, *Trends Ecol. Evol.*, 17:328–334.

James, W.P., Astrup, A., Finer, N., Hilsted, J., Kopelman, P., Rossner, S., Saris, W.H., and Van Gaal, L.F. (2000) Effect of sibutramine on weight maintenance after weight loss: a randomized trial. STORM Study Group. Sibutramine trial of obesity reduction and maintenance, *Lancet*, 356:2119–2125.

Knowler, W.C., Barrett–Connor, E., Fowler, S.E., Hamman, R.F., Lachin, J.M., Walker, E.A., and Nathan, D.M., Diabetes Prevention Program Research Group (2002) Reduction in the incidence of type 2 diabetes with life-style intervention or metformin, *N. Engl. J. Med.*, 346:393–403.

O'Rahilly, S. (2002) Insights into obesity and insulin resistance from the study of extreme human phenotypes, *Eur. J. Endocrinol.*, 147:435–441.

Scheen, A.J. (2002) Prevention of type 2 diabetes in obese patients: first results with orlistat in the XENDOS study, *Rev. Med. Liege*, 57:617–621.

Törnell, J. and Snaith, M. (2002) Transgenic systems in drug discovery: from target identification to humanized mice, *DDT*, 7:461–470.

Tuomilehto, J., Lindstrom, J., Eriksson, J.G., Valle, T.T., Hamalainen, H., Ilanne-Parikka, P., Keinanen-Kiukaanniemi, S., Laakso, M., Louheranta, A., Rastas, M., and Salminen, V., Finnish Diabetes Prevention Study Group (2001) Prevention of type 2 diabetes mellitus by changes in lifestyle among subjects with impaired glucose tolerance, *N. Engl. J. Med.*, 344:1343–1350.

Vastag, B. (2003) Experimental drugs take aim at obesity, *JAMA*, 289: 1763–1764.

Yanovski, S.Z. and Yanovski, J.A. (2002) Drug therapy: obesity, *N. Engl. J. Med.*, 346:591–603.

Index

473

B

C